S0-AIF-947

Clinical Applications of Nursing Diagnosis

Adult, Child, Women's, Psychiatric, Gerontic, and Home Health Considerations

HELEN C. COX, RN, C, EdD, FAAN
EXECUTIVE ASSOCIATE DEAN, PROFESSOR OF NURSING
TEXAS TECH UNIVERSITY HEALTH SCIENCES CENTER SCHOOL OF NURSING
LUBBOCK, TEXAS

MITTIE D. HINZ, RN, C, MSN
PERINATAL CLINICAL SPECIALIST
DOCTOR'S MEDICAL CENTER
MODESTO, CALIFORNIA

MARY ANN LUBNO, RN, PhD, CNAA
ASSOCIATE PROFESSOR OF NURSING, GRADUATE ADVISOR
UNIVERSITY OF TEXAS AT EL PASO SCHOOL OF NURSING AND ALLIED HEALTH
EL PASO, TEXAS

SUSAN A. NEWFIELD, RN, MSN, CS
ASSISTANT PROFESSOR OF NURSING
WEST VIRGINIA UNIVERSITY SCHOOL OF NURSING
MORGANTOWN, WEST VIRGINIA

NANCY A. RIDENOUR, RN, C, PhD, FNP, FAAN
ASSOCIATE DEAN FOR EDUCATION, PROFESSOR OF NURSING
TEXAS TECH UNIVERSITY HEALTH SCIENCES CENTER SCHOOL OF NURSING
LUBBOCK, TEXAS

MARY McCARTHY SLATER, RN, C, MSN
ASSOCIATE PROFESSOR OF NURSING
EASTERN KENTUCKY UNIVERSITY AD PROGRAM
RICHMOND, KENTUCKY

KATHRYN L. SRIDAROMONT, RN, C, MSN
ASSOCIATE PROFESSOR OF CLINICAL NURSING
TEXAS TECH UNIVERSITY HEALTH SCIENCES CENTER SCHOOL OF NURSING
LUBBOCK, TEXAS

Clinical Applications of Nursing Diagnosis

Adult, Child, Women's, Psychiatric, Gerontic, and Home Health Considerations

Third Edition

NO LONGER THE PROPERTY
OF THE
UNIVERSITY OF R. I. LIBRARY

 F. A. DAVIS COMPANY • *Philadelphia*

F. A. Davis
1915 Arch Street
Philadelphia, PA 19103

Copyright © 1997 by F. A. Davis Company

Copyright © 1989, 1993 by F. A. Davis Company. All rights reserved. This book is protected by copyright. No part of it may be reproduced, stored in a retrieval system, or transmitted in any form or by any means, electronic, mechanical, photocopying, recording, or otherwise, without written permission from the publisher.

Printed in the United States of America

Last digit indicates print number: 10 9 8 7 6 5 4 3 2 1

Publisher, Nursing: Robert G. Martone
Production Editors: Glenn L. Fechner, Nancee A. Morelli
Cover Designer: Steven R. Morrone

As new scientific information becomes available through basic and clinical research, recommended treatments and drug therapies undergo changes. The authors and publisher have done everything possible to make this book accurate, up to date, and in accord with accepted standards at the time of publication. The authors, editors, and publisher are not responsible for errors or omissions or for consequences from application of the book, and make no warranty, expressed or implied, in regard to the contents of the book. Any practice described in this book should be applied by the reader in accordance with professional standards of care used in regard to the unique circumstances that may apply in each situation. The reader is advised always to check product information (package inserts) for changes and new information regarding dose and contraindications before administering any drug. Caution is especially urged when using new or infrequently ordered drugs.

Library of Congress Cataloging-in-Publication Data

Clinical applications of nursing diagnosis : adult, child, women's, psychiatric, gerontic,
    and home health considerations / Helen C. Cox
    . . . [et al.]. — 3rd ed.
       p.   cm.
    Includes bibliographical references and index.
    ISBN 0-8036-0177-8
    1. Nursing diagnosis.   2. Nursing assessment.   3. Nursing.
   I. Cox, Helen C.
    [DNLM: 1. Nursing Diagnosis. 2. Nursing Process.   WY 100.4 C641 1997]
   RT48.6.C6   1997
   610.73—DC20
   DNLM/DLC
   for Library of Congress   96-34957

Authorization to photocopy items for internal or personal use, or the internal or personal use of specific clients, is granted by F. A. Davis Company for users registered with the Copyright Clearance Center (CCC) Transactional Reporting Service, provided that the fee of $.10 per copy is paid directly to CCC, 222 Rosewood Drive, Danvers, MA 01923. For those organizations that have been granted a photocopy license by CCC, a separate system of payment has been aranged. The fee code for users of the Transactional Reporting Service is: 8036-0177/97 0 + $.10.

To the administration, faculty, students, and staff of
Texas Tech University Health Sciences Center School of Nursing
for support and encouragement above and beyond the usual.

PREFACE TO THE THIRD EDITION

The North American Nursing Diagnosis Association (NANDA) has continued its work in nursing diagnostic nomenclature. The preface to the second edition of this book explains this work and remains accurate.

The third edition focuses on adding the diagnoses accepted in 1994 and updating information in each chapter. The chapter formats remain the same. We do want to point out that the expected outcomes, target dates, and evaluation flowcharts dovetail very well with today's emphasis on critical (or clinical) pathways.

At the 1994 Conference in Nashville, a preconference was held and attendees were invited to continue NANDA's work in the refinement of diagnoses. Ten diagnoses were selected for refinement and a work group assigned to each diagnosis. The work of these groups is being accepted into the taxonomy, and modifications have been made in this text to reflect the results generated by these workgroups.

We deeply appreciate the feedback from nursing faculty, nursing staff, and nursing students who are currently using this book. Your input assists us in being sure the book continues to meet your needs. We are grateful you took the time to give us the information.

Helen Cox, RN, C, EdD, FAAN

PREFACE TO THE SECOND EDITION

The North American Nursing Diagnosis Association (NANDA) has been identifying, classifying, and testing diagnostic nomenclature since the early seventies. In our opinion, use of nursing diagnosis helps to define the essence of nursing and to give direction to care that is uniquely nursing care.

In this second edition, we have made numerous changes to stay abreast of changes in national standards and criteria. In doing so, we have moved from talking about specific care plan forms to talking about the process of planning care. This allows the reader to adapt information in this book to a variety of care documentation formats and to focus on the full process of planning care to meet the individual needs of the patient.

If nurses (in all instances we are referring to registered nurses) enter the medical diagnosis of, for example, acute appendicitis as the patient's problem, they have met defeat before they have begun. A nurse cannot intervene for this medical diagnosis; intervention requires a medical practitioner who can perform an appendectomy. However, if the nurse enters the nursing diagnosis "Pain," then a number of nursing interventions come to mind.

Several books use nursing diagnosis to contribute to planning care. However, these books generally focus outcome and nursing interventions on the related factors; that is, nursing interventions deal with resolving, to the extent possible, the causative and contributing factors that result in the nursing diagnosis. We have chosen to focus nursing intervention on the nursing diagnosis. To focus on the nursing diagnosis promotes the use of concepts in nursing rather than worrying about a multitude of specifics; for example, there are common nursing measures that can be used to relieve pain regardless of the etiologic pain factor involved. Likewise, the outcomes focus on the nursing diagnosis. The main outcome nurses want to achieve when working with the nursing diagnosis "Pain" is control of the patient's response to pain to the extent possible. Again, the outcome allows the use of a conceptual approach rather than a multitude-of-specifics approach. To clarify further, we ask you to look again at the medical diagnosis of appendicitis. The physician's first concern is not related to whether the appendicitis is caused by a fecalith, intestinal helminths, or *Escherichia coli* run amok. The physician focuses first on intervening for the appendicitis, which usually results in an appendectomy. The physician will deal with etiologic factors following the appendectomy, but the appendectomy is the first level of intervention. Likewise, the nurse can deal with the related factors through nursing actions, but the first level of intervention is directed to resolving the patient's problem that is reflected by the nursing diagnosis. With the decreasing length of stay for the majority of patients entering a hospital, we may indeed do well to complete the first level of nursing actions.

Additionally, there is continuing debate among NANDA members as to whether the current list of diagnoses that are accepted for testing are nursing diagnoses or a list of diagnostic categories or concepts. We therefore have chosen to focus on concepts. Using a conceptual approach allows focus on independent nursing functions and helps avoid focusing on medical intervention. This book has been designed to serve as a guide to using NANDA accepted nursing diagnoses as the primary base for the planning of care. The expected outcomes, target dates, nursing actions, and evaluation algorithms (flowcharts) are not meant to serve as standardized plans of care but rather as guides and references in promoting the visibility of nursing's contribution to health care.

Marjory Gordon's "Functional Health Patterns" are used as an organizing framework for the book. The Functional Health Patterns allow grouping of the nursing diagnoses into specific groups, which, in our opinion, promotes a conceptual approach to assessment and formulation of a nursing diagnosis.

Chapter 1 serves as the overview/introductory chapter and gives basic content related to the process of planning care and information regarding the relationship between nursing process and nursing models (theories). Titles for Chapters 2 through 12 are taken from the functional patterns. Included in each of these chapters is a list of diagnoses within the pattern, a pattern description, pattern assessment, conceptual information, and developmental information related to the pattern.

The pattern description gives a succinct summary of the pattern's content and assists in explaining how the diagnoses within the pattern are related. The list of diagnoses within the pattern is given to simplify location of the diagnoses. The pattern assessment serves to pinpoint information from the initial assessment base and was specifically written to direct the reader to the most likely diagnosis within the pattern. Each assessment factor is designed to allow an answer of yes or no. If the patient's answer or signs are indicative of a diagnosis within the pattern, the reader is directed to the most likely diagnosis or diagnoses. The conceptual and developmental information is included to provide a quick, ready reference to the physiologic, psychological, sociological, and age-related factors that could cause modification of the nursing actions in order to make them more specific for your patient. The conceptual and developmental information can be used to determine the rationale for each nursing action.

Each nursing diagnosis within the pattern is then introduced with accompanying information of definition, defining characteristics, and related factors. We have added a section titled "Related Clinical Concerns." This section serves to highlight the most common medical diagnoses or cluster of diagnoses that could involve the individual nursing diagnosis. Immediately after the related clinical concerns section is a section titled "Have you selected the correct diagnosis?"

The "Have you selected the correct diagnosis?" section was included as a validation check because we realize that several of the diagnoses appear to be very closely related and that it can be difficult to distinguish among them. A part of this problem is related to the fact that the diagnoses have been accepted for testing, not as statements of absolute, discrete diagnoses. Thus, having this section assists the reader in learning how to pinpoint the differences among diagnoses and in feeling more comfortable in selecting a diagnosis that most clearly reflects a patient's problem area that can be helped by nursing actions.

After the diagnosis validation section are expected outcomes. Expected outcomes serve as the end point against which progress can be measured. Also called "objectives," "patient goals," and "outcome standards," the expected outcomes are connected by the words *and/or,* signifying that the reader may choose to use only one of the outcomes or to use both of the outcomes. Readers might also choose to design their own patient-specific expected outcomes using the given expected outcomes as guidelines.

Target dates are suggested following the expected outcomes. The target dates **do not** indicate the time or day the outcome must be fully achieved; instead, the target date signifies the time or day when evaluation should be completed in order to measure the patient's progress **toward** achievement of the expected outcome. Target dates are given in reference to short-term care. For home health, particularly, the target date would be in terms of weeks and months rather than days.

Nursing actions/interventions and rationales are the next information given. In most instances, the adult health nursing actions serve as the generic nursing actions. Subsequent sets of nursing actions (child health, women's health, psychiatric health, gerontic health, and home health) show only the nursing actions that are different from the generic nursing actions. The different nursing actions make each set specific for the target population, but **must be** used in conjunction with the adult health nursing actions to be complete. Gerontic health nursing actions are new to the second edition in recognition of our aging population. Gerontology will be a major practice arena for nurses in the very near future. Rationales have been included to assist the student in learning the reason for particular nursing actions. While some of the rationales are scientific in nature, that is, supported by documented research, other rationales could be more appropriately termed "common sense" or "usual practice rationales." These rationales are reasons nurses have cited for particular nursing actions and result from nursing experience, *but* research has not been conducted to document these rationales. After the home health actions, evaluation algorithms are shown for monitoring the patient's progress toward achieving the expected outcomes.

Evaluation of the patient's care is based on the degree of progress the patient has made toward achieving the expected outcome. For each stated outcome, there is an evaluation flowchart (algorithm). The flowcharts provide minimum information, but they demonstrate the decision-making process that must be used.

In all instances, the authors have used the definitions, major and minor defining characteristics, and related factors that have been accepted by NANDA for testing. A grant was provided to NANDA by F. A. Davis for the use of these materials. All of these materials may be ordered from NANDA (1211 Locust Street, Philadelphia, PA 19107).

In some instances, additional information is included following a set of nursing actions. The additional information includes material that either needs to be highlighted or does not logically fall within the defined outline areas.

Throughout the nursing actions, we have used the words *patient* and *client* interchangeably. The terms refer to the system of care and include the individual as well as the family and other social support systems. The nursing actions are written very specifically. This specificity aids in communication between and among nurses and promotes consistency of care for the patient.

We have written this book for any nurse or nursing student who is beginning to work with nursing diagnosis. We hope to promote the use of nursing diagnosis to the end that nursing itself is advanced. If you, our readers, begin to feel more comfortable with using nursing diagnosis nomenclature and begin to use nursing diagnosis more in your practice, then our hope will have become reality.

Helen Cox, RNC, EdD, FAAN

ACKNOWLEDGMENTS

The publication of a book necessitates the involvement of many people beyond the authors. We wish to acknowledge the support and assistance of the following people who indeed made this book possible:

Our families, who supported our taking time away from family activities

Bob Martone, Publisher, Nursing, whose enthusiasm for a new edition and belief in the book were most gratifying and helpful

Ruth De George, Executive Secretary, F. A. Davis, for her careful attention to and care for this book AND

A special acknowledgment to Dr. Marjory Gordon, a most gracious lady who freely shared ideas, materials, support, and encouragement

To each of these people we wish to say a heartfelt "Thank you." Please accept our deepest gratitude and appreciation.

CONTENTS

Introduction

Why This Book?

At the time the first edition of this book was written, all of the authors were faculty members at the same school of nursing. We had become frustrated with the books available for teaching nursing diagnosis to students and found that the students were also expressing some of the same frustrations.

The students felt they needed to bring several books to the clinical area because the books for nursing diagnosis had limited information on pathophysiology, psychosocial, or developmental factors that definitely impacted individualized care planning. The students were also confused about the different definitions, defining characteristics, and related factors each of the authors used. The students were having difficulty in writing individualized nursing actions for their patients because the various authors appeared to focus on specifics related to the etiology or signs and symptoms of the nursing diagnosis rather than the concept represented by the nursing diagnosis that had been emphasized to our students. The authors were also concerned about the number of books our students had to buy since the majority of the books focused on just one clinical area such as adult health or pediatrics. Thus, as the students progressed through the school, they had to buy different books for different clinical areas even though each of the books had the common theme of the use of nursing diagnosis. Another concern we, as faculty, had was the lack of information in the various books on the final phase of the nursing process, evaluation. This most vital phase was briefly mentioned but very little guidance was given on how to proceed through this phase. For these reasons we have written this book particularly geared to student use. The final concern that led to the writing of the book was our desire to have a book focused on nursing actions and nursing care, not medical care and medical diagnosis. We strongly believe and support the vital role of nurses in the provision of health care for our nation, and so we have focused in this book strictly on nursing. After all, statistics show that the largest number of health care providers are nurses and that the general public has a high respect for nurses. Therefore, let us work on developing our profession and its contributions.

Specifically, we wrote this book to assist students to learn how to apply nursing diagnosis in the clinical area. By using the framework of the nursing process and the materials generated by the North American Nursing Diagnosis Association (NANDA),* we believe this book makes it easier for you, the student, to learn and use nursing diagnosis in planning care for your patients.

The Nursing Process

PURPOSE

Gordon[1] indicates that Lydia Hall was one of the first nurses to use the term "nursing process" in the early 1950s. Since that time the term "nursing process" has been used to describe the accepted method of delivering nursing care. Iyer[2] states, "The major purpose of the nursing process is to provide a framework within which the individualized needs of the client, family, and community can be met."

It may be easier to think of a "framework" as a blueprint or an outline which guides the planning of care for a patient.†

As Doenges and Moorhouse write,[3] "The nursing process is central to nursing actions in any setting because it is an efficient method of organizing thought processes for clinical decision making and problem solving." Use of the nursing process framework is beneficial for both the patient and the nurse because it helps ensure that care is planned, individualized, and reviewed over the period of time that the nurse and patient have a professional relationship. It must be emphasized that the nursing process requires the involvement of the patient throughout all the phases. If the patient is not involved in all phases, then the plan of care is not individualized.

DEFINITION

Alfaro[4] defines nursing process as "an organized, systematic method of giving individualized nursing care that focuses on identifying and treating unique responses of individuals or groups to actual or potential alterations in health." This definition fits very nicely with the American Nurses' Association (ANA) Social Policy Statement[5]: "Nursing is the diagnosis and treatment of human responses to actual and potential health problems." Alfaro's definition is further supported by the ANA Standards of Clinical Nursing Practice[6] (Table 1–1), practice standards written by several boards of nursing,[7] and the definition of nursing that is written into the majority of nurse practice acts in the United States. (The Board of Nurse Examiners for the State of Texas Nursing Practice Standards are used as an example. See Table 1–2.)

Basically, the nursing process provides each nurse with a framework to use in working with a patient. The process begins at the time the patient needs assistance with health care

---

*Permission for nursing diagnoses from North American Nursing Diagnosis Association (1994). NANDA Nursing Diagnoses: Definitions and Classification 1995–1996. Philadelphia: NANDA. Copyright 1994 by the North American Nursing Diagnosis Association.

†*Note:* Throughout this book we use the terms "patient" and "client" interchangeably. In most instances these terms refer to the individual who is receiving nursing care; however, a patient can also be a community, such as in the community–home health nursing actions, or the patient can be a family, such as the nursing diagnosis Ineffective Family Coping, Compromised.

Table 1–1 STANDARDS OF CARE

Standard I. Assessment: The nurse collects client health data.

Standard II. Diagnosis: The nurse analyzes the assessment data in determining diagnoses.

Standard III. Outcome Identification: The nurse identifies expected outcomes individualized to the client.

Standard IV. Planning: The nurse develops a plan of care that prescribes interventions to attain expected outcomes.

Standard V. Implementation: The nurse implements the interventions identified in the plan of care.

Standard VI. Evaluation: The nurse evaluates the client's progress toward attainment of outcomes.

Source: Reprinted with permission from Standards of Clinical Nursing Practice,[6] © 1991, American Nurses Association, Kansas City, MO, p 9.

Table 1–2 STANDARDS OF NURSING PRACTICE

The registered professional nurse shall:

1. Know and conform to the laws and regulations governing the practice of professional nursing in the State of Texas.

2. Utilize the nursing process to provide individualized, goal-directed nursing care by:
   a. Performing nursing assessments regarding the health status of the patient or client
   b. Making nursing diagnoses which serve as the basis for the strategy of care
   c. Developing a plan of care based on assessment and nursing diagnoses
   d. Implementing nursing care
   e. Evaluating the patient's or client's responses to nursing interventions

3. Institute appropriate nursing intervention which might be required to stabilize a patient's or client's condition and/or prevent complications.

4. Know the rationale for, the effects of, and the proper administration of the medications and/or treatments he or she administers.

5. Accurately report and document the patient's or client's symptoms, responses, and progress.

6. Respect the patient's or client's right to privacy by protecting confidential information unless obligated or allowed by law to disclose the information.

7. Promote and participate in patient or client education and counseling based on health needs.

8. Collaborate with members of health disciplines in the interest of the patient's or client's health care.

9. Consult and utilize community agencies and resources for continuity of patient or client care.

10. Consult with the appropriate licensed practitioner to clarify any order or treatment regimen that the nurse has reason to believe is inaccurate and/or contraindicated.

11. Make assignments to other nursing personnel that take into consideration patient safety and that are commensurate with the personnel's educational preparation, experience, and knowledge.

12. Supervise nursing care provided by nursing personnel for which he or she is administratively responsible.

13. Accept only those nursing assignments that are commensurate with his of her educational preparation, experience, and knowledge of patient safety.

14. Be responsible for his or her continuing competence in nursing practice and individual professional growth.

Source: Adapted from Board of Nurse Examiners for the State of Texas,[7] p 37, with permission.

---

through the time the patient no longer needs assistance to meet health care maintenance. The nursing process represents the cognitive (thinking and reasoning), psychomotor (physical), and affective (emotions and values) skills and abilities used by the nurse to plan care for a patient.

ROLE IN PLANNING CARE

Perhaps the important question is why do we need to plan care? There are several answers to this question that range from considerations of the individual needs of a patient to the legal aspects of nursing practice.

First, the patient has a right to expect that the nursing care received will be complete and of high quality. If care plan-

ning is not done, then gaps are going to exist in the patient's care. At this time, we are seeing patients being admitted to the hospital more acutely ill than in the past. We are now caring for patients on a general medical-surgical unit who would have been in a critical care unit 10 years ago. We are now sending patients home in 1 to 3 days that we would have kept in the hospital another 5 to 10 days 10 years ago. Procedures that required a 3- to 5-day hospital stay in the past are now being performed via day surgery or outpatient facilities. A variety of factors has led to this situation including the advent of the use of diagnosis related groups (DRGs) for patient billing, managed care insurance plans, prospective payment insurance plans, capitated payment insurance plans, movement from acute care to longer-term care settings such as home health, nursing homes, and rehabilitation units, and, most importantly, the desire to contain the rapidly rising costs of health care. These problems, which together have been labeled the "quicker, sicker phenomenon," in combination with a national sporadic shortage of registered nurses have created a situation in which contact time with a patient is being cut to a minimum. If care planning is not done, given this set of circumstances, then there is no doubt that gaps will exist in the nursing care given to a patient and that such care will be incomplete, inconsistent, and certainly not of high quality.

Second, care planning and its documentation provide a means of professional communication. This communication promotes consistency of care for the patient and provides a comfort level for the nurse. Any patient admitted to a health care agency is going to have some level of anxiety. Imagine how this anxiety increases when each nurse who enters the room does each procedure differently, answers questions differently, or uses different time lines for care (e.g., a surgical dressing that has been changed in the morning every day since surgery is not changed until the afternoon). Care planning provides a comfort level for the nurse because it gives the nurse a ready reference to help ensure that care is complete. Care planning also provides a guideline for documentation and promotes practicing within legally defined standards.

Third, care planning provides legal protection for the nurse. We are practicing in one of the most litigious societies that has ever existed. In the past, nurses were not frequently named in legal actions; however, this has changed as a brief review of suits being filed these days would show. In a legal suit, the nursing care is measured against the idea of what a reasonably prudent nurse would do in the same circumstances. The accepted standards of nursing practice, as published by ANA[6] (Table 1–1) and the individual boards of nursing[7] (Table 1–2), are the accepted definitions of reasonable, prudent nursing care.

Finally, accrediting and approval agencies such as the Joint Commission on Accreditation of Healthcare Organizations (JCAHO), the National League for Nursing (NLN), Medicare, and Medicaid have criteria that specifically require documentation of planning of care. The accreditation status of a health care agency can depend on consistent documentation that planning of care has been done. Particularly with the third-party payors such as Medicare, Medicaid, and insurance companies, lack of documentation regarding the planning and implementation of care means no reimbursement for care. Ultimately, nonreimbursement for care leads to lack of new equipment, no pay raises, and in some extreme cases, hospital closures.

CARE PLAN VERSUS PLANNING OF CARE

Recent revisions of nursing standards by the JCAHO created questions regarding the necessity of nursing care plans. Some have predicted the rapid demise of the care plan, according to Brider,[8] but review of the revised nursing standards shows that the standards require not less but more detailed care planning documentation in the patient's medical record.

Review of the new criteria indicates that the standards require documentation related to the nursing process. For example, JCAHO[9] Nursing Care Standard 1.3.5 requires that:

> Nursing care data related to patient assessments, the nursing care planned, nursing interventions, and patient outcomes are permanently integrated into the clinical information system (for example, the medical record).

Rather than eliminating care plans, the new JCAHO requirements call for a more specific as well as a more permanent documentation of the plan of care. This documentation must be in the medical record. The standard indicates that a separate care plan form is no longer necessary; however, the standard also still allows a separate care plan form. Various institutions are now testing flexible ways of documenting care planning. The care plan is not dead; rather, it is revised to more clearly reflect the important role of nursing in the patient's care. No longer a separate, often discarded, and irrelevant page, the plan of care must be part of the permanent record. The flow sheets developed for this book offer guidelines for computerizing information regarding nursing care.

Faculty can use the revised JCAHO standards to assist students in developing expertise beyond writing extensive nursing care plans. This additional expertise requires the new graduate to integrate all phases of the nursing process into the permanent record. Rather than eliminating the need for care planning and nursing diagnosis, the new standards have reinforced the importance of nursing care and nursing diagnosis.

Nursing Process Steps

There are five steps, or phases, in the nursing process: assessment, diagnosis, planning, implementation, and evaluation. These steps are not discrete steps, but rather, they overlap and build on each other. To carry out the entire nursing process, you must be sure to accurately complete each step and then use the information in that step to build upon to complete the next step.

ASSESSMENT

The first step, or phase, of the nursing process is assessment. During this phase you are collecting data (factual information) from several sources. The collection and organization of this data allows you to:

1. Determine the patient's current health status
2. Determine the patient's strengths and problem areas (both actual and potential)
3. Prepare for the second step of the process — diagnosis

Data Sources and Types

The sources for data collection are numerous, but it is essential to remember that the patient is the primary data source. No one else can explain as accurately as the patient the start of the problem, the reason for seeking assistance or the exact nature of the problem, and the effect of the problem on the patient. Other sources include the patient's family or significant others, the patient's admission sheet from the admitting office, the physician's history, physical, and orders, laboratory and x-ray results, information from other caregivers, and current nursing literature.

Assessment data can be further classified as types of data. According to Iyer[2] the data types are subjective, objective, historical, and current.

Subjective data are the facts presented by the patient that show his or her perception, understanding, and interpretation of what is happening. An example of subjective data is the patient's statement, "The pain begins in my lower back and runs down my left leg."

Objective data are those facts that are observable and measurable by the nurse. These data are gathered by the nurse through physical assessment, interviewing, and observing and involve the use of the senses of seeing, hearing, smelling, and touching. An example of objective data is the measurement and recording of vital signs. Objective data are also gathered through such diagnostic examinations as laboratory tests, x-rays, and other diagnostic procedures.

Historical data are those health events that happened prior to this admission or health problem episode. An example of historical data is the patient statement, "The last time I was in a hospital was 1984 when I had an emergency appendectomy."

Current data are those facts specifically related to this admission or health problem episode. An example of this type of data is vital signs on admission—T 99.2°F, P 78, R 18, BP 134/86. Please note that just as there is overlapping of the nursing process steps, there is also overlapping of the data types. Both historical and current data may be either subjective or objective. Historical and current data assist in establishing time references and can give an indication of the patient's usual functioning.

Essential Skills

Assessment requires use of the skills needed for interviewing, conducting a physical examination, and observing. As with the nursing process itself, these skills are not used one at a time. While you are interviewing the patient, you are also observing and determining physical areas that require a detailed physical assessment. While completing a physical assessment, you are asking questions (interviewing) and observing the patient's physical appearance as well as the patient's response to the physical examination.

Interviewing generally starts with gathering data for the nursing history. In this interview, you ask for general demographic information such as name, address, date of last hospitalization, age, allergies, current medications, and the reason the patient was admitted. Depending on the agency's admission form, you may then progress to other specific questions or a physical assessment. An example of an admission assessment specifically related to the Functional Health Patterns is given in the Instructor's Manual.

The physical assessment calls for four skills: inspection, palpation, percussion, and auscultation. *Inspection* means careful and systematic observation throughout the physical examination such as observation for and recording of any skin lesions. *Palpation* means assessment by feeling and touching. Assessing the differences in temperature between a patient's upper and lower arm would be an example of palpation. Another common example of palpation is breast self-examination. *Percussion* involves touching, tapping and listening. Percussion allows determination of the size, density, locations, and boundaries of the organs. Percussion is usually performed by placing the index or middle finger of one hand firmly on the skin and striking with the middle finger of the other hand. The resultant sound is dull if the body is solid under the fingers (such as at the location of the liver) and hollow if there is a body cavity under the finger (such as at the location of the abdominal cavity). *Auscultation* involves listening with a stethoscope and is used to help assess respiratory, circulatory, and gastrointestinal status.

The physical assessment may be performed using a head-to-toe approach, a body system approach, or a Functional Health Patterns approach. In the *head-to-toe approach*, you begin with the patient's general appearance and vital signs. You would then progress, as the title indicates, from the head to the extremities.

The *body system approach* to physical assessment focuses on the major body systems. As the nurse is conducting the nursing history interview, she or he will get a firm idea of which body systems will need detailed examination. An example of this type of examination is a cardiovascular examination where the apical and radial pulses, blood pressure (BP), point of maximum intensity (PMI), heart sounds, and peripheral pulses are examined.

The *Functional Health Pattern approach* is based on Gordon's Functional Health Pattern typology and allows the collection of all types of data according to each pattern. This is the approach used by this book and leads to three levels of assessment. First is the overall admission assessment, where each pattern is assessed through the collection of objective and subjective data. This assessment will indicate patterns that need further attention, which requires implementation of the second level of pattern assessment. The second level of pattern assessment indicates which nursing diagnoses within the pattern might be pertinent to this patient, which leads to the third level of assessment, the defining characteristics for each individual nursing diagnosis. Having a three-tiered assessment might seem complicated, but each assessment is so closely related that completion of the assessment is easy. A primary advantage in using this type of assessment is the validation it gives to the nurse that the resulting nursing diagnosis is the most correct diagnosis. Another benefit to using this type of assessment is that grouping of data is already accomplished and does not have to be a separate step.

Data Grouping

Data grouping simply means organizing the information into sets or categories that will assist you to identify the patient's strengths and problem areas. A variety of organizing frameworks are available such as Maslow's Hierarchy of Needs, NANDA's Human Response Patterns, and Gordon's Functional Health Patterns. Each of the nursing theorists (e.g., Roy, Levine, and Orem) speak to assessment within the framework of their theories.

Organizing the information allows you to identify the appropriate Functional Health Pattern and will also allow you to spot any missing data. If you cannot identify the pertinent Functional Health Pattern, then you need to collect further data. The goal of data grouping is to arrive at a nursing diagnosis.

DIAGNOSIS

Diagnosis means reaching a definite conclusion regarding the patient's strengths and problems. The problems are the primary focus for planning care, and the strengths are used to assist you in implementing this care. In this book, we concentrate the diagnosis phase of the nursing process on nursing diagnosis and use the diagnoses accepted by NANDA for testing.

Nursing Diagnosis

The North American Nursing Diagnosis Association (NANDA), formerly the National Conference Group for Classification of Nursing Diagnosis, has been meeting since 1973 to identify, develop, and classify nursing diagnoses. Setting forth a nursing diagnosis nomenclature articulates nursing language, thus promoting the identification of nursing's contribution to health, and facilitates communication among nurses. In addition, the use of nursing diagnosis provides a clear distinction between nursing diagnosis and medical diagnosis and provides clear direction for the remaining aspects of the planning of care.

NANDA accepted its first working definition of nursing diagnosis in 1990[10]:

> A nursing diagnosis is a clinical judgment about individual, family, or community responses to actual or potential health problems/life processes. Nursing diagnoses provide the basis for selection of nursing interventions to achieve outcomes for which the nurse is accountable.

Much debate occurred during the Ninth Conference regarding this definition, and it is anticipated this debate will continue. The debate centers on a multitude of issues related to the definition, which are beyond the scope of this book. Readers are urged to consult the official journal of NANDA, *Nursing Diagnosis*, to keep up to date on this debate.

The definition of nursing diagnosis distinguishes nursing diagnosis from medical diagnosis. For example, nursing diagnosis is different from medical diagnosis in its focus. Kozier and Erb[11] write that nursing diagnoses focus on the patient response while medical diagnoses focus on the disease process. As indicated by the definition of nursing diagnosis, nurses also identify potential problems while physicians place primary emphasis on identifying the current problem.

Nursing diagnosis and medical diagnosis are similar in that the same basic procedures are used to derive the diagnosis (i.e., physical assessment, interviewing, and observing). Likewise, according to Kozier and Erb,[11] both types of diagnosis are designed for essentially the same reason—planning care for a patient.

A nursing diagnosis is based on the presence of defining characteristics. According to NANDA,[12] defining characteristics are clinical criteria that represent the presence of the diagnostic category (nursing diagnosis). For actual nursing diagnoses (the problem is present), a majority of the defining characteristics must be present. For risk diagnoses (risk factors indicate the problem might develop), the risk factors must be present.

Diagnostic Statements

According to the literature, complete nursing diagnostic statements include, at a minimum, the human response and an indication of the factors contributing to the response. The following is a rationale for the two-part statement[13]:

Each nursing diagnosis, when correctly written, can accomplish two things. One, by identifying the unhealthy response, it tells you what should change. . . . And two, by identifying the probable cause of the unhealthy response, it tells you what to do to effect change.

While there is no consensus on the phrase that should be used to link the response and etiologic factors, perusal of current literature indicates that the most commonly used phrases are *related to, secondary to,* and *due to.*

The phrase *related to* is gaining the most acceptance because it does not imply a direct cause-and-effect relationship. Kieffer[14] believes using the phrases *due to* and *secondary to* could reflect such a cause-and-effect relationship, which could be hard to prove. Thus a complete nursing diagnostic statement would read: Pain related to surgical incision.

Gordon[1] identifies three structural components of a nursing diagnostic statement: The problem (P), the etiology (E), and signs and symptoms (S). The *problem* describes the patient's response or current state (the nursing diagnosis). The *etiology* describes the cause or causes of the response (related to), and the *symptoms* delineate the defining characteristics or observable signs and symptoms demonstrated or described by the patient. The S component can be readily connected to the P and E statements through the use of the phrase *as evidenced by*. Using this format, a complete nursing diagnostic statement would read, "Pain related to surgical incision as evidenced by verbal comments and body posture."

As discussed in the preface, we recommend starting with stating the nursing diagnosis only. Therefore, the nursing diagnosis would be listed in the patient's chart in the same manner as it is given in the nomenclature: Pain. Remember that the objective and subjective data related to the patient's pain have already been recorded in the health record in the assessment section so there is no need to repeat it.

The nursing diagnostic statement examples given previously describe the existence of an actual problem. Professional nurses are strong supporters of preventive health care—cases in which a problem does not yet exist and measures that can be taken to ensure that the problem does not arise. In such instances the nursing diagnostic statement is prefaced by the words "Risk for." Nursing diagnoses that carry the preface "Risk for" also carry with them "Risk Factors" rather than "Defining Characteristics."

While the other books include a variety of nursing diagnoses, this book will use only the actual and risk (formerly labeled "potential") diagnoses accepted by NANDA for testing. Probable related factors (formerly "etiologic factors") will be grouped, as will the defining characteristics (formerly "signs and symptoms"), under each specific nursing diagnosis. As indicated in the preface, nursing actions in this book reflect a conceptual approach rather than a specific (to related factors or defining characteristics) approach.

To illustrate this approach, let us use the diagnosis Pain. There are common nursing orders related to the incidence of pain regardless of whether the pain is caused by surgery, labor, or trauma. You can take this conceptual approach and make an individualized adaptation according to the etiologic factors affecting your patient and the reaction your patient is exhibiting to pain.

Identifying and specifying the nursing diagnoses leads to the next phase of the process—planning. Now that you know what the problems and strengths are, you can decide how to resolve the problem areas while building on the strength areas.

PLANNING

Planning involves three subsets: setting priorities, writing expected outcomes, and establishing target dates. Planning sets the stage for writing nursing actions by establishing where we are going with our plan of care. Planning further assists in the final phase of evaluation by defining the standard against which we will measure progress.

Setting Priorities

With the sicker, quicker problem discussed earlier, you are going to find yourself in the situation of having identified many more problems that can possibly be resolved in a 1- to 3-day (today's average length of stay) hospitalization. In the long-term care facilities, such as home health, rehabilitation, and nursing homes, long-range problem solving is possible, but setting priorities of care is still necessary.

Several methods of assigning priorities are available. Some nurses will assign priorities based on the life threat posed by a problem. For example, Ineffective Airway Clearance would pose more of a threat to life than the diagnosis Risk for Impaired Skin Integrity. Some nurses will base their prioritization on Maslow's hierarchy of needs. In this instance, physiologic needs would require attention before social needs. One way to establish priorities is to simply ask the patient which problem he or she would like to pay attention to first. Another way to establish priorities is to analyze the relationships between problems. For example, a patient has been admitted with a medical diagnosis of headaches and possible brain tumor. The patient exhibits the defining characteristics of both Pain and Anxiety. In this instance we might want to implement nursing actions to reduce anxiety, knowing that if the anxiety is not reduced, pain control actions will not be successful. Once priorities have been established, you are ready to establish expected outcomes.

Expected Outcomes

Outcomes, goals, and *objectives* are terms that are frequently used interchangeably because all indicate the end point we will use to measure the effectiveness of our plan of care. Because so many published sets of standards and the JCAHO talk in terms of *outcome standards* or *criteria* we have chosen to use the term "expected outcomes" in this book.

Several authors[11,15,16] give guidelines for writing clinically useful expected outcomes:

1. Expected outcomes are clearly stated in terms of patient behavior or observable assessment factors.
   EXAMPLE
   POOR   Will increase fluid balance by time of discharge.

GOOD   Will increase oral fluid intake to 1500 mL per 24 hours by 9/11.

2. Expected outcomes are realistic, achievable, safe, and acceptable from the patient's viewpoint.

   EXAMPLE
   Mrs. Braxton is a 28-year-old female who has delayed healing of a surgical wound. She is to receive discharge instructions regarding a high-protein diet. She is a widow with three children under the age of 10. Her only source of income is Social Security.
   POOR   Will eat at least two 8-oz servings of steak daily. [unrealistic, nonachievable, unacceptable, etc.]
   GOOD   Will eat at least two servings from the following list each day:
   Lean ground meat
   Eggs
   Cheese
   Pinto beans
   Peanut butter
   Fish
   Chicken

3. Expected outcomes are written in specific, concrete terms depicting patient action.

   EXAMPLE
   POOR   Maintains fluid intake by 9/11.
   GOOD   Will drink at least 8 oz of fluid every hour from 7 a.m. to 10 p.m. by 9/11.

4. Expected outcomes are directly observable by use of at least one of the five senses.

   EXAMPLE
   POOR   Understands how to self-administer insulin by 9/11.
   GOOD   Accurately return-demonstrates self-administration of insulin by 9/11.

5. Expected outcomes are patient centered rather than nurse centered.

   EXAMPLE
   POOR   Teaches how to measure blood pressure by 9/11.
   GOOD   Accurately measures own blood pressure by 9/11.

Establishing Target Dates

Writing a target date at the end of the expected outcome statement facilitates the plan of care in several ways[11,15]:

1. Assists in "pacing" the care plan. Pacing helps keep the focus on the patient's progress.
2. Serves to motivate both patients and nurses toward accomplishing the expected outcome.
3. Helps patient and nurse to see accomplishments.
4. Alerts nurse when to evaluate care plan.

Target dates can be realistically established by paying attention to the usual progress and prognosis connected with the patient's medical and nursing diagnoses. Additional review of the data collected during the initial assessment will help indicate individual factors to be considered in establish-

ing the date. For example, one of the previous expected outcomes was stated as "Accurately return-demonstrates self-administration of insulin by 9/11."

The progress or prognosis according to the patient's medical and nursing diagnosis will not be highly significant. The primary factor will be whether diabetes mellitus is a new diagnosis for the patient or is a recurring problem for a patient who has had diabetes mellitus for several years.

For the newly diagnosed patient, we would probably want our deadline day to be 5 to 7 days from the date of learning the diagnosis. For the recurring problem, we might establish the target date to be 2 to 3 days from the date of diagnosis. The difference is, of course, the patient's knowledge base.

Now look at an example related to the progress issue. Mr. Kit is a 19-year-old college student who was admitted early this morning with a medical diagnosis of acute appendicitis. He has just returned from surgery following an appendectomy. One of the nursing diagnoses for Mr. Kit would, in all probability, be Pain. The expected outcome could be "Will have decrease in number of requests for analgesics by (date)." In reviewing the general progress of a young patient with this medical and nursing diagnosis, we know that generally analgesic requirements start decreasing within 48 to 72 hours. Therefore, we would want to establish our target date as 2 to 3 days following the day of surgery. This would result in the objective reading (assume date of surgery was 11/1): "Will have decrease in number of requests for analgesics by 11/3."

To further emphasize the target date, it is suggested that the date be underlined, highlighted by using a different-colored pen, or circled to make it stand out. Pinpointing the date in such a manner emphasizes that evaluation of progress toward achievement of the expected outcome should be made on that date. In assigning the dates, be sure not to schedule all of the diagnoses and expected outcomes for evaluation on the same date. Such scheduling would require a total revision of the plan of care which could contribute to not keeping the plan of care current. Being able to revise single portions of the plan of care facilitates use and updating of the plan. Remember the target date does not mean the expected outcome must be totally achieved by that time; instead, the target date signifies the evaluation date.

Once expected outcomes have been written, you are then ready to focus on the next phase—implementation. As previously indicated, the title supported by this book for this section is "Nursing Actions."

IMPLEMENTATION

Implementation is the action phase of the nursing process; hence, we chose the term "nursing actions." Two important steps are involved in implementation: The first is determining the specific nursing actions that will assist the patient to progress toward the expected outcome, and the second is documenting the care administered.

Nursing action is defined as nursing behavior that serves to help the patient achieve the expected outcome. Nursing actions include both independent and collaborative activities. *Independent actions* are those activities the nurse performs using his or her own discretionary judgment and that require no validation or guidelines from any other health care practitioner, for example, deciding which noninvasive technique to use for pain control or deciding when to teach the patient self-care measures. *Collaborative actions* are those activities that involve mutual decision making between two or more health care practitioners, for example, a physician and nurse's deciding which narcotic to use when meperidine is ineffective in controlling the patient's pain or a physical therapist and nurse's deciding on the most beneficial exercise program for a patient. Implementing a physician's order or referring a patient to a dietitian are other common examples of collaborative actions.

Written nursing actions guide both actual patient care and proper documentation, and they must therefore be detailed and exact. Written nursing actions should be even more definite than what is generally found in physician orders. For example, a physician writes the order "Increase ambulation as tolerated" for a patient who has been immobile for 2 weeks. The nursing actions should reflect specified increments of ambulation as well as ongoing assessment:

11/2	1.a. Prior to activity, assess BP, P, and R. After activity assess: (1) BP, P, R; (2) presence/absence of vertigo; (3) circulation; (4) presence/absence of pain.
	b. Assist to dangle on bedside for 15 minutes at least 4 times a day on 11/2.
	c. If BP, P, or R changes significantly or vertigo is present or circulation is impaired or pain is present, return to supine position immediately. Elevate head of bed 30 degrees for 1 hour; then 45 degrees for 1 hour; then 90 degrees for 1 hour. If tolerated with no untoward signs or symptoms, initiate order 1b again.
	d. Assist up to chair at bedside for 30 minutes at least 4 times a day on 11/3.
	e. Assist to ambulate to bathroom and back at least 4 times a day on 11/4.
	f. Supervise ambulation of one-half length of hall at least 4 times a day on 11/5 and 11/6.
	g. Supervise ambulation of length of hall at least 4 times a day on 11/7.

S. J. Smith, RN

Nursing actions further differ from physician orders in that the patient's response is directly related to the implementation of the action. It is rare to see a physician's order that includes alternatives if the first order has minimal, negative, or no effect on the patient.

A complete written nursing action incorporates at least the following five components according to Bolander[15]:

1. Date the action was initially written
2. A specific action verb that tells what the nurse is going to do (e.g., "assist" or "supervise")
3. A prescribed activity (e.g., ambulation)
4. Specific time units (e.g., for 15 minutes at least 4 times a day)
5. Signature of the nurse who writes the initial action order (i.e., accepting legal and ethical accountability)

A nursing action should not be implemented unless all five components are present. A nurse would not administer a medication if the physician's order read, "Give Demerol"; neither should a nurse be expected to implement a nursing action that reads, "Increase ambulation gradually."

Additional criteria that should be remembered to ensure complete, high-quality nursing action include:

1. Consistency between the prescribed actions, the nursing diagnosis, and expected outcome (including numbering).

   EXAMPLE
   Nursing diagnosis 1: Impaired physical mobility, level 2.
   Expected outcome 1: Will ambulate length of hall by 11/8.
   Nursing action 1:

11/2	1.a. Prior to activity, assess BP, P, and R. After activity, assess: (1) BP, P, R; (2) presence/absence of vertigo; (3) circulation; (4) presence/absence of pain.
	b. Assist to dangle on bedside for 15 minutes at least 4 times a day on 11/2.
	c. If BP, P, or R changes significantly or vertigo is present or circulation is impaired or pain is present, return to supine position immediately. Elevate head of bed 30 degrees for 1 hour; then 45 degrees for 1 hour; then 90 degrees for 1 hour. If tolerated with no untoward signs or symptoms, initiate order 1b again.
	d. Assist up to chair at bedside for 30 minutes at least 4 times a day on 11/3.
	e. Assist to ambulate to bathroom and back at least 4 times a day on 11/4.
	f. Supervise ambulation of one-half length of hall at least 4 times a day on 11/5 and 11/6.
	g. Supervise ambulation of length of hall at least 4 times a day on 11/7.

S. J. Smith, RN

2. Consideration of both patient and facility resources. It would be senseless to make referrals to physical and occupational therapy services if these were not available. Likewise, from a patient's resource viewpoint, it would be foolish to teach him and his family how to manage his care in a hospital bed if this bed would not be available to the patient at home.
3. Careful scheduling to include the patient's significant others and to incorporate his or her usual activities of daily living (i.e., rest, meals, sleep, and recreation).
4. Incorporation of patient teaching and discharge planning from the first day of care.
5. Individualization and updating in keeping with the patient's condition and progress.

Including the key components and validating the quality of the written nursing actions helps to promote improved documentation. In essence, the written nursing actions can give an outline for documentation.

Properly written nursing actions demonstrate to the nurse both nursing actions and documentation to be done. Referring to the preceding example, we can see that the nurse responsible for this patient's care should chart the patient's BP, P, and R rates prior to the activity, the patient's BP, P, and R rates after the activity, the presence or absence of vertigo, the presence or absence of pain, and the results of a circulatory check. Additionally, the nurse knows to chart that the patient dangled, sat up, or ambulated for a certain length of time or distance. Further, the nurse has guidelines of what to do and chart if an untoward reaction occurs in initial attempts at ambulation.

EXAMPLE

1000 BP 132/82, P 74, R 16. Up on side of bed for 5 minutes. Complained of vertigo and nausea. Returned to supine position with head of bed elevated to 30-degree angle. BP 100/68, P 80, R 24.

1100 BP 122/74, P 76, R 18. No complaints of vertigo or nausea. Head of bed elevated to 45-degree angle.

Writing nursing actions in such a manner automatically leads to reflection of the quality of care planning in the chart. Documentation of care planning in the patient's chart is essential to meet national standards of care and criteria for agency accreditation.

DOCUMENTATION

Just as development of the nursing process as a framework for practice has evolved, so documentation of that process has become an essential link between the provision of nursing care and the quality of the care provided. Several nursing documentation systems have emerged that make it easier to document the nursing process. Four of these systems will be discussed here. You will note that the narrative system is not discussed as it tends to be fragmented and disjointed, and it presents problems in retrieval of pertinent information about the patient response to and outcomes of nursing care.

The *Problem Oriented Record (POR)* with its format for documenting progress notes provides a system for documenting the nursing process. Additionally, POR is an interdisciplinary documentation system that can be used to coordinate care for all health care providers working with the patient.

The POR consists of four major components:

1. The database
2. The problem list
3. The plan of care
4. The progress notes

The *database* is that information that has been collected through patient interview, observation, and physical assessment and the results of diagnostic tests. The database provides the basis for developing the problem list.

The *problem list* is an inventory of numbered, prioritized patient problems. Patient problems may be written as nursing or medical diagnoses. Problems may be actual or risk diagnoses. Because each problem is numbered, information about each problem is easily retrieved.

The *plan of care* incorporates the expected outcomes, target dates, and prescribed nursing actions as well as other interventions designed to resolve the problem. The plan of care reflects multidisciplinary care and should be agreed to by the health care team.

The *progress note* provides information about the patient's response to or outcomes of the care provided. The full format for documenting progress is based on the acronym *SOAPIER*

which stands for *Subjective data, Objective data, Analysis/assessment, Plan, Intervention, Evaluation, and Revision.* As the plan of care is implemented for each numbered, prioritized problem, it is documented using the SOAPIER format. For example, recall the case of Mr. Kit, the 19-year-old college student who is recovering from an appendectomy. The problem list inventory would probably show Problem #1: Pain. His plan of care would state as an expected outcome: "Will have decrease in number of requests for analgesics by 11/3." Some of the written nursing actions would read:

1. Monitor for pain at least every 2 hours and have patient rank pain on a scale of 0 to 10.
2. Administer pain medications as ordered. Monitor response.
3. Spend at least 30 minutes once a shift teaching patient deep muscle relaxation. Talk patient through relaxation every 4 hours, while awake, at (list times here) once initial teaching is done.

The progress note of 11/3 would appear as follows:

PROBLEM 1
S "I have had only 1 pain medication during the last 24 hours, and that relieved my pain." "I would rank my pain as a 1 on a scale of 0 to 10."
O Relaxation exercises taught, and return-demonstration completed on 11/2. No request for pain medication within past 12 hours.
A Pain relieved.
P None.
I None.
E Expected outcome met. Problem resolved. Discontinue problem.
R None.

The POR with its SOAPIER progress note emphasizes the problem-solving component within the nursing process and provides documentation of the care provided. For further information about the POR system, you are directed to the Weed[17] reference.

FOCUS charting, which is actually an offshoot of POR, is a documentation system that uses the nursing process to document care. Unlike the interdisciplinary POR, FOCUS charting is entirely oriented to nursing documentation. Like the POR system, FOCUS charting has a database, a problem list (FOCUS), a plan of care, and progress notes. However, the FOCUS (problem list) is broader than the problem list in the POR. In addition to nursing and medical diagnoses, the FOCUS of care may also be treatments, procedures, incidents, patient concerns, changes in condition, or other significant events. The medical record incorporates the plan of care in a three-column format (in addition to date and signature) labeled FOCUS, expected patient outcomes, and nursing interventions. To illustrate, again with Mr. Kit:

Date/Signature	FOCUS	Expected Patient Outcome	Nursing Intervention
11/1 J. Jones, RN	Pain	Will have decrease in number of requests for analgesics by 11/3	Monitor for pain at least every 2 hours. Have pt rate pain on 0–10 scale. Administer pain med as ordered. Monitor response. Teach pt use of noninvasive pain relief techniques as appropriate.

The progress notes incorporate a flow sheet for documenting daily interventions and treatments and a narrative progress note using, again, a three-column format. The three-column format for the progress note includes a column for date, time, and signature, a FOCUS column, and a patient care note column. When the progress note is written in the patient care note column, it is organized using the acronym *DAR—Data, Action, and Response.* To illustrate, again using Mr. Kit:

Date/Time Signature	FOCUS	Patient Care Note	
11/1 1500 J. Jones, RN	Pain	**D**	C/o pain, "My side hurts. It is a 9 on a 0–10 scale." BP 130/84, P 88, R 22.
11/1 1530 J. Jones, RN		**A**	Demerol 100 mg given in rt gluteus. Turned to left side. Back rub given.
11/1 1615 J. Jones, RN		**R**	States pain is better. Rates it 2 on a 0–10 scale. BP 120/80, P 82, R 18.

FOCUS charting provides a succinct system for documenting the nursing process. It reflects all the elements required by JCAHO. It is flexible, provides cues to documentation with its DAR format, and makes it easy to retrieve pertinent data. For more information on FOCUS, use the information written by Lampe.[18]

The *PIE documentation system* emphasizes the nursing process and nursing diagnosis. PIE is the acronym for *Problem, Intervention, and Evaluation.* A time-saving aspect of this system is that PIE does not require a separate plan of care. The initial database and ongoing assessments are recorded on special forms or flow sheets. Assessment data are not included in the progress note unless a change in the patient's condition occurs. If a change occurs, A for Assessment would be recorded in the progress note. Routine interventions are recorded on a flow sheet, and the progress note is used for specific numbered problems.

When a problem is identified, it is entered into the progress note as a nursing diagnosis. Each problem is numbered consecutively during a 24-hour period, for example, P#1, and P#2. Therefore, the nurse may refer to the number rather than having to restate the problem. Interventions (I) directed to the problem are documented relative to the problem number (e.g., IP#1 or IP#2). Evaluation (E) reflects patient response to or outcomes of nursing interventions and is labeled according to the problem number (e.g., EP#1 or EP#2). To illustrate, again using Mr. Kit:

Date	Time	Nurse's Notes	
11/1	1500	P#1 IP#1	Pain. BP 130/84, P 88, R 22. J. Jones, RN
11/1	1530	IP#1	Demerol 100 mg given IM in rt gluteus. Turned to left side. Back rub given. J. Jones, RN
11/1	1615	EP#1	States pain relieved. Rates pain as 2 on a 0–10 scale. BP 120/80, P 82, R 18. J. Jones, RN

Each problem is evaluated at least every 8 hours, and all problems are reviewed and summarized every 24 hours. Continuing problems with appropriate interventions and evaluation are renumbered and redocumented daily, thus promoting continuity of care. When a problem is resolved, it no longer is documented.

The PIE documentation system reflects the nursing process and simplifies documentation by integrating the plan of care into the progress notes. This saves time and promotes easy retrieval of pertinent data. Siegrist, Deltor, and Stocks[19] are the originators of the PIE system.

Charting by Exception was developed by nurses at Saint Luke's Hospital in Milwaukee, Wisconsin.[20] Documenting in this system differs significantly from traditional systems in that nurses chart only significant findings or exceptions to a predetermined norm.

This system centers on the development of clinical standards that describe accepted norms. The system makes extensive use of flow sheets and is becoming increasingly popular due to its streamlined format and cost-effectiveness.

A patient care plan is established based on described standards. Nursing actions are used as the base for documentation. Flow sheets are used to highlight significant findings and define assessment parameters and findings. For example, for the postpartum patient, the standard for the cardiovascular assessment is:

Cardiovascular assessment: Apical pulse, CRT, peripheral pulses, edema, calf tenderness.
Standard: Regular apical pulse, CRT < 3 s, peripheral pulses palpable, no edema, no calf tenderness, nailbeds and mucous membranes pink.

If the assessment findings are the same as the standard, the nurse simply makes a checkmark on the flow sheet by cardiovascular assessment. If the assessment findings are different from the standard, the nurse marks an asterisk by cardiovascular assessment and explains the deviation from the standard in the narrative notes.

Charting by Exception has been shown to reduce documentation time and costs and increase attention to abnormal data. Additionally, documentation is more consistent.

More information about this system and examples of flowcharts can be found in the publication *Charting by Exception.*[20]

To complete the nursing process cycle and, depending on its outcome, perhaps start another cycle, the final phase of the process, evaluation, must be done.

EVALUATION

Evaluation simply means assessing what progress has been made toward meeting the expected outcomes; it is the most ignored phase of the nursing process. The evaluation phase is the feedback and control part of the nursing process. Evaluation requires continuation of assessment that was begun in the initial assessment phase. In this instance, assessment is the data collection form we use to measure patient progress.

Data Collection

Initially, specific data should be collected to measure the progress made toward achieving the stated expected outcome. As an example, let us return to the outcome written for Mr. Kit, the 19-year-old college student who had an appendectomy. The expected outcome was, "Will have decrease in number of requests for analgesics by 11/3." It is now 11/3, and the nurse caring for Mr. Kit notes the date and initiates evaluation of the stated outcome. She first checks the chart and counts the number of complaints of pain, number of analgesics given, and Mr. Kit's response to the pain medication. She looks for any change in medication or a change in Mr. Kit's condition. She then interviews Mr. Kit regarding his perception of pain acuity and level of relief. At the same time the nurse completes other assessments such as observing the wound condition and the ease of ambulation, or noting the presence of any other untoward signs or symptoms. The nurse then studies the data to see what action is necessary.

Action Following Data Collection

Action following data collection simply means making a nursing judgment of what modifications in the plan of care are needed. There are essentially only three judgments that can be made:

1. Resolved
2. Revise
3. Continue

Resolved means that the evaluative data indicate that the health care problem reflected in the nursing diagnosis and its accompanying expected outcome no longer exists; that is, the expected outcome has been met. The nurse documents the data collected and records the judgment—Resolved. To illustrate, let us return to Mr. Kit.

The nurse first reviews the chart. She finds that Mr. Kit requested pain medication every 3 to 4 hours for the first 18 hours after surgery. The nurses taught Mr. Kit relaxation exercises and turned him, positioned him, and gave him a back rub immediately after the administration of each analgesic. Mr. Kit has requested only 1 analgesic in the past 24 hours and none in the past 12 hours. He can return-demonstrate relaxation exercises and states he has only a mild "twinge" when he gets out of bed. He is looking forward to returning to school next week.

The nurse returns to the patient's chart and records the following: "11/3 Data—1 analgesic in past 24 hours; none in past 12 hours. Ambulates without pain; states having no pain. Resolved." She then will draw one line through the nursing diagnosis, related expected outcome(s), and nursing actions to show that they have been discontinued.

Revise can indicate two actions. In one instance, the initial nursing diagnosis was not correct so the diagnosis itself is revised. For example, the nurse may have made an initial diagnosis of Self-Esteem Disturbance. Upon collecting evaluation data, the patient and his family share further information that indicates the more appropriate diagnosis is Powerlessness, Moderate. The plan of care is then modified to reflect the change in the nursing diagnosis. For evaluation purposes, the nurse again records the data and the word "Revised." She then adds the new nursing diagnosis and marks one line through the initial nursing diagnosis.

In the second instance, while the nurse is collecting evaluation data for one nursing diagnosis and expected outcome, she finds assessment factors that show another problem has arisen. She simply records the appropriate judgment for the initial diagnosis and expected outcome (e.g., Resolved), and revises the plan to include the new nursing diagnosis with its appropriate expected outcome and nursing actions.

Continue indicates that the expected outcome has been met. The nurse again collects the appropriate data and, based on the data, makes the nursing judgment that the expected outcome has not been met. She records the data and adds the phrase, "Continue, reevaluate on (date)." She then modifies the plan of care by going back to the stated expected outcome, marking one line through the date, and adding a new date. Likewise, the nursing actions would be modified as necessary.

With evaluation, the nursing process cycle is completed (see Fig. 1–1). Another cycle can begin with both the nurse and the patient being sure that quality care is being given and received.

Nursing Process and Conceptual Frameworks

NURSING MODELS

Many nurses do not see a direct relationship between nursing models (nursing theories) and nursing process, but a direct relationship does exist. *Nursing models* present a systematic method for assessing and directing nursing practice through promoting organization and integration of what is known

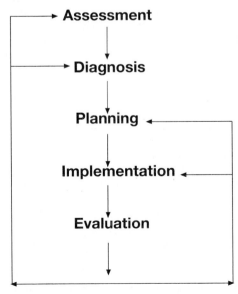

Figure 1–1 Nursing process flowchart.

about human health, illness, and nursing. Nursing models are based on purposeful orientations[21]; therefore, the *nursing process* is the action phase of a nursing model. In essence, models guide the use of the nursing process,[22] and, as previously stated, the care planning presented in this book is a result of the nursing process.

For further clarification, let us look at a few examples. If you are a supporter of Levine's conservation model, you would assess your patient in keeping with this model and then design your care plan to reflect prioritizing of the nursing diagnoses and nursing actions in a manner that would best promote conservation principles. Likewise, if you are a proponent of Roy's adaptation model, you would assess the four adaptation modes, then prioritize your diagnoses in an order that would best promote adaptive responses. In summation, current nursing models affect care planning in terms of assessment and prioritizing of nursing diagnoses rather than requiring different diagnostic statements and different nursing actions.

PATTERNS

Several typologies have emerged as a result of the work done with nursing diagnosis. The typologies are representative of another step in theory development and are designed to facilitate the use of nursing diagnosis. The typologies provide an organizational framework that enables the nurse to focus on the pattern description and assessment rather than trying to remember all the details of individual diagnoses. The nurse can easily locate the individual diagnoses by being familiar with the patterns.

Functional Health Patterns

Gordon[1] writes that the Functional Health Patterns were identified, circa 1974, to assist in the teaching of assessment and diagnosis at Boston College School of Nursing. The Functional Health Patterns organize the individual diagnoses into categories, thus providing for the organized collection of assessment data.

The advantages[1] offered by assessment according to the Functional Health Patterns include having a standardized method that does not have to be relearned if the setting, patient's age, or condition changes; having an assessment tool specifically designed to lead to identification of pertinent nursing diagnoses; and having an assessment method that is holistic in nature.

Functional Health Patterns focus on the client's usual ways of living[1] and direct attention to all the factors that impact the individual in these ways of living. Gordon[1] defines a pattern as "a sequence of behaviors across time." The Functional Health Patterns allow the nurse to assess these behaviors by promoting the patient's describing his or her own perception as well as incorporating the nurse's observations. Both the patient's description and the nurse's observations must be included to ensure a complete assessment.

Use of the Functional Health Patterns for assessment allows identification of three major types of data:

1. **Functional patterns:** The Functional Patterns are client strengths that can be used to deal with either dysfunctional or potentially dysfunctional patterns, for example, Assessment of the Coping–Stress Tolerance Pattern shows no problem areas. The nurse can then use this functional pattern to assist the patient in learning to cope with the identified problem areas.

2. **Dysfunctional patterns:** The Dysfunctional Health Patterns identify problem areas and the nursing diagnoses related to the problem areas, for example, in assessing the Elimination Pattern, the nurse identifies problems with urination and specifically with Urinary Retention. Knowing that the patient has effective individual coping, the nurse then plans teaching that will utilize this strength rather than interventions that are totally nursing focused such as intermittent catheterization. The nurse could teach the patient to use Crede's maneuver, pouring warm water over the genital area, running tap water, and so on to use the client's already demonstrated strength.

3. **Potential dysfunctional patterns:** The Potential Dysfunctional Patterns are risk conditions, for example, a client who has urinary retention is at risk for the development of Excess Fluid Volume. Utilizing this knowledge, the nurse would identify areas of observation to monitor and to teach the patient to monitor.

Use of the Functional Health Patterns in assessment stresses focus on a nursing model of assessment, diagnosis, planning, intervention, and evaluation rather than a medical model. Thus, the nurse can readily differentiate between areas for independent nursing intervention and areas requiring collaboration or referral.

Table 1–3 lists the Functional Health Patterns along with a brief description of each pattern as designed by Gordon.[23] The titles of the patterns are, in essence, self-explanatory. Because the titles are self-explanatory, the Functional Health Patterns are easy to use. The chapters in this book are organized using the Functional Health Patterns, and each chapter includes more detail regarding each Functional Health Pattern as introductory information for the specific chapter.

Human Response Patterns

Patterns of Unitary Persons was first presented at the Fourth National Conference of NANDA. A group of nursing theorists met in between, as well as during, conferences to design a framework for classification of nursing diagnoses.[24,25] The NANDA Taxonomy Committee and Special Interest Group on Taxonomy[26] reviewed, clarified, and relabeled the patterns as Human Response Patterns. These revisions were presented at the Fifth and Sixth National Conferences. The patterns proposed by the theorist group describe clustering factors that represent person-environment interaction.[27] The Unitary Persons categories were not mutually exclusive; that is, one nursing diagnosis might relate to one, two, or even three of the patterns. From the Fifth through the Ninth National Conferences, refinement of the Human Response Patterns has continued. At the Seventh National Conference the Human Response Patterns were presented as the framework for the "NANDA Nursing Diagnosis Taxonomy I,"[28] and the taxonomy was endorsed by NANDA members attending this conference. To assist you in applying this typology, each diagnosis has information regarding its category and coding place in the Human Response Pattern.

This endorsement indicated acceptance of Taxonomy I as a working document that would require further testing, revision, refinement, and expansion. Additional input regarding Taxonomy I Revised was solicited at the Eighth National Conference. Much of the discussion at the Eighth Con-

Table 1–3 **FUNCTIONAL HEALTH PATTERNS**

Pattern	Description
Health perception—health management	The patient's awareness of personal health and well-being; health practices; understanding of how health practices contribute to health status
Nutritional—metabolic	The patient's description of food and fluid intake; relationship of intake to metabolic needs; includes indicators of ineffectual nutrition on metabolic functioning, for example, healing
Elimination	Description of all routes and routines of output; includes any aids to excretion
Activity—exercise	Patient's overall activities of daily living, including recreational activity
Sleep—rest	Patient's 24-h routine of rest, relaxation, and sleep
Cognitive—perceptual	Cognitive functional performance and sensory performance
Self-perception—self-concept	Patient's self-assessment; attitudes, ability, worth; verbal and nonverbal communication
Role relationship	Patient's assessment of all roles, related responsibilities, and interrelatedness between these factors and other people
Sexuality—reproductive	Satisfaction-dissatisfaction with sexuality; any dysfunction in sexuality or reproduction
Coping—stress tolerance	Effectiveness or noneffectiveness in dealing with difficult situations; how handles; reaction to; support available
Value—belief	Ideas held in esteem by patients; guiding principles for overall lifestyle

Source: From Gordon,[23] p 2, with permission.

ference focused on the various levels of the taxonomy with specific question of the clinical usefulness of Level I.

The first level of abstraction in Taxonomy I is the Human Response Patterns. The second level is alterations in functions. Levels II through V become increasingly concrete, with Levels IV and V reflecting the diagnostic labels. Table 1–4 lists the Human Response Patterns with accompanying brief definitions. In this book we have focused on Level II and include levels IV and V in the conceptual information and Have You Selected the Correct Diagnosis? sections.

Diagnostic Divisions

Doenges, Moorhouse, and Geissler[29] designed the Diagnostic Divisions for use in their book *Nursing Care Plans: Guidelines for Planning Patient Care*. The Diagnostic Divisions group nursing diagnoses by related categories. These related categories are the result of a blending of Maslow's hierarchy of needs and a self-care philosophy. Table 1–5 demonstrates the diagnostic divisions with an explanation of each division.

Valuing Planning of Care and Care Plans

The nursing process and the resultant plan for nursing care have not been given the attention or credit that they deserve. Part of the problem is that planned nursing care has not had value attached to it. All of us will make time or a place for those things that are of value to us. It is only recently that completing and evaluating the quality of care planning has begun to show up on employee evaluation forms. Likewise, it is still rare to see "complete nursing care plan" or "update care plan" on the patient assignment form.

With the changes that are occurring in health care, due to federal and state legislated mandates, completion and use of nursing care planning is going to increase in importance. Several insurance companies now audit charts, care plans, and the like in detail. No documentation of care means no reimbursement for care. Likewise, one of the first places a lawyer looks when hunting evidence for health-related court cases is the patient's

chart. The basic principle in lawsuits has been "not charted, not done." Planning care as we propose in this book would furnish additional documentation that reasonably prudent care was given as well as providing a guideline for better charting.

Use of nursing diagnosis helps ensure that teaching and discharge planning are considered from the start of care. As we increase our knowledge and begin to think in terms related to nursing nomenclature, nursing actions for many of the diagnoses will relate to teaching and planning for home care.

Many of the standards supported by the JCAHO, the ANA, and state boards of nursing are automatically implemented when the nursing process is completed, implemented, and documented. A review of these standards by the reader will show that the nursing process and careful planning of care can meet several standards just by writing a nursing care plan.

It is not uncommon to hear, "I don't do care plans because I don't have time to do them." It is true that there is an investment of time in completing and documenting the nursing process, but in the long-range view, such planning of care actually saves time. To illustrate, one nurse, known to the authors, works full time in nursing education but works part time at a local hospital to keep her clinical skills current. One afternoon she went to work at the hospital, received her patient assignments and a brief report, then began to implement patient care. One nursing order read, "Change dressing as needed." Assessment of the dressing showed a change was needed. In the patient's room were all kinds of dressings, fluids, and ointments. There were no instructions for changing the dressing on the care plan or the patient's chart. The nurse then requested information from the patient who stated, "I don't like to look at it, so I don't know." The nurse then began to search for a staff member who had cared for this patient and could teach her the routine for the special dressing change. After 30 minutes, she finally found a nurse who had cared for the patient. Learning the proper dressing change took only a few minutes. The nurse then went back to the care plan, and in 3 minutes recorded the way to change the dressing under nursing orders.

Comparing the time it took to locate the information and

Table 1–4 HUMAN RESPONSE PATTERNS

Pattern	Description
Exchanging	To give, relinquish, or lose something while receiving something in return; the substitution of one element for another; the reciprocal act of giving and receiving
Communicating	To converse; to impart, confer, or transmit thoughts, feelings, or information, internally or externally, verbally or nonverbally
Relating	To connect, to establish a link between, to stand in some association to another thing, person, or place; to be borne or thrust in between things
Valuing	To be concerned about, to care; the worth or worthiness; the relative status of a thing, or the estimate in which it is held, according to its real or supposed worth, usefulness, or importance; one's opinion of like for a person or thing; to equate in importance
Choosing	To select between alternatives; the action of selecting or exercising preference in regard to a matter in which one is a free agent; to determine in favor of a course; to decide in accordance with inclinations
Moving	To change the place or position of a body or any member of the body; to put and/or keep in motion; to provoke an excretion or discharge; the urge to action or to do something; leave in; to take action
Perceiving	To apprehend with the mind; to become aware of by the senses; to apprehend what is not open or present to observation; to take in fully or adequately
Knowing	To recognize or acknowledge a thing or person; to be familiar with by experience or through information or report; to be cognizant of something through observation, inquiry, or information; to be conversant with a body of facts, principles, or methods of action; to understand
Feeling	To experience a consciousness, sensation, apprehension, or sense; to be consciously or emotionally affected by a fact, event, or state

Source: From Fitzpatrick, JJ: Taxonomy II: Definitions and development. In Carroll-Johnson, RM (ed): Classification of Nursing Diagnosis: Proceedings of the Ninth Conference. Lippincott, Philadelphia, 1991, with permission.

the time it took to record the information gives a graphic example of how time can be saved by completing and documenting the nursing process. Consider the time saved if the written nursing actions are used as an outline for charting or the time that could be saved in between shift reports if documentation of the nursing process was complete. Lastly, consider the time that could be saved by not having to go to court when questions arise over reasonable prudent care. Making time to use and document the nursing process because we can see its value to us actually saves us time in the long run.

Summary

The nursing process provides a strong framework that gives direction to the practice of nursing. By completing each phase, you can reassure yourself that you are providing quality, individualized care that meets local, state, and national standards. By using the NANDA nomenclature and by providing feedback to NANDA, you can help develop this nomenclature and help ensure that nursing is recognized for the contributions it makes to our nation's health.

Table 1–5 DIAGNOSTIC DIVISIONS AND NURSING DIAGNOSES

Diagnostic Divisions	Description
Activity/rest	Ability to engage in necessary/desired activities of life (work and leisure), and to obtain sleep/rest
Circulation	Ability to transport oxygen and nutrients necessary to meet cellular needs
Ego integrity	Ability to develop and use skills and behaviors to integrate and manage life experiences
Elimination	Ability to excrete waste products
Food/fluid	Ability to maintain intake of and utilize nutrients and liquids to meet physiologic needs
Hygiene	Ability to perform activities of daily living
Neurosensory	Ability to perceive, integrate, and respond to internal and external cues
Pain/comfort	Ability to control internal/external environment to maintain comfort
Respiration	Ability to provide and utilize oxygen to meet physiologic needs
Safety	Ability to provide safe, growth-promoting environment
Sexuality (component of ego integrity and social interaction)	Ability to meet requirements/characteristics of male/female role
Social interaction	Ability to establish and maintain relationships
Teaching/learning	Ability to incorporate and use information to achieve health lifestyle/optimal wellness

Source: From Doenges, Moorhouse, and Geissler,[29] p 13, with permission.

Health Perception – Health Management Pattern

Pattern Description

Nurses assist individuals, families, and communities who have limited knowledge or understanding of:

1. Their current health status
2. How to achieve a good health status
3. How to maintain a good health status

This lack of perception (awareness) leads to problems for the individual or family in the management (control) of their health status. The nursing diagnoses in this pattern result from this lack of perception and management.

Pattern Assessment

1. Review the patient's vital signs. Is the temperature within normal limits?
   a. Yes
   b. No (Risk for Infection; Altered Protection)
2. Review the results of the complete blood cell (CBC) count. Are the cell counts within normal limits?
   a. Yes
   b. No (Risk for Infection; Altered Protection)
3. Review sensory status (sight, hearing, touch, smell, and taste). Is the patient's sensory-status within normal limits?
   a. Yes
   b. No (Risk for Injury)
4. Was patient and family satisfied with the usual health status?
   a. Yes
   b. No (Health-Seeking Behavior; Altered Health Maintenance)
5. Did the patient, family, or community describe the usual health status as good?
   a. Yes
   b. No (Health-Seeking Behavior; Altered Health Maintenance)
6. Had the patient, family, or community sought any health care assistance in the past year?
   a. Yes (Health-Seeking Behavior)
   b. No (Altered Health Maintenance)
7. Did the patient, or family follow the routine the (doctor, nurse, dentist, etc.) prescribed?
   a. Yes (Effective Management of Therapeutic Regimen)
   b. No (Noncompliance, Ineffective Management of Therapeutic Regimen)
8. Did the patient or family have any accidents or injuries in the past year?
   a. Yes (Risk for Injury)
   b. No
9. Is there a disruption (change in temperature, color, field, movement, or sound) of the flow of energy surrounding the person?
   a. Yes (Energy Field Disturbance)
   b. No
10. Was the patient, family, or community able to meet therapeutic needs of all members?
    a. Yes (Effective Management of Therapeutic Regimen, [Individual, Family, Community])
    b. No (Ineffective Management of Therapeutic Regimen, [Individual, Family, Community])
11. Is the patient scheduled for surgery, or has he or she recently undergone surgery?
    a. Yes (Risk for Perioperative Positioning Injury)
    b. No

Conceptual Information

A person who practices health management techniques, for example, exercises regularly, pays attention to diet, and maintains a balance of rest and activity, has an accurate view of his or her, or his or her family's personal health status and will also identify other ways to maintain health. These people will be accurate in reporting their current health status. They also will readily identify alterations (changes) in health status and will take active steps to correct these changes to increase their movement toward optimal health. Additionally, they will also initiate measures to prevent further alterations in health status. The goal in health management is to assist all patients to achieve this level of health maintenance.

Various factors influence a person's ability to achieve optimal health perception (understanding) and health management (control). Human beings are described by Martha Rogers as energy fields.[1] Disturbance in these fields can produce symptoms. Another major factor affecting health is individual and/or family interaction with the environment.[1] This interaction increases the likelihood that environmental hazards will play a role in health management by increasing exposure to problem areas. Health protection activities can reduce environmental hazards and increase optimal health management. Examples of such activities include individual and community efforts to clean up air pollution, ensure a safe water supply, and manage sewage and hazardous waste disposal.

Another major factor is an intact sensory system. Sensory organs provide information to the individual regarding the environment. An intact nervous system is also required since it provides for optimum functioning of sensory, motor, and cognitive activities. An accurate cognitive-perceptual pattern and self-perception—self-concept pattern are also necessary to achieve the optimal level of health perception and management. The ability to think and understand greatly impacts basic knowledge of health and illness. Likewise the individual's feeling of self-worth and interpretation of the meaning of health and illness to the self will influence his or her health practices. Knowledge related to health promotion and disease prevention is essential for the individual to fully maintain health management.

Cultural, societal, and familial values and beliefs also influence the capacity to achieve positive health perception and health management. Values and beliefs influence what is identified as optimal health. Availability of appropriate health care resources in a community impacts the health care delivery system and the ability of the community to manage a therapeutic regimen. The development of nursing diagnoses for communities requires nurses to also develop interventions to influence health policy and to work with advocacy groups.[2]

The Health Belief Model[3] (see Fig. 2–1) provides a framework in which to study actions taken by individuals to avoid illness. A basic assumption of the model is that the subjective state of the individual is more important in determin-

Individual Perception	**Modifying Factors**	**Likelihood of Action**

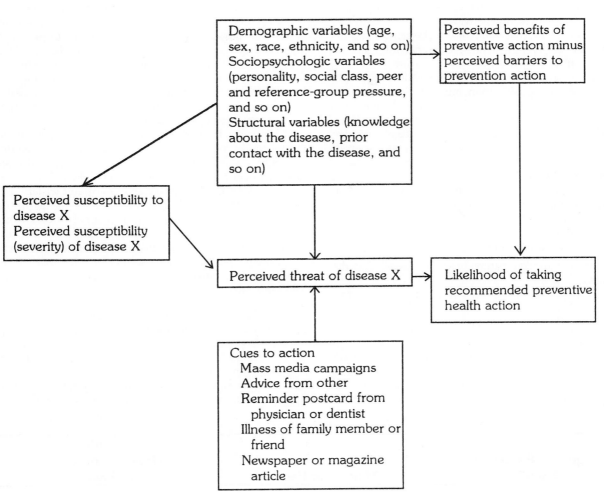

Figure 2–1 The Health Belief Model. (From Becker, MH, et al: Selected psychosocial models and correlates of individual health-related behaviors. Medical Care 15:27, 1977 [Suppl], with permission.)

ing actions than is the objective reality of the situation. The health belief model states that for an individual to take action to avoid a disease, she or he needs to believe the following:

1. That she or he is personally susceptible to disease
2. That the occurrence of the disease will have at least a moderate impact on some part of her or his life
3. That taking action will be beneficial
4. That such action will not involve overcoming psychological barriers such as cost, pain, or embarrassment

These beliefs can be described as variables under the headings of "perceived susceptibility" and "severity" and as the variables that define perceived benefits and barriers to taking action. Because these variables do not account for the activation of the behavior, the originators of the health belief model have added another class of variable called "cues to action." The individual's level of readiness provides the energy to act, and the perception of benefits provides a preferred manner of action that offers the path of least resistance. A cue to action is required to set off this appropriate action. The model suggests that by manipulating any combi-

nation of variables affecting action, the inclination to seek preventive care can be altered.

The Health Belief Model does not contain concepts related to knowledge of disease as a potential factor in determining an individual's decision to engage in preventive behavior. Several authors point out that knowledge of health consequences has only a limited relationship to the occurrence of the desired health behavior.[4–6] Yet, quite often, imparting knowledge about diseases to the patient, in an effort to encourage future preventive behavior, is the main method employed by nurses.

The Health Belief Model is disease specific. The model does not adequately explain positive health actions designed to maximize wellness, fulfillment, and self-actualization. Although the health belief model is useful in predicting preventive behavior, it does not fully explain behavior motivated by health promotion.[7] More research is needed to identify the determinants of health-promoting behavior to increase our ability to assist the patient in achieving health promotion. Preventing energy field disturbances, for example, is an area of research appropriate to nursing practice.

The Health Belief Model does provide the nurse with the conceptual notion that by working with the patient's perception of the situation, increasing the patient's cues to action, and decreasing the patient's barriers to action, the nurse can enhance the possibility that the patient will engage in disease prevention and early detection activities.

Pender[7] points out that while health promotion and disease prevention are complementary concepts, they are not congruent (identical). Health promotion is directed toward growth and improvement in well-being, while disease prevention conceptually operates to maintain the status quo.[8]

The Health Belief Model as developed by Pender[7] (see Fig. 2–2) provides the framework for nursing research and practice. This model emphasizes the importance of cognitive-perceptual factors in behavior regulation. Cognitive-perceptual factors, for example, understanding of the importance of health, understanding of the definition of health, perceived self-competency, and perceived control of health, are primary motivational mechanisms for health-promoting behavior.

Healthy People 2000[9] describes the national health promotion and disease prevention objectives. Three major goals are addressed by this document:

1. To prevent the premature onset of disease and disability.
2. To help all Americans achieve healthier, more productive lives.
3. To reduce health care costs.

The document presents baseline epidemiologic data and projected goals for health promotion, health protection, and preventive services. Special emphasis is placed on vulnerable populations, for example, lower socioeconomic status, disabled, elderly, and ethnic. This document is recommended as a guide for identifying factors that influence the health perception–health management pattern. Strategies for intervention and evaluation are also included in this document.

Whether working with individuals, families, or communities, the nurse should plan interventions appropriate for the learning needs of those being targeted. Mass-media campaigns are useful when conveying general information to large groups of people, but one-to-one communication is more effective for instructing individuals in their particular circumstances. *Put Prevention into Practice*[10] is a comprehensive system developed to assist the clinician and the patient and his or her family to establish a routine of preventive behaviors and services. The kit includes a clinician's handbook, preventive care timelines, office reminders, and patient-oriented materials to promote preventive behaviors.

The concepts of primary, secondary, and tertiary prevention[11] are also useful to the nurse when using the health management pattern. It is important for the nurse to recognize that a focus on the patient's strengths, not just the patient's problems, is an integral part of health promotion.[12, 13]

Primary prevention consists of activities that prevent a disease from occurring. A patient engaging in primary prevention activities would:

1. Maintain up-to-date immunizations
2. Have adequate water supply and sanitation facilities
3. Use seat belts and infant car seats and properly store household poisons to minimize accident fatalities
4. Eliminate tobacco products
5. Maintain adequate nutrition, elimination, exercise, social and personal relationships, and so on

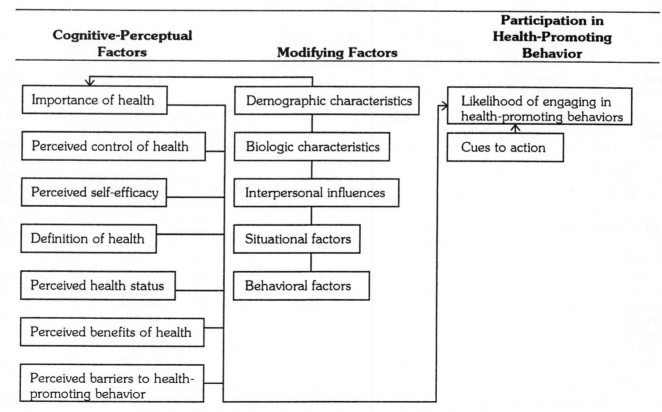

Figure 2–2 Health Promotion Model. (From Pender,[7] p 58, with permission.)

6. Employ regular oral care and dental examinations
7. Use protection against excessive sun exposure
8. Maintain weight within normal range for age, sex, and height
9. Maintain an environment free of chemical, biological, and physical hazards
10. Maintain regular sleep and rest patterns
11. Practice healthy nutritional intake (e.g., low salt, sugar, and fat intake with balanced intake of basic four food groups and total calories as appropriate for age, sex, and condition)
12. Maintain regular relaxation, recreation, and exercise activities

Secondary prevention indicates those activities designed to detect disease before symptoms are recognized. These activities include:

1. Glaucoma screening
2. Hypertensive screening
3. Hearing and vision testing
4. Pap smears
5. Breast examinations
6. Prostate and testicle examinations
7. Well-baby examinations
8. Colon and rectal examinations

Tertiary prevention refers to the treatment, care, and rehabilitation of current illness. This area indicates the patient needs to:

1. Adhere to medical and nursing treatments
2. Make lifestyle changes necessitated by condition
3. Seek consultation from experts in area requiring intervention, for example, individual practitioners and support groups

Developmental Considerations

Care providers can encourage the acceptance of responsibility for health-promoting activities and adherence to agreed-on treatment plans by giving appropriate attention to the impact developmental levels have on the individual or the primary caregiver. Publications such as *Prevention Across the Lifespan*[14] and *Put Prevention into Practice*[10] can assist the nurse, patient, family, and community to establish a routine of health-promoting behaviors and practices.

INFANT AND TODDLER

Since the neonate is totally dependent on others for care, it is the primary caregiver who is entrusted with carrying out the therapeutic interventions. As the infant grows and develops, self-care abilities increase. The following information outlines developmental milestones from birth to approximately 24 months as described by Piaget's sensorimotor stage of cognitive development.[15] During this period of development the individual must be protected from hazards in the environment, and the primary caregiver must assume the major share of responsibility for compliance with the treatment program.

Providing a safe environment includes the following accident prevention strategies: (a) turning pot handles away from edge of stove; (b) storing medicines, matches, alcohol, plastic bags, and house and garden chemicals in child-proofed areas; (c) using cold-water, not hot-water, humidifier; (d) avoiding heating formula in microwave; (e) using protection screens on heaters, fireplaces, and electrical outlets; (f) using nonflammable clothing; (g) gating stairways and windows; (h) supervising children at play, while bathing, in car, or in shopping cart; (i) controlling pets or stray animals; (j) avoiding hanging items around neck; (k) providing a smoke-free environment; (l) avoiding small objects that can be inserted in mouth or nose; (m) avoiding pillows and plastic in crib; (n) removing poisonous plants from house and garden; and (o) removing lead-based paint.

Children should be screened at birth for congenital anomalies, phenylketonuria (PKU), thyroid function, cystic fibrosis, vision, and hearing. A newborn assessment should be performed, and anticipatory guidance should be provided for patients regarding growth and development, safety, health promotion, and disease prevention.

Well-baby examinations and developmental assessments are recommended at 2, 4, 6, 15, and 18 months.[10, 16] Height and weight should be recorded on growth charts with hemoglobin and hematocrit checked at least once during infancy. Parent counseling includes discussion of nutrition with attention paid to iron-rich foods, safety and accident prevention, oral, perineal, and perirectal hygiene, sensory stimulation of the infant, baby bottle tooth decay, and the effects of passive smoking. Immunizations are given during the well-baby checks according to the following schedule[17,18]:

1. Diphtheria, pertussis, tetanus (DPT) at 2, 4, 6, and 12 to 18 months or DtaP at 15 months.
2. Oral polio vaccine at 2, 4, and 6 to 18 months.
3. Measles, mumps, and rubella (MMR) vaccine and tuberculin test at 12 to 15 months.
4. Varicella vaccine is recommended for children between 12 and 18 months, preferably at the same visit that the MMR vaccine is administered.[19]
5. *Haemophilus* influenza type b conjugate vaccine (HibCV) should be given at 2, 4, 6, and 12 to 15 months.[18, 20, 21]

For children who have not been immunized during the first year of life, you will need to consult the latest established standards for appropriate timetables.[17,22] Hepatitis B vaccine (HBv) should be given at birth, 2 to 4 months, and 6 to 18 months.[18,23] HBv can be administered at the same time as DTP and/or HibCV.[23]

Host factors such as age and behavior will affect the susceptibility to infectious disease. In general, most infectious diseases produce the greatest morbidity and mortality in the very old and the very young.[24] It is also important to note that the normal newborn will have a white blood cell count that is higher than that of the normal adult. The normal white blood cell count decreases gradually throughout childhood until reaching the adult norms.[25] It is essential that the nurse be very familiar with the blood cell count norms for this age group.

During fetal life, the fetus is protected by maternal antibodies (assuming the mother has developed antibodies to these diseases) to diseases such as diphtheria, tetanus, measles, and polio. This temporary immunity lasts 3 to 6 months. Colostrum contains antibodies that provide protection against enteric pathogens. Some infections can cross the placental barrier, leading to the development of congenital (present at birth) infections. Syphilis, HIV, and rubella are examples of such infections. Pathogenic organisms such as herpes simplex may be acquired during passage through the birth canal. Because the infant does not begin to produce its own immunoglobulins until 2 to 3 months after birth, he or she is susceptible to infections for which he or she has not gained passive immunity.

TORCH infections (toxoplasmosis, hepatitis B, rubella, cytomegalovirus, herpes) can be of serious concern during the perinatal period.[26] When caring for a pregnant female or a newborn, it is important to teach techniques to prevent acquisition and transmission of these disorders and to recognize early signs and symptoms so that early interventions can be instituted. For newborns the HBv series should be initiated at birth before discharge from the hospital.[23]

Child care practices must include hygienic disposal of soiled diapers and cleaning of the perineum. Proper handwashing technique is required of the care provider. Proper formula preparation and storage are also critical if the newborn is to be bottle-fed. Anatomically the newborn and infant's eustachian tube facilitates the passage of infection-causing organisms into the middle ear. It is important for care providers not to prop bottles but rather to hold the newborn or infant while feeding. Passive exposure to tobacco smoke irritates the bronchial tree and increases the possibility of respiratory infection.

The infant may respond to an infection with a very high fever. Care providers should be taught how to take axillary temperatures, to provide hydration to an ill infant, to give tepid baths when a fever is elevated, and to seek professional evaluation when an infant has a febrile illness.

TODDLER AND PRESCHOOLER

During the preoperational period, children learn how to teach themselves through trial and error, exploration, and repetition. From age 2 to 4, the child is egocentric, using himself or herself as a standard for others; he or she can categorize on the basis of a single characteristic. Because of the child's curiosity and exploration of the environment, it is important for the care provider to provide a safe environment. During this period the words "no," "hot," "sharp," and "hurt" should be introduced and repeatedly reinforced by the care provider. Safety rules should be taught and reinforced frequently.

From age 4 to 7, the child can begin to see simple relationships and has the beginning ability to think in logical classes. The child can learn his or her own address and can follow directions of three steps. Rules need to be reinforced. The child can be responsible for personal hygiene with instruction and coaching.

Strategies used to provide a safe environment for the infant should also be employed during childhood. Discipline, accident prevention, and the development of self-care proficiency related to eating, dressing, bathing, and dental hygiene are important areas of concern. Developmental assessments with emphasis on hearing, vision, and speech are recommended. DPT or DTaP and OPV are given once between the ages of 4 and 6, at or before school entry. Consult guidelines if the child has not been immunized during the first year of life.[17,22] The Immunizations Practices Advisory Committee (ACIP) of the U.S. Public Health Service[27] recommends that a second dose of MMR be given at 4 to 5 years, when the child enters kindergarten.

Anticipatory guidance should be given to parents on the development of initiative and guilt, nutrition and exercise, safety and accident prevention, toothbrushing and dental care, effects of passive smoking, and skin protection from ultraviolet light.[15] Additionally, the parents should be taught that, as the child begins to explore the environment and put objects and foods into his or her mouth, it will be important to ensure that contact with infectious pathogens or foreign bodies is controlled. Foreign-object-induced infection should be considered in childhood infections of the external ear, nose, and vagina.

If the preschooler has been exposed to other children, he or she most likely will have experienced several middle ear, gastrointestinal, and upper respiratory tract infections. If the child has not been around other children, he or she will likely experience such infections when entering preschool or kindergarten. Preventing injuries will also assist in the prevention of infection. The adenoidal and tonsillar lymphoid tissue may normally enlarge during the early school years partly in response to the exposure to pathogens in school.

The child will require assistance with toileting hygiene until 4 to 5 years of age. Handwashing techniques can be introduced along with toilet training and followed with consistent role modeling by the adults and older children with assistance to the child. Bubble baths and other scented soaps and toilet tissue may irritate the urethra in the female and lead to urinary tract or vaginal infections. Parents, grandparents, and the child should be taught to avoid such items. In addition, proper dental hygiene can be taught to the child to help in preventing tooth and gum infections.

SCHOOL-AGE CHILD

This period is characterized by developing logical approaches to concrete problems; the concepts of reversibility and conservation are developed, and the child can organize objects and events into classes and arrange them in order of increasing values. The child can be responsible for personal hygiene and simple household tasks. The child will need assistance when ill, but he or she can be taught self-care activities as required such as insulin injections or taking medications on a regular basis. The child can distinguish and describe physical symptoms and report them to the appropriate caregiver, and he or she can follow instructions.

Strategies employed by care providers to provide a safe environment, prevent disease, and promote health can be taught to the child. The child can perform many of these functions with supervision. Emphasis is placed on health education of the child in safety and accident prevention, nutrition, substance abuse, and anticipated changes with puberty. Anticipatory guidance for both the parents and their child should include the development of industry and inferiority. A preadolescent immunization status check is recommended at age 11 to 12.[18,19] Hepatitis B vaccine is recommended for those who did not receive the vaccine as a child. Screening of high-risk groups for tuberculosis is recommended.[10]

ADOLESCENT

True logical thought is developed and abstract concepts can be manipulated by the person in this developmental level. A scientific approach to problem solving can be planned and implemented. The adolescent can develop, with guidance, responsibility for total self-care. With experience the adolescent requires less guidance and can assume full decision-making responsibility and total responsibility for self-care.

Emphasis should be placed on health education of the adolescent in healthy living habits, safe driving, sex education, skin care, substance abuse, career choices, relationships, dating and marriage, breast self-examination for females, and testicular self-examination for males. Screening for pregnancy, sexually transmitted diseases, depression, high blood pressure, and substance abuse can be done. Anticipatory guidance should be given to parents and adolescents about the development of identity, role confusion, and formal operational thought.[15]

The hormonal changes of puberty may lead to acne vulgaris. If severe, proper hygiene and dermatologic evaluation will prevent serious complications. The changes in the vaginal tissue secondary to hormonal changes provide an environment conducive to yeast infections. If the adolescent is engaging in sexual activity, he or she is at risk for exposure to sexually transmitted diseases. Irritants such as soap and bubble bath may increase the possibility of urinary tract infection in females. Improper genital hygiene also predisposes the female to urinary tract infection.

Persons born after 1956 who lack evidence of immunity to measles should receive the MMR vaccine.[18,27] The MMR vaccine should not be given during pregnancy. Individuals susceptible to mumps should be vaccinated.[28] A diphtheria and tetanus vaccination (TD) should be given at age 14 to 16. Hepatitis B vaccine should be given to anyone who did not receive immunizations as a child.[19] Screening of high-risk groups for tuberculosis is recommended.[10] Adolescents may be living in group settings, for example, a dormitory, which increases the risk of contracting a communicable disease. Good personal hygiene is important to decrease this risk.

Risk-taking behavior of adolescents[29] may increase the risk of infection and accidents. Examples of these risk-taking behaviors include sexual intercourse; IV drug use; use of alcohol and tobacco; traumatic injury that breaks the skin allowing a portal of entry for pathogenic organisms; fad diets or other activities that decrease the overall health status; improper technique or equipment in water sports; motor vehicle accidents; running a vehicle or other combustion engines when not properly ventilated; substance abuse; choking on food; smoke inhalation; improper storage and handling of guns, ammunition, and knives; excessive risk-taking behavior; smoking in bed; improper use or storage of flammable items, hazardous tools, and equipment; drug ingestion; playing or working around toxic vegetation; improper preparation and storage of food; and improper precautions and use of insecticides, fertilizers, cleaning products, medications, alcohol, and other toxic substances.

ADULT

Adult thought is more refined than adolescent thought because experience and education allow the adult to differentiate among many points of view and potential outcomes in an objective and realistic manner. The adult can consider more options and can apply inductive as well as deductive approaches to problem solving. The adult assumes total responsibility for the care of a child. In middle adult years, the adult may also care for an elderly parent.

The adult is concerned about many of the same health promotion and disease prevention issues the adolescent worries about. Emphasis should be placed on lifestyle counseling related to family planning, parenting, stress management, career advancement, relationship enhancement, hazards at work, and development of intimacy and generativity.

Regular breast self-examination (females) and testicular self-examination (males) should be taught and encouraged. Females should be advised to have Pap smears regularly. Screening for glaucoma, high blood pressure, blood cholesterol, rubella antibodies, sexually transmitted diseases, and colon, endometrial, oral, or breast cancer should be done if the patient is in a risk category.

As the body develops more and more antibodies to pathogens, the adult may find that he or she does not have as many colds as he or she used to. Some viral infections (mumps, for example) may present serious consequences to adults (males in the case of mumps). The adult female is as susceptible to genitourinary infections as the adolescent. Sexually active adults are at risk for sexually transmitted diseases.

Tetanus-diphtheria (Td) boosters should be given every 10 years. Hepatitis B vaccine should be given to people at risk to exposure. Remember, persons born after 1956 who lack evidence of immunity to measles should receive the MMR vaccine, but the MMR vaccine should not be given during pregnancy. Individuals susceptible to mumps should be vaccinated. Pneumococcal and influenza vaccines are given based upon susceptibility and at-risk status.[30] Advanced age, conditions associated with decline in antibody levels, Native American ethnicity, and institutional settings such as military training camps, jails, and boardinghouses are all identified as risk factors[30–32] for the development of pneumonia and influenza. Tuberculosis screening of high-risk populations is recommended.[10]

OLDER ADULT

In the absence of illness affecting cognitive functioning, the older adult maintains formal operational abilities. The older adult can assume total responsibility for decision making and self-care. The older adult also often assumes responsibility for the care of others such as a spouse, child, or grandchild. As with other developmental levels, illness or physical disability can alter the cognitive functioning and lead to self-care deficits.

Emphasis is on health education related to grandparenting, retirement, and home safety. Anticipatory guidance is related to the development of ego integrity. The importance of regularly scheduled breast self-examinations, Pap smears, mammographies (females), and testicular self-examinations (males) should be taught and encouraged. Glaucoma, blood pressure, and colon cancer screening should also be done. Podiatry care should be given as needed. Tetanus-diphtheria (Td) boosters, hepatitis B vaccine, and pneumococcal and influenza vaccines are given according to the same conditions discussed in the Adult Health section.[28,30–33] Lack of achievement of adult immunization recommendations is a serious problem in this country. Less than half of the 65 or older population receive the influenza vaccine, and only 20 percent receive the pneumococcal vaccine. Influenza vaccine should be given yearly to people 65 or older and to younger people in high-risk groups. Pneumococcal vaccine should be given one time to people 65 or older or to younger people in high-risk groups.[34–37] The elderly as a group demonstrate a low immunity to tetanus based on population-based serologic surveys.[38] Inadequate immunization and waning immunity after immunization are both thought to contribute to the low rate of immunity. Tuberculosis may also be a problem in the elderly.[39]

Elderly people may have a decreased ability to remove themselves from hazardous situations due to decreased mobility. They also may have a decreased ability to recognize smoke- or gas-related odors secondary to a decreased olfactory sense. Sensory, motor, and perceptual deficits as well as orthostatic hypotension may increase the risk for injury and increase self-care deficits.

There is an increase in frequency and severity of infections with aging. Normally the immunologic defenses decline with aging.[24] Skin changes may provide easier access to infecting organisms since increased dryness and thinning of the dermis makes the skin more injury prone. Motility and secretion, for example, hydrochloric acid, decrease in the GI tract. Esophageal and gastric peristalsis are decreased. Renal filtration, absorption, and excretion diminish. Incomplete emptying of the bladder provides a medium for the growth of organisms. The respiratory muscles are weaker, and there is decreased elasticity of lung tissue. Diminished cough and gag reflexes may increase the possibility of aspiration. The skin becomes thinner and less elastic. Poor circulation related to vascular insufficiency, peripheral neuropathy, and the increased fragility of the skin increase the possibility of tissue trauma and resulting invasion by microorganisms.

There is decreased production of T lymphocytes leading to impaired ability to destroy infectious organisms. The production of antibodies by B lymphocytes is also decreased. These changes make the elderly more susceptible to infection and unable to recover as quickly as they did when they were younger; some may not develop immunity after an infection.

Chronic illness and hospitalization or nursing home placement additionally increase the risk of infection.[24] An important point to remember is that the elderly adult may not demonstrate an increased body temperature in response to an infection. An additional point to emphasize is that infection in the older adult may be manifested by mental status changes such as confusion or restlessness.

APPLICABLE NURSING DIAGNOSES

Energy Field Disturbance

DEFINITION

A disruption of the flow of energy surrounding a person's being which results in a disharmony of the body, mind, and/or spirit.[40]

NANDA TAXONOMY: EXCHANGING 1.8

DEFINING CHARACTERISTICS[40]

1. Major defining characteristics
   a. Temperature change (warmth, coolness)
   b. Visual changes (image, color)
   c. Disruption of the field (vacant, hold, spike, bulge)
   d. Movement (wave, spike, tingling, dense, flowing)
   e. Sounds (tone, words)
2. Minor defining characteristics
   None given.

RELATED FACTORS[40]

None given.

RELATED CLINICAL CONCERNS

1. Chronic or catastrophic illness
2. Trauma
3. Autoimmune deficiency syndrome
4. Insomnia
5. Chronic fatigue syndrome
6. Cancer
7. Recent surgery
8. Sensory or perceptual disorders
9. Pain

HAVE YOU SELECTED THE CORRECT DIAGNOSIS?

Fatigue   For this diagnosis, the client will report exhaustion and lack of energy. Assessment will document an overall reduction of energy, not a disruption of energy.

Activity Intolerance   The client will relate, via interview, specific activities that cannot be accomplished. Specific physical findings, such as abnormal pulse and respiration rates, will be present during activity.

Ineffective Thermoregulation   This diagnosis relates to temperature fluctuations only. Energy field disruption will demonstrate other defining characteristics in addition to temperature change.

Sleep Pattern Disturbance   A problem in the sleep-rest pattern could result in alterations in the energy field. Interviewing the person regarding sleep habits will assist in clarifying if the primary diagnosis is Sleep Pattern Disturbance or Energy Field Disturbance.

Sensory or Perceptual Alterations   Determining the person's orientation to time and place, his or her ability to discern objects in the environment via vision, touch, sound, or smell, and his or her problem-solving abilities will assist in distinguishing Energy Field Disturbance from Sensory or Perceptual Alterations.

Pain   Observing for signs and symptoms of pain (facial mask, guarding behavior, moaning, or crying) will distinguish Pain from Energy Field Disturbance.

EXPECTED OUTCOMES

1. Patient will verbalize a perception of consistent energy level by (date), and/or
2. Assessment will demonstrate a consistent energy field by (date).

TARGET DATE

Locating the reason(s) for Energy Field Disturbance may require several days or even weeks. Due to complexities involved in accepting this diagnosis for both the client and the nurse, frequent evaluation is required. It is recommended that target dates be no further than 3 days from the date of initial diagnosis.

NURSING ACTIONS/INTERVENTIONS WITH RATIONALES

Adult Health

ACTIONS/INTERVENTIONS	RATIONALES

• Establish trusting relationship with patient.
• Allow patient to talk about condition.
• Assess energy field.
 	
• Center self:
  ○ Imagine self as open system with energy flow content in, through, and out of the system.
  ○ Consciously quiet your mind; put aside or detach from inward and outward distractions.
  ○ Focus full attention and *intention* on *helping* patient.
• Assess for heat or tingling over specific body areas:
  ○ Glide hands, palm down, and slowly move over body, head to toe, 2−4 in above body.
• Be sensitive to any images that come to mind: words, symbols, pictures, colors, sound, mood, emotion, etc.[43]
 	
• Attempt to get a sense of the dynamics of the energy field. Synthesize assessment data into an understandable format.
• Redirect areas of accumulated energy, reestablish the energy flow, and direct energy to depleted areas. Repattern or rebalance patient's energy field.
• Do therapeutic touch for no longer than 10 min.
• Assess patient's subjective reaction to therapeutic touch. Patient should feel more relaxed, less anxious, and less pain (if there were complaints of pain prior to therapeutic touch).
• Teach patient relaxation exercises using some of the same techniques as therapeutic touch:
  ○ Assist patient to center self.
  ○ Teach patient to imagine a peaceful place. Help patient to visualize place through all the senses and to allow the energy of the imagined place to bring about a state of calmness.
  ○ Teach patient to scan his or her body to self-assess areas of body or muscle tension.
  ○ Assist patient to consciously relax that tense area of the body.
• Practice relaxation at least 10−20 min a day.
	Promotes accurate assessment.
	Promotes nurse-patient relationship.
	Alterations, variations, and/or asymmetry in the energy field is detected through assessment.[41]
	Promotes accurate assessment.
	
	There may be a loss of energy, disruption or blockage in the flow of energy, or an accumulation of energy in a part of the body.[42]
	
	Energy transfer or transformation can occur without direct physical contact between two systems.[41] Hands are focal points for the direction and modulation of energy.[41] Could disrupt the energy field of the therapist.
	Nurse acts as a conduit through which the environmental or universal energy passes to the patient.[41]
	
	Relaxation requires the patient to stop trying and to step outside of self and adopt a nontrying attitude. This allows the person to release and use the inherent energy of self.[44]
	
	Rebalances energy flow through the body.[44]

Child Health

ACTIONS/INTERVENTIONS	RATIONALES
• Monitor for reciprocity of maternal-infant dyad. • Identify developmentally appropriate parameters to determine the most conducive and therapeutic method for monitoring child's energy field.[45]	Provides assessment for causative factors. Energy field disturbance may be related to numerous other altered patterns due to the infant or child's basic coping repertoire, especially altered thermoregulation—altered neurological status.
• Monitor energy field with a focus on maintaining self-comforting activities for child. May begin with soft music and/or soothing voice.[46]	Will enhance assessment of energy field.
• Begin with gentle but firm pressure of hands on one another.	Warms hands.
• Assess energy field from head to toe. Focus on determining sites where differences are present.	Routine assessment.
• Attempt to redirect areas of lesser flow or greater flow within an overall free-flowing energy field, allowing ½–1 in between nurse's hand and child.	Restores balance. The infant or child has a small energy field.
• Monitor client's responses to therapeutic touch. Focus on identifying stimulus response.	Permits evaluation of success of therapy.
• Teach client (or family, depending on client's age) to note physical and mental cues that alter energy field, especially stressors.[47,48]	Promotes early intervention.
• Offer age-appropriate relaxation techniques, e.g., imaginary floating like a feather to suggest lightness for a school-ager vs. gentle rocking to rhythmic music for an infant.[49,50]	Pays attention to developmental level.
• Be mindful of contributing factors of self. Offer ways to assist caregiver in learning techniques for maintenance of energy field balance.	Provides long-term assistance.
• As appropriate, assist family to develop ways to reduce sensitivity to external triggering cues.	Provide long-term balance.

Women's Health

Same as Adult Health except for the following:

ACTIONS/INTERVENTIONS	RATIONALES
• Instruct in use of therapeutic touch and stress reduction as a means of coping with labor pain.	Provides a natural source of dealing with the discomfort of labor.[51] Allows the woman and her newborn to experience a drug-free labor and delivery.

Psychiatric Health

ACTIONS/INTERVENTIONS	RATIONALES
• Explain intervention to client in terms that facilitate reality orientation and do not exacerbate thought disorders. ○ Use examples that elicit client's past experience with personal energy fields that do not reinforce delusional beliefs, e.g., EEG and EKG measure electrical energy that flows from the body; walking across the floor and then touching something releases this build-up of energy that can be seen or felt as a mild shock.	Prevents reinforcement of delusional system and facilitates the development of a trusting relationship.[52]

Rubbing a balloon over the hair and watching it stand up when the balloon is moved away is another example.
- ○ Instruct client that these techniques facilitate their own healing potential and are used in conjunction with other treatments.
- Discuss with the client his or her perceptions or concerns about their alterations.

- Select one of the following methods for altering energy fields based on the assessment:
  - ○ Therapeutic touch
  - ○ Foot or hand reflexology
  - ○ Visual imagery
  - ○ Visualization with relaxation techniques
  - ○ Acupressure
  - ○ TENS
  - ○ Biofeedback
- Note referral information here with date and time of appointment with practitioner.
- Prepare the client and environment for the application of the intervention:
  - ○ Provide private, quiet environment.
  - ○ Teach client about the intervention.
  - ○ Obtain client's permission to utilize the intervention.
  - ○ Provide appropriate music that increases client's feelings of comfort.
  - ○ Provide essential oils or other odors that enhance client's sense of well-being.
- Focus own attention on the intent of the interaction.

- Inform client that he or she should tell practitioner if he or she notices any difference in the way he or she feels during the application of the technique. This could include feelings of relaxation, warmth, or change in breathing patterns.

- Assist client into a comfortable position that will facilitate treatment.
- Utilize selected technique (number) times a day for (number) minutes. Observe client for signs that indicate that the desired effect has occurred. This could include:
  - ○ Sigh
  - ○ Relaxation in muscles
  - ○ Slower, deeper breathing
  - ○ Drop in voice volume
  - ○ Peripheral flush on the face and neck
  - ○ Client's report of feeling different
  - ○ Reassessment indicates balance has occurred
- Assist client into comfortable, relaxed position after treatment.
- Teach client those techniques that can maintain balance between treatments and that do not require the assistance of a practitioner. These include:
  - ○ Relaxation
  - ○ Cross crawl exercises
  - ○ Stress reduction
  - ○ Cognitive reframing
  - ○ Visualization
  - ○ Improved nutrition
  - ○ Decreasing use of tobacco and alcohol
- Note teaching schedule and content here.

Understanding the client's cognitive map facilitates the development of interventions that facilitate client change.[52]

All of these techniques have been demonstrated to have effects on the body's energy fields.[42,44,53-58] Application of these interventions by the nurse is related to having appropriate training in the technique. If the nurse is unskilled in the techniques, efforts should be made for appropriate referrals at this point. Additional information on these techniques can be found in the references.

Increases client's level of comfort.[52,56]

Builds trust and promotes client's sense of control.[52] Sound that is loud and irritating can have a negative impact on psychological and physiological well-being.[43] Odors have impact on the limbic system and impact affect.

The nurse's intention provides a crucial basis for these interventions.[42,55]

Change that occurs with alterations in the energy fields may be perceived by the client before the practitioner notices a difference. The goal of these interventions is to promote balance so the treatment should stop when these differences are observed by the client or practitioner.[42,44,54] Also promotes client's sense of control.[44,45]

It is important that client is well supported because the techniques do promote the relaxation response.

The ability of the client to maintain balance is based on general levels of wellness, lifestyle, and stressors.[54]

Maintenance of energy field balance involves a holistic approach to care.[54]

Gerontic Health

ACTIONS/INTERVENTIONS	RATIONALES
• Obtain medication profile (prescription and over the counter) to determine if drug actions or reactions contribute to the disturbance.	Medications may contribute to energy field disturbances.
• Ensure adequate padding and proper position for any sessions.	Proper positioning will prevent pain, pressure, and thus disturbances in concentration.
• Adjust massage efforts and pressure to compensate for changes in older patient's tactile sensation.	Older adults with aging changes in the nervous system may have a decreased perception of being touched.
• Use teaching materials, as needed, that are appropriate for the patient (such as printed information of a size that is easily read or quality audiotapes that are not distorted or high pitched).	Uncompensated sensory changes of aging can affect the ability to use audiovisual sources if the information is not adjusted to meet the older adult's needs.

Home Health

ACTIONS/INTERVENTIONS	RATIONALES
• Assist the client and family to identify disturbances in energy field.	Early identification assists in providing early intervention.

• Teach the client and family techniques to prevent and/or treat energy field disturbance:
  ○ Therapeutic touch.
  ○ Foot or hand reflexology
  ○ Visual imagery
  ○ Visualization with relaxation techniques
  ○ TENS
  ○ Biofeedback
	Involvement improves motivation and improves the outcome. Self-care is enhanced.

• Assist the client and family in providing a private, quiet environment.	Client comfort is increased and response to intervention is enhanced.[52,56]

• Teach the client and family techniques to maintain balance between treatments requiring the assistance of a practitioner:
  ○ Relaxation
  ○ Cross crawl exercises
  ○ Stress reduction
  ○ Cognitive reframing
  ○ Visualization
  ○ Improved nutrition
  ○ Decreased use of tobacco and alcohol
	These techniques have been demonstrated to have effects on human energy fields.[42,44,53,54,56,57,59]

• Assist the client and family in identifying resources in the community, e.g.:
  ○ Massage therapists
  ○ Reflexologists
  ○ Stress reduction classes
	Use of existing community services is efficient use of resources.

Energy Field Disturbance

FLOWCHART EVALUATION: EXPECTED OUTCOME 1

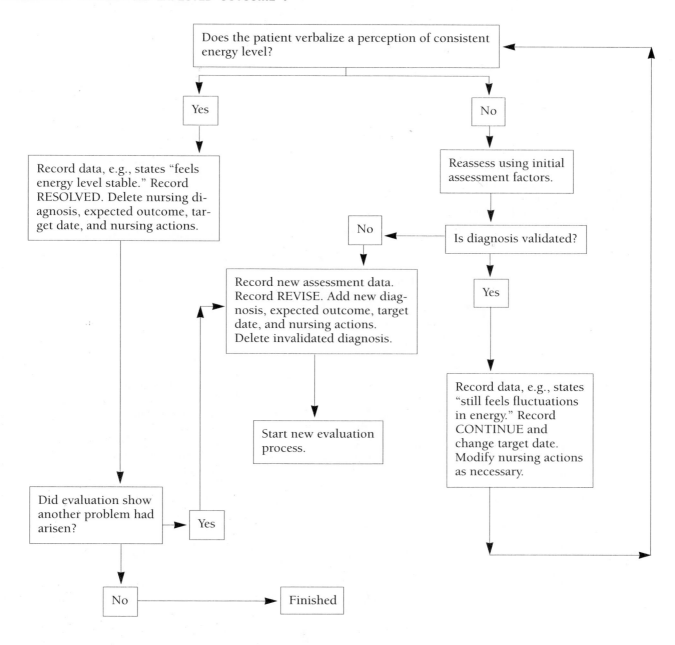

Energy Field Disturbance

FLOWCHART EVALUATION: EXPECTED OUTCOME 2

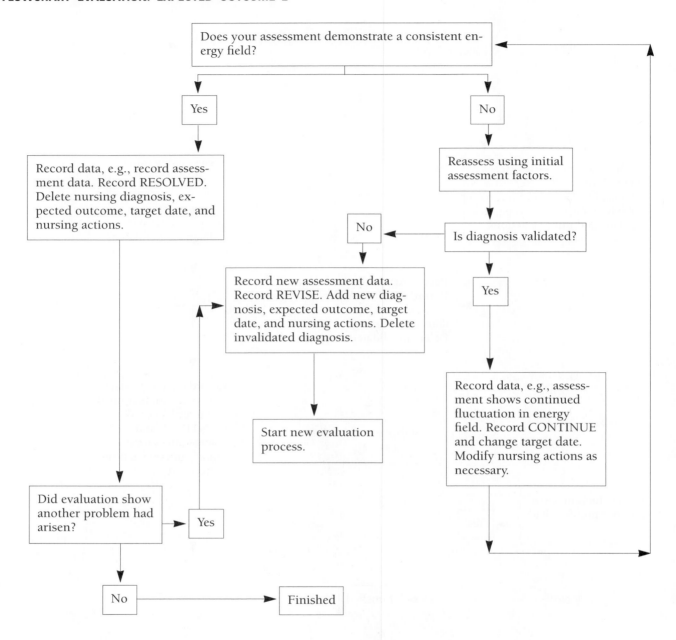

Health Maintenance, Altered

DEFINITION

Inability to identify, manage, and/or seek out help to maintain health.[40]

NANDA TAXONOMY: MOVING 6.4.2

DEFINING CHARACTERISTICS[40]

1. Major defining characteristics
   a. Demonstrated lack of knowledge regarding basic health practices
   b. Demonstrated lack of adaptive behaviors to internal or external environmental changes
   c. Reported or observed inability to take responsibility for meeting basic health practices in any or all functional pattern areas
   d. History of lack of health-seeking behavior
   e. Expressed interest in improving health behaviors
   f. Reported or observed lack of equipment or financial and/or other resources
   g. Reported or observed impairment of personal support systems
2. Minor defining characteristics
   None given.

RELATED FACTORS[40]

1. Lack of or significant alteration in communication skills (written, verbal, and/or gestural)
2. Lack of ability to make deliberate and thoughtful judgments
3. Perceptual or cognitive impairment (complete or partial lack of gross and/or fine motor skills)
4. Ineffective individual coping
5. Dysfunctional grieving
6. Unachieved developmental tasks
7. Ineffective family coping
8. Disabling spiritual distress
9. Lack of material resources

RELATED CLINICAL CONCERNS

1. Dementias such as Alzheimer's disease and multi-infarct
2. Mental retardation
3. Any condition causing an alteration in level of consciousness, for example, closed head injury, carbon monoxide poisoning, or cerebrovascular accident
4. Any condition impacting the person's mobility level, for example, hemiplegia, paraplegia, fractures, or muscular dystrophy
5. Chronic diseases, for example, rheumatoid arthritis, cancer, chronic pain, or multiple sclerosis

HAVE YOU SELECTED THE CORRECT DIAGNOSIS?

Spiritual Distress   A problem in the Value-Belief Pattern could result in variance in health maintenance. If the therapeutic regimen causes conflict with cultural or religious beliefs or with the individual's value system, then it is likely some alteration in health maintenance will occur. Interviewing the patient regarding individual values, goals, or beliefs that guide personal decision making will assist in clarifying whether the primary diagnosis is Altered Health Maintenance or a problem in the Value-Belief Pattern.

Ineffective Coping   Either Ineffective Coping or Ineffective Family Coping could be suspected if there are major differences between the patient and family reports of health status, health perception, and health care behavior. Ineffective Community Coping may be present if there are inadequate resources for problem solving or deficits in social support services for community members. Verbalizations by the patient or family member regarding inability to cope also indicate ineffective coping. Community members may express dissatisfaction with meeting community needs.

Altered Family Process   Through observing family interactions and communication, the nurse may assess that Altered Family Process exists. Rigidity of family functions and roles, poorly communicated messages, and failure to accomplish expected family developmental tasks are a few observations to alert the nurse to this possible diagnosis.

Activity Intolerance or Self-Care Deficit   The nursing diagnosis of Activity Intolerance or Self-Care Deficit should be considered if the nurse observes or validates reports of inability to complete the required tasks because of insufficient energy or because of the patient's inability to feed, bathe, toilet, dress, and groom himself or herself.

Powerlessness   The nursing diagnosis of Powerlessness is considered if the patient reports or demonstrates having little control over situations, expresses doubt about ability to perform, or is reluctant to express his or her feelings to health care providers.

Knowledge Deficit   A Knowledge Deficit may exist if the patient or family verbalizes less-than-adequate understanding of health management or recalls inaccurate health information.

Impaired Home Maintenance Management   This diagnosis is demonstrated by the inability of the patient or family to provide a safe living environment.

EXPECTED OUTCOMES

1. Will describe at least (number) contributing factors that lead to health maintenance alteration and at least one measure to alter each factor by (date) and/or
2. Will design a positive health maintenance plan by (date)

TARGET DATE

Assisting patients to adapt their health maintenance will require a significant investment of time and will also require close collaboration with home health caregivers. For these reasons it is recommended the target date be no less than 7 days from the date of admission.

NURSING ACTIONS/INTERVENTIONS WITH RATIONALES
Adult Health

ACTIONS/INTERVENTIONS	RATIONALES

• Assist patient to identify factors contributing to health maintenance alteration through one-to-one interviewing and value clarification strategies. Factors may include:
  ○ Stopping smoking[60–63]
  ○ Ceasing drug and alcohol use
  ○ Establishing exercise patterns[64]
  ○ Following good nutritional habits
  ○ Using stress management techniques
  ○ Using family and community support systems
  ○ Using over-the-counter medications
  ○ Using herbs, vitamins, food supplements, or cleansing programs[65]
	Healthy living habits reduce risk. Assistance is often required to develop long-term change. Identification of the factors significant to the patient will provide the foundation for teaching positive health maintenance.

• Develop with the patient a list of assets and deficits as he or she perceives them. From this list, assist the patient in deciding what lifestyle adjustments will be necessary.	Increases patient's sense of control and keeps the idea of multiple changes from being overwhelming.
• Identify, with patient, possible solutions, modifications, etc., to cope with each adjustment.	The more the patient is involved with decisions, the higher the probability that the patient will incorporate the changes.
• Develop a plan with the patient which shows both short-term and long-term goals. For each goal specify the time the goal is to be reached.	Avoids overwhelming the patient by indicating that not all goals have to be accomplished at the same time.
• Have patient identify at least two support persons. Arrange for these persons to come to the unit and participate in designing the health maintenance plan.	Provides additional support for patient in maintaining plan.
• Assist patient and significant others to develop a list of *potential* strategies that would assist in the development of the lifestyle changes necessary for health maintenance. (This list should be a brainstorming process and include those solutions that appear to be very unrealistic as well as those that appear most realistic). After the list is developed, review each item with the patient, combining and eliminating strategies when appropriate.	People most often approach change with "more of the same" solutions. If an individual does not think that the strategy will have to be implemented, he or she will be more inclined to develop creative strategies for change.[66]
• Develop with the patient a list of the benefits and disadvantages of behavior changes. Discuss each item with the patient as to the strength of motivation that each item has.	Placing items in priority according to patient's motivation increases probability of success.
• Develop a behavior change contract with the patient, allowing the patient to identify appropriate rewards and consequences. Remember to establish modest goals and short-term rewards. Note reward schedule here.	Positive reinforcement enhances self-esteem and supports continuation of desired behaviors. This also promotes patient control which in turn increases motivation to implement the plan.[52]

- Teach patient appropriate information to improve health maintenance (e.g., hygiene, diet, medication administration, relaxation techniques, and coping strategies).

  Provides the patient with the basic knowledge needed to enact the needed changes.

- Review activities of daily living (ADL) with patient and support person. Incorporate these activities into the design for a health maintenance plan. (*Note:* May have to either increase or decrease ADL).

  Incorporation of usual activities personalizes the plan.

- Assist patient and support person to design a monthly calendar that reflects the daily activities needed to succeed in health maintenance.

  Provides a visual reminder.

- Have patient and support person return-demonstrate health maintenance procedures at least once a day for at least 3 days before discharge. Times and types of skills should be noted here.

  Permits practice in a nonthreatening environment where immediate feedback can be given.

- Set a time to reassess with the patient and support person progress toward the established goals. This should be on a frequent schedule initially and can then gradually decrease as the patient demonstrates mastery. Note evaluation times here.

  Provides an opportunity to evaluate and to give the patient positive feedback and support for achievements.

- Provide the patient with appropriate positive feedback on goal achievement. Remember to keep this behaviorally oriented and specific.

- Communicate the established plan to the collaborative members of the health care team.

  Provides continuity and consistency in care.

- Refer patient to appropriate community health agencies for follow-up care. Be sure referral is made at least 3–5 days before discharge.

  Ensures the service can complete their assessment and initiate operations before the patient is discharged from the hospital. Use of the network of existing community services provides for effective utilization of resources. Facilitates patient's keeping of appointments and reinforces importance of health maintenance.

- Schedule appropriate follow-up appointments for patient before discharge. Notify transportation service and support persons of these appointments. Write appointment on brightly colored card for attention. Include date, time, appropriate name (physician, physical therapist, nurse practitioner, etc.), address, telephone number, and name and telephone number of person who will provide transportation.

Child Health

NOTE: Developmental consideration should always guide the health maintenance planned for the child patient. Also, identification of primary defects is stressed to reduce the likelihood of secondary and tertiary delays.

ACTIONS/INTERVENTIONS	RATIONALES
• Teach patient and family essential information to establish and maintain health according to age, development, and status.	An individualized plan of care will more definitively reflect specific health maintenance needs and will increase the value of the plan to the patient and his or her family. Reinforcement in a more tangible mode facilitates compliance with the plan of health maintenance, especially with long-term situations.
• Assist patient and family in designing a calendar to monitor progress in meeting goals. Offer developmentally appropriate methods, e.g., toddlers enjoy stickers of favorite cartoon or book characters.	
• Identify risk factors that will impact health care maintenance, e.g., prematurity, congenital defects, altered neurosensory functioning, errors of metabolism, or altered parenting.	Identification of risk factors allows for more appropriate anticipatory planning of health care, assists in minimizing crises and escalation of simple needs, and serves to reduce anxiety.
• Begin to prepare for health maintenance on initial meeting with child and family.	A holistic plan of care realistically includes futuristic goals, not merely immediate health needs.
• Provide appropriate phone numbers for health team members and clinics to child and parents to assist in follow-up.	Anticipatory planning for potential need for communication allows the patient or family realistic methods for assuming health care while enjoying the back-up of resources.

Women's Health

ACTIONS/INTERVENTIONS	RATIONALES
• Assist the patient to describe her perception and understanding of essential information related to her individual lifestyle and the adjustment necessary to establish and maintain health in each cycle of reproductive life.	Allows assessment of the patient's basic level of knowledge so that a plan can begin at the patient's current level of understanding.
• Develop with the patient a list of stress-related problems at work and at home as she perceives them. From this list, assist the patient in deciding what lifestyle adjustments will be necessary to establish and maintain health.	Provides essential information to assist patient in planning a healthy lifestyle.
• Identify with the patient possible solutions and modification to facilitate coping with adjustments. Develop a plan that includes short-term and long-term goals. For each goal specify the time the goal is to be reached.	Provides sequential steps to alternate health maintenance within a defined time period. Keeps the patient from being overwhelmed by all the changes that might be necessary.
• Provide factual information to the patient about menstrual cycle patterns throughout the lifespan. Include prepubertal, menarcheal, menstrual, premenopausal, menopausal, and postmenopausal phases.	Provides basic information and knowledge that is needed throughout lifespan.
• Teach patient how to record accurate menstrual cycle, obstetric, and sexual history. Assist patient in recognizing lifestyle changes that occur as a part of normal development.	Provides the patient with the information necessary to cope with changes throughout the reproductive cycle.
• Discuss pregnancy and the changes that occur during pregnancy and childbearing. Stress the importance of a physical examination *before* becoming pregnant to include a Pap smear, rubella titer, AIDS profile, and genetic workup (if indicated by family history).	Provides patient with the information needed to plan for a healthy pregnancy.
• Describe and assist the patient in planning routines that will maintain well-being for the mother and fetus during pregnancy, e.g., reducing fatigue, eating a nutritionally adequate diet, exercising properly, obtaining early prenatal care, and attending classes to obtain information about infant nutrition, infant care, and the birthing experience.	Provides the expectant family with information to enable them to make informed choices about pregnancy, childbirth, and beginning parenting.
• Provide information and support during postpartum period to assist the new mother in establishing and maintaining good infant nutrition, whether breast-feeding or formula feeding.	
• Refer patient to appropriate groups for support and encouragement after birth of baby, e.g., La Leche League and parenting groups.	
• Teach terminology and factual information related to spontaneous abortion or the interruption of pregnancy. Encourage expression of feelings by the patient and her family. Provide referrals to appropriate support groups within the community.	Allows patient to grieve and reduces fear regarding subsequent pregnancies.
• Provide contraceptive information to the patient, including describing different methods of contraception and their advantages and disadvantages.	Allows patient to plan appropriate contraceptive measures according to personal values and beliefs.
• Emphasize the importance of lifestyle changes necessary to cope with postmenopausal changes in the body, such as estrogen replacement therapy, calcium supplements, balanced diet, exercise, and routine sleep patterns.	Provides patient with basic information that will assist in planning a healthy lifestyle during and following menopause.

- Teach the patient the importance of routine physical assessments throughout the reproductive life cycle including breast self-examination, Pap smears, and routine exams by the health care provider of her choice, e.g., nurse midwife, nurse practitioner, or physician.

Provides knowledge that allows the patient to plan a healthy lifestyle.

Psychiatric Health

ACTIONS/INTERVENTIONS	RATIONALES
• Include the client in group therapy to provide positive role models and peer support and to permit assessment of goals and exposure to differing problem solutions.	Group provides opportunities to relate and react to others while exploring behavior with each other.

Gerontic Health

NOTE: Major emphasis here is on educating the client. Due to stereotypes about aging, there is a misconception that older adults cannot learn new information. This is untrue. The majority of elderly people are quite capable of cognitive growth and intellectual development, and there are ways to enhance the learning experience for older adults.[67]

ACTIONS/INTERVENTIONS	RATIONALES
• Ensure privacy, comfort, and rapport prior to teaching sessions.	Reduces anxiety and provides a nondistracting environment that enhances learning ability.
• Avoid presenting large amounts of information at one time.	This allows patient an increased opportunity to process and store new information. The most ideal way to present new material to the older adult is through self-paced instruction.
• Monitor energy level as teaching session progresses.	
• Present small units of information, with repetition, and encourage patient to use cues that enhance ability to recall information.	The cues should be highly personalized for the individual patient. An older woman learning to do a dressing change might relate the steps involved to a recipe for baking, first I do this, then this, etc.

Home Health

ACTIONS/INTERVENTIONS	RATIONALES
• Assist the client and family to identify home and workplace factors that can be modified to promote health maintenance, e.g., ramps instead of steps, tacking down throw rugs, and maintaining a nonsmoking environment.[68,69]	This action will enhance safety and assist in preventing accidents. Promoting a nonsmoking environment helps reduce the damaging effects of passive smoke.
• Involve the client and family in planning, implementing, and promoting a health maintenance pattern through: ○ Helping to establish family conferences ○ Teaching mutual goal setting ○ Teaching communication ○ Assisting family members in specified tasks as appropriate (e.g., cooking, cleaning, transportation, companionship, or support person for exercise program)	Involvement improves motivation and the outcome.

Continued

ACTIONS/INTERVENTIONS	RATIONALES

• Teach the client and family health promotion and disease prevention activities:
  ○ Relaxation techniques
  ○ Nutritional habits to maintain optimal weight and physical strength
  ○ Techniques for developing and strengthening support networks (e.g., communication techniques or mutual goal setting)
  ○ Physical exercise to increase flexibility, cardiovascular conditioning, and physical strength and endurance[70]
  ○ Evaluation of occupational conditions[69]
  ○ Control of harmful habits (e.g., control of substance abuse)
  ○ Therapeutic value of pets[71]
	These activities promote a healthy lifestyle.

Health Maintenance, Altered

FLOWCHART EVALUATION: EXPECTED OUTCOME 1

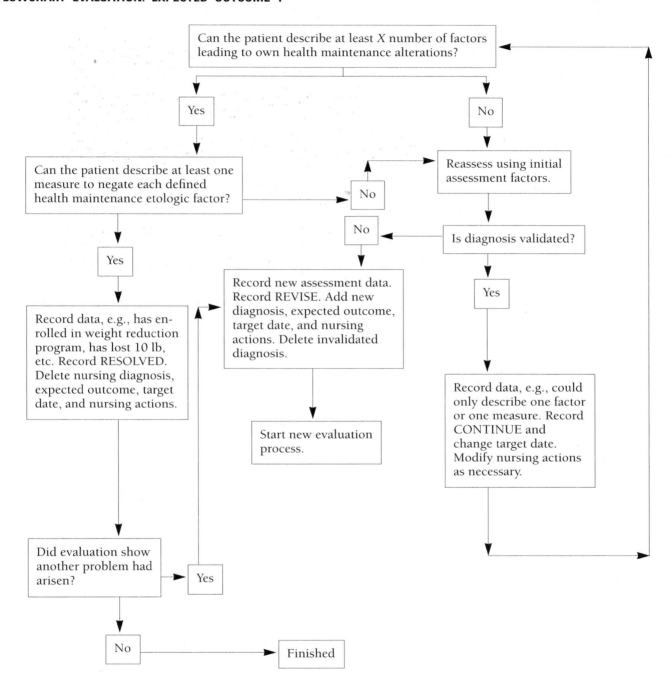

Health Maintenance, Altered

FLOWCHART EVALUATION: EXPECTED OUTCOME 2

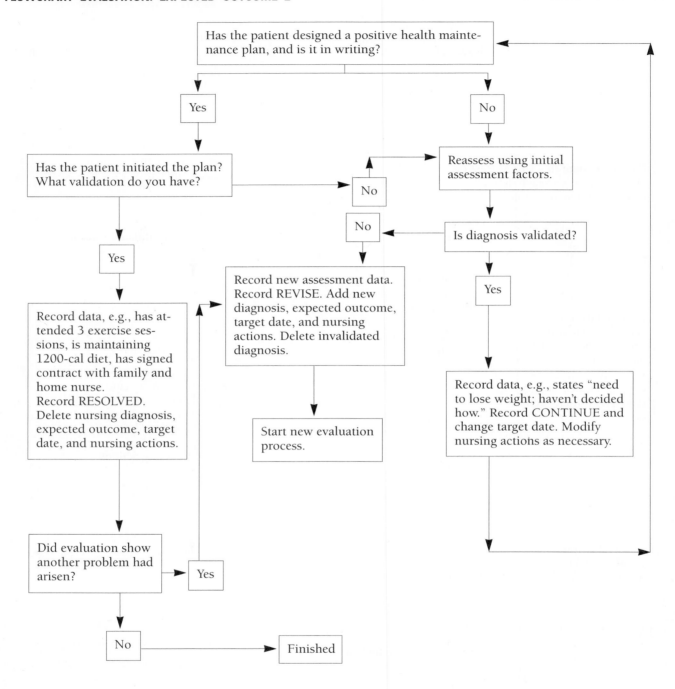

Health-Seeking Behaviors (Specify)

DEFINITION

A state in which an individual in stable health is actively seeking ways to alter personal health habits and/or the environment in order to move toward a higher level of health.[40]*

NANDA TAXONOMY: CHOOSING 5.4

DEFINING CHARACTERISTICS[40]

1. Major defining characteristics
   a. Expressed or observed desire to seek a higher level of wellness
2. Minor defining characteristics
   a. Expressed or observed desire for increased control of health practice

b. Expression of concern about impact of current environmental conditions on health status
c. Stated (or observed) unfamiliarity with wellness community resources
d. Demonstrated or observed lack of knowledge in health promotion behaviors

RELATED FACTORS[40]

None given.

RELATED CLINICAL CONCERNS

Since this diagnosis, as indicated by the definition, relates to individuals in stable health, there are no related medical diagnoses.

HAVE YOU SELECTED THE CORRECT DIAGNOSIS?

Impaired Home Maintenance Management This diagnosis may be involved if the individual or family is unable to independently maintain a safe, growth-promoting immediate environment.

Powerlessness If the client expresses the perception of lack of control or influence over the situation and potential outcomes or does not participate in care or decision making when opportunities are provided, the diagnosis of Powerlessness should be investigated. Community powerlessness may be an indicator of Ineffective Community Coping.

EXPECTED OUTCOMES

1. Will describe or write realistic plans to modify habit (name) by (date) and/or
2. Will (increase or decrease) (habit) by (amount) by (date)

EXAMPLE
Will decrease smoking by 75 percent by (date).
Will increase exercise by walking 2 miles three times per week by (date).

TARGET DATE

Changing a habit involves a significant investment of time and energy regardless of whether the change involves starting a new habit or stopping an old habit. Therefore, the target dates should be expressed in terms of weeks and months.

NURSING ACTIONS/INTERVENTIONS WITH RATIONALES
Adult Health

ACTIONS/INTERVENTIONS	RATIONALES
• Initiate discharge plans soon after admission to facilitate posthospital follow-up.	Allows adequate time to complete discharge planning and teaching required for home care.
• Note potential risk factors that should be dealt with regarding actual health status (e.g., financial status, coping strategies, or resources).	Provides basic knowledge that will contribute to individualized discharge planning.
• Teach patient about activities for promotion of health and prevention of illness (e.g., well-balanced diet including restricted sodium and cholesterol intake, need for adequate rest and exercise, effects of air pollutants including smoking, and stress management techniques).	Provides the patient and family with the essential knowledge needed to modify behavior.

Continued

Stable health status is defined as age-appropriate illness prevention measures have been achieved, client reports good or excellent health, and signs and symptoms of disease, if present, are controlled.

ACTIONS/INTERVENTIONS	RATIONALES
• Review patient's problem-solving abilities, and assist patient to identify various alternatives, especially in terms of altering his or her environment.	Promotes shared decision making and enhances patient's feeling of self-control.
• Provide appropriate teaching to assist patient and family in becoming confident in self-seeking health care behavior, e.g., teach assertiveness techniques to patient and family.	Increases sense of self-control and reduces feelings of powerlessness.
• Assist patient and family to list benefits of high-level wellness and health-seeking behavior.	Makes visible the reasons these activities will help the family.
• Help patient and family develop a basic written plan for achieving individual high-level wellness. Provide time for questions before dismissal to solidify plans for follow-up care. At a minimum 30 min per day for 2 days prior to discharge should be allowed for this question-and-answer period. Note times here.	Demonstrates importance of follow-up care.
• Give and review pamphlets about wellness community resources.	Reinforces teaching and provides ready reference for patient and family after discharge from agency.
• Support patient in his or her health-seeking behavior. Advocate when necessary.	Provides supportive environment and underlines the importance of health-seeking activities.
• Refer to appropriate health-care providers and various community groups as appropriate for assistance needed by the patient and her or his family.	Provides professional support systems that can assist in health-seeking behavior.

Child Health

ACTIONS/INTERVENTIONS	RATIONALES
• Monitor child and family for perceived value of health. Incorporate into any plan personal and family needs identified through this monitoring.	Values are formulated in the first 6 years of life and will serve as primary factors in how health is perceived and enjoyed by the individual and family. If values are in question, there is greater likelihood that how health is able to be maintained will be subject to this values conflict. Until health-seeking behavior is identified as a value, follow-up care will not be deemed to be beneficial. Knowing available resources and incorporating these resources into the plan for health care will facilitate long-term attention to health.
• Assist child and family to identify appropriate health maintenance needs and resources, e.g., immunizations, nutrition, daily hygiene, basic safety, how to obtain medical services when needed (including health education), how to take temperature on an infant, basic skills, and care for health problems, health insurance, Medicaid, and Crippled Children's Services.	

Women's Health

ACTIONS/INTERVENTIONS	RATIONALES
• Teach the patient the importance of seeking information and support during the reproductive life cycle. Include information about prepubertal, menarcheal, menstrual, childbearing, parenting, menopause, and postmenopausal periods of the life cycle.	Provides the basic information needed to support health-seeking behaviors.

Psychiatric Health

ACTIONS/INTERVENTIONS	RATIONALES
• Assign client a primary care nurse.	Provides increased individuation and continuity of care facilitating the development of a therapeutic relationship. The nursing process requires that a trusting and functional relationship exist between nurse and client.[52] Promotes client's perception of control.
• Primary care nurse will spend 30 min twice a day with client (note times here). The focus of these interactions will conform to the following schedule: ∘ *Interaction 1:* Have the client identify specific areas of concern. List the identified concerns on the care plan. Also identify the primary source of this concern (i.e., client, family member, member of the health care team, or other members of the client's social system).	
∘ *Interaction 2:* List *specific* goals for each concern the client has identified. These goals should be achievable within a 2- to 3-day period. (One way of setting realistic, achievable goals is to divide the goal described by the client by 50 percent.)	Promotes client's self-esteem when goals can be accomplished.
∘ *Interaction 3:* Have the client identify steps that have been previously taken to address the concern.	Promotes client's self-esteem and provides motivation for continued efforts.
∘ *Interaction 4:* Determine the client's perceptions of abilities to meet established goals and areas where assistance may be needed. (If client indicates a perception of inability to pursue goals without a great deal of assistance, the alternative nursing diagnoses of Powerlessness and Knowledge Deficit may need to be considered.) • All future interactions will be spent assisting the client in developing strategies to achieve the established goals, developing action plans, evaluating the outcome of these plans, and then revising future actions. • Provide positive verbal reinforcement for client's achievements of goals. This reinforcement should be specific to the client's goals. Note those things that are rewarding to the client here and the kind of behavior to be rewarded.	

Gerontic Health

ACTIONS/INTERVENTIONS	RATIONALES
• Nursing actions for this diagnosis and the older adult are essentially the same as those in adult health. • Encourage patient to participate in health-screening and health promotion programs such as Senior Wellness Programs. These programs are often offered by hospitals and senior citizens' centers.	Provides a cost-effective, easily accessible, long-term support mechanism for the patient.

Home Health

ACTIONS/INTERVENTIONS	RATIONALES
• Help the client identify his or her personal definition of health, perceived personal control, perceived self-efficacy, and perceived health status. • Assist the client in identifying required lifestyle changes. Assist the client to develop potential strategies that would facilitate the lifestyle changes required. • Refer to Altered Health Maintenance for additional actions that would also be applicable with this diagnosis.	Awareness of definition of health, locus of control, perceived efficiency, and health status is helpful in identifying potential facilitators and barriers to action. Lifestyle changes require change in behavior. Self-evaluation and support facilitate these changes.

Health-Seeking Behaviors (Specify)

FLOWCHART EVALUATION: EXPECTED OUTCOME 1

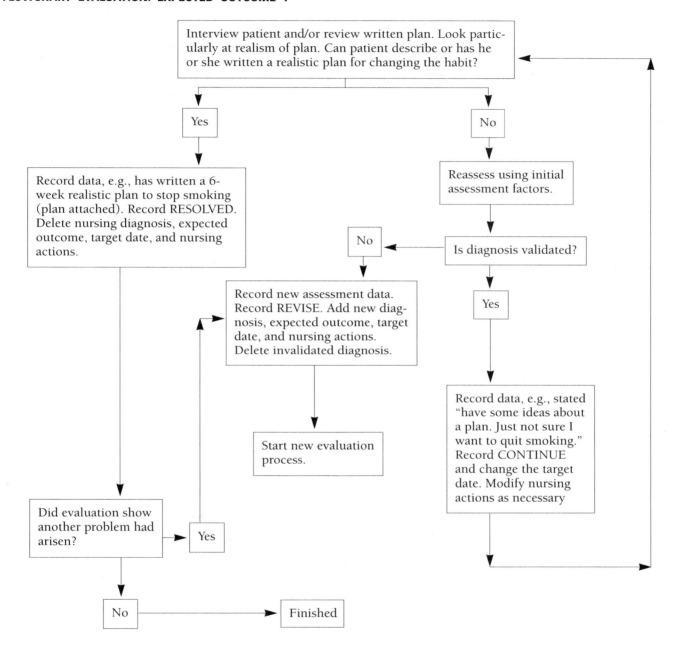

Health-Seeking Behaviors (Specify)

FLOWCHART EVALUATION: EXPECTED OUTCOME 2

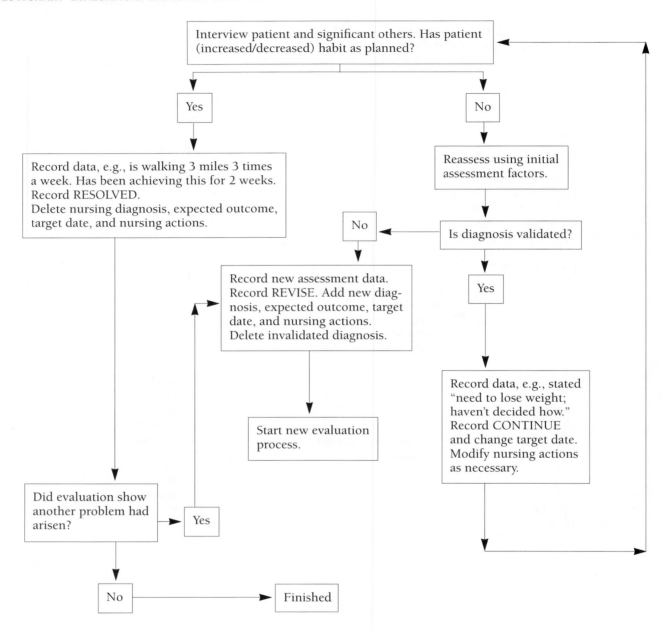

Infection, Risk for

DEFINITION

The state in which an individual is at increased risk for being invaded by pathogenic organisms.[40]

NANDA TAXONOMY: EXCHANGING 1.2.1.1

DEFINING CHARACTERISTICS[40]

1. Major risk factors
   a. Inadequate primary defenses (broken skin, traumatized tissue, decrease of ciliary action, stasis of body fluids, change in pH secretions, altered peristalsis)
   b. Inadequate secondary defenses (e.g., decreased hemoglobin, leukopenia, suppressed inflammatory response) and immunosuppression
   c. Inadequate acquired immunity
   d. Tissue destruction and increased environmental exposure
   e. Chronic disease
   f. Invasive procedures
   g. Malnutrition
   h. Pharmaceutical agents
   i. Trauma
   j. Rupture of amniotic membranes
   k. Insufficient knowledge to avoid exposure to pathogens
2. Minor risk factors
   None given.

RELATED FACTORS[40]

The risk factors serve also as the related factors.

RELATED CLINICAL CONCERNS

1. AIDS
2. Burns
3. COPD
4. Diabetes mellitus
5. Any surgery and any condition where steroids are used as a part of the treatment regimen
6. Substance abuse or dependence
7. Premature rupture of membranes

HAVE YOU SELECTED THE CORRECT DIAGNOSIS?

Self-Care Deficit Self-Care Deficit, especially in the areas of toileting, feeding, and bathing-hygiene, may need to be considered if improper handwashing, personal hygiene, toileting practice, or food preparation and storage have increased the risk of infection.

Impaired Skin Integrity; Impaired Tissue Integrity; Altered Nutrition, Less Than Body Requirements; Altered Oral Mucous Membrane These factors may be predisposing the client to infection.

Impaired Physical Mobility This diagnosis should be considered if skin breakdown is secondary to lack of movement. Skin breakdown always predisposes the patient to High Risk for Infection.

Altered Body Temperature, Risk for or Hyperthermia These diagnoses should be considered when the body temperature increases above normal, which is common in infectious processes.

Ineffective Management of Therapeutic Regimen (Noncompliance) This diagnosis may be occurring in cases of inappropriate antibiotic usage or inadequate treatment of wounds or chronic diseases.

EXPECTED OUTCOMES

1. Will return-demonstrate measures to decrease the risk for infection by (date) and/or
2. Will remain free from any symptoms of an infection by (date)

TARGET DATE

An appropriate target date would be within 3 days from the date of diagnosis.

NURSING ACTIONS/INTERVENTIONS WITH RATIONALES
Adult Health

ACTIONS/INTERVENTIONS	RATIONALES
• Monitor vital signs every 4 h around the clock. State times here.	Provides a baseline that allows quick recognition of deviations in subsequent measurements.
• Use universal precautions, and teach patient and family the purpose and techniques of universal precautions.[72–76]	Protects patient and family from infection.
• Maintain adequate nutrition and fluid and electrolyte balance. Provide a well-balanced diet with increased amounts of vitamin C, sufficient iron, and 2400–2600 mL of fluid daily.	Helps prevent disability that would predispose patient to infection.
• Collaborate with physician regarding screening specimens for culture and sensitivity, e.g., blood, urine, and spinal fluid.	Allows accurate determination of the causative organism and identification of the antibiotic that will be most effective against the organism.
• Monitor the administration of antibiotics for maintenance of blood levels and for side effects, e.g., diarrhea.	Antibiotics have to be maintained at a consistent blood level, usually 7–10 days, to kill causative organisms. Antibiotics may destroy normal bowel flora, predisposing the patient to the development of diarrhea and increasing the chance of infection in the lower GI tract.
• Maintain a neutral thermal environment.	Avoids overheating or overcooling of room that would contribute to complications for the patient.
• Assist patient with a thorough shower at least once daily (dependent on age) or total bed bath daily.	Reduces microorganisms on the skin.
• Wash your hands thoroughly between each treatment. Teach patient the value of frequent handwashing.	Prevents cross contamination and nosocomial infections.
• Provide good genital hygiene, and teach patient how to care for the genital area.	Prevents spread of opportunistic infections.
• Use reverse or protective isolation as necessary.	Protects the patient from exposure to pathogens.
• Use sterile technique when changing dressings or performing invasive procedures.	Protects the patient from exposure to pathogens.
• Turn every 2 h on (odd/even) hour.	Prevents inadequate tissue perfusion and stasis of blood.
• Cough and deep breathe every 2 h on (odd/even) hour	Mobilizes static pulmonary secretions.
• Perform passive exercises or have patient perform active ROM exercises every 2 h on the (odd/even) hour. Remember patient may have decreased tolerance of activity.	Prevents inadequate tissue perfusion and stasis of blood.
• Teach the patient and family about the infectious process, routes, pathogens, environmental and host factors, and aspects of prevention.	Provides basic knowledge for self-help and self-protection.
• Consult with appropriate assistive community resources as indicated.	Appropriate use of existing community service is efficient use of resources.

Child Health

ACTIONS/INTERVENTIONS	RATIONALES
• Monitor axillary temperature every 2 h on the (odd/even) hour.	Most appropriate route for frequent measurements for the very young child. Oral temperature measurements would not be accurate.
• Encourage child and parents to verbalize fears, concerns, or feelings related to infection by scheduling at least 30 min per shift to counsel family. Note times here.	Provides support, decreases anxiety and fears, and provides teaching opportunity.

Women's Health

ACTIONS/INTERVENTIONS	RATIONALES
• In the presence of ruptured amniotic membranes, monitor for signs of infection at least every 4 h at (state times here), e.g., elevated temperature or vaginal discharge odor	Provides clinical data needed to quickly recognize the presence of infection.
• Use aseptic technique when performing vaginal examinations, and limit the number of vaginal examinations during labor.	Reduce the opportunities to introduce infection.
• Teach mother to take only showers (no tub baths) and to monitor and record temperature. Have her take temperature at least every 4 h on a set schedule.	Teaches patient basic information to recognize and prevent infection.
• Keep linens and underpads clean and changed as necessary during labor.	Reduces the likelihood of nosocomial infections.
• Monitor incisions (C-section or episiotomy) at least every 4 h at (state times here) for redness, drainage, oozing, hematoma, or loss of approximation.	Provides clinical data needed to quickly recognize the presence of infection.
• During postpartum period, monitor fundal height at least every 4 h at (state times here) around the clock for 48 h.	Provides database necessary to screen for infection.
• During postpartum period, monitor patient, at least every 4 h at (state times here), for any signs of foul-smelling lochia, uterine tenderness, or increased temperature.	Provides clinical data needed to quickly recognize the presence of infection.
• In instances of abortion, obtain a complete obstetric history.	
• Monitor abdomen at least every 4 h at (state times here) for any swelling, tenderness, or foul-smelling vaginal discharge following an abortion.	
• If meconium present in amniotic fluid, immediately clear airway of infant by suctioning (preferably done by physician immediately upon delivery of infant's head).	Helps prevent aspiration pneumonia in infant.
• Suction gastric contents immediately. Observe for sternal retractions, grunting, trembling, jitters, or pallor. If any of these signs are present, notify the physician at once.	Indicates development of respiratory complications secondary to meconium.
• Wash hands each time before and after you handle the baby.	Prevents development of nosocomial infections.
• Avoid wearing sharp jewelry that could scratch the baby.	
• Keep umbilical cord clean and dry by cleansing at each diaper change or at least every 2 h on (odd/even) hour.	
• Monitor circumcision site for swelling, odor, or bleeding each diaper change or at least every 2 h on (odd/even) hour.	

• Demonstrate and have parent return-demonstrate:
  ○ How to take baby's temperature measurement
  ○ How to properly care for umbilical cord and circumcision
	Gives parents basic information regarding prevention of infection and monitoring for the development of infection.

Psychiatric Health

ACTIONS/INTERVENTIONS	RATIONALES
• Monitor the temperature of clients receiving antipsychotic medications twice a day, and report any elevations to physician. Note times for temperature measurement here.	These clients are at risk for developing agranulocytosis. The greatest risk is 3–8 wk after therapy has begun.

Continued

• Monitor the client for the presence of a sore throat in the absence of a cold or other flu-like symptoms at least daily. Report any occurrence.	These clients are at risk for developing agranulocytosis. The greatest risk is 3–8 wk after therapy has begun.
• Teach the client to report temperature elevations and sore throats in the absence of other symptoms to the physician.	This could be a symptom of agranulocytosis.
• During the first 8 wk of treatment with an antipsychotic, report any signs of infection in the client to the physician for assessment of white cell count.	Provides a baseline for comparison after the client has begun antipsychotic therapy.
• Review the client's CBC before antipsychotics are started, and report any abnormalities on this and any subsequent CBCs to the physician.	
• Teach the client and family handwashing techniques, nutrition, appropriate antibiotic use, hazards of substance abuse, and universal precautions.	These measures can help prevent or decrease the risk of infection.

Gerontic Health

ACTIONS/INTERVENTIONS	RATIONALES
• Avoid shearing forces when repositioning patient.	Dermal fragility leads to frequent skin tears when patients are repositioned or transferred from bed to chair, etc.
• Monitor any incidents of nausea, vomiting, or diarrhea.	The GI tract of the older adult is more sensitive to the effects of contaminated food; therefore, he or she is more susceptible to GI infections.
• Encourage frequent handwashing by the patient.	Hands may serve as fomites due to more frequent contact with contaminated items, e.g., wheelchair wheels.

Home Health

ACTIONS/INTERVENTIONS	RATIONALES
• Teach client and family measures to prevent transmission of infectious disease to others. Assist patient and family with lifestyle changes that may be required: 　○ Handwashing 　○ Isolation as appropriate 　○ Proper disposal of infectious waste (e.g., bagging) 　○ Proper use of disinfectants 　○ Appropriate medical intervention (e.g., antibiotics or antipyretics) 　○ Immunization 　○ Signs and symptoms of infection 　○ Treatment for lice and removal of nits 　○ Asepsis for wound care NOTE: Items can be sterilized at home by immersing in boiling water for 10 min. The water needs to be boiling for the entire 10 min.	Many infectious diseases can be prevented by appropriate measures. Client and family members require this information and the opportunity to practice these skills.

- Participate in tuberculosis screening and prevention program.[77]
- Monitor for factors contributing to the high risk for infection.
- Involve the client and family in planning, implementing, and promoting reduction in the high risk for infection:
  ○ Family conference
  ○ Mutual goal setting
  ○ Communication
- Teach the client and family measures to prevent or decrease potential for infection:
  ○ Handwashing techniques
  ○ Universal precautions for blood and body fluids
  ○ Personal hygiene and health habits
  ○ Nutrition; immunization schedule
  ○ Proper food storage and preparation
  ○ Elimination of environmental hazards such as rodents or insects
  ○ Proper sewage control and trash collection
  ○ Appropriate antiobiotic use
  ○ Hazards of substance abuse
  ○ Preparation and precautions when traveling to areas in which infectious diseases are endemic
  ○ Signs and symptoms of infectious diseases for which the client and family are at risk
  ○ Preparation for disaster (water storage, canned or dried food, and emergency waste disposal).

This action serves as the database to identify the need for interventions to prevent infections.

Family involvement is important to ensure success. Communication and mutual goals improve the outcome.

These measures reduce the risk of infection.

Infection, Risk for

FLOWCHART EVALUATION: EXPECTED OUTCOME 1

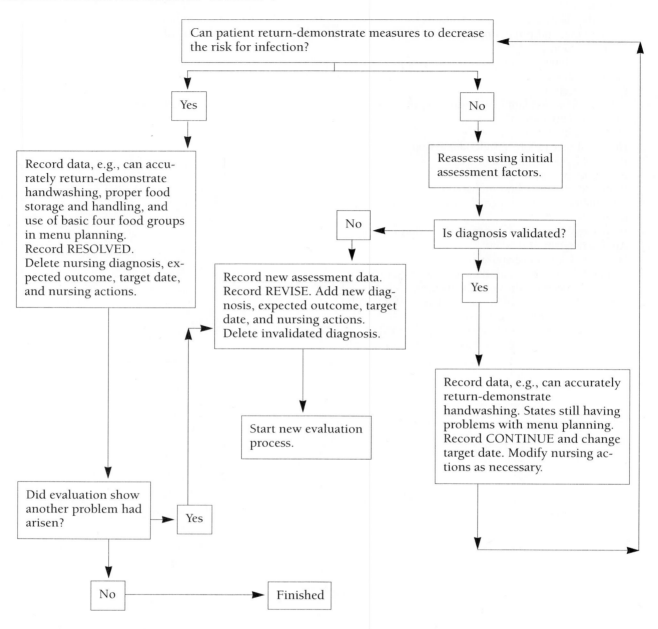

Can patient return-demonstrate measures to decrease the risk for infection?

Yes

No

Record data, e.g., can accurately return-demonstrate handwashing, proper food storage and handling, and use of basic four food groups in menu planning.
Record RESOLVED.
Delete nursing diagnosis, expected outcome, target date, and nursing actions.

Reassess using initial assessment factors.

No

Is diagnosis validated?

Yes

Record new assessment data. Record REVISE. Add new diagnosis, expected outcome, target date, and nursing actions. Delete invalidated diagnosis.

Record data, e.g., can accurately return-demonstrate handwashing. States still having problems with menu planning. Record CONTINUE and change target date. Modify nursing actions as necessary.

Start new evaluation process.

Did evaluation show another problem had arisen?

Yes

No

Finished

Infection, Risk for

FLOWCHART EVALUATION: EXPECTED OUTCOME 2

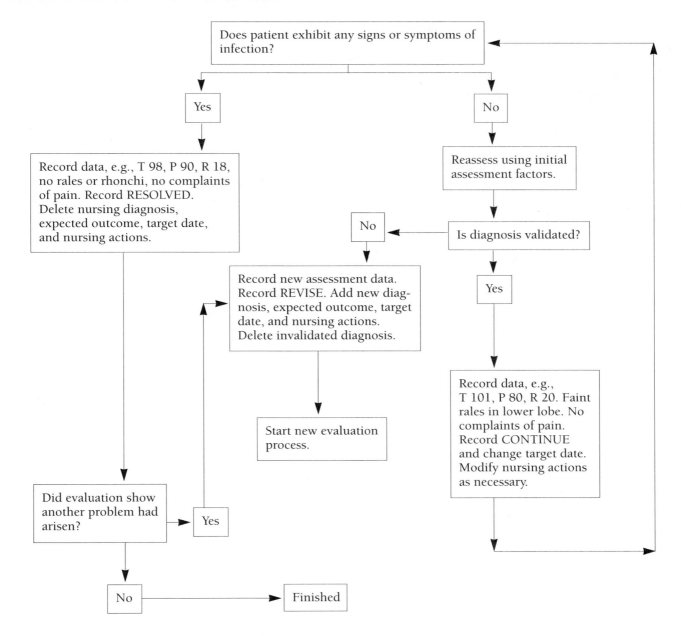

Injury, Risk for

DEFINITION

A state in which the individual is at risk for injury as a result of environmental conditions interacting with the individual's adaptive and defensive resources.[40]

NANDA TAXONOMY: EXCHANGING 1.6.1

DEFINING CHARACTERISTICS (RISK FACTORS)[40]

NOTE: According to the NANDA Taxomony, Risk for Injury is a Level 3 diagnosis. Level 4 diagnoses under Risk for Injury are Suffocation, Poisoning, and Trauma. To assist you in making the most specific diagnosis, the definitions, defining characteristics, and related factors for these Level 4 diagnoses are also included.

A. Risk for Injury

1. Major risk factors
   a. Internal
      (1) Biochemical, regulatory function: Sensory dysfunction, integrative dysfunction, effector dysfunction, tissue hypoxia
      (2) Malnutrition
      (3) Immunoautoimmune dysfunction
      (4) Abnormal blood profile: Leukocytosis-leukopenia, altered clotting factors, thrombocytopenia, sickle cell, Thalassemia, decreased hemoglobin
      (5) Physical: Broken skin, altered mobility
      (6) Developmental age: Physiologic, psychosocial
      (7) Psychological: Affective, orientation
   b. External
      (1) Biological: Immunization level of community, microorganism
      (2) Chemical: Pollutants, poisons, drugs, pharmaceutical agents, alcohol, caffeine, nicotine, preservatives, cosmetics and dyes
      (3) Nutrients: Vitamins, food types
      (4) Physical: Design, structure, and arrangement of community building, and/or equipment
      (5) Mode of transport or transportation
      (6) People, provider: Nosocomial agents, staffing patterns, cognitive, affective and psychomotor factors
2. Minor risk factors
   None given.

B. Risk for Injury, Suffocation

Definition: Accentuated risk of accidental suffocation (inadequate air available for inhalation)[40]

1. Major risk factors
   a. Internal (individual)
      (1) Reduced olfactory sensation
      (2) Reduced motor abilities
      (3) Lack of safety education
      (4) Lack of safety precautions
      (5) Cognitive or emotional difficulties
      (6) Disease or injury process
   b. External (environmental)
      (1) Pillow placed in an infant's crib
      (2) Propped bottle placed in an infant's crib
      (3) Vehicle warming in closed garage
      (4) Children playing with plastic bags or inserting small objects into their mouths or noses
      (5) Discarded or unused refrigerators or freezers without removed doors
      (6) Children left unattended in bathtubs or pools
      (7) Household gas leaks
      (8) Smoking in bed
      (9) Use of fuel-burning heater not vented to outside
      (10) Low-strung clothesline
      (11) Pacifier hung around infant's head
      (12) Eating large mouthfuls of food
2. Minor risk factors
   None given.

C. Risk for Injury, Poisoning

Definition: Accentuated risk of accidental exposure to or ingestion of drugs or dangerous products in doses sufficient to cause poisoning[40]

1. Major risk factors
   a. Internal (individual)
      (1) Reduced vision
      (2) Verbalization of occupational setting without adequate safeguards
      (3) Lack of safety or drug education
      (4) Lack of proper precaution
      (5) Cognitive or emotional difficulties
      (6) Insufficient finances
   b. External (environmental)
      (1) Large supplies of drugs in house
      (2) Medicines stored in unlocked cabinet accessible to children or confused persons
      (3) Dangerous products placed or stored within the reach of children or confused persons
      (4) Availability of illicit drugs potentially contaminated by poisonous additives
      (5) Flaking, peeling paint or plaster in presence of young children
      (6) Chemical contamination of food and water
      (7) Unprotected contact with heavy metals or chemicals
      (8) Use of paint, lacquer, or other substances that emit noxious fumes in poorly ventilated areas or without effective protection
      (9) Presence of poisonous vegetation
      (10) Presence of atmospheric pollutants
2. Minor risk factors
   None given.

D. Risk for Injury, Trauma

Definition: Accentuated risk of accidental tissue injury, for example, wound, burn, fracture[40]

1. Major risk factors
   a. Internal (individual)
      (1) Weakness
      (2) Poor vision
      (3) Balancing difficulties
      (4) Reduced temperature or tactile sensation
      (5) Reduced large or small muscle coordination
      (6) Reduced hand-eye coordination
      (7) Lack of safety education

(8) Lack of safety precautions

(9) Insufficient finances to purchase safety equipment or effect repairs

(10) Cognitive or emotional difficulties

(11) History of previous trauma

b. External (environmental)

(1) Slippery floors (e.g., wet or highly waxed)

(2) Snow or ice collected on stairs or walkways

(3) Unanchored rugs

(4) Bathtub without handgrip or antislip equipment

(5) Use of unsteady ladders or chairs

(6) Entering unlighted rooms

(7) Unsteady or absent stair rails

(8) Unanchored electric wires

(9) Litter or liquid spills on floors or stairways

(10) High beds

(11) Children playing without a gate at the top of the stairs

(12) Obstructed passageways

(13) Unsafe window protection in homes with young children

(14) Inappropriate call-for-aid mechanisms for bed-resting patient

(15) Pot handles facing toward front of stove

(16) Bathing in very hot water (e.g., unsupervised bathing of young children)

(17) Potential igniting of gas leaks

(18) Delayed lighting of gas burner or oven

(19) Experimenting with chemical or gasoline

(20) Unscreened fires or heaters

(21) Wearing plastic apron or flowing clothes around open flame

(22) Children playing with matches, candles, or cigarettes

(23) Inadequately stored combustibles or corrosives (e.g., matches, oily rags, or lye)

(24) Highly flammable children's toys or clothing

(25) Overloaded fuse boxes

(26) Contact with rapidly moving machinery, industrial belts, or pulleys

(27) Sliding on coarse bed linen or struggling within bed restraints

(28) Faulty electrical plugs, frayed wires, or defective appliances

(29) Contact with acids or alkalis

(30) Playing with fireworks or gunpowder

(31) Contact with intense cold

(32) Overexposure to sun, sunlamps, or radiotherapy

(33) Use of cracked dinnerware or glasses

(34) Knives stored uncovered

(35) Guns or ammunition stored unlocked

(36) Large icicles hanging from roof

(37) Exposure to dangerous machinery

(38) Children playing with sharp-edged toys

(39) High-crime neighborhood and vulnerable clients

(40) Driving a mechanically unsafe vehicle

(41) Driving after partaking of alcoholic beverages or drugs

(42) Driving at excessive speed

(43) Driving without necessary visual aid

(44) Children riding in the front seat in car

(45) Smoking in bed or near oxygen

(46) Overloaded electrical outlet

(47) Grease waste collected on stoves

(48) Use of thin or worn potholders

(49) Misuse of necessary headgear for motorized cyclists or young children carried on adult bicycles

(50) Unsafe road or road-crossing conditions

(51) Play or work near vehicle pathways (e.g., driveways, laneways, or railroad tracks)

(52) Nonuse or misuse of seat restraints

2. Minor risk factors
   None given.

RELATED FACTORS[40]

The risk factors serve as the related factors for risk diagnoses.

RELATED CLINICAL CONCERNS

1. AIDS
2. Dementias such as Alzheimer's disease or multi-infarct
3. Diseases of the eye such as cataracts or glaucoma
4. Medications, for example, hallucinogens, barbiturates, opioids, or benzodiazepines
5. Epilepsy
6. Substance abuse or dependence

HAVE YOU SELECTED THE CORRECT DIAGNOSIS?

Activity Intolerance This diagnosis should be considered if the nurse observes or validates reports of the patient's inability to complete required tasks because of insufficient energy. Insufficient energy could lead to accidents through, for example, falling or dropping items.

Impaired Physical Mobility This diagnosis is appropriate if the patient has difficulty with coordination, range of motion, muscle strength and control, or activity restrictions related to treatment. This could be manifested by the frequent occurrence of accidents or injury.

Knowledge Deficit This diagnosis may exist if the client or family verbalizes less-than-adequate understanding of injury prevention.

Continued

Impaired Home Maintenance Management This diagnosis is demonstrated by the inability of the patient or the family to provide a safe living environment.

Altered Thought Process This diagnosis should be considered if the patient exhibits impaired attention span, impaired ability to recall information, impaired perception, judgment, and decision making, or impaired conceptual reasoning abilities. This diagnosis could certainly be reflected in increased accidents or injuries.

Risk for Violence This diagnosis exists if the accidents or injuries can be related to the risk factors for self-inflicted or other-directed physical trauma (e.g., self-destructive behavior, substance abuse, rage, or hostile verbalizations).

EXPECTED OUTCOMES

1. Will identify hazards (list) contributing to risk for injury and at least one corrective measure (list) for each hazard by (date) and/or
2. Will have no incidents of injury by (date)

TARGET DATE

While preventing injury may be a lifelong activity, establishing a mindset to avoid injury can be begun rapidly. An appropriate target date would be within 3 days of admission.

NURSING ACTIONS/INTERVENTIONS WITH RATIONALES

Adult Health

ACTIONS/INTERVENTIONS	RATIONALES
• Check on patient at least once an hour. If risk for injury exists, do not leave patient unattended. Schedule sitters around the clock. If the patient has been identified as being at risk for injury, e.g., falls, place green dot on armband, chart, and head of bed.	Primary preventive measures to ensure patient safety. Green dot serves to alert other health care personnel of patient's status.
• Check respiratory rate, depth, and chest sounds at least every 4 h at (state times here).	Ongoing monitoring of risk factors.
• Do not leave medications, solutions, or any type of liquids in the room. Use only paper cups and containers that can be disposed of immediately in patient's room. Use "Mr. Yuk" on bottle labels of poisonous substances. Teach patient and family to use this type of labeling at home.	Basic safety measures to prevent poisoning.
• Keep continuous check on airway patency. Keep suctioning equipment, ventilation equipment, and lavage setup on standby.	Ongoing monitoring of risk factors.
• Keep bed wheels locked and bed in low position. Keep head of bed elevated at least 30 degrees at all times.	
• Pad siderails and keep siderails up when patient is in bed.	
• Make sure handrails are in place in the bathroom and that safety strips are in tub and shower. Do not leave patient unattended in bathtub or shower.	
• Keep the patient's room free of clutter.	Basic safety measures to prevent injury.
• Orient the patient to time, person, place, and environment at least once a shift.	Keep patient aware of environment.
• Provide night light.	Safety measure to prevent falling at night.
• Assist in correcting, to the extent possible, any sensory-perceptual problems through appropriate referrals.	Correction of sensory-perceptual problems, vision, for example, will assist in accident prevention.
• Assist the patient with all transfer and ambulation. If the patient requires multiple pillows for rest or positioning, tape the bottom layer of pillows to prevent dislodging.	Assists in preventing suffocation or tripping on pillows.

- Teach patient and family safety measures for use at home:
  - Use nonskid rugs or tack down throw rugs.
  - Use handrails.
  - Install ramps.
  - Use color contrast for steps, door knobs, electrical outlets, and light switches.
  - Avoid surface glare (e.g., floors or table tops).
  - Maintain clean, nonskid floors, and keep rooms and halls free of clutter.
  - Change physical position slowly.
  - Use covers for electrical outlets.
  - Position pans with handles toward back of stove.
  - Have family post poison control number for ready reference.
  - Provide extra lighting in room and night light.
- Teach patient and significant other: Basic safety measures.
  - Alterations in lifestyle that may be necessary (e.g., stopping smoking, stopping alcohol ingestions, decreasing or ceasing drug ingestion, or ceasing driving)
  - Use of assistive devices (e.g., walkers, canes, crutches, or wheelchairs)
  - Heimlich maneuver
  - CPR
  - Recognition of signs and symptoms of choking and carbon monoxide poisoning
  - Necessity of chewing food thoroughly and cutting   Allows time for checking and correction of problem areas.
    food into small bites
- Refer to appropriate agency for safety check of home. Make referral at least 3 days prior to discharge.

Child Health

ACTIONS/INTERVENTIONS	RATIONALES
• Maintain appropriate supervision of infant at all times. Allow respite time for parents. **Do not** leave infant unattended. Have bulb syringe available in case of need to suction oropharynx. If regular equipment for suctioning is required, validate by checking label that all safety checks have been completed on equipment. Be aware of potential for young children to answer to any name. Validate identification for procedures in all young children.	Will prevent medication or treatment errors.
• Keep siderails of crib up, and monitor safety of all attachments for crib or infant's bassinet.	Infants and small children are prone to putting small pieces in mouth, nose, or ears. Basic safety measures. Helps prevent scalding or chilling of infant.
• Check temperature of water before bathing and formula or food before feeding. **Do not** microwave formula.	
• Maintain contact at all times during bathing. Infants unable to sit must be held constantly. Older children should be monitored as well, with special attention given mental or physical needs for a handicapped child.	
• Place infant on back or side or as physician orders. Special instructions may be required with preterm infants and/or those with special conditions, e.g., gastric esophageal reflux.	Helps prevent aspiration in case of vomiting. New updates regarding SIDS now provide this mandate from the American Academy of Pediatrics.

Continued

ACTIONS/INTERVENTIONS	RATIONALES

• Investigate any signs and symptoms that warrant potential child protective service referral.
 • Teach family basic safety measures:
   ○ Store plastic bags in cabinet out of child's reach.
   ○ Do not cover mattress or pillows of infant or child with plastic.
   ○ Make certain crib design follows federal regulations and that mattress has appropriate fit with crib frame.
   ○ Discourage sleeping in bed with infant.
   ○ Avoid use of homemade pacifiers (use only those of one-piece construction with loop handle).
   ○ **Do not** tie pacifier around infant's neck.
   ○ Untie bibs, bonnets, or other garments with snug fit around neck of infant before sleep.
   ○ Inspect toys for removable parts and check for safety approval.
   ○ **Do not** feed infant foods which do not readily dissolve such as grapes, nuts, and popcorn.
   ○ Keep doors of large appliances, especially refrigerators, closed at all times.
   ○ Maintain fence and constant supervision with swimming pool.
   ○ Exercise caution while cleaning with attention to pails of water and cleaning solutions.
   ○ As infant or child is able, encourage swimming lessons with supervision and foster water safety.
   ○ Use caution in exposure to sun for periods greater than 10 min at a time.
   ○ Use appropriate seat belts and car seats according to weight and development.
   ○ Keep matches and pointed objects, such as knives, in a safe place out of child's reach.
   ○ Use lead-free paint on child's furniture and environment.
   ○ Keep toxic substances locked in cabinet and out of child's reach.
   ○ Hang plants and avoid placement on floor and tables.
   ○ Discard used poisonous substances.
   ○ **Do not** store toxic substances in food or beverage containers.
   ○ Administer medication as a drug, not as candy.
   ○ Use child-proof medication containers.
   ○ Keep syrup of ipecac on hand in case of accidental poisoning.
   ○ As applicable, use any special monitoring equipment as recommended for child.
   ○ Monitor meal times to prevent aspiration with giggling.
	Provides assistance for child and family in instances of child abuse.
	 Ensures environmental safety for infant or child.

Women's Health

ACTIONS/INTERVENTIONS	RATIONALES
• Teach patient and family the risk for injury to the fetus and patient when the pregnant women smokes, is exposed to secondhand smoke, or engages in substance abuse, e.g., alcohol and drugs (legal or illegal).	Provides initial safety information regarding the well-being of the fetus.

• Report to proper authorities any suspicion of family violence (see Chaps. 9 and 10 for more detailed nursing actions).	A legal requirement in most states.
• Provide atmosphere that allows the patient considering abortion to relate her concerns and experiences and to obtain detailed information about the method of abortion that is being considered.	Allows patient to receive nonjudgmental information about the pros and cons of all choices available.
• Encourage questions and verbalization of patient's life expectations.	
• Provide information on options available to patient.	
• Assist patient in identifying lifestyle adjustments that decision could entail.	
• Involve significant others, if so desired by patient, in discussion and problem-solving activities regarding lifestyle adjustments.	
• In instances where the patient has performed a self-induced abortion, obtain detailed information regarding the method used. Provide atmosphere that allows patient to relate her experience.	In self-induced abortion, there is high probability of injury and subsequent infection. This information will provide the health team with basic data to begin assessing the degree of injury.
• Ascertain if abortifacients (castor oil, turpentine, lye, ammonia, etc.) were used or if mechanical means (coat hanger, knitting needles, broken bottle, or knife).	
• Regardless of the type of abortion, obtain a history from patient that includes: 　○ Date of last menstrual period 　○ Method of contraception, if any 　○ Previous obstetric history 　○ Known allergies to anesthetics, analgesics, antibiotics, or other drugs 　○ Current drug usage 　○ Past medical history	Provides basic database to initiate planning of care.
• Note patient's mental state, e.g., anxious, frightened, or ambivalent.	
• Perform physical assessment with special notice of: 　○ Amount and character of vaginal discharge 　○ Temperature elevation 　○ Pain 　○ Bleeding: Consistency, amount, and color	
• Teach patient importance of proper storage of birth control pills, spermicides, and medications.	
• Assist patient in identifying drugs that are teratogenic to the fetus.	Provides information that allows the patient to plan for safety during pregnancy.
• Assist patient in becoming aware of environmental hazards when pregnant, such as x-rays, people with infections, cats (litter boxes), and hazards on the job (surgical gases, industrial hazards).	

Psychiatric Health

ACTIONS/INTERVENTIONS	RATIONALES
• Orient client to person, place, and time on each interaction.	Disorientation can increase the client's risk for injury if the environment is perceived as dangerous.
• Provide appropriate assistance to client as he or she moves about the environment.	Prevent falls and possible injury.

Continued

ACTIONS/INTERVENTIONS	RATIONALES

• Monitor level of consciousness every 15 min when the client is acutely disoriented following special treatments or when consciousness is affected by drugs or alcohol. If level of consciousness is impaired, place client on side to prevent aspiration of vomitus, and withhold solid food until level of consciousness improves. Place client in bed with siderails and keep siderails raised.
• Do not allow client to smoke without supervision when disoriented or when consciousness is clouded.
• Provide supervision for clients using new tools that could precipitate injury in special activities such as occupational therapy.
• Teach client and support system:
  ○ Risks associated with excessive use of drugs and alcohol
  ○ Appropriate methods for compensating for sensory-perceptual deficits (e.g., use of pictures or colors to distinguish environmental cues when ability to read is lost)
• Remove all environmental hazards (e.g., personal grooming items that could produce a hazard, cleaning agents, foods that produce a hazard when taken with certain medicines, plastic bags, clothes hangers, belt and ties, or shoestrings). Remove unnecessary pillows and blankets from the bed.
• Maintain close supervision of client. (If client is suicidal, refer to nursing actions for Risk for Violence, Chap. 9, for specific interventions.)
• Check client's mouth carefully after oral medicines are given for any amounts that might be held in the mouth to be used at a later date.
• If client is at risk for holding pills in the mouth to be used later, collaborate with physician to have doses changed to liquids or injections.
• Keep lavage setup and airway and oxygen equipment on standby.
• Talk with client and support system about situations that increase the risk for poisoning and develop a list of these situations.
• Label all medicines and poisonous substances appropriately.
	Patient safety is of primary importance. Provides information about client's current status so interventions can be adapted appropriately. Prevents aspiration by facilitating drainage of fluids away from airway, and prevents falls and possible injury.
	
	Prevents client from acting impulsively to injure self with items easily found in environment. This allows staff time to offer alternative coping strategies when clients are experiencing difficulty with coping.
	
	Prevents client from acting impulsively.
	
	Basic safety precautions.

Gerontic Health

ACTIONS/INTERVENTIONS	RATIONALES
• Refer the independent elder to home health for home safety assessment at least 3 days prior to discharge from hospital.	Provides timely home care planning, and allows implementation of safety measures before patient is discharged.

- Instruct patient on safe administration of medication. Monitor for knowledge of drug dosage, reason for medication, expected effect, and possible side effects. Reinforce teaching on a daily basis.

- If patient suffers from dementia, teach the caregiver the following safety adaptations[78]:
  - Place in a locked closet articles such as power tools, medications, or appliances that the individual may misuse and injure self or others.
  - Ensure that water temperature is low enough to prevent scalding.
  - Remove knobs from stove if cooking is a fire hazard.
  - Install gates at the top of stairs to prevent falls.
  - Tape door latches or remove tumblers from locks to prevent patient from accidentally locking himself or herself in rooms.
  - Place 2 locks on entry and exit doors if the individual is prone to wandering.
  - Ensure that furnishings do not have sharp edges or large areas of glass that could cause injury during a fall.

Basic medication safety measures.

Older adults with the diagnosis of dementia often display signs of poor judgment. The above teaching factors decrease the risk for injury in the home setting.

Home Health

ACTIONS/INTERVENTIONS	RATIONALES

• Involve client and family in planning, implementing, and promoting reduction in the risk for injury:
  ○ Arrange family conferences.
  ○ Assist family to define mutual goals.
  ○ Promote communication.
  ○ Assist family members with specific tasks as appropriate to reduce the risk for injury. (*Note:* Restraining the client may increase, not decrease, the risk for injury.[79]) It is important to arrange the environment so that the client can avoid injury, e.g., use bedside commode or raised toilet seat, remove unnecessary furniture, pick up objects that may be blocking pathways,[80–82] remove unsafe or improperly stored chemicals, weapons, cooking utensils, and appliances, use and store safely toxic substances, obtain certification in first aid and CPR, properly store food, obtain knowledge of poisonous plants, learn to swim, remove fire hazards from environment, design and practice an emergency plan for action if fire occurs, and properly use machines powered by petroleum products.
	Involvement of the client and family enhances motivation and increases the possibility of positive outcomes and the long-term lifestyle changes required.

• Teach client and family injury prevention activities as appropriate:
  ○ Proper lifting techniques
  ○ Back exercises to prevent back injury
  ○ Removal of hazardous environmental conditions such as improper storage of hazardous substances, improper use of electrical appliances, smoking in bed, open heaters and flames, and congested walkways
	Prevention activities reduce the risk of injury. Many people either do not know these prevention strategies or need to have them reinforced.

Continued

ACTIONS/INTERVENTIONS	RATIONALES
○ Proper ventilation when using toxic substances ○ First aid for poisoning ○ Proper labeling, storage, and disposal of toxic materials such as household cleaning products, lawn and garden chemicals, and medications ○ Proper food preparation and storage ○ Proper skin, lung, and eye protection when using toxic substances ○ Toxic substances out of reach of infants and young children ○ Recognition of toxic plants and removal from environment as indicated ○ Plan of action if accidental poisoning occurs	
• Assist client and family in lifestyle adjustments that may be required.	For long-term change, lifestyle adjustments are often required. Many people require assistance with these changes.
• Refer to appropriate assistive community resources as indicated.	Use of existing community services is efficient use of resources.
• Participate in early-return-to-work programs.[83]	Such programs lead to better client outcomes.
• Participate in local, state, and national immunization initiatives.[83]	Community participation in immunization initiatives improves the rate of appropriate immunization and reduces the risk of outbreak of the diseases for which vaccines are available.

Injury, Risk for

FLOWCHART EVALUATION: EXPECTED OUTCOME 1

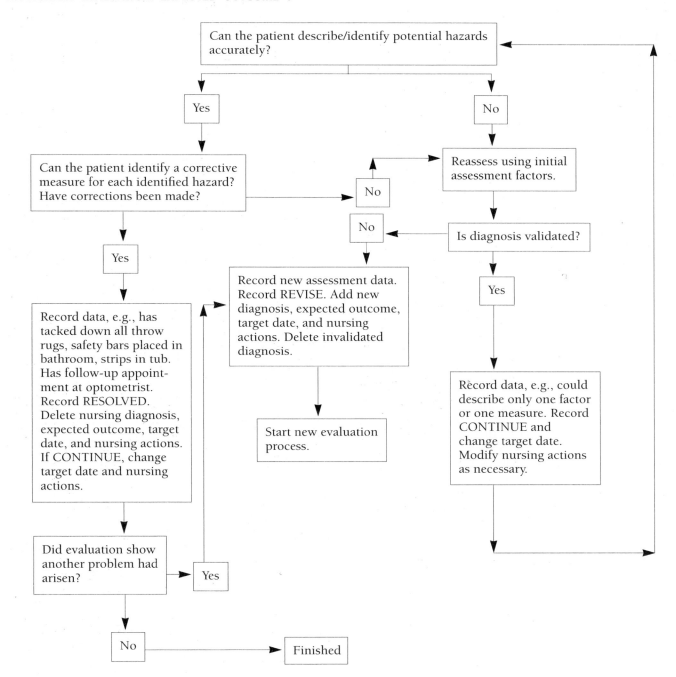

Injury, Risk for

FLOWCHART EVALUATION: EXPECTED OUTCOME 2

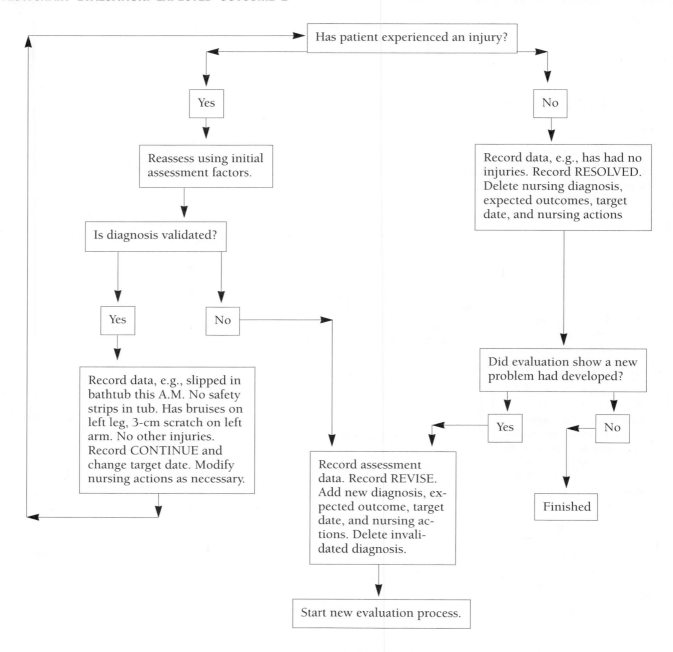

Management of Therapeutic Regimen (Individual), Effective

DEFINITION

A pattern of regulating and integrating into daily living a program for treatment of illness and its sequelae that is satisfactory for meeting specific health goals.[40]

NANDA TAXONOMY: CHOOSING 5.2.1.1; 5.2.2

DEFINING CHARACTERISTICS[40]

1. Major defining characteristics
   a. Appropriate choices of daily activities for meeting the goals of a treatment or prevention program
   b. Illness symptoms within a normal range of expectation
   c. Verbalized desire to manage the treatment of illness and prevention of sequelae
   d. Verbalized intent to reduce risk factors for progression of illness and sequelae
2. Minor defining characteristics
   None given.

RELATED FACTORS[40]

None given.

RELATED CLINICAL CONCERNS

Any condition requiring long-term management; for example, cardiovascular diseases and diabetes mellitus.

HAVE YOU SELECTED THE CORRECT DIAGNOSIS?

There are currently no other diagnoses this diagnosis could be compared to or that are close to the concept of this diagnosis. This diagnosis could be classified as a wellness diagnosis; that is, the patient with this diagnosis is progressing toward wellness and appropriate health maintenance.

EXPECTED OUTCOMES

1. Will demonstrate continued commitment, as evidenced by (specific actions of patients, for example, continued exercise program), to prevent sequelae by (date).
2. Subsequent assessments document continued progress toward health by (date).

TARGET DATE

Effective management of a therapeutic regimen will require a lifelong commitment by the client. Therefore, target dates will vary from weeks to years. It would be appropriate to set the first target date, after the patient's discharge, for 1 month.

NURSING ACTIONS/INTERVENTIONS WITH RATIONALES

Adult Health

ACTIONS/INTERVENTIONS	RATIONALES
• Allow time for patient to discuss his or her feelings about the therapeutic regimen.	
• Support patient in choices made to effectively manage therapeutic regimen.	Encourages patient's sense of control and strengthens support systems.
• Review availability and use of resources and support groups.	
• Answer questions about disease process and therapeutic regimen. Provide teaching for any new components of therapeutic regimen.	
• Assist patient to solve problems as they arise.	Encourages patient's sense of self-control.
• Allow and monitor self-care while in the hospital.	Promotes independence.
• Have patient return-demonstrate activities associated with therapeutic regimen, i.e., dressing changes, glucose testing; blood pressure checks; counting calories, fat grams, carbohydrates, and sodium intake; and self-administering medications. Supervise performance, critique, and reteach as necessary.	Provides feedback for skills, reaffirms motivation.

Continued

ACTIONS/INTERVENTIONS	**RATIONALES**
• Review self-reported plan of activities with patient, and continue to encourage its use and the sharing of the plan with patient's employer and physician.	Provides visual record of plan that is integrated into patient's lifestyle.
• Review accomplishment of goals of therapeutic regimen, and praise patient for even small accomplishments.	Improves motivation and gives the patient a sense of achievement.
• Allow at least 30 min a day for patient to verbalize possible conflicts with therapeutic regimen. Role-play possible scenarios.	Provides an opportunity for patient to verbalize and act out alternate coping strategies in a nonthreatening environment.
• Have patient make follow-up appointments with appropriate resources or health care providers prior to discharge.	Facilitates continuity and consistency of plan.
• Continue to coordinate care with other health care providers or community resources.	Promotes patient advocacy.

Child Health

ACTIONS/INTERVENTIONS	**RATIONALES**
• Utilize appropriate age and developmental communication.	Assists in developing a trusting relationship with client and primary caregiver.
• Determine client's and primary caregiver's perception of condition.	Provides starting point for discussing and teaching therapeutic regimen.
• Assist family to determine when and where follow-up care will be utilized.[45,46]	Promotes long-term management.
• Offer verbal and emotional reinforcement for appropriate attendance to mutually agreed-to criteria. State criteria here; e.g., maintain immunizations.	Provides positive reinforcement.
• Acknowledge need for caregiver to be relieved (at regular intervals) of total responsibilities of dependent infant or child. Encourage caregiver to express feelings regarding responsibility. Delineate community resources that can augment care.[45,46]	Assists in preventing caregiver role strain. Promotes effective management.
• Identify subsequent factors that are likely to resurface over time, e.g., developmental concerns.	

Women's Health

ACTIONS/INTERVENTIONS	**RATIONALES**
• Utilize Prenatal Risk Indicator Tools to identify women who are high risk for pregnancy and birth. Assess and counsel those mothers identified as high risk. Assist patient to plan changes necessary in her lifestyle to maintain pregnancy and health of mother and fetus until birth.[84–87]	Provides patient with information needed to make informed choices and necessary lifestyle changes in order to maximize health for self and fetus.
• Provide new mother with information about various support groups and health care programs when early postpartum discharge occurs. Provide teaching and support on an ongoing basis from time of conception until end of postpartum period for the new mother, her family, and her baby. Provide new parents with written handouts, help-line telephone numbers, follow-up appointments with advanced practice nurse, pediatrician, and obstetrician following postpartum discharge.	

Psychiatric Health

ACTIONS/INTERVENTIONS	RATIONALES

• Sit with client (number) minutes (number) times a day to discuss:
  ○ His or her understanding of the current situation
  ○ Strategies that assist the client in this management
  ○ Support systems
  ○ Stressors.
  Note important data from these discussions here.
	Promotes the development of a trusting relationship by communicating respect for the client.[57,58] Provides assessment data that will assist in the development of a plan to support client's current behaviors.

• Discuss with the client signs and symptoms that would indicate that assistance is needed with management.	Promotes client's sense of control.[52]
• Develop, with the client, a plan for obtaining the necessary assistance when needed.	
• Provide positive social reinforcement and other behavioral rewards for demonstration of adaptive management. (Those things that the client finds rewarding should be listed here with a schedule for use. The kinds of behaviors that are to be rewarded should also be listed.)	Positive reinforcement encourages adaptive behavior and enhances self-esteem.[56]

• Discuss with the client the impact of stress on physiologic and psychological well-being. Develop with the client a plan for learning relaxation techniques, and have client practice technique for 30 min 2 times a day at (times) while hospitalized. Remain with client during practice session to provide verbal cues and encouragement as necessary. These techniques can include:
  ○ Meditation
  ○ Progressive deep muscle relaxation
  ○ Visualization techniques that require the client to visualize scenes that enhance the relaxation response
  ○ Biofeedback
  ○ Prayer
  ○ Autogenic training
	Anxiety decreases coping abilities and physiologic well-being.[56] Repeated rehearsal of a behavior internalizes and personalizes it.[56]

• Develop with the client a plan for integrating relaxation techniques into daily schedule at home.	Having a concrete plan increases the probability that the behavior will be implemented in the new environment.
• Develop with the client a plan to include play into daily activities. Note the plan and specific activities here.	Play provides a sense of joy and rejuvenates inner vitality, enhancing coping abilities.[56]

• Establish a time to meet with the client and those members of his or her support system identified as most important. Note time here. Utilize this time to discuss:
  ○ Support system's understanding of the client's situation
  ○ Support system's perceptions of their involvement with the management of the illness
  ○ Support system's perceptions of their needs at this time
	Interactions between the support system and the individual can impact individual health and coping.[58] Provides opportunity to assess support system's perspective to assist in developing interventions and further their acceptance of the intervention.[52]

• Develop with the support system a plan to meet the perceived needs. Note this plan here.	Increases support system's sense of control while enhancing self-esteem. Provides opportunities for increasing support system coping by recognizing that the illness has an impact on this system.[56,58]
• Identify, with the client, community support groups that can be utilized when he or she returns home. Note those groups identified here with a plan for contacting them before the client leaves the hospital.	Groups can provide hope, information, and role models for coping and support.[56]

Gerontic Health

ACTIONS/INTERVENTIONS	RATIONALES
• Monitor at each subsequent contact for continued ability to effectively manage regimen.	Physiologic aging or exacerbation of chronic illness may, over time, diminish continued ability to implement regimen.

Home Health

See Home Health plan for Management of Therapeutic Regimen (Individual), Ineffective. The difference is the nurse has assessed Effective and uses the plan of care in a preventive mode to make possible earlier identification of problems. For the individual who is effectively managing care, the nurse supports the current effective behavior.

Management of Therapeutic Regimen (Individual), Effective

FLOWCHART EVALUATION: EXPECTED OUTCOME 1

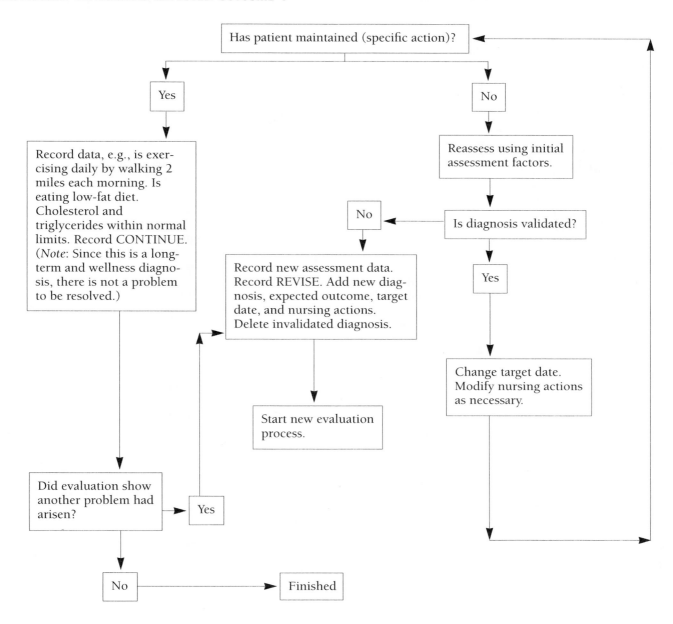

Management of Therapeutic Regimen (Individual), Effective

FLOWCHART EVALUATION: EXPECTED OUTCOME 2

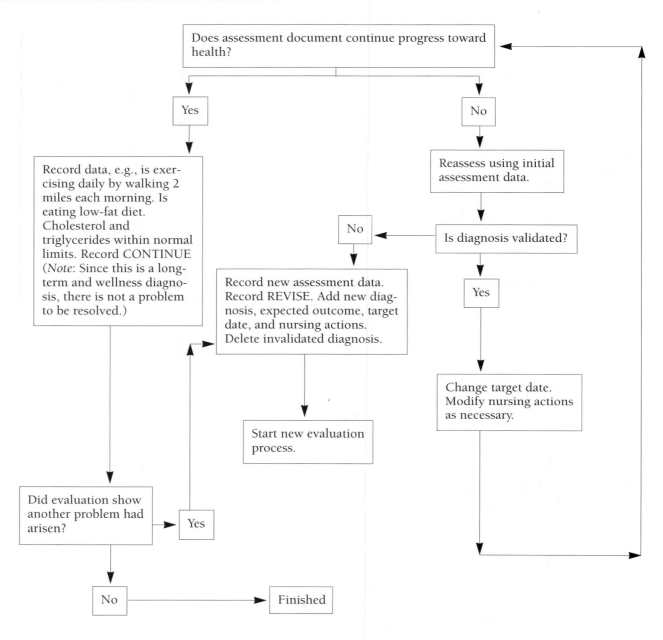

Management of Therapeutic Regimen (Individuals, Families, Communities, Ineffective)

NOTE: This diagnosis was proposed at the Tenth NANDA Conference with the result that a proposal to delete Noncompliance was expected to be presented at the next conference; however, this has not occurred to date. As discussed in the conceptual section of this chapter and in the additional information later in this section, there are many people who object to the diagnosis of Noncompliance. For this reason, we will not provide nursing actions for Noncompliance but will provide the definition, defining characteristics, and related factors for this diagnosis until it is officially deleted. In 1994, the categories of Families and Communities were added.

DEFINITION

Ineffective Management of Therapeutic Regimen (Individuals): A pattern of regulating and integrating into daily living a program for treatment of illness and the sequelae of illness that is unsatisfactory for meeting specific health goals.[40]

Noncompliance (Specify): A person's informed decision not to adhere to a therapeutic recommendation.[40]

Ineffective Management of Therapeutic Regimen (Families): A pattern of regulating and integrating into family processes a program for treatment of illness and the sequelae of illness that is unsatisfactory for meeting specific health goals.[40]

Ineffective Management of Therapeutic Regimen, Communities: A pattern of regulating and integrating into community processes programs for treatment of illness and the sequelae of illness that is unsatisfactory for meeting health-related goals.[40]

NANDA TAXONOMY: CHOOSING 5.2.1, 5.2.1.1, 5.2.2, AND 5.2.3

DEFINING CHARACTERISTICS[40]

1. Ineffective Management of Therapeutic Regimen, Individual
   a. Major defining characteristics
      (1) Choices of daily living ineffective for meeting the goals of a treatment or prevention program
   b. Minor defining characteristics
      (1) Acceleration (expected or unexpected) of illness symptoms
      (2) Verbalized desire to manage the treatment of illness and prevention of sequelae
      (3) Verbalized difficulty with regulation and/or integration of one or more prescribed regimens for treatment of illness and its effects or prevention of complications
      (4) Verbalized that he or she did not take action to include treatment regimens in daily routines
      (5) Verbalized that he or she did not take action to reduce risk factors for progression of illness and sequelae

2. Noncompliance
   a. Major defining characteristics
      (1) Behavior indicative of failure to adhere (by direct observation or by statements of patient or significant others) **Note:** This is a critical characteristic.
      (2) Objective tests (physiologic measures or detection of markers)
      (3) Evidence of development of complications
      (4) Evidence of exacerbation of symptoms
      (5) Failure to keep appointments
      (6) Failure to progress
   b. Minor defining characteristics
      None given.
3. Ineffective Management of Therapeutic Regimen; Families
   a. Major defining characteristics
      (1) Inappropriate family activities for meeting the goals of a treatment or prevention program
   b. Minor defining characteristics
      (1) Acceleration (expected or unexpected) of illness symptoms of a family member
      (2) Lack of attention to illness and its sequelae
      (3) Verbalized desire to manage the treatment of illness and prevention of the sequelae
      (4) Verbalized difficulty with regulation and/or integration of one or more effects or prevention of complication
      (5) Verbalizes that family did not take action to reduce risk factors for progression of illness and sequelae
4. Ineffective Management of Therapeutic Regimen; Communities
   a. Major defining characteristics
      (1) Deficits in people and programs to be accountable for illness care of aggregates
      (2) Deficits in advocates for aggregates
      (3) Deficits in community activities for secondary and tertiary prevention
      (4) Illness symptoms above the norm expected for the number and type of population
      (5) Number of health care resources insufficient for the incidence or prevalence of illness(es)
      (6) Unavailable health care resources for illness care
      (7) Unexpected acceleration of illness(es)
   b. Minor defining characteristics
      None given.

RELATED FACTORS[40]

1. Ineffective Management of Therapeutic Regimen, Individual
   a. Complexity of health care system
   b. Complexity of therapeutic regimen
   c. Decisional conflicts
   d. Economic difficulties
   e. Excessive demands made on individual or family
   f. Family patterns of health care
   g. Inadequate number and types of cues to action
   h. Knowledge deficits
   i. Mistrust of regimen and/or health care personnel
   j. Perceived seriousness
   k. Perceived susceptibility
   l. Perceived barriers

m. Perceived benefits
n. Powerlessness
o. Social support deficits
2. Noncompliance
    a. Patient value system: Health beliefs, cultural influences, spiritual values
    b. Client-provider relationships
3. Ineffective Management of Therapeutic Regimen; Families
    a. Complexity of health care system
    b. Complexity of therapeutic regimen
    c. Decisional conflict
    d. Economic difficulties
    e. Excessive demands made on individual or family
    f. Family conflict

4. Ineffective Management of Therapeutic Regimen, Communities
    None given.

RELATED CLINICAL CONCERNS

1. Any diagnosis new to the patient, that is, patient does not have education or experience in dealing with this disorder.
2. Any diagnosis of a chronic nature, for example, pain, migraine headaches, or rheumatoid arthritis.
3. Any diagnosis that has required a change in health care providers, for example, referred from long-time family physician to cardiologist.

HAVE YOU SELECTED THE CORRECT DIAGNOSIS?

Knowledge Deficit   This is the most appropriate diagnosis if the patient or family verbalizes less-than-adequate understanding of health management or recalls inaccurate health information.

Ineffective Individual Coping or Ineffective Family Coping   These diagnoses are suspected if there are major differences between the patient and family reports of health status, health perception, and health care behavior. Verbalizations by the patient or family regarding inability to cope also indicate this differential nursing diagnosis.

Altered Family Processes   Through observing family interactions and communication, the nurse may assess that Altered Family Processes is a consideration. Poorly communicated messages, rigidity of family functions and roles, and failure to accomplish expected family developmental tasks are a few observations to alert the nurse to this possible diagnosis.

Activity Intolerance or Self-Care Deficit   These diagnoses should be considered if the nurse observes or validates reports of inability to complete the tasks required because of insufficient energy or because of inability to feed, bathe, toilet, dress, and groom self.

Altered Thought Process   If the patient exhibits impaired attention span, impaired ability to recall information, impaired perception, judgment, and decision making, or impaired conceptual and reasoning abilities, the nursing diagnosis of Altered Thought Process should be considered.

Impaired Home Maintenance Management   This diagnosis is demonstrated by the inability of the patient or family to provide a safe living environment.

ADDITIONAL INFORMATION

Some nursing authors object to the term "Noncompliance."[88–91] Compliance can become the basis for a power-oriented relationship in which one is judged and labeled compliant or noncompliant based on the hierarchical position of the professional in relation to the patient. The diagnosis of Noncompliance is to be used for those patients who wish to comply with the therapeutic recommendations but are prevented from doing so by the presence of certain factors. The nurse can in such situations strive to lessen or eliminate the factors that preclude the willing patient from complying with recommendations.

The principles of informed consent and autonomy[92] are critical to the appropriate use of this diagnosis. A person may freely choose not to follow a treatment plan. The nursing diagnosis Noncompliance does not mean that a patient is not willing to obey but rather that a patient has attempted a prescribed plan but has found it difficult to follow through with it. The area of noncompliance must be specified. A patient may follow many aspects of a treatment program very well and find only a small part of the plan difficult to manage. Such a patient is noncompliant only in the area of difficulty.

Several nursing authors have recognized the interdependent nature of illness and healing.[90,92–95] This interdependence is especially pronounced in chronic illness. As a patient and his or her family adapts to a chronic condition, noncompliance with prescribed treatment regimens may actually be constructive and therapeutic, not detrimental.[94] The nurse who learns to listen to the patient and plan treatments in collaboration with the patient will benefit from the wisdom of people experiencing illness.[96,97]

EXPECTED OUTCOMES

1. Will identify barriers to implementing regimen and devise at least one way to overcome each barrier (list) by (date) and/or
2. Will return-demonstrate appropriate technique or procedures (list) for self-care by (date)

TARGET DATE

The specific target dates for these objectives will be directly related to the barriers identified, the patient's entering level of knowledge, and the comfort the patient feels in expressing satisfaction or dissatisfaction. The target date could range from 1 to 5 days following the date of admission.

NURSING ACTIONS/INTERVENTIONS WITH RATIONALES

Adult Health

ACTIONS/INTERVENTIONS	RATIONALES
• Help the patient and/or family identify potential areas of conflict, e.g., values, religious beliefs, cultural mores, or cost.	Assesses motivation and decreases risk of ineffective management of therapeutic regimen.
• Start instructions for self-care within 24 h of admission.	Provides time to incorporate changes into lifestyle and to practice as necessary before day of discharge from hospital.
• Assist the patient and/or family in identifying factors that actually or potentially may impede the desired therapeutic regimen plan: ○ Sense of control ○ Language barriers (provide translators, assign nursing personnel to care for patient who speak the patient's language) ○ Cultural concerns (cultural mores, religious beliefs, etc.; design a plan that will allow incorporation of the therapeutic regimen within the cultural norms of the patient) ○ Financial constraints ○ Knowledge deficits ○ Time constraints ○ Level of knowledge and skill related to treatment plan ○ Resources available to meet treatment plan objectives ○ Complexity of treatment plan ○ Current response to treatment plan ○ Use of nonprescribed interventions ○ Entry to health care system	Assesses motivation and decreases risk of diagnosis development.
• Make a list of these potential areas of conflict and help patient and family problem solve each area one at a time.	
• Allow opportunities for the patient and family to vent feelings about therapeutic regimen. Schedule at least 30 min at least once per day for this activity. Note times here.	
• Teach the patient and significant others knowledge and skills needed to implement the therapeutic regimen (e.g., measuring blood pressure, counting calories, administering medications, or weighing self).	
• Have the patient and significant others return-demonstrate or restate principles at least daily for at least 3 consecutive days prior to discharge.	Allows sufficient practice time that provides immediate feedback on skills, etc.
• Design a chart to assist the patient to visually see the effectiveness of therapeutic regimen (e.g., weight-loss chart, days without smoking, blood pressure measurements). Begin the chart in hospital within 1 day of admission. Follow up 1 wk after discharge.	Visualization of actual progress promotes implementation of prescribed regimen.

Continued

ACTIONS/INTERVENTIONS	RATIONALES
• Assist in the development of a schedule that will allow the patient to keep appointments and not miss work. Forward plan to employer and physician.	Demonstrates importance of schedule to patient, employer, and physician. Coordinated effort encourages adherence to regimen.
• Assist the patient in developing time-management skills to incorporate time for relaxation and exercise. Have patient develop a typical 1-wk schedule, then work with patient to adapt schedule as needed.	Individualizes schedule and highlights need for relaxation and exercise.
• Contract, in writing, with the patient and/or significant others for specifics regarding regimen. Have patient and family establish mutual-goal-setting sessions. Assign specific family members specific tasks. Follow-up 1 wk after discharge; recheck 6 wk following discharge.	Demonstrates, in writing, the importance of the plan and by listing definitive follow-up times, enhances the probability of regimen implementation. Involvement increases motivation and improves the probability of success.
• Design techniques that encourage the patient's or family's implementation of the regimen, such as setting single, easy-to-accomplish, short-term goals first and progressing to long-term goals as the short-term goals are met. For example, if the idea of stopping smoking is too overwhelming, help patient design a personal adaptive program; for example, change to a lower tar and nicotine cigarette, timed smoking (only 1 cigarette per 30 or 60 min), stabilize, then make further reductions.	Prevents multiple changes from overwhelming patient, thus avoiding one major contributor to ineffective management of therapeutic regimen.
• Teach the patient and significant others assertive techniques that can be used to deal with dissatisfaction with caregivers.	Long waiting periods in offices, unanswered questions, being rushed, etc., increase the likelihood of abandoning the regimen. Assertiveness helps the patient and family overcome the feelings of powerlessness and increases the sense of control.
• Allow time for the patient and family to verbalize fears related to therapeutic regimen (e.g., body image, cost, side effects, pain, or dependency) by devoting at least 30 min per day to this activity. List times here.	Increases patient's sense of control. Facilitates continuity and consistency of plan.
• Assist in correction of sensory, motor, etc., deficits to the extent possible through referrals to appropriate consultants (e.g., occupational therapist, physical therapist, ophthalmologist, or audiologist).	
• Have patient and/or family design a home care plan. Assist the patient to modify the plan as necessary. Forward the plan to home health service, social service, physician, etc.	
• Relate any information regarding dissatisfaction to appropriate caregiver (e.g., to physician—problems with the time spent in waiting room, cultural needs, privacy needs, costs, or need for generic prescriptions).	
• Make follow-up appointments prior to the patient's leaving the hospital. Do it from the patient's room, and put appropriate information regarding appointment on brightly colored card (i.e., name, address, time, date, and telephone number).	Demonstrates exactly how to make appointments for patient.
• Refer the patient and/or family to appropriate follow-up personnel, e.g., nurse practitioner, visiting nurse service, social service, or transportation service. Make referral at least 3 days prior to discharge.	Allows time for home care assessment and initiation of service.
• Request follow-up personnel to remind the patient of appointments via card or telephone.	Shares the responsibility for implementing the regimen and demonstrates the importance attached to follow-up care by those providers.
• For the last 2–3 days of hospitalization, let the patient perform all of his or her own care. Supervise performance, critique, and reteach as necessary.	

NOTE: For Ineffective Management of Therapeutic Regimen, Communities, see Home Health.

Child Health

NOTE: Due to the dependency of the infant or child, ineffective management will **always** include both the individual and the family.

ACTIONS/INTERVENTIONS	RATIONALES
• Assist in developing health values of regimen adherence before the infant's birth through emphasis of these aspects in childbirth education classes.	Initiates idea of individual health management for child's health before birth. Allows sufficient time for parents to incorporate these ideas.
• Allow for the infant's or child's schedule in appointment scheduling (e.g., respect for naps, mealtimes). Involve the family in planning care for the infant or child.	Facilitates comfort for child, parents, and health care provider. Demonstrates individuality and increases likelihood of regimen implementation.
• Provide appropriate criteria for monitoring follow-up of infant's or child's status, especially in instance of chronic condition, to also demarcate when to call doctor or case manager.	Anticipatory specific planning and knowledge of condition will enhance self-management behaviors, thereby valuing self-esteem and likelihood of continued appropriate follow-up.
• Reward progress in the appropriate manner for age and development.	
• Depending on needs of infant or child, may, when services cannot be procured, require a change in location with the goal of seeking effective therapeutic regimen services. This may depend on state and/or local funding with referral on regional basis. Language or educational needs must also be addressed.	The weakest component of many communities relates to care of the young, thus making consideration of the child a critical component.

Women's Health

ACTIONS/INTERVENTIONS	RATIONALES
• Develop a sensitivity for cultural differences of women's roles and the impact on their implementation of a therapeutic regimen.[98]	Demonstration of understanding of the patient's culture and inclusion of these differences in planning increase the probability of effective management of the therapeutic regimen.
• Encourage family to share views of childbirth with health care personnel through classes and interviews.[98]	
• Discuss with family their traditions and taboos for mother and baby during transitional period after childbirth, e.g., in some Far Eastern cultures, the mother does not touch the infant for several days after birth. The grandmother or aunts become the primary caregivers for the infant.[98]	Increases patient satisfaction and compliance and allows the childbirth instructor and nursing personnel to plan with patient and family appropriate care during childbearing.
• Assess pregnant woman's and her family's perception of the tasks of pregnancy complicated by high-risk factors such as premature rupture of membranes, premature labor, maternal or fetal illness, and social-economic hardships.[85–87]	Provides basis for plan of care and allows family to make informed choices about care needs during and after pregnancy.
### FAMILY	
• Assess pregnant woman's and her family's perception of the tasks of pregnancy complicated by high-risk factors such as premature rupture of membranes, premature labor, maternal or fetal illness, and social-economic hardships.[85–87]	Provides basis for plan of care and allows family to make informed choices about care needs during and after pregnancy.

Continued

ACTIONS/INTERVENTIONS	RATIONALES
• Encourage family to share concerns of the changes and restrictions on family lifestyle as a result of the high-risk pregnancy. (Example: Restrictions on pregnant woman involving changes in homemaking, childrearing, sexuality, social and recreational activities, disruptions in career, and financial commitments.) Help the family identify community agencies and resources that can assist them to better follow the treatment regimen.	Allows caregivers to determine importance of compliance with treatment regimen to the family and to refer them to the proper resources.

COMMUNITY

ACTIONS/INTERVENTIONS	RATIONALES
• Inform appropriate agencies when new mothers (parents) exhibit signs and symptoms of nonattachment to their newborn, substance abuse, homelessness, and dysfunctional family dynamics that could become violent.[85–87]	Allows for appropriate support and follow-up for the new mother and her newborn infant.
• Inform (network with) appropriate community agencies (home visiting nurses, public health nurses, child protective agencies, etc.) to provide new mothers and their infants transitional care during postpartum (particularly after early discharge).	Assures smooth, safe transition for new mother and her family into parenting roles. Assures physical and psychological stability for the new mother and her infant. Provides continuity of care from the hospital to the home to the primary caregiver (physician, advanced practice nurse, etc.).

Psychiatric Health

NOTE: It is important to remember that the mental health client is influenced by a larger social system and that this social system plays a crucial role in the client's ongoing participation with the health care team. The conceptualization that may be most useful in intervention and assessment of the client who does not follow the recommendations of the health care team in this area may be *system persistence*. Hoffman[99] uses this concept to communicate the idea that the system is signaling that it desires to continue in its present manner of organization. This could present a situation in which the individual client indicates to the health care team that he or she desires change, and yet change is not demonstrated due to the constraints placed on the individual by the larger social system (i.e., the family). This places the responsibility on the nurse to initiate a comprehensive assessment of the client system when the diagnosis of Ineffective Management of the Therapeutic Regimen or Noncompliance is considered.

ACTIONS/INTERVENTIONS	RATIONALES
• Involve the client system in discussions on the treatment plan. This should include: ◦ Family ◦ Individuals the client identifies as important in making decisions related to health (i.e., cultural healers, social institutions such as probation officers, public welfare workers, officials in the school system, etc.)	Promotes client's perceived control and increases potential for client's involvement in the treatment plan.
• Discuss with the family their perception of the current situation. This should include each family member, and each should be given an opportunity to present his or her perspective. Questions to ask the family include: ◦ What do you think is the difficulty here? ◦ Who is most affected by the current situation? ◦ Who is least affected?	Communicates respect of the family and their experience of the situation, which promotes the development of a trusting relationship, provides information about the family's strengths, and provides the nurse with an opportunity to support these strengths in a manner that will facilitate the development of a treatment program that the family will implement.[52]

- ○ What have you done that has helped the most?
- ○ The least?
- ○ What happened when you tried to work on the situation?
- ○ What has changed in the family since the beginning of the current situation?
- ○ What is the best advice you have received about this situation?
- ○ What is the worst?

For further guidance in the process, refer to Wright and Leahey[58] (1994).

- Discuss with the identified system those factors that inhibit system reorganization:
  - ○ Knowledge and skills related to necessary change
  - ○ Resources available
  - ○ Ability to use these resources
  - ○ Belief system about treatment plan
  - ○ Cultural values related to the treatment plan

Recognition of those factors that inhibit change can facilitate the development of a plan that eliminates these problems.

- Assess the involvement of other systems, such as social services, school systems, health care providers, in the family situation.

Larger systems often impose "rules" on families that maintain the larger system by sacrificing the families' coping abilities or becoming overinvolved to the degree that families feel in a one-down position. The primary "rule" blames the family for problems.[58]

- Assist the system in making the appropriate adjustments in system organization.

Affirms and promotes client's strengths.

- Enhance current patterns that facilitate system reorganization.
- Role-model effective communication by:
  - ○ Seeking clarification
  - ○ Demonstrating respect for individual, family members, and the family system
  - ○ Listening to expression of thoughts and feelings
  - ○ Setting clear limits
  - ○ Being consistent
  - ○ Communicating with the individual being addressed in a clear manner
  - ○ Encouraging sharing of information among appropriate system subgroups

Models for the family effective communication that can enhance their problem-solving abilities.

- Demonstrate an understanding of the complexity of family problems by:
  - ○ Not taking sides in family problem solving
  - ○ Providing alternative explanations of behavior patterns that recognize the contributions of all persons involved in the situation, including health care providers, if appropriate.

Promotes the development of a trusting relationship while developing a positive orientation.[52,58]

- Make small changes in those patterns that inhibit system changes. For example, ask the client to talk with the family in the group room instead of in an open public area on the unit, or ask the client who washes his or her hands frequently to use a special soap and towel and then gradually introduce more changes in the patterns.

Promotes client's control and provides realistic achievable goals for the client, thus preserving self-esteem when change can be accomplished.

- Advise the client to make changes slowly. It is important not to expect too much too soon.

Increases self-esteem and increases desire to continue those behaviors that elicit this response.

- Provide the appropriate positive verbal feedback to all parts of the system involved in assisting with the changes. It is important not to focus on the demonstration of old patterns of behavior at this time. The smallest change should be recognized.

Continued

ACTIONS/INTERVENTIONS	RATIONALES
• Develop goals with the family that are based on the data obtained in the assessment. These goals should be specific and behavioral in nature.	Promotes the family's sense of control and the development of a trusting relationship by communicating respect for the client system. Accomplishment of goals provides positive reinforcement, which motivates continued behavior and enhances self-esteem.[52,58]
• Provide positive reinforcement to families for the strengths observed during the assessment and subsequent interviews.	Positive reinforcement motivates continued behavior and enhances self-esteem.[58]
• Encourage communication between family members by: ○ Having family members discuss alternative solutions and goal setting ○ Having each family member indicate how he or she might contribute to resolution of the concerns ○ Having family members identify strengths of one another and how these can contribute to the resolution of the situation	Assists the family in developing problem-solving skills that will serve in future situations and promotes healthy family functioning.[58]
• Develop teaching plan to provide the family with information that will enhance their problem solving. Note the content and schedule for this plan here.	Lack of information about the situation can interfere with problem solving.[58]
• Provide opportunities for the expression of a range of affect; this can mean having the family discuss situations that promote laughing and crying together. Express to the family that their emotional experiences are normal.	Validates family members' emotions and helps to identify appropriateness of their affective responses. Persistent, intense emotions can inhibit problem solving.[58] Normalizing decreases sense of isolation and assists in making connections between family members.[58] Suggesting specific tasks can provide the family with new ways to interact that can improve problem solving.[58]
• Contract with the family for specific behavioral homework assignments that will be implemented before the next meeting. These should be concrete and involve only minor changes in the family's normal patterns. For example, have them start with calling a resource for the information they may need to do something different. If it is difficult for the family to accomplish these tasks, the family system may be having unusual problems with the change process and should be referred to an advanced practitioner for further care.	
• If the task is not completed, do not chastise the family. Indicate that the nurse misjudged the complexity of the task, and assess what made it difficult for the family to complete the task. Develop a new, less complex task based on this information. If the nurse and family continue to have difficulty developing a plan of cooperation, a referral may need to be made to a nurse with advanced training in family systems work.	Promotes positive orientation and recognizes that the development of change strategies is an interactive process between the family and the health care system.[52,58]
• Communicate the plan to all members of the health care team.	Promotes continuity of care and builds trust.
• Refer family to community resources for continued support. Assist family in making these contacts by developing a specific plan. Note the specific plan here with the types of support needed.	Community resources can provide ongoing support. A specific plan increases opportunities for success.[52,58]
• Develop, with the family, opportunities for them to have time together and in various subgroupings (parents, parents with children, children) that involve activities other than those directly related to the current problem. This could include respite activities, family play time, relaxation, and other stress reduction activities. Note this plan here.	Provides families with positive experiences with one another and opportunities to rebuild resources for coping. Also assists them in developing a broader identity of the family. They are more than the problem or illness.[52,58]
• Before termination, praise the family's accomplishments. Give the family credit for the change.	Reinforces family's strengths and promotes self-esteem. Reminds family of the new skills they have acquired.[52,58]

NOTE: Refer to Home Health for primary interventions for Ineffective Management of Therapeutic Regimen, Communities. The primary agencies that are available to assist with community mental health resources are the Mental Health Association and National Alliance for the Mentally Ill (NAMI). NAMI publishes a journal titled *Innovations & Research*. Both of these associations open their membership to professionals, consumers, families of consumers, and members of the community interested in mental health issues. The purpose of these organizations is to provide community resources and support for mental health consumers and their families and advocate for mental health consumers.

Gerontic Health

ACTIONS/INTERVENTIONS	RATIONALES
• Refer to mental health specialist to rule out depression.	Depression in the elderly is frequently underdiagnosed and undertreated.
• Refer to community resources.	The older patient may have concerns related to availability of support systems, financial concerns regarding medication costs, and availability of transportation. Use of already available community resources provides a long-term, cost-effective support system.
• Establish communication link with primary caregiver and family.	Family members may not be geographically available.
• Advise family members of availability of managed care resources present in the community where older client resides.	Provides care options for family to consider.
• Provide follow-up support via home visits and phone contacts.	Presents opportunities for continued problem solving and increasing trust.
• Assist caregivers in establishing and meeting their needs.	Enables continuation of care while decreasing the potential for burnout.
• Review with client and family the therapeutic regimen.	Helps determine possible areas of difficulty for client or caregiver.
• Provide written or audiotaped or videotaped information on therapeutic regimen to assist client and caregiver in adhering to regimen.	Provides quick access to information to the caregiver or client.
• Incorporate a variety of local, regional, or state social services to ensure that needed information about the regimen is available to older patients.	Information flow may be impeded due to temporary relocation or social isolation.
• Identify older community leaders, via age-related groups or associations, who can identify strengths or weaknesses of the community (such as senior citizen center members, church groups, support groups focused on problems common to older adults).	Peer or cohort influences may assist in identifying and promoting problem solving.

Home Health

ACTIONS/INTERVENTIONS	RATIONALES
• Assist the client, family, or community to delineate factors contributing to ineffective therapeutic regimen management by helping them to assess: ◦ Level of knowledge and skill related to treatment plan ◦ Resources available to meet treatment plan objectives ◦ Appropriate use of resources to meet treatment plan objectives ◦ Complexity of treatment plan ◦ Current response to treatment plan ◦ Use of nonprescribed interventions ◦ Barriers to compliance	Barriers and facilitators to ineffective management can be altered to improve outcomes.
• Involve the client, family, and community in planning, implementing, and promoting the treatment plan through [91,97,99]:	Involvement increases motivation and improves the probability of success.

Continued

ACTIONS/INTERVENTIONS	RATIONALES
○ Assisting with family conferences ○ Coordinating mutual goal setting ○ Promoting increased communication ○ Assigning family members specific tasks as appropriate to assist in maintaining the therapeutic regimen plan (e.g., support person for patient, transportation, or companionship in meeting mutual goals) ○ Identifying deficits in community resources ○ Population surveillance to detect changes in illness patterns for the community • Support the client, family, or community in eliminating barriers to implementing the regimen by: ○ Providing for privacy. ○ Referring to community services (e.g., church, home health volunteer, transportation service, or financial assistance). ○ Alerting other health care providers and social service personnel of the problem that long waiting periods create. ○ Providing for interpreters and for community-based language classes for English speakers to learn other languages as well as for non-English-speakers to learn English. ○ Identify community leaders to develop coalitions to address the problems identified ○ Serve as social activist to encourage necessary participants to complete their tasks. This may include fund-raising, testifying before governing bodies, or coordinating efforts of several groups and organizations. • Assigning one health care provider or social service worker, as much as possible, to avoid lack of continuity in care provision. • Assisting health care providers and social service workers to understand the constructive nature of noncompliance in chronic illness.[100] • Make timely phone calls to clients to discuss care (e.g., one day after being seen in clinic for minor acute infection, or weekly or monthly on a routine schedule for a chronically ill person[101]). • Collaborating with other health care professionals and social service workers to reduce the number and variety of medications for chronically ill clients.[102] • Reteach the client and family appropriate therapeutic activities as the need arises. • Identify unmet needs of the community. • Involve community leaders and representative sampling of the community population in focus groups to identify issues and to develop action plan to meet the unmet needs. • Identify resources available and those needed to implement action plan. • Create marketing plan to disseminate information and generate interest in plan. • Foster community partnerships to ensure the continuation of the plan.	Many barriers are institutional and can be eliminated or reduced. Reinforcement of information and continued assistance may be required to improve implementation of the therapeutic regimen.[103] Accurate community needs assessment provides data to set community goals. Collaboration among community leaders and citizens provides support for long-term change. Appropriate use of existing resources. Provides direction for development of needed resources. Communication of the plan is necessary to sustain interest and increase participation. Long-term maintenance of the plan will require commitment and collaboration among many groups.

Management of Therapeutic Regimen (Individuals, Families, Communities), Ineffective

FLOWCHART EVALUATION: EXPECTED OUTCOME 1

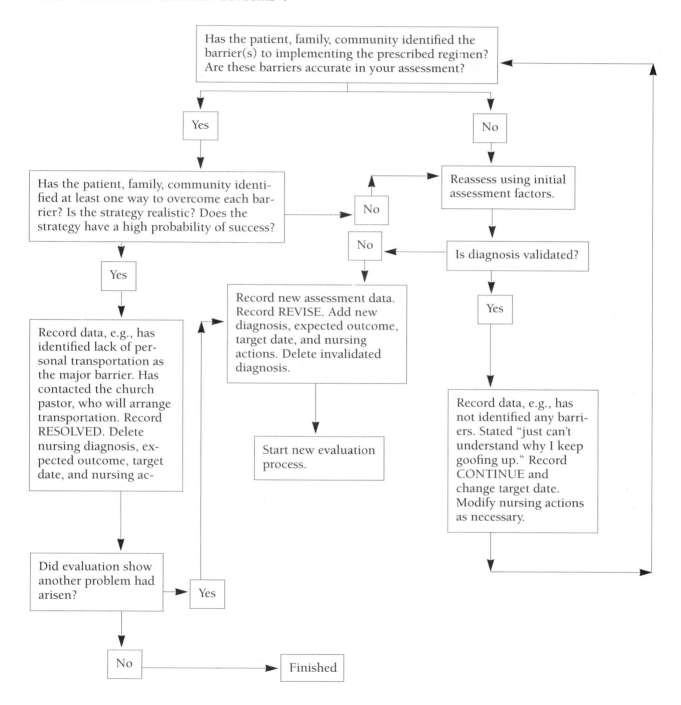

Has the patient, family, community identified the barrier(s) to implementing the prescribed regimen? Are these barriers accurate in your assessment?

Yes

No

Has the patient, family, community identified at least one way to overcome each barrier? Is the strategy realistic? Does the strategy have a high probability of success?

No

Reassess using initial assessment factors.

No

Is diagnosis validated?

Yes

Record new assessment data. Record REVISE. Add new diagnosis, expected outcome, target date, and nursing actions. Delete invalidated diagnosis.

Yes

Record data, e.g., has identified lack of personal transportation as the major barrier. Has contacted the church pastor, who will arrange transportation. Record RESOLVED. Delete nursing diagnosis, expected outcome, target date, and nursing ac-

Start new evaluation process.

Record data, e.g., has not identified any barriers. Stated "just can't understand why I keep goofing up." Record CONTINUE and change target date. Modify nursing actions as necessary.

Did evaluation show another problem had arisen?

Yes

No

Finished

Management of Therapeutic Regimen (Individuals, Families, Communities), Ineffective

FLOWCHART EVALUATION: EXPECTED OUTCOME 2

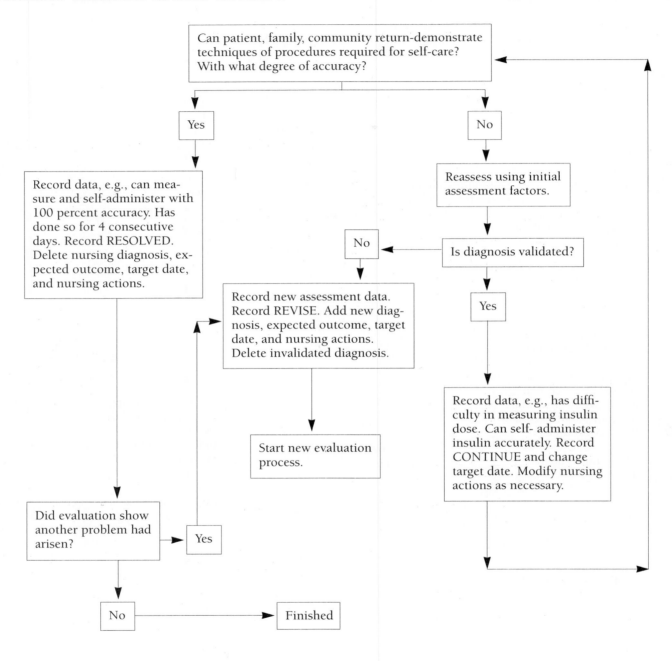

Can patient, family, community return-demonstrate techniques of procedures required for self-care? With what degree of accuracy?

Yes

Record data, e.g., can measure and self-administer with 100 percent accuracy. Has done so for 4 consecutive days. Record RESOLVED. Delete nursing diagnosis, expected outcome, target date, and nursing actions.

Did evaluation show another problem had arisen?

Yes

No → Finished

Record new assessment data. Record REVISE. Add new diagnosis, expected outcome, target date, and nursing actions. Delete invalidated diagnosis.

Start new evaluation process.

No

Reassess using initial assessment factors.

No ← Is diagnosis validated?

Yes

Record data, e.g., has difficulty in measuring insulin dose. Can self- administer insulin accurately. Record CONTINUE and change target date. Modify nursing actions as necessary.

Perioperative Positioning Injury, Risk for

DEFINITION

A state in which the client is at risk for injury as a result of the environmental conditions found in the perioperative setting.[40]

NANDA TAXONOMY: MOVING 6.1.1.1.2

DEFINING CHARACTERISTICS[40]

1. Major risk factors
   a. Disorientation
   b. Immobilization
   c. Muscle weakness
   d. Sensory or perceptual disturbances due to anesthesia
   e. Obesity
   f. Emaciation
   g. Edema
2. Minor risk factors
   None given.

RELATED FACTORS[40]

The risk factors also serve as the related factors.

RELATED CLINICAL CONCERNS

1. Any condition requiring surgical intervention
2. Peripheral vascular disease
3. Diabetes mellitus
4. Malnutrition
5. Arthritis deformans
6. Dementias, such as Alzheimer's disease or multi-infarct

HAVE YOU SELECTED THE CORRECT DIAGNOSIS?

Risk for Injury   This diagnosis is broader based than Risk for Perioperative Positioning Injury. The latter would be used only when surgery is involved.

Risk for Peripheral Neurovascular Dysfunction   This diagnosis is broader based than Risk for Perioperative Positioning Injury. A comparison of risk factors documents a wider variety of risk factors for peripheral neurovascular dysfunction.

EXPECTED OUTCOMES

1. Will remain free from any signs or symptoms of perioperative positioning injury by (date) and/or
2. Will return-demonstrate measures to decrease the risk for perioperative positioning injury by (date)

TARGET DATE

Due to the emergency nature of this diagnosis, target dates should be set in terms of hours for the first 2 days postoperatively. For the outcome related to the patient's role in prevention (outcome #2), all activities should be completed prior to surgery.

NURSING ACTIONS/INTERVENTIONS WITH RATIONALES

Adult Health

ACTIONS/INTERVENTIONS	RATIONALES
GENERAL PRINCIPLES (GENERALLY APPLIES TO ALL POSITIONS, INCLUDING SUPINE)	
• Keep siderails up on stretcher.	Basic safety measures.
• The patient should be in a comfortable position whether aware or asleep; assure that OR bed is dry and free from wrinkles.	Prevents softening of the skin and indentations of skin.
• Length of operative procedure should *always* be considered in positioning and supporting patient during the operation.	Certain complications can arise with extended length of operation, e.g., low back pain for patient in supine position, or pressure on heels and/or toes from drapes.
• Provide adequate exposure of the operative site.	
• Maintain good anatomical alignment. Pad bony prominences and pressure points.	Prevents impaired circulation, awkward position, or undue pressure.
• Ensure good respiration with no restrictions.	Avoids respiratory complications and assists in providing good oxygenation.

Continued

ACTIONS/INTERVENTIONS	**RATIONALES**
• Nerves should be protected—arm, hands, legs, ankles, and feet; use a footboard.	Maintains alignment; relieves pressure.
• The elderly, very thin, or obese should have special consideration; assess nutritional status, level of hydration, vascular disease, etc.	Reduces the risk of complication.
• Check mobility and range of motion prior to positioning. Note any physical abnormalities and/or injuries and how they may affect the proposed position.	Avoids unnecessary strain on already compromised joints, etc.
• Move patient only when anesthetist indicates patient can be moved, and have a sufficient number of people available to move the patient safely.	Avoids startling semiconscious patient and provides basic safety.
• Assure that no metal is touching the patient.	Reduces pressure risk and risk of injury if cautery is used. Basic safety measures.
• The dispersion pad should be on a fatty area, i.e., mid to upper thigh, depending on operative site. Recheck dispersion pad if patient has to be repositioned.	
• Place arms at right angles to the patient. Do not hyperextend the arms. Secure the arms with a restraint around the wrist.	Avoids strain on arms.
• Place the safety belt above the patient's knees (depending on operative site).	Avoids compromising circulation in popliteal area.
• Assure that all supports are padded.	Basic safety measures.

SPECIFIC POSITIONS

Lithotomy

• Raise legs at the same time.	Reduces strain on hip joints.
• Lower legs, slowly at the same time.	
• Adjust height of stirrups to fit patient's legs.	
• Be sure that no part of the legs touches metal.	Prevents electrical burns.
• Cover stirrups with linen, or place long leg booties on patient's legs (up to mid thigh).	Protects nerves and circulation.
• Pad popliteal space.	
• Assure that patient's buttock is over lower break in table.	

Nephro or Thoracic Surgery

• Move patient slowly and carefully, as a unit; have sufficient assistance.	Basic safety measure.
• Patient will be on side over the middle break of the table.	
• Position lower arm at a 90-degree angle away from body.	
• Place upper arms parallel to each other on a separate and high armboard or straight above the head. Restrain as needed. Protect nerves and muscles.	Facilitates respirations; maintains circulation.
• Support patient's sides with padded kidney rests.	Provides support for side and back.
• Bend bottom leg 45–90 degrees. Top leg should be straight.	Stabilizes the patient.
• Place pillow(s) between knees and legs and feet.	Protects pressure points.

Jacksonian (Modified Knee-Chest)

NOTE: Patient will probably be put to sleep on the stretcher and then rolled onto the OR table.

• Have sufficient assistance to move the patient.	Basic safety measure.
• Extend arms on armboards above the head.	Facilitates respiration; maintains circulation.
• Place pillow under ankles.	Protects pressure points.
• Support chest.	Stabilizes patient's position.
• Turn head to side; assure an adequate airway.	Allows good expansion of chest and promotes gas exchange.

Prone (Upper and Lower Back Surgery)

NOTE: Patient will probably be put to sleep on the stretcher and then rolled onto a back frame. This allows the back to be hyperextended and supports the chest for good respirations. Actions are the same as Jacksonian position except:

- Place pillows under upper chest, thighs, legs, ankles, and feet.

Trendelenburg

- Support shoulders with padded shoulder rests.

Avoid pressure strains. Provides good anatomical alignment.

Provides stabilization of patient's position.

Child Health

NOTE: Any procedure requiring prolonged stabilization in a fixed position places neonates and children at risk for this diagnosis; e.g., ECMO (extracorporeal membranous oxygenation) with cannulation of major vessels requires fixed positioning for several days to 1 week.

ACTIONS/INTERVENTIONS	RATIONALES
• Monitor skin integrity from head to toes with specific attention to head, ears, elbows, back, and heels, or other body parts in direct contact with surface of mattress or lines from monitoring equipment.[45]	Decreases likelihood of impact of shearing forces.

Women's Health

Same as for Adult Health except for the following:

ACTIONS/INTERVENTIONS	RATIONALES
• Determine proper alignment and positioning of mother during the C-section. Place a wedge cushion under the left buttock when positioning mother on surgical table. • Assist the mother's chosen partner (support person) to prepare for the C-section by describing the events that will take place, explaining his role and where he will sit (a stool or chair next to the mother's head) during the surgery, and identifying who will assist him.	Enhances circulation and oxygen supply to the placenta and the fetus. Reassures and supports the partner (support person) during surgery, allowing him to be supportive to the pregnant woman.

Psychiatric Health

Nursing interventions and rationales for this diagnosis are the same as Adult Health. Mental health clients that are most commonly at risk for this diagnosis are those receiving electroconvulsive therapy treatments (ECT).

Gerontic Health

ACTIONS/INTERVENTIONS	RATIONALES
• Provide head and neck support that prevents head rotation or hyperextension. • Ensure adequate padding over pressure-prone areas. • Observe, especially intraoperatively, for external pressure caused by leaning on patient. • Position extremities with caution.	Hyperextension or rotation may cause vertebral circulatory compromise in older patients. Decreases potential for circulatory compromise as well as nervous system or skin injury in older patients at risk for these problems. Compromised circulation or increased skin pressure can result in patient injury. Older patients have an increased risk for osteoporosis and, consequently, fractures.

Home Health

ACTIONS/INTERVENTIONS	RATIONALES
• Preoperative teaching to client and family concerning the need for early ambulation, deep-breathing exercises, and adequate pain control as soon as possible postoperatively to prevent complications. • Involve home caregiver in developing plan of care to decrease risk of complications.	Involvement of the client and family increases motivation. Correct knowledge supports the behavior. Involvement in the planning increases motivation and success of the intervention.

Perioperative Positioning Injury, Risk for

FLOWCHART EVALUATION: EXPECTED OUTCOME 1

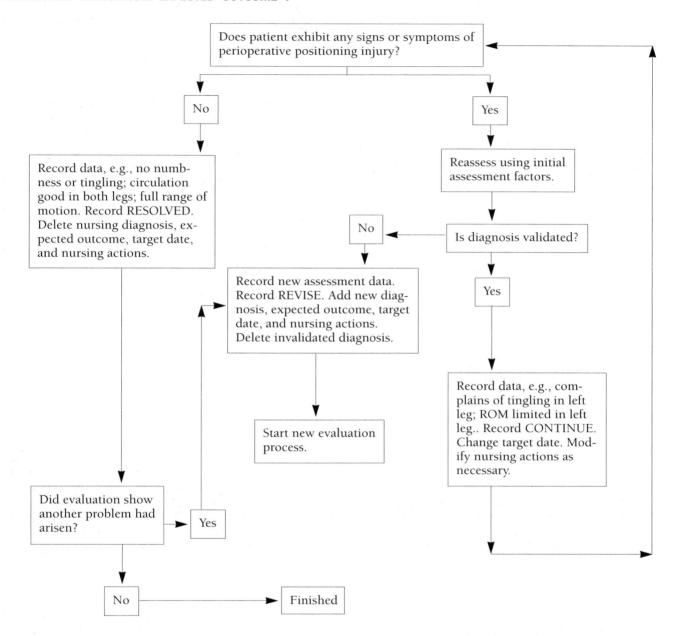

Perioperative Positioning Injury, Risk for

FLOWCHART EVALUATION: EXPECTED OUTCOME 2

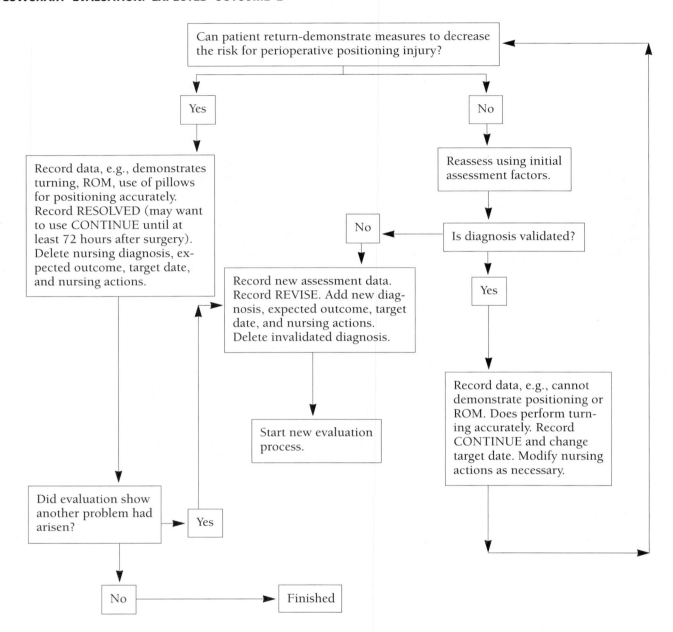

Protection, Altered

DEFINITION

The state in which an individual experiences a decrease in the ability to guard the self from internal or external threats such as illness or injury.[40]

NANDA TAXONOMY: EXCHANGING 1.6.2

DEFINING CHARACTERISTICS[40]

1. Major defining characteristics
   a. Deficient immunity
   b. Impaired healing
   c. Altered clotting
   d. Maladaptive stress response
   e. Neurosensory alterations
2. Minor defining characteristics
   a. Chilling
   b. Perspiring
   c. Dyspnea
   d. Cough
   e. Itching
   f. Restlessness
   g. Insomnia
   h. Fatigue
   i. Anorexia
   j. Weakness
   k. Immobility
   l. Disorientation
   m. Pressure sores

RELATED FACTORS[40]

1. Extremes of ages
2. Inadequate nutrition
3. Alcohol abuse
4. Abnormal blood profiles (leukopenia, thrombocytopenia, anemia, coagulation)
5. Drug therapies (antineoplastic, corticosteroid, immune, anticoagulant, thrombolytic)
6. Treatments (surgery, radiation)
7. Disease such as cancer and immune disorders

RELATED CLINICAL CONCERNS

1. AIDS
2. Diabetes mellitus
3. Anorexia nervosa
4. Cancer
5. Clotting disorders, e.g., disseminated intravascular coagulation, thrombophlebitis, anticoagulant medications.
6. Substance abuse or dependence
7. Any disorder requiring use of steroids

HAVE YOU SELECTED THE CORRECT DIAGNOSIS?

Risk for Infection   This diagnosis would most likely be a companion diagnosis. Risk means the individual is not presenting the actual defining characteristics of the diagnosis; but there are indications the diagnosis could develop. Altered Protection is an actual diagnosis.

EXPECTED OUTCOMES

1. Will return-demonstrate measures to increase self-protection by (date) and/or
2. Will exhibit, via lab tests, no worsening of condition by (date)

TARGET DATE

Altered Protection is a long-lasting diagnosis. Therefore, a date to totally meet the expected outcome could be weeks and months. However, since the target date signals the time to check progress, a date 3 days from the date of the original diagnosis would be appropriate.

NURSING ACTIONS/INTERVENTIONS WITH RATIONALES

Adult Health

ACTIONS/INTERVENTIONS	RATIONALES
• Place patient in protective isolation but **do not** promote an isolated feeling for the patient. Encourage frequent telephone calls and visits from significant others.	Lessens sense of isolation and maintains therapeutic relationships.
• Check patient at least every 30 min while awake. Spend 30 min with client every 2 h on (odd/even) hour while awake to answer questions and provide emotional support while in reverse isolation. Note times for these interactions here.	

Continued

ACTIONS/INTERVENTIONS	RATIONALES
• Collaborate with occupational therapist regarding diversionary activity.	
• Protect patient from injury and infection. (See appropriate nursing actions and rationales under the diagnoses Risk for Injury and Risk for Infection.)	Protects patient from infection or spread of infection.
• Use universal precautions in caring for the patient.	
• Monitor:	Allows comparison to baseline at admission and evaluation of effectiveness of therapy.
◦ Vital signs, mucous membranes, skin integrity, and response to medications at least once per shift.	
◦ Unexplained blood in urine.	
◦ Prolonged bleeding after blood has been drawn or from injection sites.	
◦ Side effects of blood and blood products: Monitor for possibility of blood reaction. Take vital signs every 15 min × 4, then every 30 min until transfusion completed. In the event of transfusion reaction, stop the transfusion immediately, maintain IV line with saline, and notify the physician while monitoring patient for further anaphylactic signs and symptoms.	
◦ Effects and side effects of steroids: Improved general status, decreased inflammatory signs and symptoms versus untoward effects including bleeding, Na or K imbalance. Calculate and record intake and output at least once per shift.	
◦ Effects and side effects of antineoplastics such as nausea, cardiac arrhythmias, extrapyramidal signs and symptoms. These side effects will vary according to the specific agents used. Take vital signs every 5–10 min during actual administration, and use a cardiac monitor.	
◦ Signs and symptoms of infection such as lymphoid interstitial pneumonia or recurrent oral candidiasis.	
• Apply pressure after each injection and after removal of IV needle.	Assists in stopping of bleeding.
• Provide oral hygiene or assist patient with oral hygiene at least 3 times per day.	Prevents opportunistic infection.
• Provide body hygiene or assist patient with body hygiene at least once daily at time of patient's choosing.	
• Measure and record intake and output at end of each shift.	Monitors effectiveness of bowel and bladder function.
• Encourage patient to eat nutritious meals. Collaborate with diet therapist regarding patient's likes, dislikes, and planning for dietary needs after hospital discharge.	Ensures balanced intake of necessary vitamins, minerals, etc., to assist in tissue repair. Assists in lessening impact of infections.
• Collaborate with physician regarding repeat laboratory examinations (CBC, blood coagulation studies, urinalyses, drug levels, etc.)	Gives guidelines for future therapeutic regimen as well as assessing effectiveness of current regimen.
• Collaborate with psychiatric nurse practitioner as necessary.	Provides source for assistance with interventions for maladaptive stress response.
• Teach patient and significant others:	Provides basic knowledge needed for patient and family to make modifications necessitated by alteration in protective mechanisms.
◦ Medication administration	
◦ Signs and symptoms to be reported	
◦ Special laboratory or other procedures to be done at home	
◦ Anticipatory safety needs	
◦ Routine daily care	
◦ Appropriate clean and sterile technique	
◦ Isolation or reverse-isolation technique	
◦ Common antigens and/or allergens and seasonal variations	

○ How to avoid or reduce exposure to antigens and/or allergens (alteration of environment)
○ Type and use of protective equipment
○ Universal precautions
○ Rationale for compliance with prescribed regimen
○ Resources available for assistance with health care, legal questions, or ethical questions
• Collaborate with other health professionals regarding ongoing care.
• Identify community resources for patient and family. Make referrals at least 3 days before discharge from hospital.

Care required is interdisciplinary in nature.

Allows time for agencies to initiate service. Use of existing community services is effective use of resources.

Child Health

NOTE: Infants at risk for this diagnosis are premature infants, infants with family history of hemophilia or sickle cell anemia, infants whose mothers have a history of drug abuse or HIV, and children who have histories of medication reaction. In infants especially, incubation for HIV depends on acquisition time. The infant may be exposed any time during pregnancy, but sero-con/retroversion to a negative HIV status may occur, with a later positive HIV again. The more symptomatic the mother, the greater the effect in the infant due to constant reinfection in the infant. For infants whose mothers are HIV positive, 26 percent will be HIV positive in the first 5 months of life, an additional 24 percent will be HIV positive by 12 months of life, and the remaining 50 percent will be HIV positive by 2 years of age. Key symptoms are intercurrent infection and weight loss. Other conditions noted include failure to thrive, hepatomegaly, cardiomegaly, lymphoid interstitial pneumonia, chronic diarrhea, cardiomyopathy, encephalopathy, and opportunistic infections. Even tuberculosis may be seen in these infants, with a tendency to progress from primary to miliary phase. In these infants there may be disseminated BCG infection. It is important to be aware of lab studies requiring large amounts of blood to study the course of sero HIV status. This blood drawing is problematic in the already depressed immune/reticuloendothelial systems of these infants. It is imperative that these infants **not be given** live polio vaccine due to their HIV positive status.

ACTIONS/INTERVENTIONS	RATIONALES
• Maintain monitoring for: ○ Observable lesions of ecchymotic nature or evidence of tendency toward bruising ○ Decreased absorption of nutrients (especially the premature infant because of the possibility of necrotizing enterocolitis)	Essential monitoring to avoid overwhelming of child's system by infection, etc.
• Provide at least one 30- to 60-min opportunity per day for family to ventilate feelings about the specific illness of their child.	Reduces anxiety, fear, and anger, and provides an opportunity for teaching.
• Teach child and family essential care.	Basics of home care for child with diagnosis of altered protection.
• As applicable, exercise caution for any medications or blood products to be administered.	
• Provide diversionary therapy according to child's status, developmental level, and interests.	Prevents boredom and restlessness, and fosters continued development of child in spite of illness.
• Be aware of current frustration with use of DDS (dideocytidene) and AZT (zidovudine) in children. At this time, protocols dictate doses.	Avoid unrealistic hope. Ideally toxicity is balanced against the need to reach therapeutic CNS dosage levels.
• Remind family that current treatment for AIDS is only palliative. Be sensitive to the unique nature of this health concern for all involved. Promote attention to the need for:	Avoids unrealistic hope while providing knowledge and support necessary to deal with a fatal illness.

Continued

ACTIONS/INTERVENTIONS	RATIONALES
○ Spiritual and emotional support ○ Nutritional support ○ Treatment of HIV–related infections ○ Administration of IV immune globulin ○ Treatment of tumors and end organ failure ○ Chronic pain. • Acknowledge potential loss of mother for infant with HIV, and plan appropriately for foster care status as indicated.	Anticipatory planning will assist in health maintenance in best interest of infants in event of need for separation from mother.

Women's Health

ACTIONS/INTERVENTIONS	RATIONALES
• Maintain monitoring for defining characteristics of Altered Protection: ○ HELLP Syndrome (a severe form of pregnancy-induced hypertension): Monitor lab results for low platelets (less than 100,000/cc), elevated liver enzymes, elevated SGOT/SGPT, intravascular hemolysis, schistocytes or burr cells on peripheral smear, low HCT (without evidence of significant blood loss) and hypertension.[85,104]	Provides basic knowledge base for planning of care.
○ Other high-risk history in the mother such as history of preterm labor, chronic hypertension, sickle cell anemia, and other blood disorders. ○ Signs and symptoms of infection.	Allows nursing staff time and information to plan individual care for mother and her newborn infant.
○ Mother's history of drug abuse, alcohol abuse, HIV, or domestic violence.	Safety of mother and infant is of utmost importance. Provides opportunity for assessment of home environment and provision of assistance.

Psychiatric Health

NOTE: Clients receiving antipsychotic neuroleptic drugs are at risk for development of agranulocytosis. This can be a life-threatening side effect and usually occurs in the first 8 weeks of treatment. Any rapid onset of sore throat and fever should be immediately reported and actively treated. Tricyclic antidepressants can cause blood dyscrasias with long-term therapy. Initial symptoms of these dyscrasias include fever, sore throat, and aching

ACTIONS/INTERVENTIONS	RATIONALES
• Immediately report client's complaint of sore throat or development of temperature elevation to physician. Institute nursing actions for hyperthermia (Chap. 3).	Alterations could be symptoms of agranulocytosis or blood dyscrasias, which would place client at risk for infection. Prompt recognition and intervention prevent progression and improve client outcome.
• Teach client who has had this type of response to antipsychotic neuroleptics or tricyclic antidepressants that he or she should not take this drug again. • If client is experiencing severe alterations in thought processes, provide one-to-one observation until mental status improves or until client can again participate in unit activities.	Client safety is of primary importance. Provides opportunity for ongoing assessment of the quality of the content of the client's thought and provides ongoing reality orientation.

Gerontic Health

ACTIONS/INTERVENTIONS	RATIONALES
• Monitor sensory status. Ensure that adaptive equipment (glasses, hearing aids, etc.) is functioning and used appropriately.	Pyrexia and elevated WBCs may not be present with infection. The first indicator of infection may be restlessness, confusion, an alteration in mental status, incontinence, irritability, or falls.
• Monitor mobility level. Ensure that adaptive equipment (brace, walker, etc.) is available.	
• Monitor for subtle changes in condition.	
• Avoid use of soaps that may cause dry skin.	Daily bathing may not be appropriate due to skin dryness associated with aging.
• Initiate measures to maintain skin integrity such as an egg crate mattress or specialized bed.	Assists in preventing skin breakdown.

Home Health

ACTIONS/INTERVENTIONS	RATIONALES

• Develop with client, family, and caregiver plans for dealing with emergency situations, e.g.:
  ○ Decision making regarding calling ambulance
  ○ Decision tree for calling nurse or physician
	Advanced planning improves the response and outcomes in crisis situations.

• Assist client and family to identify learning needs such as:
  ○ Universal precautions
  ○ How to disinfect surfaces contaminated with blood or body fluids (use 1:10 solution of bleach)
  ○ Protective isolation
  ○ Proper handwashing
  ○ Use of separate razors, toothbrushes, eating utensils, etc.
  ○ Proper cooking of food
  ○ Avoidance of pet excrement
  ○ Avoidance of others with infection
  ○ Skin care, oral hygiene, and wound care
  ○ Use of protective equipment
  ○ Signs and symptoms of infection, fluid and electrolyte imbalance, malnutrition, pathologic changes in behavior, and underlying disease process
  ○ CPR and first aid
  ○ Hazardous waste disposal, e.g., soiled dressings, needles, or chemotherapy vials
  ○ Advance directive, e.g., living wills and durable power of attorney for health care
  ○ Financial and/or estate planning
  ○ Symptom management and pain control
  ○ Administration of required medications
  ○ Nutrition
  ○ Care of catheters, IVs, respiratory therapy equipment, etc.
  ○ Laundry and dishwashing
  ○ Environmental cleanliness
	This action describes knowledge required to protect the client and the family.

• Assist client and family to identify resources to meet identified learning needs.	Involvement of the client and the family improves their ability to identify resources and to function more independently.

Continued

ACTIONS/INTERVENTIONS	RATIONALES
• Involve client and family in planning and implementing environmental, social, and family adaptations to protect the client.	Involvement of the client and the family improves motivation and outcomes.
• Plan with family and client for safe as well as meaningful activities according to client's level of functioning and interests.	Provides for activity while protecting the client and family.
• Assist client and family in lifestyle adjustments that may be required.	Lifestyle changes often require support.

Protection, Altered

FLOWCHART EVALUATION: EXPECTED OUTCOME 1

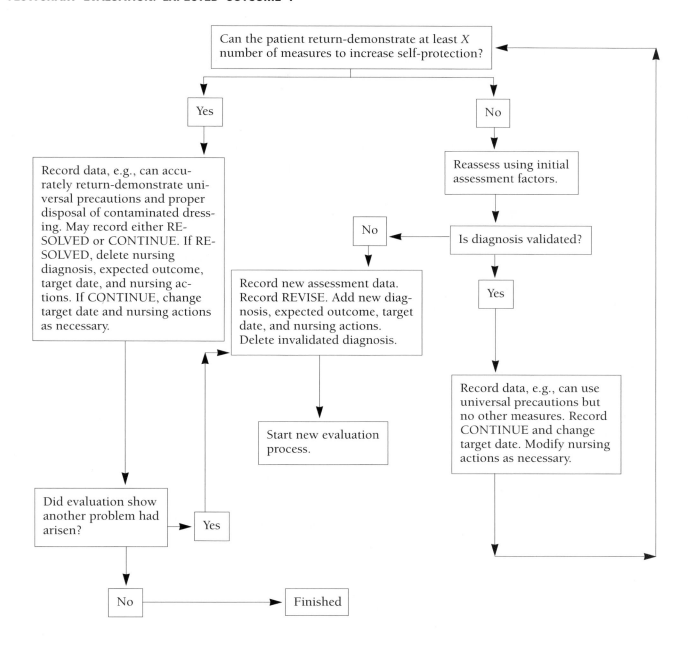

Protection, Altered

FLOWCHART EVALUATION: EXPECTED OUTCOME 2

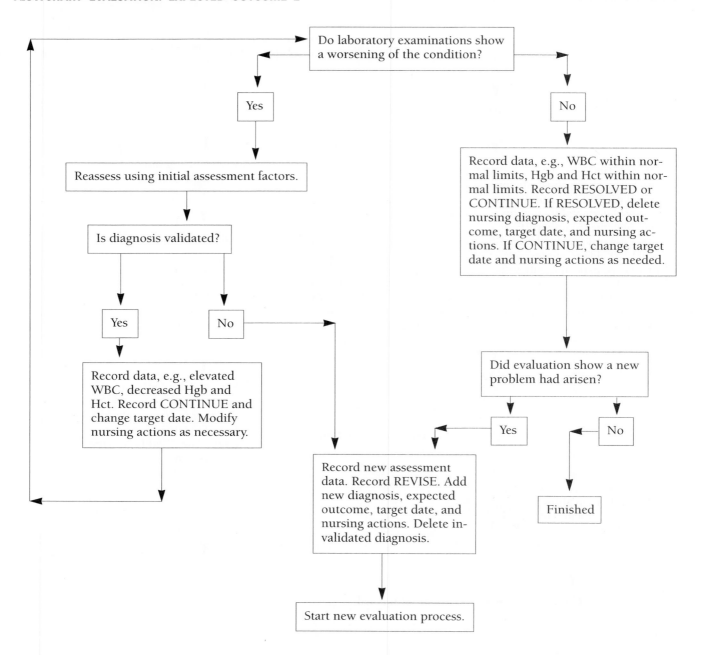

Do laboratory examinations show a worsening of the condition?

Yes

No

Reassess using initial assessment factors.

Record data, e.g., WBC within normal limits, Hgb and Hct within normal limits. Record RESOLVED or CONTINUE. If RESOLVED, delete nursing diagnosis, expected outcome, target date, and nursing actions. If CONTINUE, change target date and nursing actions as needed.

Is diagnosis validated?

Yes

No

Record data, e.g., elevated WBC, decreased Hgb and Hct. Record CONTINUE and change target date. Modify nursing actions as necessary.

Did evaluation show a new problem had arisen?

Yes

No

Record new assessment data. Record REVISE. Add new diagnosis, expected outcome, target date, and nursing actions. Delete invalidated diagnosis.

Finished

Start new evaluation process.

Nutritional-Metabolic Pattern

Pattern Description

This pattern focuses on food and fluid intake, the body's use of this intake (metabolism), and problems that might influence intake. Problems in this pattern may arise from a physiologic, psychologic, or sociologic base. Physiologic problems may be primary in nature, for example, vitamin deficiency, or they may arise secondary to another pathophysiologic state such as a peptic ulcer. Psychologic problems, such as stress, may result in an alteration, such as overeating or anorexia nervosa, in the nutritional-metabolic pattern. Sociologic factors, for example, low income, inadequate storage facilities, social isolation, and cultural food preferences, may result in an altered nutritional-metabolic state.

A popular saying is "You are what you eat." This is a truism; what we eat is converted to our cellular structure and affects its functioning. The nutritional-metabolic pattern allows us to look at the whole of this relationship.

Pattern Assessment

1. Weigh patient. Does patient weigh more than the recommended range for his or her height, age, and sex?
   Yes (Altered Nutrition, More Than Body Requirements, Risk for or Actual; Fluid-Volume Excess; Altered Body Temperature, Risk for)
   No
2. Does the patient weigh less than the recommended range for his or her height, age, and sex?
   Yes (Altered Nutrition, Less Than Body Requirements; Fluid-Volume Deficit, Risk for or Actual; Altered Body Temperature, Risk for)
   No
3. Have the patient describe a typical day's intake of both food and fluid, including snacks and the pattern of eating. Is the patient's food intake above the average for his or her age, sex, height, weight, and activity level?
   Yes (Altered Nutrition, More Than Body Requirements, Risk for or Actual)
   No
4. Is the patient's food intake below the average for his or her age, sex, height, weight, and activity level?
   Yes (Altered Nutrition, Less Than Body Requirements)
   No
5. Is the patient's fluid intake sufficient for his or her age, sex, height, weight, activity level, and fluid output?
   Yes
   No (Fluid-Volume Deficit, Risk for or Actual; Altered Body Temperature, Risk for)
6. Does the patient show evidence of edema?
   Yes (Fluid-Volume Excess)
   No
7. Is the patient's gag reflex present?
   Yes
   No (Impaired Swallowing, Risk for Aspiration)
8. Does the patient cough or choke during eating?
   Yes (Impaired Swallowing, Risk for Aspiration)
   No

9. Assess the patient's mouth, eyes, and skin. Are these assessments within normal limits (e.g., no lesions, soreness, or inflamed areas)?
   Yes
   No (Impaired Tissue Integrity, Altered Oral Mucous Membrane)
10. Is the patient able to move freely in bed? Ambulate easily?
    Yes
    No (Impaired Tissue Integrity; Impaired Skin Integrity, Risk for or Actual)
11. Review the patient's temperature measurement. Is the temperature within normal limits?
    Yes
    No (Ineffective Thermoregulation, Hyperthermia, Hypothermia)
12. Is the patient's temperature above normal?
    Yes (Ineffective Thermoregulation, Hyperthermia)
    No
13. Is the patient's temperature below normal?
    Yes (Ineffective Thermoregulation, Hypothermia)
    No
14. Is the patient exhibiting signs or symptoms of infection? Vasoconstriction? Vasodilation? Dehydration?
    Yes (Altered Body Temperature, Risk for)
    No
15. Ask the patient: "Do you have any problems swallowing food? Fluids?"
    Yes (Impaired Swallowing, Risk for Aspiration)
    No

The next questions pertain only to a mother who is breast-feeding.

16. Weigh the infant. Is his or her weight within normal limits for his or her age?
    Yes (Effective Breast-Feeding)
    No (Ineffective Breast-Feeding)
17. Ask the patient: "Do you have any problems or concerns about breast-feeding?"
    Yes (Ineffective Breast-Feeding)
    No (Effective Breast-Feeding)

Conceptual Information

The nutritional-metabolic pattern requires looking at four separate but closely aligned aspects: nutrition, fluid balance, tissue integrity, and thermoregulation. All four functionally interrelate to maintain the integrity of the overall nutritional-metabolic functioning of the body.

Food and fluid intake provides carbohydrates, proteins, fats, vitamins, and minerals, which are metabolized by the body to meet energy needs, maintain intracellular and extracellular fluid balances, prevent deficiency syndromes, and act as catalysts for the body's biochemical reactions.[1]

NUTRITION

Nutrition refers to the intake, assimilation, and use of food for energy, maintenance, and growth of the body.[2] Assisting the patient in maintaining a good nutritional-metabolic status facilitates health promotion and illness prevention and provides dietary support in illness.[1]

Swallowing is associated with the intake of food or fluids. *Swallowing* is a complex activity that integrates sensory, muscular, and neurologic functions that generally occur in four phases: (1) *oral preparatory phase*, during which the food is chewed, mixed with saliva, and prepared for digestion; (2) *oral phase*, during which food is moved backward past the hard palate and downward to the pharynx; (3) *pharyngeal phase*, when the larynx closes and the food enters the esophagus; and (4) *esophageal phase*, during which the food passes through the esophagus, in peristaltic movement, to the stomach. The first two phases are voluntarily controlled, and the last two phases are involuntarily controlled.

Many factors affect a person's nutritional status, such as food availability; food cost; the meaning food has for an individual; cultural, social, and religious mores; and physiologic states that might alter a person's ability to eat.[3]

In essence, we are initially concerned with the adequacy or inadequacy of the patient's nutritional state. If the diet is adequate, there is no major reason for concern, but we must be sure that all are defining "adequacy" in a similar manner. Most people probably define an adequate diet as lack of hunger; however, professionals look at an adequate diet as being one in which nutrient intake balances with body needs. The diet is adequate if it meets either minimum daily requirements (MDR) or recommended dietary allowances (RDA) standards. The MDR standards are lower for nutrient amounts than the RDA standards, but they do provide enough nutrients to prevent deficiency problems. The RDA standards are the ones more widely used and are based on the well-known "basic four food groups."[3] The guidelines incorporating the basic four food groups were recently revised and represented as the Food Guide Pyramid, which is currently the best standard to use in assessing dietary adequacy. The revised standard calls for:

Bread, cereals, rice, pasta	Enriched or whole-grain products; 6–11 servings per day
Vegetables	3–4 servings per day
Fruits	2–4 servings per day
Milk, yogurt, cheese	Milk, ice cream, yogurt, and cheese; 2–3 servings per day
Meat, poultry, fish, dry beans, eggs, nuts	Meat, eggs, fish, and poultry; 2–3 servings of 2–3 oz per day
Fats, oils, sugars	Used sparingly

NOTE: Many adults may be lactose intolerant. Lactase enzymes are now available over the counter as a digestive aid for lactose intolerance.

An inadequate nutritional state may be reflective of intake (calories) or use of the intake (metabolism) or a change in activity level. Underweight and overweight are the most commonly seen conditions that reflect alteration in nutrition.[4]

Underweight can be caused by inadequate intake of calories. In some instances, the intake is within the RDA, but there is malabsorption of the intake. The malabsorption or inadequate intake can be due to physiologic causes (pathophysiology), psychologic causes (anorexia, bulimia), or cultural factors (lack of resources or religious proscriptions).[4]

Special notice needs to be given to maternal nutritional needs during the postpartum period. New mothers need optimal nutrition to promote healing of the tissues traumatized during labor and delivery, to restore balance in fluid and electrolytes created by all the rapid changes in the body, and, if the mother is breast-feeding, to produce adequate amounts of milk containing fluid and nutrients for the infant.[5]

The breast-feeding woman can generally meet the nutritional needs of herself and her infant through adequate dietary intake of food and fluids; however, since the energy demand is greater during lactation, RDA standards recommend an additional 500 cal/day above the norm to prevent catabolism of lean tissue.[5] Studies have shown that the caloric intake of breast-feeding women ranges from 2460 to 3060 Kcal/day and that successful breast-feeding may be related to the nutritional status during pregnancy.[6]

An overweight condition is rarely due to a physiologic disturbance, although a genetic predisposition may exist. Overweight is most commonly due to an imbalance between food and activity habits (i.e., increased intake and decreased activity).[4] However, recent research has indicated there is a metabolic set point and in actuality, overweight people may be eating less than normal-weight people.

Either underweight or overweight may be a sign of malnutrition (inadequate nutrition), with the result that the patient exhibits signs and symptoms of more than body requirements or less than body requirements. In either instance, the nurse must assess the patient carefully for his or her overall concept of malnutrition.

FLUID VOLUME

Fluid volume incorporates the aspects of actual fluid amount, electrolytes, and metabolic acid-base balance. Regardless of how much or how little a patient's intake or how much or how little a patient's output is, the fluid, electrolyte, and metabolic acid-base balances are maintained within a relatively narrow margin. This margin is essential for normal functioning in all body systems, and so it must receive close attention in providing care.

Approximately 60 percent of an adult's weight is body fluid (liquid plus electrolytes plus minerals plus cells), and approximately 75 percent of an infant's weight is body fluid. The various parts of body fluid are taken in daily through food and drink and are formed through the metabolic activities of the body.[1,3] The body fluid distribution includes *intracellular* (within the cells), *interstitial* (around the cells), and *intravascular* (in blood cells) fluids. The combination of interstitial and intravascular fluids is known as *extracellular* (outside the cells) *fluid*. Distribution of body fluid is influenced by both the fluid volume and the concentration of electrolytes. Body fluid movement, between the compartments, is constant and occurs through the mechanisms of osmosis, diffusion, active transport, and osmotic and hydrostatic pressure.[1,3]

Body fluid balance is regulated by intake (food and fluid), output (kidney, gastrointestinal tract, skin, and lungs), and hormones (antidiuretic hormones, glucocorticoids, and aldosterone). The largest amount of fluid is located in the intracellular compartment, with the volume of each compartment being regulated predominantly by the solute (mainly the electrolytes).

Electrolytes are either positively or negatively charged particles (ions). The major positively charged electrolytes (cations) are sodium (the main extracellular electrolyte), potassium (the most common intracellular electrolyte), calcium, and magnesium. The major negatively charged electrolytes (anions) are chloride, bicarbonate, and phosphate. The electrolyte compositions of the two extracellular compartments (interstitial and intravascular) are nearly identical. The intracellular fluid contains the same number of electrolytes as the extracellular fluid does, but the intracellular electrolytes carry opposite electrical charges from the electrolytes in the extracellular fluid. This difference between extracellular and intracellular electrolytes is necessary for the electrical activity of nerve and muscle cells.[1,3] Therefore, the electrolytes help regulate cells functioning as well as the fluid volume in each compartment.

Usually the body governs intake through thirst and output through increasing or decreasing body fluid excretion via the kidneys, gastrointestinal tract, and respiration. Because of the way the body governs intake and output, in addition to the effects of pathophysiologic conditions such as shock, hemorrhage, diabetes, and vomiting on intake and output, the patient may enter a state of metabolic acidosis or alkalosis.

Acid-base balance reflects the acidity or alkalinity of body fluids and is expressed as the pH. In essence, the pH is a function of the carbonic acid:bicarbonate ratio.[3] Acid-base balance is regulated by chemical, biologic, and physiologic mechanisms. The chemical regulation involves buffers in the extracellular fluid, while the biologic regulation involves ion exchange across cell membranes. The physiologic regulation is governed in the lungs by carbon dioxide excretion and in the kidneys through metabolism of bicarbonate, acid, and ammonia.[1]

Metabolic acidosis is caused by situations in which the cellular production of acid is excessive (e.g., diabetic ketoacidosis), high doses of drugs have to be metabolized (e.g., aspirin), or excretion of the produced acid is impaired (e.g., renal failure).[3] Weight reduction practices can contribute to the development of acidosis (fad diets or diuretics) as can chemical substance abuse.[1]

Fluid volume is affected by regulatory mechanisms, body fluid loss, or increased fluid intake. Because fluid volume is so readily affected by such a variety of factors, continuous assessment for alterations in fluid volume must be made.

TISSUE INTEGRITY

Nutrition and fluid are vitally important to tissue maintenance and repair. Underlying tissues are protected from external damage by the skin and mucous membranes. Thus, the integrity of the skin is extremely important in the promotion of health because the skin and mucous membranes are the body's first line of defense. The skin also plays a role in temperature regulation and in excretion.

The skin and mucous membranes act as protection through their abundant supply of nerve receptors that alert the body to the external environment (e.g., temperature, pressure, or pain). The skin and mucous membranes also act as barriers to pathogens, thus protecting the internal tissues from these organisms.[3]

The skin's superficial blood vessels and sweat glands (eccrine and apocrine) assist in thermoregulation. As the body temperature rises, the superficial blood vessels dilate and the sweat glands increase secretion. These two actions result in increased perspiration which, through evaporation, cools the body. During instances of excessive perspiration, water, sodium chloride, and nonprotein nitrogen are excreted through the skin; this affects fluid volume and osmotic balance. As the body temperature drops, the opposite reactions occur; there is vessel constriction and decreased sweat gland secretion so that body heat is retained internally.

To fulfill its protective function of the underlying tissues, the skin and mucous membranes must be intact. Any change in skin or mucous membrane integrity can allow pathogen invasion and will also allow fluid and electrolyte loss. Skin and mucous membrane integrity relies on adequate nutrition and removal of metabolic wastes internally and externally, cleanliness, and proper positioning. A recent study[7] found that the length of a surgical procedure and extracorporeal circulation were associated with increased risk of skin breakdown for elective procedures. In emergency surgical settings or in cases of patients in poor health (very elderly and medically indigent), age and serum albumin levels might also be predictive of increased risk for skin breakdown.[7] Any factor that compromises nutrition, fluid, or electrolyte balance can result in impairment of skin or mucous membrane integrity or, at least, a high risk for impairment of skin integrity or mucous membrane integrity.

THERMOREGULATION

Thermoregulation refers to the body's ability to adjust its internal core temperature within a narrow range. The core temperature must remain fairly constant for metabolic activities and cellular metabolism to function for the maintenance of life. The core temperature rarely varies more than 1°C (less than 2°F). In fact, the range of temperature that is compatible with life ranges only from approximately 32.2 to 40°C (90 to 104°F).

Both the hypothalamus and the thyroid gland are involved in thermoregulation. The hypothalamus regulates temperature by responding to changes in electrolyte balances. Both the extracellular cations sodium and calcium affect the action potential and depolarization of cells. When there is an imbalance of sodium and calcium within the hypothalamus, hypothermia or hyperthermia can result. The thyroid glands regulate core body temperature by increasing or decreasing metabolic activities and cellular metabolism, thus altering heat production.

Many factors influence thermoregulation. The skin has previously been mentioned as a thermoregulatory organ. Heat is gained or lost to the environment by evaporation, conduction, convection, and radiation. Evaporation occurs when body heat transforms the liquid on a person's skin to vapor. Conduction is the loss of heat to a colder object through direct contact. When heat is lost to the surrounding cool air, it is called *convection*. *Radiation* occurs when heat is given off to the environment, helping to warm it.

A person generally loses approximately 70 percent of heat from radiation, convection, and conduction. Another 25 percent is lost through insensible mechanisms of the lungs and evaporation from the skin, and about 5 percent is lost in urine and feces. When the body is able to produce and dissipate heat within a normal range, the body is in "heat balance."[8]

The interrelationship of nutrition, fluid balance, thermoregulation, and tissue integrity explains the nursing diagnoses that have been accepted in the nutritional-metabolic pattern. Indeed, if there is an alteration in any one of these four factors, it would be wise for the nurse to assess the other three factors to ensure a complete assessment.

Developmental Considerations

INFANT

Swallowing is a reflex present before birth, since during intrauterine life the fetus swallows amniotic fluid. Following the transition to extrauterine life, the infant learns very rapidly (within 12 to 24 hours) to coordinate sucking and swallowing. There are really no developmental considerations for the act of swallowing since it is a reflex.

The normal process for swallowing involves both the epiglottis and the true vocal cords. These two structures move together to close off the trachea and to allow saliva or solid and liquid foods to pass into the esophagus. The respiratory system is thus protected from foreign bodies.

Salivation is adequate at birth to maintain sufficient moisture in the mouth. However, maturation of many salivary glands does not occur until the third month and corresponds with the baby's learning to swallow at other than a reflex level.[9] Tooth eruption begins at about 6 months of age and stimulates saliva flow and chewing. The infant has a small amount of the enzyme ptyalin, which breaks down starches.

Water constitutes the greatest proportion of the infant's body weight. Approximately 75 to 78 percent of an infant's body weight is water with about 45 percent of this water found in the extracellular fluid. The newborn infant loses significant water through insensible methods (approximately 35 to 45 percent) because of relatively greater body surface area to body weight. The respiratory rate of an infant is approximately two times that of the adult; therefore, the infant is also losing water through insensible loss from the lungs. The newborn also loses water through direct excretion in the urine (50 to 60 percent) and through fairly rapid peristalsis due to the immaturity of the GI tract.

The newborn is unable to concentrate urine well so is more sensitive to inadequate fluid intake or uncompensated water loss.[10] The body fluid reserve of the infant is less than that of the adult, and since the infant excretes a greater volume per kilogram of body weight than the adult, infants are very susceptible to fluid-volume deficit. The infant needs to consume fluids equal to 10 to 15 percent of body weight. Fluid and electrolyte requirements for the newborn are 70 to 100 mL/kg per 24 hours, 2 mEq of sodium and potassium per kilogram per 24 hours, and 2 to 4 mEq of chloride per kilogram per 24 hours.

The kidney function of the infant does not reach adult levels until 6 months to 1 year of age.[10] The functional capacity of the kidneys is limited, especially during stress. In addition, the glomerular filtration rate is low, tubular reabsorption or secretory capacity is limited, sodium reabsorption is decreased, and the metabolic rate is higher. Therefore, there is a greater amount of metabolic wastes to be excreted. The infant's kidney is less able to excrete large loads of solute-free water than the more mature kidney.[11]

Feeding behavior is important not only for fluid but also for food. The caloric need of the infant is 117 cal per kilogram of body weight.[4]

Breast milk contains adequate nutrients and vitamins for approximately 6 months of life. Some bottle formulas are overly high in carbohydrates and fat (especially cholesterol), which may lead to a potential for increasing fat cells.

The introduction of solid foods should not occur until 4 to 6 months of age. Studies have indicated that there is a relationship between the early introduction of solid food (less than 4 months of age) and overfeeding of either milk or food, leading to infant and adult obesity.[4] The infant should be made to feel secure, loved, and unhurried at feeding time. Skin contact is very important for the infant for both physiologic and psychologic reasons.

The skin of an infant is functionally immature, and thus the baby is more prone to skin disorders. Both the dermis and the epidermis are loosely connected, and both are relatively thin, which easily leads to chafing and rub burns.[9] Epidermal layers are permeable, resulting in greater fluid loss. Sebaceous glands, which produce sebum, are very active in late fetal life and early infancy, causing milia and cradle cap, which goes away at about 6 months of age. Dry, intact skin is the greatest deterrent to bacterial invasion. Sweat glands (eccrine or apocrine) are not functional in response to heat and emotional stimuli until a few months after birth, and function remains minimal through childhood. The inability of the skin to contract and shiver in response to heat loss causes ineffective thermal regulation.[4] Also, the infant has no melanocytes to protect against the rays of the sun. This is true of dark-skinned infants as well as light-skinned infants.

Core body temperature in the infant ranges from 97 to 100°F. Temperature in the infant fluctuates considerably because the regulatory mechanisms in the hypothalamus are not fully developed. (It is not considered abnormal for the newborn infant to lose 1 to 2°F immediately after birth.) The infant is unable to shiver to produce heat, nor does the infant have much subcutaneous fat to insulate the body. However, the infant does have several protective mechanisms by which he or she is able to conserve heat to keep the body temperature fairly stable. These mechanisms include vasoconstriction so that heat is maintained in the inner body core, an increased metabolic rate which increases heat production, a closed body position (the so-called fetal position) which reduces the amount of exposed skin, and the metabolism of adipose tissue.

This particular adipose tissue is called "brown fat" because of the rich supply of blood and nerves. Brown fat composes 2 to 6 percent of body weight of the infant. Brown fat aids in adaptation of the thermoregulation mechanisms.[9] The ability of the body to regulate temperature at the adult level matures at approximately 3 to 6 months of age.

TODDLER AND PRESCHOOLER

By the end of the second year, the child's salivary glands are adult size and have reached functional maturity.[9] The toddler is capable of chewing food, so it stays longer in his or her mouth and the salivary enzymes have an opportunity to begin breaking down the food. The saliva also covers the teeth with a protective film that helps prevent decay. Drooling no longer occurs since the toddler easily swallows saliva.

Dental caries occur infrequently in children under 3 years, but rampant tooth decay in very young children is almost always related to prolonged bottle feeding at nap time and bedtime (bottle mouth syndrome). The toddler should be weaned from the bottle or at least not allowed to fall asleep with the bottle in her or his mouth.[12] Parents should be taught that the adverse effects of bedtime feeding are greater than thumb sucking or the use of pacifiers.

Affected teeth remain susceptible to decay after nursing stops. If deciduous teeth decay and disintegrate early, spacing of the permanent teeth is affected, and immature speech patterns develop. Discomfort is felt, and emotional problems may result.[12]

The first dental examination should be between the ages of 18 and 24 months. Dental hygiene should be started when the first tooth erupts by cleansing the teeth with gauze or cotton moistened with hydrogen peroxide and flavored with a few drops of mouthwash. After 18 months, the child's teeth may be brushed with a soft or medium toothbrush.[12] Fluoride supplements are believed to prevent caries.

In the toddler there is beginning to be the appropriate proportion of body water to body weight (62 percent water).[13] The extracellular fluid is about 26 percent, whereas the adult has about 19 percent extracellular fluid. Toddlers have less reserve of body fluid than adults and lose more body water daily, both from sensible and insensible loss. This age group is highly predisposed to fluid imbalances.[14] These imbalances relate to the fact that the kidney still is immature so water conservation is poor and the toddler still has an increased metabolic rate and therefore greater insensible water loss than the adult. However, GI motility slows so this age group is better able to tolerate fluid loss through diarrhea. The 2- to 3-year-old needs 1100 to 1200 mL (4 to 5 8-oz glasses) of fluid every 24 hours, whereas the preschooler needs 1300 to 1400 mL of fluid every 24 hours.

The caloric need in the toddler is 1000 cal/day or 100 cal/kg at 1 year and 1300 to 1500 cal/day at 3 years. A child should not be forced to "clean the plate" at mealtime, and food should not be viewed as a reward or punishment. Instead, caloric intake should be related to the growing body and energy expenditures.

The caloric need of the preschooler is 85 cal/kg. Eating assumes increasing social significance and continues to be an emotional as well as a physiologic experience.[4] Frustrating or unsettled mealtimes can influence caloric intake, as can manipulative behavior on the part of the child or parent. The child may also be eating empty calories between meals.

In the toddler functional maturity of skin creates a more effective barrier against fluid loss; the skin is not as soft as the infant's, and there is more protection against outside bacterial invasion. The skin remains dry because sebum secretion is limited. Eccrine sweat gland function remains limited, eczema improves, and the frequency of rashes declines.

Skin, as a perceptual organ, experiences significant development during this period. Children like to "feel" different objects and textures and like to be hugged. Melanin is formed during these years, and thus the toddler, preschooler, and school-age child is more protected against sun rays.[9]

In addition, small capillaries in the periphery become more capable of constriction and thus thermoregulation. Also, the child is able to sense and interpret that he or she is hot or cold and can voluntarily do something about it.

SCHOOL-AGE CHILD

The child at this age begins losing baby teeth as permanent teeth erupt. The child should not be evaluated for braces until after all 6-year molars have erupted. The permanent teeth are larger than the baby teeth and appear too large for the small face, causing some embarrassment. Good oral hygiene is important.

For the school-age child, the percentage of total body water to total body weight continues to decrease until about 12 years of age when it approaches adult norms.[14] Changes occur in extracellular fluid from 22 percent at 6 years to 17.5 percent at age 12 due to the proportion of body surface area to mass, increasing muscle mass and connective tissue, and increasing percentage of body fat.

Water is needed for excretion of the solute load. Balance is maintained through mature kidneys leading to mature concentration of urine and acidifying capacities. Fluid requirements can be calculated by height, weight, surface area, and metabolic activity. The school-age child needs about 1.5 to 3 qt of fluid a day. Additionally, the child needs a slightly positive water balance. The electrolyte values are similar to those for the adult except for phosphorus and calcium (due to bone growth).[14]

The caloric need of the school-age child is greater than that of an adult (approximately 80 cal/kg or 1600 to 2200 cal/day). The ages of 10 to 12 reflect the peak ages of caloric and protein needs of the school-age child (need 50 to 60 cal/kg per day) due to the accelerated growth, muscle development, and bone mineralization. "The school-age child reflects the nutritional experiences of early childhood and the potential for adulthood."[4]

ADOLESCENT

By age 21, all 32 permanent teeth have erupted. The adolescent needs frequent dental visits because of cavities and also for orthodontic work that may be in progress. There is a growth spurt and sexual changes. A total increase in height of 25 percent and a doubling of weight are normally attained.[15] Muscle mass increases and total body water declines with increasing sexual development.[16] The adolescent needs 34 to 45 cal/kg per day and tends to have eating patterns based on external environmental cues rather than hunger. Eating becomes more of a social event. There is a high probability of eating disorders such as anorexia and bulimia arising during this age period.

The basal metabolic rate increases, lung size increases, and maximal breathing capacity and forced expiratory volume increase, leading to increased insensible loss of fluid through the lungs. Total body water decreases from 61 percent at age 12 to 54 percent by age 18 due to an increase in fat cells. Fat cells do not have as much water as tissue cells.[16] The water intake need of the adolescent is about 2200 to 2700 mL per 24 hours.

Sebaceous glands become extremely active during adolescence and increase in size. Eccrine sweat glands are fully developed and are especially responsive to emotional stimuli (and are more active in males); apocrine sweat glands also began to secrete in response to emotional stimuli.[17] Stopped-up sebaceous glands lead to acne, and the adolescent's skin is usually moist.

YOUNG ADULT

The amount of ptyalin in the saliva decreases after 20 years of age; otherwise the digestive system remains fully functioning. The appearance of "wisdom teeth" or third molars occurs at 20 to 21 years. There are normally four third molars, although some individuals may not fully develop all four. Third molars can create problems for the individual. Eruptions are unpredictable in time and presentation, and molars may come in sideways or facing any direction. This can force other teeth out of alignment, which makes chewing difficult and painful. Often these molars need to be removed to prevent irreparable damage to proper occlusion of jaws. Even normally erupting third molars may be painful. The young adult must see a dentist regularly.

Total body water in the young adult is about 50 to 60 percent. There is a difference between males and females due to the difference in the number of fat cells. Most water in the young adult is intracellular with only about 20 percent of fluid being extracellular. Growth is essentially finished by this developmental age.

ADULT

Ptyalin has sharply decreased by age 60 as well as other digestive enzymes. Total body water is now about 47 to 54.7 percent. Diet and activity indirectly influence the amount of body water by directly altering the amount of adipose tissue. In the adult the activity level is stable or is beginning to decline. The basal metabolic rate gradually decreases along with a reduced demand for calories. The adult needs to reduce calorie intake by approximately 7.5 percent.[18]

Tissues of the integumentary system maintain a healthy, intact, glowing appearance until age 50 or 55 if the individual is receiving adequate vitamins, minerals, other nutrients, and fluids and maintains good personal hygiene. Wrinkles do become more noticeable, however, and body water (from integumentary tissues) decreases, leading to thinner, drier skin that bruises more easily. Fat increases, leading to skin that is not as elastic and will not recede with weight loss, so bags develop readily under the eyes.[9] Also, skin wounds heal more slowly because of decreased cell regeneration.

OLDER ADULT

In the older adult the mouth undergoes changes associated with aging that can affect nutrition. Tooth decay, loss of teeth, degeneration of jaw bone, progressive gum recession, and increased reabsorption of the dental arch can make eating and chewing a difficult task for the elderly person if good dental health has not been maintained. Reduced chewing ability, decrease in salivation, and perhaps poorly fitting dentures compound the problem of poor nutrition of the aged. Aging causes an atrophy of olfactory organs and a loss of taste buds. Usually salt and sweet taste buds are lost first with bitter and sour taste buds remaining intact; therefore,

food has little flavor. This leads to aged persons having a characteristic unpleasant bitter taste in their mouths called *dysgeusia*.[19]

Loss of taste is compounded by gum disease, poor teeth, or dentures. Fifty percent of the elderly have lost their teeth. Ninety percent who have natural teeth have periodontal disease.[20] The aged are especially vulnerable to oral carcinoma.[4]

Total body water of the older adult is about 45 to 50 percent. Although values are within normal, the elderly cannot tolerate extremes of temperature well because of slower response time to adapt to change. Excess heat and overexertion are not tolerated well by the older adult. The older adult naturally has drier, wrinkled skin so assessment of skin in the elderly for alteration in fluid volume needs to be interpreted carefully. The recommended sites to use in assessing skin turgor in the older adult include the abdomen, sternum, and forehead. There is a decrease in the number of body cells and adipose tissue, leading to a decrease in total body water. However, cell size increases.

Serum protein (albumin) production is decreased, but globulin is increased. Therefore, there is not much difference in blood volume. However, the nurse needs to consider the proportion of blood volume to body weight.

There is a decrease in nephrotic tubular functioning, which affects removal of waste, urine concentration, and dilution. This in turn leads to a decrease in specific gravity and urine osmolarity. There is decreased bladder capacity, leading to nocturia. Therefore, the elderly may limit fluid in the evening to offset nocturia, but limiting fluids may lead to nocturnal dehydration. Sodium and chloride levels remain constant, but potassium decreases. In the older adult the blood level and excretion of aldosterone decrease 50 percent if sodium is depleted.[21]

Gonadal hormones may influence fluid and electrolyte balance in terms of sodium and water retention. Therefore, with the loss of hormones in aging, there is a decrease in sodium and water retention.

Many changes are occurring in the GI tract (decreased enzyme secretion, general gastric irritation, decreased nutrient and drug absorption, decreased HCl secretion, decreased peristalsis and elimination, and decreased sphincter muscle tone) of the older adult that make nutrition a primary concern.[4] The older adult needs decreased calories but needs an increase in vitamins and trace elements as well as an adequate intake of protein, fat, carbohydrates, bulk, and electrolytes (sodium, potassium, calcium, and magnesium). However, financial concerns may lead the elderly to buy inappropriate foods containing empty calories.

The skin of the older adult becomes drier and thinner; skin lesions or discoloration and scaliness (keratosis) may appear. Integumentary changes in the older adult are readily noticeable because of our society's emphasis on youth and beauty.[9] The older adult has wrinkles, mostly in the face; exposure to the sun also produces and hastens formation of wrinkles. Fatty layers are lost in the trunk, face, and extremities, leading to the appearance of increased joint size throughout the body. The skin is nonelastic and may lose water to the air in low-humidity situations, which results in chapping.

Extremes of temperature are difficult for the elderly. Body temperature may increase because of a decrease in size, number, and functioning of the sweat glands; or the person may need a sweater because of decreased fat and peripheral circulation. Fragile blood vessels lead to bruising. The older adult loses melanocytes, leading to pale, light skin; hair turns gray, and the elderly lose hair. Older women may have hair on the face or chin due to androgen-estrogen imbalances.

There is an absolute decrease in intracellular water and a decrease in both sebaceous and sweat glands. With age, skin becomes less effective as a tactile organ (touch, pressure, pain, and local temperature changes) because of the slowing of impulses to the brain and a decrease in the number of receptors.[22] Therefore, an elderly person may have a burn or frostbite and not be aware of it.

APPLICABLE NURSING DIAGNOSES

Aspiration, Risk for

DEFINITION

The state in which an individual is at risk for entry of gastrointestinal secretions, oropharyngeal secretions, or solids or fluids into tracheobronchial passages.[23]

NANDA TAXONOMY: EXCHANGING 1.6.1.4

DEFINING CHARACTERISTICS (RISK FACTORS)[23]

1. Major defining characteristics
   a. Reduced level of consciousness
   b. Depressed cough and gag reflexes
   c. Presence of tracheostomy or endotracheal tube
   d. Incompetent lower esophageal sphincter
   e. Gastrointestinal tubes
   f. Tube feedings
   g. Medication administration
   h. Situations hindering elevation of upper body
   i. Increased intragastric pressure
   j. Increased gastric residual
   k. Decreased gastrointestinal motility
   l. Delayed gastric emptying
   m. Impaired swallowing
   n. Facial, oral, or neck surgery or trauma
   o. Wired jaws
2. Minor defining characteristics
   None given.

RELATED FACTORS[23]

The risk factors also serve as the related factors for this nursing diagnosis.

RELATED CLINICAL CONCERNS

1. Closed head injury
2. Any diagnosis with presenting symptoms of nausea and vomiting
3. Bulimia
4. Any diagnosis requiring use of a nasogastric tube
5. Spinal cord injury

HAVE YOU SELECTED THE CORRECT DIAGNOSIS?

Impaired Swallowing *Swallowing* means that when food or fluids are present in the mouth, the brain signals both the epiglottis and the true vocal cords to move together to close off the trachea so that the food and fluids can pass into the esophagus and thus into the stomach. Impaired Swallowing implies that there is a mechanical or physiologic obstruction between the oropharynx and the esophagus that prevents foods or fluids from passing into the esophagus. In Risk for Aspiration there may or may not be an obstruction between the oropharynx and the esophagus. The major pathophysiologic dysfunction that occurs in Risk for Aspiration is the inability of the epiglottis and true vocal cords to move to close off the trachea. This inability to close off the trachea may occur because of pathophysiologic changes in the structures themselves or because messages to the brain are absent, decreased, or impaired.

Ineffective Airway Clearance In Ineffective Airway Clearance, the patient is unable to effectively clear secretions from the respiratory tract due to some of the same related factors as are found with Risk for Aspiration. However, in Ineffective Airway Clearance, the defining characteristics (abnormal breath sounds, cough, change in rate or depth of respirations, etc.) are associated directly with respiratory function, whereas the defining characteristics of Risk for Aspiration are directly or indirectly related to the oropharyngeal mechanisms that protect the tracheobronchial passages from the entrance of foreign substances.

EXPECTED OUTCOMES

1. Will demonstrate no risk factors of aspiration by (date) and/or
2. Will implement plan to offset Risk for Aspiration by (date)

TARGET DATE

Aspiration is life-threatening. Initial target dates should be stated in hours. After the number of risk factors has been reduced, the target date can be moved to 2- to 4-day intervals.

NURSING ACTIONS/INTERVENTIONS WITH RATIONALES

Adult Health

ACTIONS/INTERVENTIONS	RATIONALES
• Have suction equipment available. • Sit patient up or elevate head of bed, especially during meals, if not contraindicated. If contraindicated, place patient on right side. • Feed slowly and cut food into small bites. Instruct patient to chew thoroughly. Observe gag and cough reflexes. Monitor for food and secretion accumulation in mouth. Sit with patient during mealtime if cognitive functioning indicates a need for close observation. • Teach patient to be cognizant of closing off trachea before attempting to swallow: 　◦ Have the patient clear his or her throat by coughing and expectorating. If patient unable to expectorate, suction the secretions. 　◦ Have the patient inhale as food is put in the mouth. 　◦ Have the patient then perform a Valsalva maneuver as he or she is swallowing. 　◦ Have the patient cough, swallow again, and exhale deeply. 　◦ Start with soft, nonacidic, noncrumbly foods rather than liquids. Liquids are more difficult to control. 　◦ Discuss with the patient the purpose for any alterations in care necessitated by this diagnosis, e.g., upright position, small, frequent meals, soft foods. • Offer small, frequent feedings at least 6 times a day rather than 3 large meals a day. Offer soft foods rather than a full liquid diet. • Delay fluids associated with meals for at least 30 min after each meal. • Have the patient cough and clear secretions prior to offering any food or fluid. • Teach patient to limit conversation while either eating or drinking. • Provide calm, relaxed atmosphere during mealtime, and assist patient with relaxation exercises as needed. • Teach patient and family the Heimlich maneuver and have return-demonstrate at least daily for 3 days before discharge. • Teach patient and family suctioning technique as needed, including appropriate ordering of supplies. • Refer patient and family to appropriate resources.	Would be required for emergency relief of aspiration. Decreases risk of reflux from stomach, thus decreasing risk of aspiration. Placing patient on right side facilitates food passage into the pylorus. All of these measures are designed to reduce the risk of aspiration. Decreased sensation may allow pocketing of food in mouth. Reduces risk of aspiration and promotes compliance by involving patient in his or her plan of care. Liquids are more easily aspirated than soft food. Smaller and more frequent feedings reduce risk of aspiration while maintaining nutritional status. Decreases the likelihood of coughing, gagging, and choking. Would assist in episodes of choking and would allow patient and family to feel comfortable with level of expertise before going home. Provides long-term teaching and support.

Child Health

ACTIONS/INTERVENTIONS	RATIONALES
• Determine best position for patient as determined by underlying risk factors, e.g., head of bed elevated 30 degrees with infant propped on right side after feeding. • Check bilateral breath sounds every 30 min or with any change in respiratory status.	Natural upper airway patency is facilitated by upright position. Turning to right side decreases likelihood of drainage into trachea rather than esophagus in the event of choking. In the event of aspiration, increased gurgling and rales with correlated respiratory difficulty (from mild to severe) will be noted.

Continued

ACTIONS/INTERVENTIONS	RATIONALES
• Measure amount of residual, immediately before feeding, in nasogastric tube and report any excess beyond 10–20 percent of volume or as specified.	Monitors the speed of digestion and indicates the patient's ability to tolerate the feeding.
• Note and record the presence of any facial trauma or surgery of face, head, or neck-associated drainage.	Monitoring for these risk factors will assist in preventing unexpected or undetected aspiration.
• Monitor for risk factors that would promote aspiration, e.g., increased intracranial pressure, Reye's syndrome, nausea associated with medications, cerebral palsy, or neurologic damage.	An increased stimulation or sensitivity to the gag reflex increases the likelihood of choking and possible aspiration.
• Assist patient and family to identify factors that will help prevent aspiration, e.g., avoiding self-stimulation of gag reflex, avoiding deep oral or pharyngeal suctioning, and chewing food thoroughly.	
• Provide opportunities for patient and family to ask questions or ventilate regarding risk for aspiration by scheduling at least 30 min twice a day at (times) for discussing concerns.	Allows an opportunity to decrease anxiety, provides time for teaching, and allows individualized home care planning.
• Teach family and patient (if old enough) age-appropriate CPR, first aid, and Heimlich maneuver.	Basic safety measures for dangers of aspiration.

Women's Health

NOTE: The following actions pertain to the newborn infant in the presence of meconium in amniotic fluid.

ACTIONS/INTERVENTIONS	RATIONALES
• Alert obstetrician and pediatrician of the presence of meconium in amniotic fluid.	Presence of meconium alerts health care providers to possible complications.
• Assemble equipment and be prepared for resuscitation of the newborn at the time of delivery.	Basic emergency preparedness.
• Be prepared to suction infant's nasopharynx and oropharynx while head of infant is still on the perineum.	
• Immediately evaluate and record the respiratory status of the newborn infant.	
• Assist pediatrician in viewing the vocal cords of infant (have various sizes of pediatric laryngoscopes available). If meconium is present, be prepared to insert endotracheal tube for further suctioning.	
• Continue to evaluate and record infant's respiratory status.	There is no designated time frame for observation; however, the nurse needs to continue to evaluate the infant for at least 12–24 h for respiratory distress and the complications of pulmonary interstitial emphysema, pneumomediastinum, pneumothorax, persistent pulmonary hypertension, CNS dysfunction, and renal failure. These infants should be place in a level 2 or 3 nursery.
• Reassure parents by keeping them informed of actions.	Reduces anxiety.
• Allow opportunities for parents to verbalize fears and ask questions.	Reduces anxiety and provides teaching opportunity.

Psychiatric Health

> **NOTE:** Clients receiving electroconvulsive therapy (ECT) are at risk for this diagnosis.

ACTIONS/INTERVENTIONS	RATIONALES
• Remain with client who has had ECT until gag reflex and swallowing have returned to normal. Monitor gag reflex and swallowing every 30 min until they return to normal.	Basic safety measures until client can demonstrate control.
• Place client who has had ECT on right side until reactive.	Lessens the probability of aspiration through the influence of gravity on stomach contents.
• Clients in four-point restraint should be placed on right side or stomach. Elevate client's head to eat and remove restraints one at a time to facilitate eating. Request that oral medications be changed to liquid forms.	Lessens probability of aspiration due to difficulty in swallowing tablets or pills which might cause gagging.
• Observe clients receiving antipsychotic agents for possible suppression of cough reflex.	One side effect of these medications is suppression of the cough reflex. Loss of this reflex promotes the likelihood of aspiration.

Gerontic Health

ACTIONS/INTERVENTIONS	RATIONALES
• Older adults may develop a decreased gag reflex. To reduce the risk of aspiration: 　○ Monitor gag reflex before any procedures involving anesthesia such as bronchoscopy, EGD, or general surgery.	Establishes baseline data to use for comparison after the procedure is completed.
• Monitor gag reflex postprocedure prior to giving fluids or solids.	Ensuring return of gag reflex will decrease risk of aspiration once oral intake is resumed.

Home Health

The nursing actions for home health care for this diagnosis are the same as the actions enumerated in the Adult Health section.

Aspiration, Risk for
FLOWCHART EVALUATION: EXPECTED OUTCOME 1

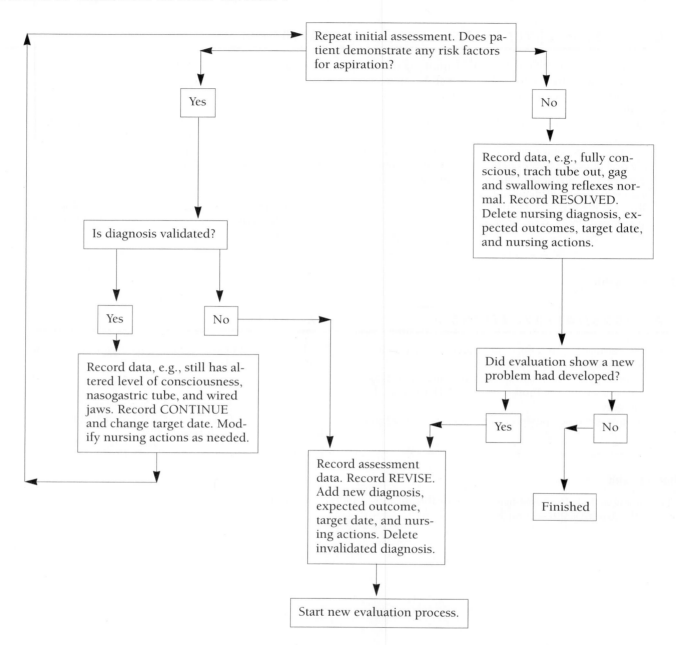

Aspiration, Risk for
FLOWCHART EVALUATION: EXPECTED OUTCOME 2

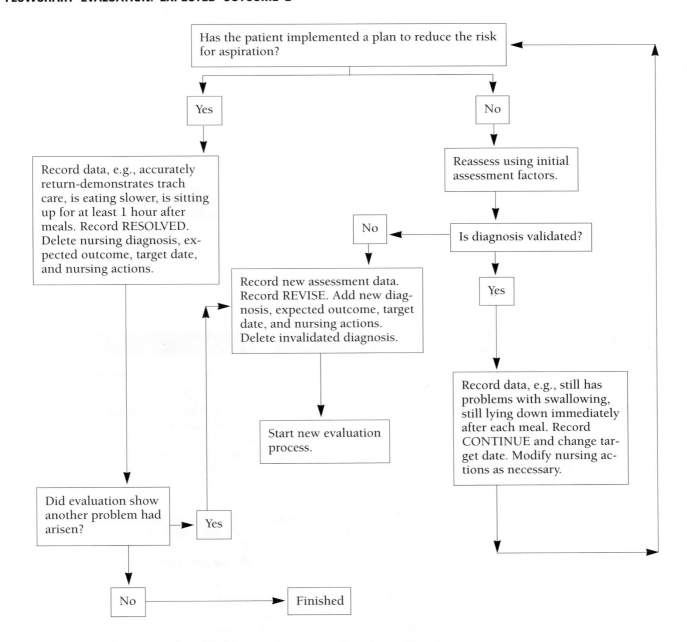

Body Temperature, Altered, Risk for

DEFINITION

The state in which the individual is at risk for failure to maintain body temperature within normal range.[23]

NANDA TAXONOMY: EXCHANGING 1.2.2.1

DEFINING CHARACTERISTICS (RISK FACTORS)[23]

1. Major defining characteristics
   a. Extremes of age
   b. Extremes of weight
   c. Exposure to cold or cool or warm or hot environments
   d. Dehydration
   e. Inactivity or vigorous activity
   f. Medications causing vasoconstriction or vasodilation
   g. Altered metabolic rate
   h. Sedation
   i. Inappropriate clothing for environmental temperature
   j. Illness or trauma affecting temperature regulation
2. Minor defining characteristics
   None given.

RELATED FACTORS[23]

The risk factors also serve as the related factors for this nursing diagnosis.

RELATED CLINICAL CONCERNS

1. Any infectious process
2. Hyperthyroidism or hypothyroidism
3. Any surgical procedure
4. Head injuries

HAVE YOU SELECTED THE CORRECT DIAGNOSIS?

Risk for Altered Body Temperature needs to be differentiated from Hypothermia, Hyperthermia, and Ineffective Thermoregulation.

Hypothermia Hypothermia is the condition under which a person maintains a temperature lower than normal for him or her. This means that the body is probably dissipating heat normally but is unable to produce heat normally. In Risk for Altered Body Temperature, both heat production and heat dissipation are potentially nonfunctional. In Hypothermia a lower-than-normal body temperature can be measured. In Risk for Altered Body Temperature, temperature measurement may not show an abnormality until the condition has changed to Hyperthermia or Hypothermia.

Hyperthermia Hyperthermia is the condition under which a person maintains a temperature higher than normal. This means that the body is probably producing heat normally but is unable to dissipate the heat normally. Both heat production and heat dissipation are potentially nonfunctional in Risk for Altered Body Temperature. As with Hypothermia, a temperature measurement will show an abnormal measurement.

Ineffective Thermoregulation Ineffective Thermoregulation means that a person's temperature fluctuates between being too high and too low. There is nothing wrong, generally, with heat production or heat dissipation; however, the thermoregulatory systems in the hypothalamus or the thyroid are dysfunctional. Again a temperature measurement will show an abnormality.

EXPECTED OUTCOMES

1. Will have no alteration in body temperature by (date) and/or
2. Will describe at least (number) measures to keep body temperature within a range of 98 to 99°F by (date)

TARGET DATE

Initial target dates would be stated in hours. After stabilization, target dates could be extended to 2 to 3 days.

NURSING ACTIONS/INTERVENTIONS WITH RATIONALES

Adult Health

ACTIONS/INTERVENTIONS	RATIONALES
• Monitor for factors contributing to Risk for Alteration in Body Temperature at least every 2 h on (odd/even) hour. (Refer to Risk Factors.)	Detects overproduction or underproduction of heat.
• Monitor temperature at least every 2 h on (odd/even) hour.	
• Note pattern of temperature for last 48 h.	Assists in ascertaining any trends. Typical viral-bacterial differentiation may be possible to detect on temperature curves.
• Monitor skin and mucous membrane integrity every 2 h on (odd/even) hour.	Allows early detection of impaired tissue integrity which can lead in infection.
• Maintain fluid and electrolyte balance. Monitor intake and output every hour.	Adequate hydration assists in maintaining normal body core temperature.
• If temperature is above or below 98.6°F (or parameters defined by physician), take appropriate measures to bring temperatures back to normal range. Refer to nursing actions for Hypothermia, page 152, or Hyperthermia, page 145.	
• Follow up with cultures for identification of causative organisms if infection is present.	Identification of organism allows determination of most appropriate antibiotic therapy.
• Maintain consistent room temperature.	Prevents overheating or overcooling due to environment.
• Teach patient to wear appropriate clothing and modify routines to prevent alterations in body temperature:	Regulates constant metabolism and provides warmth.
◦ Wear close-knit undergarments in winter to prevent heat loss.	
◦ Wear hat and gloves in cold weather because heat is lost from head and hands.	
◦ Wear wool rather than synthetic fibers because wool provides better insulation.	
◦ Wear socks or stockings at night.	
◦ Wear light, loose, but protecting clothing in hot weather.	
◦ Wear hat in hot weather to protect head.	
◦ Use sheet blankets rather than regular sheets.	
◦ Try to stay indoors on windy days.	
◦ Try to work outdoors in early morning and to work for limited periods of time.	
◦ Have frequent, small meals every 3–4 h and warm liquids every 2 h on the (odd/even) hour.	
• Avoid sedatives and tranquilizers that depress cerebral function and circulation.	Risk factors for this diagnosis.
• Assist patient to learn to assess biorhythms—generally early morning is the period of lowest body metabolic activity; add extra clothes until food and physical movement stimulate increased cellular metabolism and circulation.	Helps determine peak and trough of temperature variations.
• Alternate physical and sedentary activity every 2 h on (odd/even) hour.	Assists in maintaining consistency in metabolic functioning.
• Teach patients to use heating pads and electric blankets in safe manner.	Basic safety measure.
• Refer to nursing diagnoses Hypothermia or Hyperthermia for interventions related to these situations once the alteration has occurred.	

Child Health

ACTIONS/INTERVENTIONS	RATIONALES
• Monitor temperature at least every hour.	The young infant and child may lack mature thermoregulatory capacity. Temperatures either too high (102°F or above) or too low (below 97°F) may bring about spiraling metabolic demise for acid-base status. Seizures and shock may follow.

• If temperature is less than 97°F rectally (or parameters defined by physician), take appropriate measures for maintaining temperature:
  ○ Infants: Radiant warmer or isolette
  ○ Older child: Thermoblanket
  ○ Administer medications as ordered.
	Young infants and children may not be able to initiate compensatory regulation of temperature, especially in premature and altered CNS/immune conditions. These basic measures must be taken to safeguard a return to homeostatic condition.

• Be cautious to not overdose in a 24-h period. Abide by recommended dosage schedule per eight or pediatric medication recommendations.	Using caution in dosage calculation and abiding by appropriate guidelines will minimize inadvertent overdosing and subsequent untoward effects of medication.

• If temperature is above 101°F, take appropriate measures to bring temperature back to normal range (or at least 98–100°F):
  ○ Administer Tylenol, antibiotics, or other medications as ordered.
  ○ Monitor and document related symptoms with specific regard for potential febrile seizures.
  ○ Monitor for the development of febrile seizures, and check for history of febrile seizures.
	Young infants and children may have febrile seizures due to immature thermoregulatory mechanisms and must be appropriately safeguarded against further sequelae.

○ If infant or child has reduced threshold for seizures during times of fever, be prepared to treat seizures with anticonvulsants, maintain airway, and provide for safety from injury.	Anticipatory planning promotes optimal resuscitation efforts.
○ Provide appropriate teaching to child and parents related to hyperthermia and hypothermia, e.g., temperature measurement, wearing of proper clothing, use of Tylenol instead of aspirin, consuming adequate amounts of food and fluid, and use of tepid baths.	Self-care will empower and foster long-term confidence as well as reduce anxiety.
○ Be cautious to not overtax the infant or child with congestive heart failure or pulmonary problems by allowing a temperature elevation to develop. ○ Avoid use of aspirin and aspirin products.	Increased metabolic demands in the presence of an already taxed cardiopulmonary status can become severe, resulting in life-threatening conditions if left untreated. Standards of care per the American Academy of Pediatrics to decrease the potential for Reye's syndrome.
○ Avoid use of tympanic membranous thermometer in infants of 6 mo or less.	Studies indicate that tympanic thermometers are inaccurate in infants, especially those less than 3 mo of age.

Women's Health

ACTIONS/INTERVENTIONS	RATIONALES
• Assist patient in identifying lifestyle adjustments necessary to maintain body temperature within normal range during various life phases, e.g., perimenopause or menopause.	So-called hot flashes related to changes in the body's core temperature can be somewhat controlled in women by estrogen replacement therapy; however, as hormone levels fluctuate with the aging process, some hot flashes will occur. These can be helped by adjusting the environment, e.g., room temperature, amount of clothing, or temperature of fluids consumed.
• Maintain house at a consistent temperature level of 70–72°F.	

- Keep bedroom cooler at night, and layer blankets or covers that can be discarded or added as necessary.
- Have patient drink cool fluids, e.g., iced tea or cold soda.
- Have patient wear clothing that is layered so that jackets, etc., can be discarded or added as necessary.
- In collaboration with physician, assist patient in understanding role of estrogen and the amount of estrogen replacement necessary during perimenopause and menopause.

Individuals have unique, different requirements as to the amount of estrogen necessary to maintain appropriate hormone levels. It is of prime importance that each patient can recognize what her body's needs are and communicate this information to the health care provider.[5]

Psychiatric Health

ACTIONS/INTERVENTIONS	RATIONALES
• Observe clients receiving neuroleptic drugs for signs and symptoms of hyperthermia. Teach clients these symptoms and caution them to decrease their activities in the warmest part of the day and to maintain adequate hydration, especially if they are receiving lithium carbonate with these drugs.	Neuroleptic drugs may decrease the ability to sweat and therefore make it difficult for the client to reduce body temperature.[24,25]
• Observe clients receiving antipsychotics and antidepressants for loss of thermoregulation. The elderly client, especially, should be monitored for this side effect. Provide the client with extra clothing and blankets to maintain comfort. Protect this client from contact with uncontrolled hot objects such as space heaters and radiators. Heating pads and electric blankets can be used with supervision.	Antipsychotics and antidepressants can cause a loss of thermoregulation. The client's learned avoidance behavior can be altered and consciousness can be clouded due to medications.[24,25]
• Do not provide electric heating devices to the client who is on suicide precautions or who has alterations in thought processes.	Basic safety measure.
• Notify physician if client receiving antipsychotic agents has an elevation in temperature or flu-like symptoms.	Antipsychotics, especially chlorpromazine and thioridazine, can cause agranulocytosis. This risk is greatest 3–8 wk after therapy has begun.[24,25] Clients who have experienced this side effect in the past should not receive the drug again since a repeat episode is highly possible.
• Review client's CBC before drug is started, and report any abnormalities on subsequent CBCs to the physician.	Basic monitoring for agranulocytosis.
• Clients receiving phenothiazines should be monitored for hot, dry skin, CNS depression, and rectal temperature elevations (can be up to 108°F). Monitor client's temperature 3 times a day while awake at (times). Notify physician of alterations.	These medications can produce hyperthermia, which can be fatal. This hyperthermia is due to a peripheral autonomic effect.[24,25]
• Monitor clients receiving tricyclic antidepressants (TCAs) and the monoamine oxidase inhibitors (MAOIs) for alterations in temperature 3 times a day while awake (note times here). Notify physician of any alterations.	The side effect of a hyperpyretic crisis can be produced in clients receiving these medications.[24,25]

Gerontic Health

Nursing actions for gerontics are the same as those given in the Adult Health section.

Home Health

ACTIONS/INTERVENTIONS	RATIONALES
• Teach measures to decrease or eliminate Risk for Alteration in Body Temperature: ○ Wearing appropriate clothing. ○ Taking appropriate care of underlying disease. ○ Avoiding exposure to extremes of environmental temperature. ○ Maintain temperature within norms for age, sex, and height. ○ Ensure appropriate use of medications. ○ Ensure proper hydration. ○ Ensure appropriate shelter.	Appropriate environmental temperature regulation will provide support for physiologic thermoregulation.
• Assist client and family to identify lifestyle changes that may be required: ○ Learn survival techniques if client works or plays outdoors. ○ Measure temperature in a manner appropriate for the developmental age of the person. ○ Maintain ideal weight. ○ Avoid substance abuse.	Support is often helpful when individuals and families are considering lifestyle alterations.
• Involve client and family in planning, implementing, and promoting reduction or elimination of the Risk for Alteration in Body Temperature by establishing family conferences to set mutual goals and to improve communication.	Involvement of client and family provides opportunity to increase motivation and enhance self-care.
• Consult with appropriate assistive resources as indicated.	Cost-effective and appropriate use of available resources.

Body Temperature, Altered, Risk for

FLOWCHART EVALUATION: EXPECTED OUTCOME 1

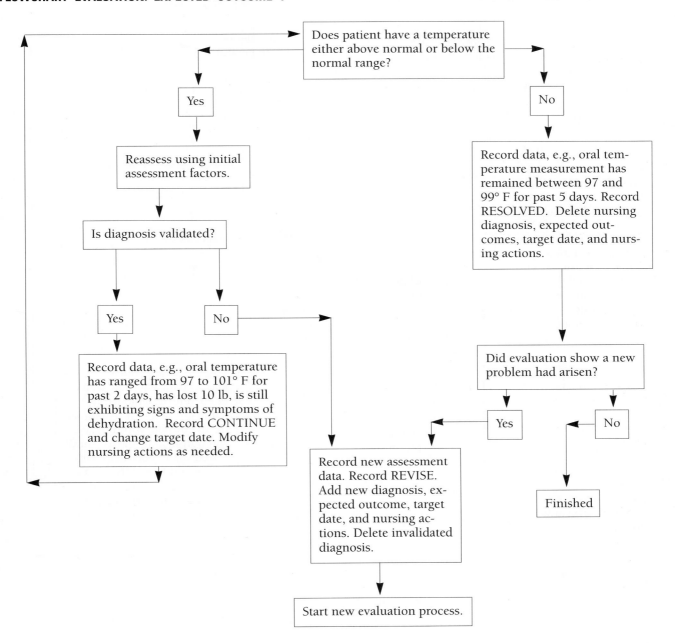

Body Temperature, Altered, Risk for

FLOWCHART EVALUATION: EXPECTED OUTCOME 2

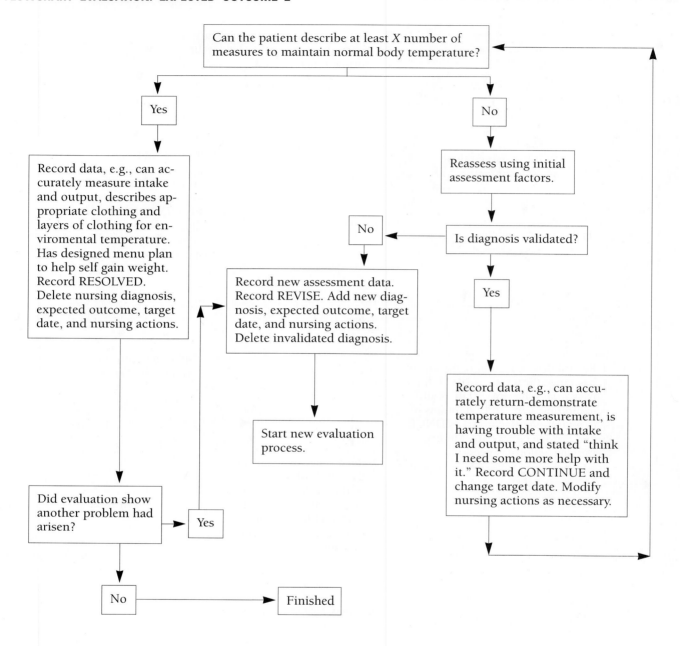

Can the patient describe at least *X* number of measures to maintain normal body temperature?

Yes

Record data, e.g., can accurately measure intake and output, describes appropriate clothing and layers of clothing for enviromental temperature. Has designed menu plan to help self gain weight. Record RESOLVED. Delete nursing diagnosis, expected outcome, target date, and nursing actions.

No

Reassess using initial assessment factors.

No

Is diagnosis validated?

Yes

Record new assessment data. Record REVISE. Add new diagnosis, expected outcome, target date, and nursing actions. Delete invalidated diagnosis.

Start new evaluation process.

Record data, e.g., can accurately return-demonstrate temperature measurement, is having trouble with intake and output, and stated "think I need some more help with it." Record CONTINUE and change target date. Modify nursing actions as necessary.

Did evaluation show another problem had arisen?

Yes

No

Finished

Breast-Feeding, Effective

DEFINITION

The state in which a mother-infant dyad-family exhibits adequate proficiency and satisfaction with the breast-feeding process.[23]

NANDA TAXONOMY: MOVING 6.5.1.3

DEFINING CHARACTERISTICS[23]

1. Major defining characteristics
   a. Mother able to position infant at breast to promote a successful latch-on response.
   b. Infant is content after feeding.
   c. Regular and sustained suckling and swallowing at the breast.
   d. Appropriate infant weight patterns for age.
   e. Mother-infant communication patterns (infant cues, maternal interpretation, and response) are effective.

2. Minor defining characteristics
   a. Signs and/or symptoms of oxytocin release (let-down or milk ejection reflex).
   b. Adequate infant elimination patterns for age.
   c. Eagerness of infant to nurse.
   d. Maternal verbalization of satisfaction with the breast-feeding process.

RELATED FACTORS[23]

1. Basic breast-feeding knowledge
2. Normal breast structure
3. Normal infant oral structure
4. Infant gestational age greater than 34 weeks
5. Support sources
6. Maternal confidence

RELATED CLINICAL CONCERNS

Since this is a wellness diagnosis, there are no related clinical concerns.

HAVE YOU SELECTED THE CORRECT DIAGNOSIS?

Ineffective Breast-Feeding   Effective Breast-Feeding is a wellness diagnosis. It signifies a successful experience for both the mother and the baby. If there is a problem with breast-feeding, then the appropriate diagnosis is Ineffective Breast-Feeding. These two diagnoses could be considered to be at opposite ends of a continuum.

Altered Parenting   Effective Breast-Feeding focuses upon the nutrition and growth of the infant rather than the degree of attachment with the infant. Although Effective Breast-Feeding contributes to the attachment of the infant to the mother and the mother to the infant, the supplying of the infant with nutrition by breast-feeding or by formula feeding should be differentiated from attachment processes, which are addressed in Altered Parenting, Risk for or Actual, Role Conflict.

EXPECTED OUTCOMES

1. The infant will have:
   a. Adequate weight gain and return to birth weight by 3 weeks of age
   b. Six or more wet diapers in 24 hours and
   c. At least 2 stools every 24 hours and/or
2. Mother will recognize hunger cues of infant and demonstrate at least 2 breast-feeding techniques by (date).

TARGET DATE

While it usually takes 2 to 3 weeks for the mother and infant to establish a mutual pattern of feeding, an initial target date of 4 days should be set to assure an effective beginning to the breast-feeding process.

NURSING ACTIONS/INTERVENTIONS WITH RATIONALES

Adult Health

For this diagnosis, Women's Health nursing actions serve as the generic actions. This diagnosis would probably not arise on an adult health unit.

Child Health

It is doubtful that this diagnosis would arise on a child health care unit. Please see nursing actions under Women's Health.

Women's Health

NOTE: If the diagnosis of Effective Breast-Feeding has been made, the most appropriate nursing action is continued support for the diagnosis. Successful lactation can be established in any woman who does not have structural anomalies of the milk ducts and who exhibits a desire to breast-feed. Adoptive mothers can breast-feed as well as birthmothers. The following actions serve to facilitate the development of Effective Breast-Feeding.

ACTIONS/INTERVENTIONS	RATIONALES
• Review the mother's knowledge base regarding breast-feeding prior to the initial breast-feeding of the infant.	To determine the basis for assistance and teaching. Avoid unessential repetition for the mother.
• Demonstrate and assist the mother and significant other with correct breast-feeding techniques, e.g., positioning and latch-on.	Successful lactation depends upon understanding the basic how-to's and correct techniques for the actual feeding act.
• Teach mother and significant other basic information related to successful breast-feeding, e.g., milk supply, diet, rest, breast care, breast engorgement, infant hunger cues, and parameters of a healthy infant.	
• Assess the mother's breasts for graspable nipples, surgical scars, skin integrity, and abnormalities prior to the initial breast-feeding of the infant.	Provides the assessment base for diagnosing of potential problems as well as the base for developing strategies for success.
• Assess the infant for ability to breast-feed prior to breast-feeding, e.g., state of awareness or physical abnormalities.	
• Place infant to breast within the first hour after birth unless contraindicated (mother or infant instability) and on cue afterward.	It is important to work with the infant's sleep-wake cycle in establishing breast-feeding after birth. If the infant can successfully suckle immediately after birth, a successful and encouraging pattern is usually established for both the mother and the infant.
• To initiate and maintain lactation when the mother is unable to breast-feed infant, encourage the mother to express breast milk either manually or by using a breast pump at least every 3 h.	This assists in establishing and maintaining the milk supply. It also allows the mother to provide emotional support as well as nutritional support to the infant who cannot breast-feed due to prematurity or illness.
• Observe the infant at breast, noting behavior, position, latch-on, and sucking technique with the initial breast-feeding and then as necessary. Document these observations in the mother's and infant's charts.	
• Encourage the mother and significant other to identify support systems to assist her with meeting her physical and psychosocial needs at home.	The majority of women who are successfully breast-feeding when leaving the hospital quit after 3 wk at home. Support systems are a critical component in the maintenance of successful lactation.[26]
• Encourage mother to drink at least 2000 mL a day, or 8 oz every hour, of fluids.	
• To provide sufficient amounts of calcium, protein, and calories, encourage the mother to eat a wide variety of foods from the 4 basic food groups.	Breast-feeding mothers should increase their caloric intake to 2000 to 2500 cal/day in order to maintain successful lactation.
• Encourage the mother to breast-feed at least every 2–3 h for a minimum of 10 min per side to establish milk supply, and then to regulate feeding according to infant's demands.	Newborns need frequent feeding to satisfy their hunger and to establish their feeding patterns. It is important that the mother understand the infant's suckling will determine the supply and demand of breast milk.
• Monitor the infant's output for number of wet diapers. Document the number of diapers and the color of urine. (Remember, there should be at least 6 in a 24-h period.)	Helps to determine intake and nutritional status of infant.
• Weigh the infant at least every third day and record.	
• Assist the mother in planning a day's activities when breast-feeding to ensure that the mother gets sufficient rest.	Helps the new mother to establish a schedule that is beneficial for both mother and infant.
• Encourage advanced planning for the working mother if she intends to continue to breast-feed after returning to work.	

- Involve the father or significant other in breast-feeding by encouraging the "provider-protector" role.

The breast-feeding mother requires a lot of support and encouragement. Fathers can supply this by providing her with time for rest and assistance with infant care. For example, the father can bring the infant to the mother at night rather than the mother having to get up each time for the feeding. Fathers can intervene with family and friends to provide nursing mothers privacy and quiet.

Psychiatric Health

This diagnosis will not be applicable in a mental health setting.

Gerontic Health

This diagnosis is not applicable in gerontic health.

Home Health

The Home Health nursing actions for this diagnosis are the same as those for Women's Health.

Breast-Feeding, Effective

FLOWCHART EVALUATION: EXPECTED OUTCOME 1

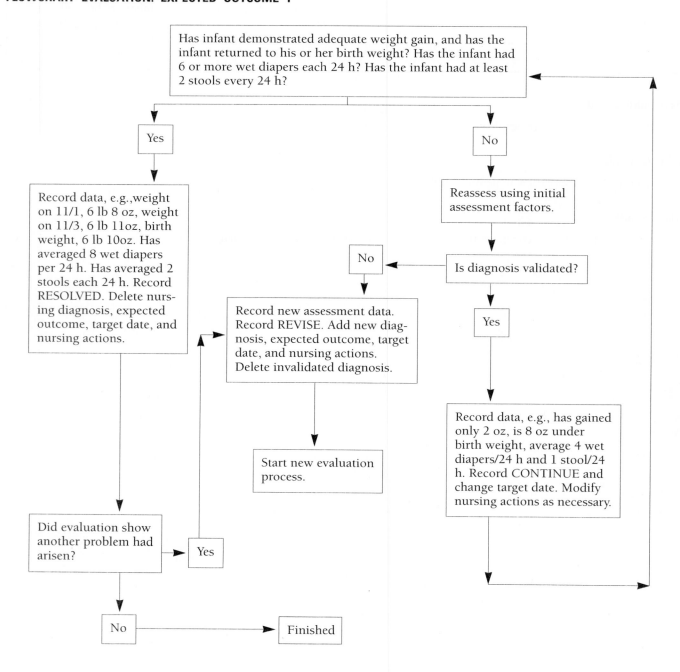

Has infant demonstrated adequate weight gain, and has the infant returned to his or her birth weight? Has the infant had 6 or more wet diapers each 24 h? Has the infant had at least 2 stools every 24 h?

Yes

No

Record data, e.g.,weight on 11/1, 6 lb 8 oz, weight on 11/3, 6 lb 11oz, birth weight, 6 lb 10oz. Has averaged 8 wet diapers per 24 h. Has averaged 2 stools each 24 h. Record RESOLVED. Delete nursing diagnosis, expected outcome, target date, and nursing actions.

Reassess using initial assessment factors.

No

Is diagnosis validated?

Yes

Record new assessment data. Record REVISE. Add new diagnosis, expected outcome, target date, and nursing actions. Delete invalidated diagnosis.

Start new evaluation process.

Record data, e.g., has gained only 2 oz, is 8 oz under birth weight, average 4 wet diapers/24 h and 1 stool/24 h. Record CONTINUE and change target date. Modify nursing actions as necessary.

Did evaluation show another problem had arisen?

Yes

No

Finished

Breast-Feeding, Effective

FLOWCHART EVALUATION: EXPECTED OUTCOME 2

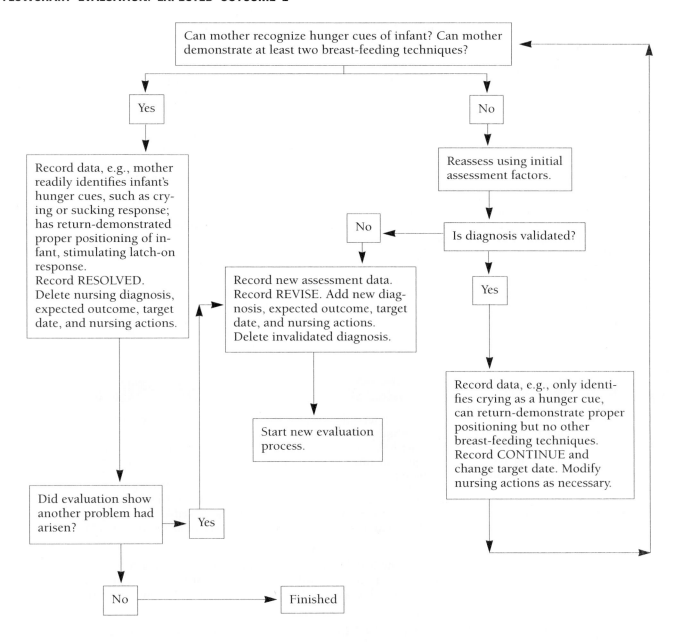

Breast-Feeding, Ineffective

DEFINITION

The state in which a mother, infant, or child experiences dissatisfaction or difficulty with the breast-feeding process.[23]

NANDA TAXONOMY: MOVING 6.5.1.2

DEFINING CHARACTERISTICS[23]

1. Major defining characteristics
   a. Unsatisfactory breast-feeding process
2. Minor defining characteristics
   a. Actual or perceived inadequate milk supply
   b. Inability of infant to attach onto maternal breast correctly
   c. No observable signs of oxytocin release
   d. Observable signs of inadequate infant intake
   e. Nonsustained sucking at the breast
   f. Insufficient emptying of each breast per feeding
   g. Persistence of sore nipples beyond the first week of breast-feeding
   h. Insufficient opportunity for sucking at the breast
   i. Infant exhibiting fussiness and crying within the first hour after breast-feeding; unresponsiveness to other comfort measures
   j. Infant arching and crying at the breast, resisting latching on

RELATED FACTORS[23]

1. Prematurity
2. Infant anomaly
3. Maternal breast anomaly
4. Previous breast surgery
5. Previous history of breast-feeding failure
6. Infant receiving supplemental feedings with artificial nipple
7. Poor infant sucking reflex
8. Nonsupportive partner or family
9. Knowledge deficit
10. Interruption in breast-feeding
11. Maternal anxiety or ambivalence

RELATED CLINICAL CONCERNS

1. Any diseases of the breast
2. Cleft lip; cleft palate
3. Failure to thrive
4. Prematurity
5. Child abuse

STOP

HAVE YOU SELECTED THE CORRECT DIAGNOSIS?

Ineffective Breast-Feeding should be differentiated from the patient's concern over whether she wants to breast-feed or not. Although a mother who does not want to breast-feed will more than likely be ineffective in her breast-feeding attempts, ineffective breast-feeding can be related to problems other than just an unwillingness to breast-feed. Other diagnoses that might need to be differentiated include:

Anxiety   Anxiety is defined as a vague, uneasy feeling, the source of which is often nonspecific or unknown to the individual. If an expression of perceived threat to self-concept, health status, socioeconomic status, role functioning, or interaction patterns is made, this would constitute the diagnosis of Anxiety.

Altered Parenting   Altered Parenting is defined as the inability of the nurturing figures to create an environment that promotes optimum growth and development of another human being. Adjustment to parenting, in general, is a normal maturation process following the birth of a child.

Altered Growth and Development: Self-Care Skills   This diagnosis is defined according to a demonstrated deviation from age-group norms for self-care. Inadequate caretaking would be defined according to specific behavior and attitudes of the individual mother or infant.

Ineffective Individual Coping   This diagnosis is defined as the inability of the individual to deal with situations that require coping or adaptation to meet life's demands and roles. All the changes secondary to the birth of a new baby could result in this diagnosis.

EXPECTED OUTCOMES

1. Will verbalize increased satisfaction with breast-feeding process by (date) and/or
2. Infant will require no supplemental feedings by (date)

TARGET DATES

Because Ineffective Breast-Feeding can be physically detrimental to the infant as well as emotionally detrimental to the mother, an initial target date of 3 days would be best.

NURSING ACTIONS/INTERVENTIONS WITH RATIONALES

Adult Health

For this nursing diagnosis, the Women's Health nursing actions serve as the generic nursing actions.

Child Health

ACTIONS/INTERVENTIONS	RATIONALES

• Monitor for factors contributing to infant's ability to suck:
  ○ Structural abnormalities, e.g., cleft lip or palate
  ○ Altered level of consciousness, seizures, or CNS damage
  ○ Mechanical barriers to sucking, e.g., endotracheal tube or ventilator
  ○ Pain or underlying altered comfort or medication
  ○ Prematurity with diminished sucking ability
	Assessment of infant's ability to suck. Will assist in meeting goals for effective breast-feeding.

• Determine the effect the altered or impaired breast-feeding has on mother and infant by providing at least one 30-min period per day for talking with mother. Monitor maternal feelings expressed, maternal-infant behaviors observed, and excessive crying or unrelenting fussiness in infant.	The maternal-infant responses will provide the essential database in determining how serious the breast-feeding issues are. This information will dictate how to approach the problem and promote realistic follow-up.
• To the degree possible, provide emotional support for infant in instances of temporary inability to breast-feed, e.g., gavage feedings with appropriate cuddling. Include parents in care. Allow infant to suck on pacifier if possible.	Provides temporary substitutions for breast-feeding that promote trust and sense of security for infant. Also, bonding with mother is still possible.
• Coordinate parents' visitation with infant to best facilitate successful breast-feeding in such areas as rest, natural hunger cycles, and comfort of all involved.	
• Assist with plan to manage impaired breast-feeding to best provide support to all involved, e.g., breast-pumping for period of time with support for this effort until normal breast-feeding can be resumed. Breast milk may be frozen or even given in gavage feeding. Support mother's choice for whatever alternatives chosen.	Maintaining the mother's confidence in breast-feeding and supporting her choice for alternative feeding demonstrate the valuing of her beliefs.

Women's Health

ACTIONS/INTERVENTIONS	RATIONALES
• Ascertain mother's desire to breast-feed infant through careful interviewing and reviewing of mother's knowledge of breast-feeding.	Provides intervention base for nursing actions. Allows planning of support, teaching, and evaluation of motives and desires to breast-feed.
• List the advantages and disadvantages of breast-feeding for the mother.	Assists the mother to make an informed decision about breast-feeding.
• Obtain a breast-feeding and bottle-feeding history from the mother, e.g., did she breast-feed before, and if so, was it successful or unsuccessful?	
• Allow for uninterrupted breast-feeding periods.	Providing the mother and infant with uninterrupted breast-feeding times allows them to become acquainted with each other and allows time for learning different breast-feeding techniques.
• Collaborate with physician, lactation consultant, perinatal clinical nurse specialist, etc., to determine ways to make abnormal breast structure amenable for breast-feeding.	Assists mother who has strong desire to breast-feed to be successful.

Continued

ACTIONS/INTERVENTIONS	RATIONALES
• Observe mother with infant during breast-feeding. Explain and demonstrate methods to increase infant sucking reflex. Demonstrate to mother various positions for breast-feeding and how to alternate positions with each feeding to prevent nipple soreness, e.g., sitting up, lying down, using football hold, holding baby "tummy to tummy," using pillows for mother's comfort, or using pillows for supporting baby.	Provides basic information and visible support to assist with successful breast-feeding.
• Ascertain mother's need for privacy during breast-feeding.	Promotes mother's comfort with the physical act of breast-feeding.

• Monitor for poor or dysfunctional sucking by checking:
  ○ Position mother is using to hold baby
  ○ Baby's mouth position on areola and nipple
  ○ Position of baby's head, e.g., inappropriate hyperextension
	Proper positioning facilitates satisfaction with breast-feeding for both mother and baby.

• Ascertain mother's support for breast-feeding from others, e.g., husband or significant other, patient's mother, obstetrician, pediatrician, and nurses on postpartum unit.	Support from others is essential in attaining successful breast-feeding.
• Discuss infant's needs and frequency of feedings.	Provides basic information and visible support to assist with successful breast-feeding.
• Assist mother in planning a day's activities when breast-feeding, ensuring that the mother gets plenty of rest.	Provides information necessary for the mother to plan the basics of her self-care.

• Teach patient:
  ○ The proper diet for the breast-feeding mother, listing important food groups and necessary calories to adequately maintain milk production
  ○ The idea of advanced planning for the working mother who plans to breast-feed
  ○ That it takes time to establish breast-feeding (usually a month)
  ○ The use of various hand pumps, battery-operated pumps, and electric pumps
  ○ How to hand-express breast milk
  ○ How to properly store expressed breast milk	

• Schedule specific times for consultation and support for the mother. Plan at least 30 min per shift (while awake) for talking with mother.	
• If baby is separated from mother, such as in NICU, involve baby's nurses in planning with mother routines and times for breast-feeding infant.	
• Refer mother to breast-feeding support groups.	Provides basic information and visible support to assist with successful breast-feeding.
• For the mother who has had a cesarean section, place a pillow over the abdomen before putting infant to breast.	Assists in keeping pressure off the incision line while breast-feeding.
• Assist the mother of a premature baby to pump breast routinely to initiate milk production.	
• Demonstrate proper storage and transportation of breast milk for the premature baby.	Basic teaching to ensure safe nutrition for infant.

• Assist mother who has to wean a premature baby from tube feedings to breast-feeding by:
  ○ Teaching mother to place infant at the breast several times a day and during tube feeding
  ○ Encouraging mother to hold, cuddle, and interact with infant during tube feedings
  ○ Allowing mother and infant privacy to begin interaction with breast-feeding
  ○ Being available to assist with infant during breast-feeding interaction
  ○ Reassuring mother it might take several attempts before baby begins to breast-feed
	Provides needed support during this process.

- Give breast-feeding mothers copies of educational materials.
- If breast-feeding is not possible due to an infant physical deformity, teach the mother how to pump breasts and how to feed infant breast milk in bottles with special nipples.
- Encourage maternal attachment behavior.

Provides a readily available information source.

Allows the mother the option of breast-feeding in the event that the deformity can be surgically corrected.

Assists mother in adjustment to parenting and effective caretaking of infant.

Psychiatric Health

Refer to Women's Health nursing actions for interventions related to this diagnosis.

Gerontic Health

This diagnosis is not appropriate for gerontic health.

Home Health

ACTIONS/INTERVENTIONS	RATIONALES
• Teach measures to promote effective breast-feeding, e.g., quiet environment, adequate nutrition and hydration, appropriate technique, and family support.	Knowledge and support increase the likelihood of a positive outcome.
• Assist client and family in identifying risk factors pertinent to the situation: ○ Premature infant ○ Infant anomaly ○ Maternal breast dysfunction ○ Infection ○ Previous breast surgery ○ Supplemental bottle feedings ○ Nonsupportive family ○ Lack of knowledge ○ Anxiety	Identification of and early interventions in high-risk situations provide the opportunity to prevent problems.
• Consult with or refer to appropriate resources as indicated.	Appropriate and cost-effective use of available resources.

Breast-Feeding, Ineffective

FLOWCHART EVALUATION: EXPECTED OUTCOME 1

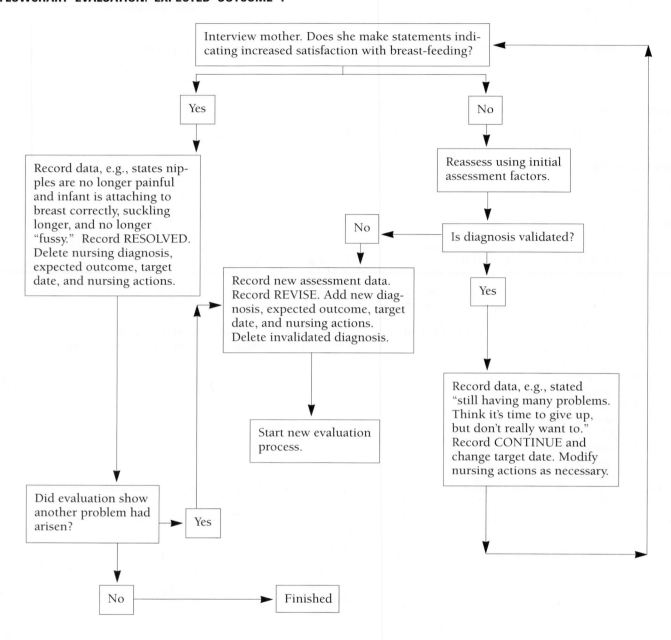

Interview mother. Does she make statements indicating increased satisfaction with breast-feeding?

Yes

No

Record data, e.g., states nipples are no longer painful and infant is attaching to breast correctly, suckling longer, and no longer "fussy." Record RESOLVED. Delete nursing diagnosis, expected outcome, target date, and nursing actions.

Reassess using initial assessment factors.

No

Is diagnosis validated?

Record new assessment data. Record REVISE. Add new diagnosis, expected outcome, target date, and nursing actions. Delete invalidated diagnosis.

Yes

Start new evaluation process.

Record data, e.g., stated "still having many problems. Think it's time to give up, but don't really want to." Record CONTINUE and change target date. Modify nursing actions as necessary.

Did evaluation show another problem had arisen?

Yes

No

Finished

Breast-Feeding, Ineffective

FLOWCHART EVALUATION: EXPECTED OUTCOME 2

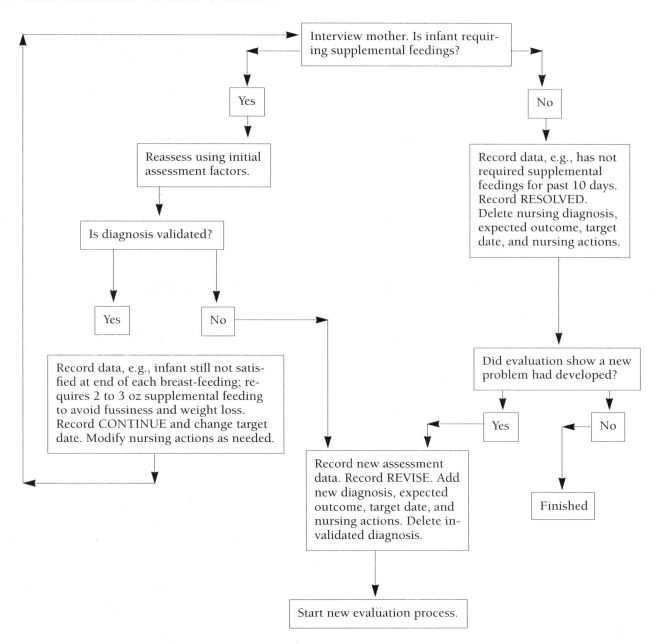

Breast-Feeding, Interrupted

DEFINITION

A break in the continuity of the breast-feeding process as a result of inability or inadvisability to put baby to breast for feeding.[23]

NANDA TAXONOMY: MOVING 6.5.1.2.1

DEFINING CHARACTERISTICS[23]

1. Major defining characteristics
   a. Infant not receiving nourishment at the breast for some or all of feedings
2. Minor defining characteristics
   a. Maternal desire to maintain lactation and provide (or eventually provide) her breast milk for her infant's nutritional needs
   b. Separation of mother and infant
   c. Lack of knowledge regarding expression and storage of breast milk

RELATED FACTORS[23]

1. Maternal or infant illness
2. Prematurity
3. Maternal employment
4. Contraindications to breast-feeding (e.g., drugs or true breast milk jaundice)
5. Need to abruptly wean infant

RELATED CLINICAL CONCERNS

1. Any condition requiring emergency admission of mother to hospital
2. Any condition requiring emergency admission of infant to hospital
3. Prematurity
4. Postpartum depression

HAVE YOU SELECTED THE CORRECT DIAGNOSIS?

Ineffective Breast-Feeding With Ineffective Breast-Feeding, there is expressed dissatisfaction or problems with breast-feeding. With Interrupted Breast-Feeding, there is no expressed dissatisfaction or major problems; however, breast-feeding has temporarily ceased due to factors beyond the mother's control.

Ineffective Infant Feeding Pattern In this diagnosis, there is a defined problem with the infant's ability to suck, swallow, and breathe. Breast-feeding for this infant has not ever been successful. With Interrupted Breast-Feeding, the infant has no problems with sucking or swallowing and the stoppage of breast-feeding can be overcome by storing breast milk and feeding the infant via a bottle.

EXPECTED OUTCOMES

1. Family will have designed a plan to overcome Interrupted Breast-Feeding by (date) and/or
2. Infant will demonstrate no weight loss secondary to adaptations for Interrupted Breast-Feeding by (date)

TARGET DATES

Since this interruption might occur as a result of an emergency, initial evaluation should occur within 24 hours after the initial diagnosis. Thereafter, target dates can be moved to every 3 days.

NURSING ACTIONS/INTERVENTIONS WITH RATIONALES

Adult Health

ACTIONS/INTERVENTIONS	RATIONALES

• Arrange care activities to facilitate mother's breast-feeding of infant according to feeding schedule of mother-infant dyad.
• Encourage continuation of breast-feeding:
  ○ Arrange special visitation privileges for infant and infant's caregiver during the time of the mother's hospitalization.
  ○ Provide privacy for family.
  ○ Collaborate with diet therapist regarding mother's nutritional needs during this time.
	Supports continued successful breast-feeding, attachment, and bonding.

- ◦ Provide breast pump for mother, and assist with breast pumping as needed every 3–4 h.
- • Collaborate with perinatal clinical nurse specialist and/or lactation consultant regarding maintenance of breast-feeding.

Helps relieve engorgement. Milk can be stored and used to feed infant.
Provides needed consultation for nurse and her patient.

Child Health

ACTIONS/INTERVENTIONS	RATIONALES
• Monitor for infant's ability to suck. Encourage sucking on a regular basis, especially if gavage feedings are a part of the therapeutic regimen.	Provides basic data critical to success. In times of non-breast-feeding, it is beneficial to encourage sucking to reinforce the feeding time as pleasurable and to enhance digestion unless contraindicated by a surgical or medical condition, e.g., cleft repair of lip or palate, prolonged NPO with concerns for air swallowing. Feedback may provide essential valuing during times of stress.

• Provide support for the mother-infant dyad to facilitate breast-feeding satisfaction.
• Monitor infant cues suggesting satisfaction:
  ◦ Weight gain appropriate for status
  ◦ Ability to sleep at intervals
	The fact that the infant's satisfaction and input are valued provides a critical component in the entire process of breast-feeding.

Women's Health

ACTIONS/INTERVENTIONS	RATIONALES

• Provide appropriate information on why breast-feeding needs to be interrupted. Be specific about length of time, e.g., days, weeks, or months, and offer options for maintaining breast milk until able to resume breast-feeding.[26–28]
• Describe routine for pumping, expressing, and storing breast milk during emergency period.
• Contact lactation consultant and/or perinatal nurse who can assist with plan of nursing care and with maintenance of breast milk during mother's illness, e.g., emergency surgery, medical regimen (medications) that contradict breast-feeding, or injury requiring hospitalization of mother.[29,30]
• Provide mother with appropriate information about breast pumps and how to obtain one (rent or buy) to aid in expression of breast milk, e.g., semiautomatic breast pump, automatic breast pump, battery-operated breast pump, or manual breast pump.
• Demonstrate and have mother return-demonstrate proper assembly and use of breast pump.
• Assist mother in learning manual expression of breast milk.[30]
  ◦ Good handwashing technique before expressing milk
  ◦ Correct positioning of hand and fingers so as not to damage breast tissue
  ◦ Sterile wide-mouth funnel and bottle for storage of breast milk
• Discuss options for maintaining breast-feeding with the mother who is returning to work. Provide assistance to help mother establish feeding schedule with work schedule, e.g., breast-feed a.m. and p.m., pumping at noon, etc.[28–30]
	Assists breast-feeding families in establishing and maintaining breast-feeding capabilities when it is inadvisable or impossible to put baby to breast for feeding.

Continued

ACTIONS/INTERVENTIONS	RATIONALES
• Discuss options for maintaining breast-feeding with the mother who is returning to work. Provide assistance to help mother establish feeding schedule with work schedule, e.g., breast-feed a.m. and p.m., pumping at noon, etc.[28-30] • Provide resources, e.g., printed materials or consultant, to assist mother when negotiating with employer for time and place to pump or breast-feed during working hours.[30] • Assist mother and family to arrange schedule to bring infant to her during working hours. • Encourage mother and significant other to verbalize their frustrations and concerns about establishing and maintaining lactation when the infant is ill or premature.[31-34] • Refer to lactation consultant or clinical nurse specialist who can support parents and assist nurse in developing a program of breast-feeding or supplementing of infant with mother's breast milk.[35]	Provides basic information that assists in promoting effective breast-feeding.

Psychiatric Health

This diagnosis will not, in all likelihood, be applicable in a mental health setting. Should a mother be admitted with a mental health–related diagnosis, the physician would probably suggest changing the infant to bottle-feedings. Should the physician agree that breast-feeding could continue, the adult health actions would be applicable for the mental health client.

Gerontic Health

This diagnosis is not appropriate for gerontic health.

Home Health

NOTE: If home care is needed because of either mother or infant illness or disability, the nurse will need to address the underlying problem in order to promote Effective Breast-Feeding. It is not likely that home health care would be initiated if the only diagnosis was Effective Breast-Feeding; however, there are lactation consultants whose entire practice is home health. This practice has been specifically designed to assist with maintenance of successful lactation.

ACTIONS/INTERVENTIONS	RATIONALES
• Support mother, infant, and family dynamics for successful breast-feeding. • Recognize cultural variations in feeding practices when assessing effectiveness of breast-feeding. • Provide additional education or referrals as requested or as situation changes.	Encouragement and support increase the potential for positive outcomes. Feeding patterns vary according to cultural norms. Community-based support is ongoing; early intervention as the situation changes increases the potential for continued effectiveness.

Breast-Feeding, Interrupted

FLOWCHART EVALUATION: EXPECTED OUTCOME 1

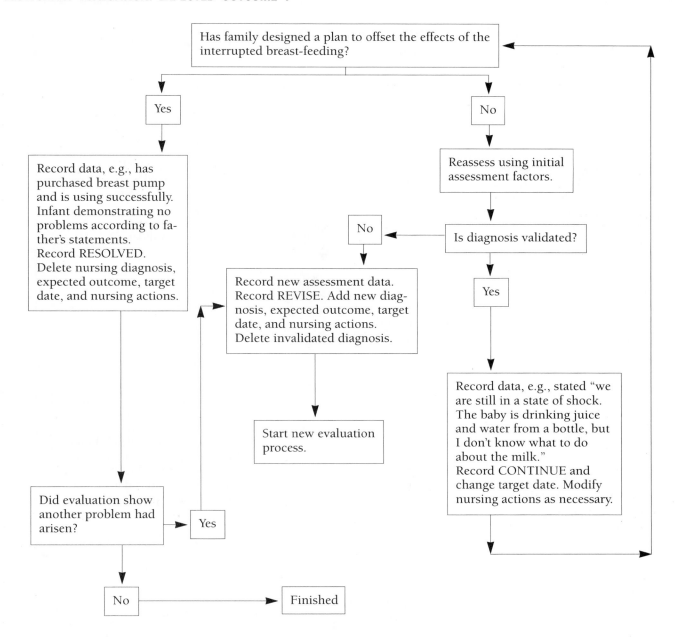

Has family designed a plan to offset the effects of the interrupted breast-feeding?

Yes

No

Record data, e.g., has purchased breast pump and is using successfully. Infant demonstrating no problems according to father's statements.
Record RESOLVED.
Delete nursing diagnosis, expected outcome, target date, and nursing actions.

Reassess using initial assessment factors.

No

Is diagnosis validated?

Record new assessment data.
Record REVISE. Add new diagnosis, expected outcome, target date, and nursing actions.
Delete invalidated diagnosis.

Yes

Start new evaluation process.

Record data, e.g., stated "we are still in a state of shock. The baby is drinking juice and water from a bottle, but I don't know what to do about the milk."
Record CONTINUE and change target date. Modify nursing actions as necessary.

Did evaluation show another problem had arisen?

Yes

No

Finished

Breast-Feeding, Interrupted

FLOWCHART EVALUATION: EXPECTED OUTCOME 2

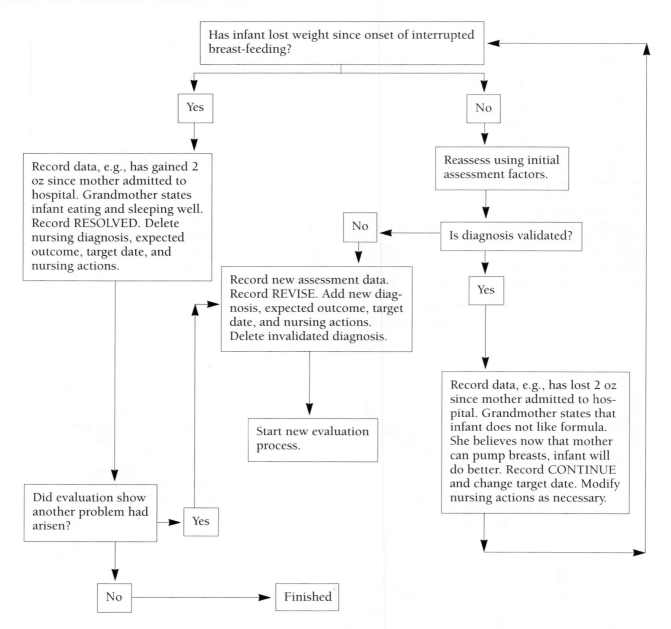

Has infant lost weight since onset of interrupted breast-feeding?

Yes

No

Record data, e.g., has gained 2 oz since mother admitted to hospital. Grandmother states infant eating and sleeping well. Record RESOLVED. Delete nursing diagnosis, expected outcome, target date, and nursing actions.

Reassess using initial assessment factors.

No

Is diagnosis validated?

Record new assessment data. Record REVISE. Add new diagnosis, expected outcome, target date, and nursing actions. Delete invalidated diagnosis.

Yes

Start new evaluation process.

Record data, e.g., has lost 2 oz since mother admitted to hospital. Grandmother states that infant does not like formula. She believes now that mother can pump breasts, infant will do better. Record CONTINUE and change target date. Modify nursing actions as necessary.

Did evaluation show another problem had arisen?

Yes

No

Finished

Fluid-Volume Deficit, Risk for or Actual

DEFINITION

The state in which an individual experiences decreased intravascular, interstitial, and/or intracellular fluid.[23]

NANDA TAXONOMY: EXCHANGING 1.4.1.2.2.1 AND 1.4.1.2.2.2

DEFINING CHARACTERISTICS[23]

1. Major defining characteristics
   A. Risk for Fluid-Volume Deficit
      (1) Extremes of age
      (2) Extremes of weight
      (3) Excessive losses through normal routes, for example, diarrhea
      (4) Loss of fluid through abnormal routes, for example, indwelling tubes
      (5) Deviations affecting access to or intake or absorption of fluids, for example, physical immobility
      (6) Factors influencing fluid needs, for example, hypermetabolic state
      (7) Knowledge deficiency related to fluid volume
      (8) Medications, for example, diuretics

   B. Actual Fluid-Volume Deficit
      (1) Decreased urine output
      (2) Increased urine concentration
      (3) Sudden weight loss or gain
      (4) Decreased venous filling
      (5) Increased hematocrit
      (6) Decreased blood pressure
      (7) Decreased skin/tongue turgor
      (8) Dry skin/mucous membranes
2. Minor defining characteristics
   None given.

RELATED FACTORS[23]

   A. Risk for Fluid-Volume Deficit:
      The risk factors also serve as the related factors for this diagnosis.
   B. Actual Fluid-Volume Deficit:
      1. Active fluid-volume loss
      2. Failure of regulatory mechanisms

RELATED CLINICAL CONCERNS

   1. Addison's disease (adrenal insufficiency or crisis)
   2. Hemorrhage
   3. Burns
   4. AIDS
   5. Crohn's disease
   6. Vomiting and diarrhea
   7. Ulcerative colitis

HAVE YOU SELECTED THE CORRECT DIAGNOSIS?

Altered Oral Mucous Membrane and Altered Nutrition, Less Than Body Requirements The client may not be able to ingest food or fluid because of primary problems in the mouth, or the client may not be ingesting enough food from which the body can absorb fluids.

Altered Bowel Elimination, Diarrhea or Altered Urinary Elimination, Incontinence This diagnosis may be causing an extreme loss of fluid before it can be absorbed and used by the body.

Impaired Skin Integrity This diagnosis could be the primary problem. For example, the patient who has been burned has grossly impaired skin integrity. The skin is supposed to regulate the amount of fluid lost from it. If there is relatively little intact skin, the skin is unable to perform its regulatory function and there is significant loss of fluid and electrolytes.

Self-Care Deficit or Altered Parenting In the infant or young child, the problem may primarily be a Self-Care Deficit or Altered Parenting. The infant or young child is not able to obtain the fluid he or she wants and must depend on others. If the parents are unable to recognize or meet these needs, then the infant or young child may have a Risk for or Actual Fluid-Volume Deficit. Even in an adult, the primary nursing diagnosis may be Self-Care Deficit. Again, if the adult is unable to obtain the fluid he or she requires because of some pathophysiologic problem, then he or she may have a Risk for or Actual Fluid-Volume Deficit.

EXPECTED OUTCOMES

1. Intake and output will balance within 200 mL by (date) and/or
2. Will describe (number) factors influencing adequate hydration and methods to prevent fluid-volume deficit by (date)

TARGET DATES

Normally, intake and output will approximately balance only every 72 hours; thus, an appropriate target date would be 3 days.

NURSING ACTIONS/INTERVENTIONS WITH RATIONALES
Adult Health

ACTIONS/INTERVENTIONS	RATIONALES

• Measure and record total intake and output every shift:
  ○ Check intake and output hourly.
  ○ Observe and document color and consistency of all urine, stools, and vomitus.
  ○ Check urine specific gravity every 4 h at (state times here)
	Determines fluid loss and need for replacement.

• Take vital signs every 2 h on (odd/even) hour, and include apical pulse.	Permits monitoring of cardiovascular response to illness state and replacement therapy.
• Monitor intravenous fluids. (See Altered Nutrition, Less Than Body Requirements, Additional Information, pp. 165).	Monitoring of fluid replacement and prevention of fluid overload.

• Monitor:
  ○ Skin turgor at least every 4 h at (state times here) while awake
  ○ Electrolytes, blood urea nitrogen, hematocrit, and hemoglobin (Collaborate with physician regarding frequency of lab tests)
  ○ Central venous pressure every hour (if appropriate)
  ○ Mental status and behavior at least every 2 h on the (odd/even) hour
  ○ For signs and symptoms of shock at least every 4 h at (state times here), e.g., weakness, diaphoresis, hypotension, tachycardia, or tachypnea
	Essential monitoring for fluid and electrolyte imbalance.

• Weigh daily at (state time here). Teach patient to weigh at same time each day in same-weight clothing.	Monitoring for fluid replacement. Allows consistent comparison of weight.

• Force fluids to a minimum of 2000 mL daily:
  ○ Ascertain patient's fluid likes and dislikes (list here).
  ○ Offer small amount of fluid (4–5 oz) at least every hour while awake and at every awakening during night.
  ○ Offer fluids at temperature that is most acceptable to patient, e.g., warm or cool.
  ○ Interspace fluids with high-fluid-content foods, e.g., popsicles, gelatin, pudding, ice cream, or watermelon. Note patient's preferences here.	

• Administer medications as ordered, e.g., antidiarrheal or antiemetics. Monitor medication effects.	
• Assist patient to eat and drink as necessary. Provide positive verbal support for patient's consuming fluid.	Prevents dehydration and easily replaces fluid loss without resorting to IVs. Frequent fluids improve hydration; variation in fluids is helpful to encourage patient to increase intake.
• Administer or assist with oral hygiene after each meal and before bedtime.	Cleans and lubricates the mouth. Encourages patient to eat and drink.
• Turn and properly position patient at least every 2 h on (odd/even) hour. • Encourage patient to alter position frequently. • Provide active and passive ROM every 4 h at (state times here) while awake.	Prevents stasis of fluids in any one part of body. Assists in circulation of fluid.
• Schedule at least 1-h rest periods for patient at least 4 times a day at (times).	Prevents overexertion and extra strain on circulatory system.

• If temperature elevation develops:
  ○ Maintain cool room temperature.
  ○ Offer cool, clear liquids.
  ○ Administer ordered antipyretics.
  ○ Give tepid sponge bath.	

ACTIONS/INTERVENTIONS	RATIONALES
o Remove heavy and excess clothing and bed covers.	Assists in reducing fluid loss due to perspiration, etc.
• If gastric tube is present:	
o Use only normal saline for irrigation.	
o Monitor amount of oral intake of water and ice chips. Avoid if at all possible. Offer commercial electrolyte replenishment solutions if permitted, e.g., Gatorade or 10K.	Avoids altering of electrolyte balance which, in turn, may alter fluid-volume balance.
• Teach patient, prior to discharge, to increase fluid intake at home during:	
o Elevated temperature episodes	
o Periods when infection and elevated temperatures are present	
o Periods of exercise	
o Hot weather	
• Measures to ensure adequate hydration:	Supports patient's self-care by pointing out measures he or she can use to control fluid imbalance. Adequate intake and early intervention will prevent undesirable outcomes.
o Need to drink fluids before feeling of thirst is experienced	
o Recognizing signs and symptoms of dehydration such as dry skin, dry lips, excessive sweating, dry tongue, and decreased skin turgor	
o How to measure, record, and evaluate intake and output	
• Refer to other health care professionals as necessary.	Provides support and fosters cost-effective collaboration through use of readily available resources.

Child Health

ACTIONS/INTERVENTIONS	RATIONALES
• Measure and record total intake every shift:	A 24-h fluid assessment will be meaningful for diagnosing deficits and also provide a basis for replacement needs. Specific gravity is a good indicator of degree of hydration.
o Check intake and output hourly (may require weighing diapers or insertion of a Foley catheter [infants may require use of a 5 or 8 feeding tube if size 10 Foley is too large]).	
o Check urine specific gravity every 2 h on (odd/even) hour or every voiding or as otherwise ordered.	
• Force fluids to a minimum appropriate for size (will be closely related to electrolyte needs and cardiac, respiratory, and renal status):	Prompt replacement and maintenance of appropriate fluids will prevent further circulatory or systemic problems. Specific attention is also required with respect to sodium, potassium, and caloric intake. Infants are subject to fluid-volume depletion because of their relatively greater surface area, higher metabolic rate, and immature renal function.[36]
o Infant: 70–100 mL/kg in 24 h	
o Toddler: 55–70 mL/kg in 24 h	
o School-age child: 20–50 mL/kg in 24 h	
• Weigh patient daily at same time of day, on same scale and in same clothing (infants without diaper).	Accuracy of weight readings cannot be overstressed. The weight often serves as a major indicator of the effectiveness of the treatment regimen. Iatrogenic problems are more likely to occur with inaccuracies.
• Assist in individualizing oral intake to best suit the patient's needs and preferences. Include parents in designing this plan.	When options exist, honoring them facilitates better compliance with goals and helps the patient and family to feel valued.

Women's Health

ACTIONS/INTERVENTIONS	RATIONALES

• Assist patient to identify lifestyle factors that could be contributing to symptoms of nausea and vomiting during early pregnancy:
  ◦ Identify patient's support system.
  ◦ Monitor patient's feelings (positive or negative) about pregnancy.
  ◦ Evaluate social, economic, and cultural conditions.
  ◦ Involve significant others in discussion and problem-solving activities regarding physiologic changes of pregnancy that are affecting work habits and interpersonal relationships (e.g., nausea and vomiting).
	Provides basis for treatment of symptoms and basis for teaching and support strategies.

• Teach patient measures that can help alleviate pathophysiologic changes of pregnancy. In collaboration with dietitian:
  ◦ Obtain dietary history.
  ◦ Assist patient in planning diet that will provide adequate nutrition for her and her fetus' needs.	

• Teach methods of coping with gastric upset, nausea, and vomiting:
  ◦ Eat bland, low-fat foods (no fried or spicy foods).
  ◦ Increase carbohydrate intake.
  ◦ Eat small amounts of food every 2 h (avoid empty stomach).
  ◦ Eat dry crackers or toast before getting up in the morning.
  ◦ Take vitamins and iron with night meal before going to bed (vitamin B, 50 mg, can be taken twice a day but never on an empty stomach).
  ◦ Drink high-protein liquids (e.g., soups or eggnog).[5]
	Provides information, education, and support for self-care during pregnancy.

• Monitor patient for:
  ◦ Variances in appetite
  ◦ Vomiting first 16 wk (beyond 12 wk) of pregnancy
  ◦ Weight loss
  ◦ Intractable nausea and vomiting
	Provides basis for therapeutic intervention if necessary as well as support of patient which can decrease fear and feelings of helplessness.

• Collaborate with physician regarding monitoring for:
  ◦ Electrolyte imbalance: Hemoconcentration, ketosis with ketonuria, hyponatremia, hypokalemia
  ◦ Dehydration (*Note:* "During pregnancy, gastric acid secretion normally is reduced because of increased estrogen stimulation. This places the women at risk for alkalosis rather than the acidosis that usually occurs in an advanced stage of dehydration."[5])
  ◦ Hydration (approximately 3000 mL/24 h) and providing vitamin supplements
  ◦ Restriction of oral intake and providing parental administration of fluids and vitamins (*Note:* "Vitamin B_6 has been found effective and safe for use in nausea and vomiting of pregnancy."[5])
	Provides support and information to increase self-awareness and self-care.

• Allow expression of feelings and encourage verbalization of fears and questions by scheduling at least 30 min with patient at least once per shift.	

• Provide patient and family with diet information for the breast-feeding mother to prevent dehydration:
  ◦ Increase daily fluid intake.
  ◦ Drink at least 20 mL of fluid daily.
	Provides information that allows for successful lactation and healthy recovery from childbirth.

- ○ Extra fluid can be taken just before each breast-feeding (e.g., water, fruit juices, decaffeinated tea, or milk).
- ○ Eat well-balanced meals that include the four basic food groups.
- Teach the parents the fluid intake needs of the newborn. The newborn should be taking in approximately 420 mL soon after birth and building to 1200 mL at the end of 3 mo.
- Monitor newborn for fluid deficit, and teach parents to monitor via the following factors:
  - ○ "Fussy baby" especially immediately after feeding
  - ○ Constipation (remember, breast-fed babies have fewer stools than formula-fed babies)
  - ○ Weight loss or slow weight gain
- Evaluate baby, mother, and nursing routine:
  - ○ Is baby getting empty calories (e.g., a lot of water between feedings)?
  - ○ Monitor infant for nipple confusion from switching baby from breast to bottle and vice versa many times.
  - ○ Count number of diapers per day (should have 6–8 really wet diapers per day).
  - ○ Monitor infant for intolerance to mother's milk or bottle formula.
- Monitor baby for illness or lactose intolerances.
- Monitor how often mother is nursing infant (infrequent nursing can cause slow weight gain).

Provides information and support for healthy growth and development of newborn.

Psychiatric Health

ACTIONS/INTERVENTIONS	RATIONALES
• If client is confused or unable to interpret signs of thirst, place on intake and output measurement, and record this information every shift.	Medications and/or clouded consciousness may effect client's ability to recognize need for fluids.
• Evaluate potential for fluid deficit resulting from medication or medication interaction, e.g., lithium and diuretics. If this presents a risk, place client on intake and output measurement every shift.	Estimated daily requirement for adults is 1500–3000 mL/day.[37]
• Evaluate mental status every shift at (times)	Basic monitoring to determine client's ability to independently take fluids.
• If client's values and beliefs influence intake: ○ Alter environment as necessary to facilitate fluid intake, and note alterations here, e.g., if client thinks fluids from cafeteria are poisonous, have client assist in making drink on unit. ○ Provide positive attention to client at additional times to avoid not drinking as a way of obtaining negative attention.	

Gerontic Health

ACTIONS/INTERVENTIONS	RATIONALES
• Encourage patient to drink at least 8 oz of fluid every hour while awake.	Older adults with cognitive deficits may forget to consume liquids. Prompting such patients to drink fluids should be an essential part of their plan of care.
• Be sure fluids are within reach of the patient confined to bed.	For those confined to bed or with restricted movement, this action is a simple, basic measure to promote fluid intake.

Home Health

ACTIONS/INTERVENTIONS	RATIONALES

• Assist client and family in identifying risk factors pertinent to the situation:
  ○ Diabetes
  ○ Protein malnourishment
  ○ Extremes of age
  ○ Excessive vomiting or diarrhea
  ○ Medication for fluid retention or high blood pressure
  ○ Confusion or lethargy
  ○ Fever
  ○ Excessive blood loss
  ○ Wound drainage
  ○ Inability to obtain adequate fluids because of pain, immobility, or difficulty in swallowing
	Early intervention in risk situations can prevent dehydration.

• Assist client and family in identifying lifestyle changes that may be required:
  ○ Avoiding excessive use of caffeine, alcohol, laxatives, diuretics, antihistamines, fasting, and high-protein diets
  ○ Use of salt tablets
  ○ Exercising without electrolyte replacement
	Avoidance of dehydrating activities will prevent excessive fluid loss.

Fluid-Volume Deficit, Risk for or Actual

FLOWCHART EVALUATION: EXPECTED OUTCOME 1

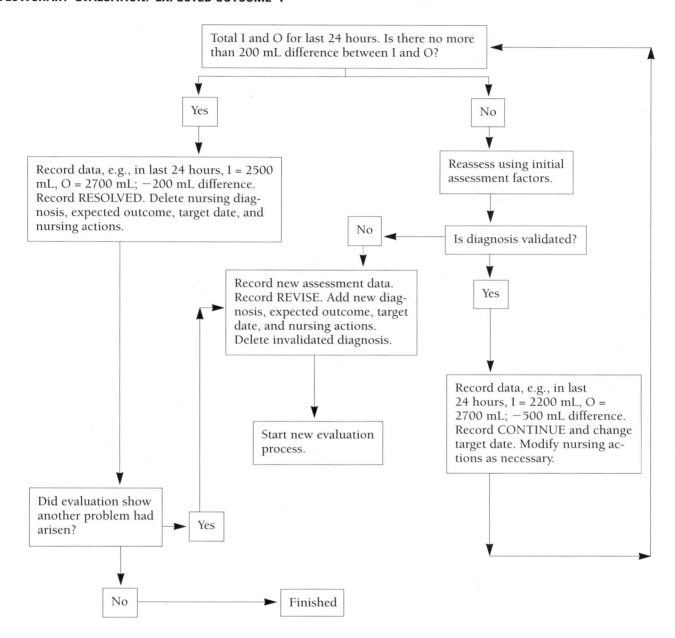

Total I and O for last 24 hours. Is there no more than 200 mL difference between I and O?

Yes

No

Record data, e.g., in last 24 hours, I = 2500 mL, O = 2700 mL; −200 mL difference. Record RESOLVED. Delete nursing diagnosis, expected outcome, target date, and nursing actions.

Reassess using initial assessment factors.

No

Is diagnosis validated?

Yes

Record new assessment data. Record REVISE. Add new diagnosis, expected outcome, target date, and nursing actions. Delete invalidated diagnosis.

Record data, e.g., in last 24 hours, I = 2200 mL, O = 2700 mL; −500 mL difference. Record CONTINUE and change target date. Modify nursing actions as necessary.

Start new evaluation process.

Did evaluation show another problem had arisen?

Yes

No

Finished

Fluid-Volume Deficit, Risk for or Actual

FLOWCHART EVALUATION: EXPECTED OUTCOME 2

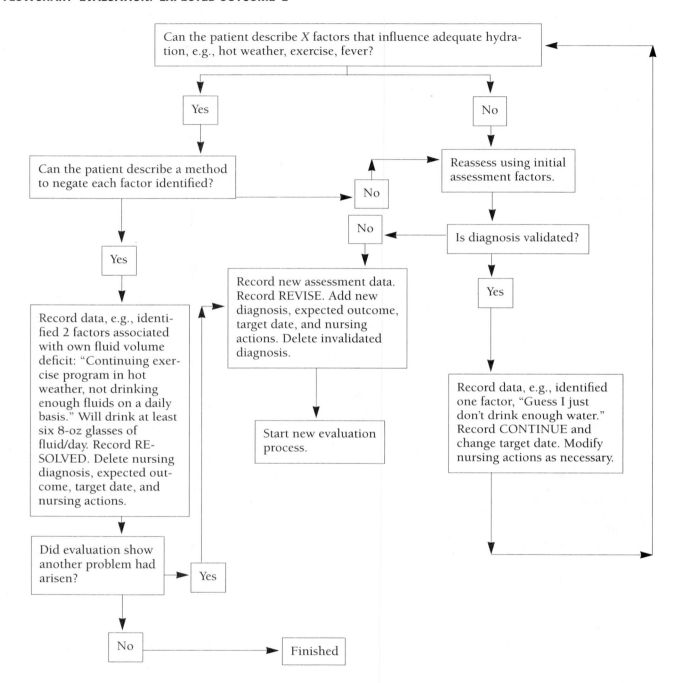

Fluid-Volume Excess

DEFINITION

The state in which an individual experiences increased isotonic fluid retention.[23]

NANDA TAXONOMY: EXCHANGING 1.4.1.2.1

DEFINING CHARACTERISTICS[23]

1. Major defining characteristics
   a. Edema
   b. Effusion
   c. Anasarca
   d. Weight gain
   e. Shortness of breath
   f. Intake greater than output
   g. Abnormal breath sounds, rales (crackles)
   h. Decreased hemoglobin and hematocrit
   i. Increased central venous pressure changes
   j. Jugular vein distention
   k. Positive hepatojugular reflex
2. Minor defining characteristics
   None given.

RELATED FACTORS[23]

1. Compromised regulatory mechanisms
2. Excess fluid intake
3. Excess sodium intake

RELATED CLINICAL CONCERNS

1. Congestive heart failure
2. Renal failure
3. Cirrhosis of the liver
4. Cancer
5. Toxemia

HAVE YOU SELECTED THE CORRECT DIAGNOSIS?

Altered Cardiac Output, Decreased and Impaired Gas Exchange The body depends on both appropriate gas exchange and adequate cardiac output to oxygenate tissues and circulate nutrients and fluid for use and disposal. If either of these is compromised, then the body will suffer in some way. One of the major ways the body suffers is in the circulation of body fluid. Fluid will be left in tissue and not absorbed into the general circulation to be redistributed or eliminated.

Altered Nutrition, More Than Body Requirements This diagnosis could be the primary problem. The person ingests more food and fluid than the body can metabolize and eliminate. The result is excess fluid volume in addition to the other changes in the body's physiology.

Impaired Urinary Elimination, Retention One way the body compensates fluid balance is through urinary elimination. If the body cannot properly eliminate fluids, then the system "backs up" so to speak, and excess fluid remains in the tissues.

Impaired Mobility Besides appropriate gas exchange and adequate cardiac output, the body also needs movement of muscles to assist in transporting food and fluids to and from the tissue. Impaired Mobility might lead to an alteration in movement of food and fluids. Waste products of metabolism and excess fluid are allowed to remain in tissues, creating a fluid-volume excess.

ADDITIONAL INFORMATION

Fluid-volume excess can occur as a result of water excess, sodium excess, or water and sodium excess.[38] Careful assessment and monitoring are needed to recognize the difference in precipitating causes.

Edema: Mild or 1+ means that the skin can be depressed 0 to 1/4 inch; moderate or 2+ means that the skin can be depressed 1/4 to 1/2 inch; severe or 3+ means that the skin can be depressed 1/2 to 1 inch; and deep pitting edema or 4+ means that the skin can be depressed more than 1 inch and it takes longer than 30 seconds to rebound.

EXPECTED OUTCOMES

1. Intake and output will balance within 200 mL by (date) (*Note:* may want difference to be only 50 mL for a child) and/or
2. Will not exhibit any signs or symptoms of fluid-volume excess by (date)

TARGET DATES

In a healthy person, intake and output reach an approximate balance over a span of 72 hours. An acceptable target date would then logically be the third day of admission.

NURSING ACTIONS/INTERVENTIONS WITH RATIONALES

Adult Health

ACTIONS/INTERVENTIONS	RATIONALES
• Take vital signs every 2 h at (state times here), and include apical pulse.	Permits monitoring of cardiovascular response to illness state and therapy.
• Check lung, heart, and breath sounds every 2 h on (odd/even) hour.	Essential monitoring for fluid collection in lungs and cardiac overload due to edema
• Elevate head of bed.	Facilitates respiration.
• Measure and record total intake and output every shift.	Assists in determining amount of fluid retention and need for fluid limitation.
• Check intake and output hourly (urinary output not less than 30 mL/h).	
• Observe and document color and character of urine, vomitus, and stools.	
• Check urine specific gravity at least every 2 h on (odd/even) hour.	
• Monitor:	Essential monitoring for fluid and electrolyte imbalance.
○ Skin turgor at least every 4 h while awake (note times here).	
○ Electrolytes, hemoglobin, and hematocrit. Collaborate with physician regarding frequency of lab tests.	
○ Mental status and behavior at least every 2 h on (odd/even) hour.	
• Weigh daily at (state times here).	Monitoring for fluid replacement. Allows consistent comparison of weight.
• Weigh at same time each day and in same-weight clothing.	
• Administer medication (e.g., diuretics) as ordered. Monitor medication effects.	
• Collaborate with physician regarding restricting intake:	Restricting fluids prevents cardiovascular system overload and reduces workload on renal system.
○ Amount	
○ Type, e.g., clear fluids only or intravenous only	
• Turn and properly position patient at least every 2 h on (odd/even) hour.	Prevents stasis of fluids in any one part of body. Assists in circulation of fluid and assists in preventing skin integrity problems.
• Check dependent parts for edema (e.g., ankles, sacral area, and buttocks).	
• Protect edematous skin from injury:	
○ Avoid shearing force.	
○ Use powder or cornstarch to avoid friction.	
○ Use pillows, foam rubber pads, etc. to avoid pressure.	
○ Encourage patient to alter position frequently.	
○ Provide active and passive ROM every 4 h while awake at (state times here).	
• Administer or assist with complete oral hygiene after each meal and at bedtime.	Cleans and lubricates the mouth. Permits patient to more fully enjoy foods and fluid allowed.
• Teach patient to monitor own intake and output at home.	Support patient's self-care by pointing out measures he or she can use to control fluid imbalance. Adequate intake and early intervention will prevent undesirable outcomes.
• In collaboration with dietitian:	Cost-effective use of readily available resources. Promotes interdisciplinary care, thus better care, for patient.
○ Obtain nutritional history.	
○ Begin high-protein diet (80–100 g of protein).	
○ Reduce sodium intake (not above 6 g daily or below 2.5 g daily).	
○ Refer patient to other health care professionals as appropriate.	

Child Health

ACTIONS/INTERVENTIONS	RATIONALES

• Measure and record total intake and output every shift:
  ◦ Check intake and output hourly, and weigh diapers.
  ◦ Monitor specific gravity at least every 2 h or as specified.
• Reposition as tolerated every half-hour.
	A strict assessment of intake and output serves to guide treatment for indication of hydration status. The specific gravity will assist in determining cardiac, renal, and respiratory function and electrolyte status.
	Prevents stasis of fluids in any one part of body. Assists in circulation of fluid and assists in preventing skin integrity problems.

• Weigh daily at same time under same conditions of dress (infant without clothes, children in underwear).	Accuracy of weight is critical, serves as a major indicator for treatment effectiveness, and is an ongoing parameter for treatment.
• Administer medications as ordered with attention to appropriate dosage and potential effect on electrolytes.	Potassium and sodium alterations may be present and must be addressed to prevent further fluid or electrolyte imbalance.
• Anticipate potential for respiratory distress and monitor appropriately by cautious checking of breath sounds, respiratory effort, and level of consciousness. • Administer fluids per IV with appropriate equipment, i.e., buretrol and clamping off main supply of fluids even while on IV pump and placing 2 h of fluid at a time in buretrol or as stated.	Fluid overload and fluid and electrolyte deviations may lead to respiratory and/or cardiac arrest if undetected or untreated. Likelihood of iatrogenic fluid overdose is lessened with appropriate safeguards.

Women's Health

NOTE: Pregnancy-induced hypertension, often called the "disease of theories," has been documented for the last 200 years. Numerous causes have been proposed but never substantiated; however, data collected during this time do support the following:

1. Chorionic villi must be present in the uterus for a diagnosis of PIH to be made.
2. Women exposed for the first time to chorionic villi are at increased risk for developing PIH.
3. Women exposed to an increased amount of chorionic villi, for example, multiple gestation or hydatidiform mole, are at greater risk for developing PIH.
4. Women with a history of PIH in a previous pregnancy are at increased risk for developing PIH.
5. Women who change partners are more likely to develop PIH in a subsequent pregnancy.
6. There is a genetic predisposition for the development of PIH which may be a single gene or multifactorial.
7. Vascular disease places the patient at greater risk for developing superimposed PIH.[37]

ACTIONS/INTERVENTIONS	RATIONALES

• Review client's history for factors associated with pregnancy-induced hypertension (PIH):
  ◦ Family and personal history such as diabetes or multiple gestation
  ◦ RH incompatibility or hypertensive disorder
  ◦ Chronic blood pressure 140/90 mm Hg or greater prior to pregnancy, or in the absence of a hydatidiform mole, that persists for 42 days postpartum
	Basic database required to assess for potential of PIH.

• During current pregnancy observe for following characteristics of PIH:
  ◦ Nulliparous women under 20 or over 35 yr of age
  ◦ Multipara with multiple gestation, renal, or vascular disease
	Increased knowledge for patient will assist the patient with earlier help-seeking behaviors.

Continued

ACTIONS/INTERVENTIONS	RATIONALES

○ Presence of hydatidiform mole
• Monitor patient for chronic hypertension[38]:
    ○ Increase in systolic blood pressure of 30 mm Hg or diastolic blood pressure of at least 15 mm Hg above baseline on 2 occasions at least 2 h apart
    ○ Development of proteinuria
• Monitor and teach patient to immediately report the following signs of PIH:
    ○ Increase of 30 mm in blood pressure or 140/90 blood pressure and above
    ○ Edema: Weight gain of 5 lb or greater in 1 wk
    ○ Proteinuria: 1 g/L or greater of protein in a 24-h urine collection (2+ by dipstick)
    ○ Visual disturbances: Blurring of vision or headaches
    ○ Epigastric pain
• Observe closely for signs of severe preeclampsia in any patient who presents with[26]:
    ○ Blood pressure greater than or equal to 160 mm Hg systolic, or greater than or equal to 110 mm Hg diastolic, on at least 2 occasions 6 h apart with the patient on bedrest
    ○ Proteinuria greater than or equal to 5 g in 24 h or 3+ or 4+ on qualitative assessment
    ○ Oliguria: Less than 400 mL in 24 h
    ○ Cerebral or visual disturbances
    ○ Epigastric pain
    ○ Pulmonary edema or cyanosis
    ○ Impaired liver function of unclear etiology
    ○ Thrombocytopenia
• Monitor, at least once per shift, for edema. Teach patient to:
    ○ Monitor swelling of hands, face, legs, or feet (**Caution:** May need to remove rings)
    ○ Be aware of a possible need to wear loose shoes or a bigger shoe size
    ○ Schedule rest breaks during the day and to elevate feet
    ○ When lying down, lie on left side to promote placental perfusion and prevent compression of vena cava
• In collaboration with dietitian:
    ○ Obtain nutritional history.
    ○ Place patient on high-protein diet (80–100 g of protein).
    ○ Place patient on reduced sodium intake (not above 6 g daily or below 2.5 g daily).
• Monitor:
    ○ Intake and output: Urinary output not less than 30 mL/h or 120 mL/4 h
    ○ Effect of magnesium sulfate ($MgSO_4$) and hydralazine hydrochloride (Apresoline) therapy (have antidote for $MgSO_4$ [calcium gluconate] available at all times during $MgSO_4$ therapy)
    ○ Deep tendon reflexes (DTR) at least every 4 h (state times here)
    ○ Respiratory rate, pulse, and BP at least every 2 h on the (odd/even) hour
	Knowledge of the complexity and multisystem nature of the disease assists with early detection and treatment.
	
	Increased knowledge for patient will assist the patient with earlier help-seeking behaviors.
	
	Basic safety measures.

- ○ Fetal heart rate and well-being at least every 2 h on the (odd/even) hour
- Institute seizure precautions.
- Ensure bedrest and reduction of noise level in patient's environment.

Decreases sensory stimuli that might increase the likelihood of a seizure.

Psychiatric Health

ACTIONS/INTERVENTIONS	RATIONALES

• Observe chronic psychiatric clients and clients with preexisting alcoholism[39] for signs and symptoms of polydipsia and/or water intoxication. The observations include[39–41]:
  ○ Frequent trips to sources of fluid and excessive consumption of fluids
  ○ Client stating "I feel as if I have to drink water all of the time" or a similar statement
  ○ Fluid-seeking behavior
  ○ Dramatic or rapid fluctuations in weight
  ○ Polyuria
  ○ Incontinence
  ○ Carrying large cups
  ○ Urine specific gravity of 1.008 or less[39]
  ○ Decreases in serum sodium
	A pattern of extreme polydipsia and polyuria can develop in clients with psychiatric disorders. This may be related to dopamine central nervous system activity and dysfunction in antidiuretic hormone activity in combination with psychosocial factors. The sense of thirst can also be increased by certain medications.[40,41]

• Discuss client's explanations for excessive drinking to determine causes of excessive fluid intake. If it is determined that drinking is a diversionary activity or an attempt to avoid interaction, implement nursing actions for Social Isolation and/or Diversional Activity Deficit as appropriate. If it is determined that fluid intake is related to testing concern of staff or testing limits, refer to nursing actions for Powerlessness or Self-Concept Disturbance.	Determining exact reason for polydipsia allows for more effective intervention.

• If it is determined client is at risk for water intoxication, implement the following actions:
  ○ Monitor and document fluid intake and output and weight fluctuations on a daily basis.
  ○ Restrict fluids as ordered by physician.
	Water intoxication can be life-threatening.[39]

• Provide small medicine cup (30 mL) for client to obtain fluids.	
• Provide fluids such as chipped ice on a schedule. Note schedule here.	
• Instruct client in need for reducing nicotine consumption. If client cannot do this, it may be necessary to initiate a "rationing" plan. If so, note plan here.	Nicotine increases release of ADH, a water-conserving hormone.[39]
• Provide client with sugarless gum and/or hard candy to decrease dry mouth. Note client's preference.	
• Identify with client those activities that would be most helpful in diverting attention from fluid restriction. Note specific activities here with schedule for use.	
• Refer to occupational and recreational therapists.	
• If client continues to have difficulty restricting fluids, provide increased supervision by limiting client to day area or other group activity rooms where he or she can be observed. Note restrictions here. If necessary, place client on one-to-one observation.	

Continued

ACTIONS/INTERVENTIONS	RATIONALES
• Talk with client about feelings engendered by restrictions for 15 min per shift. Note times here. • Discuss client's restriction in community meeting if: ○ Restrictions are impacting others on the unit ○ Support from peers would facilitate client's maintaining restrictions • Provide positive verbal support for client's maintaining restriction(s). • Identify with client appropriate rewards for maintaining restrictions and reaching goals. Describe rewards and behaviors necessary to obtain rewards here.	Promotes client's self-esteem and provides motivation for continued efforts. Promotes client's self-esteem, sense of control, and motivation for continuing his or her efforts.

Gerontic Health

Nursing actions for the gerontic health patient with this nursing diagnosis are the same as those for Adult Health and Home Health.

Home Health

ACTIONS/INTERVENTIONS	RATIONALES
• Teach methods to protect edematous tissue. ○ Practice proper body alignment. ○ Use pillows, pads, etc., to relieve pressure on dependent parts. ○ Avoid shearing force when moving in bed or chair. ○ Alter position at least every 2 h.	Tissue is at risk for injury. Client and family can be taught to minimize risks and damage.
• Assist client and family to set criteria to help them to determine when a physician or other intervention is required.	Plan decision making to prepare for potential crisis.
• Assist client and family in identifying risk factors pertinent to the situation, e.g., heart disease, kidney disease, diabetes mellitus, diabetes insipidus, liver disease, pregnancy, or immobility.	Identification of risk factors and understanding of relationship to fluid excess provide for intervention to reduce or prevent negative outcomes.
• Teach signs and symptoms of fluid excess: ○ Peripheral and dependent edema ○ Shortness of breath ○ Taut and shiny skin	Early recognition of signs and symptoms provides data for early intervention.
• Assist client and family in identifying lifestyle changes that may be required: ○ Avoid standing or sitting for long periods of time; elevate edematous limbs. ○ Avoid crossing legs. ○ Avoid constrictive clothing (girdles, garters, knee-highs, rubber bands to hold up stockings, etc.). ○ Consider wearing antiembolism stockings. ○ Avoid excess salt. Teach patient and family to read labels for sodium content. Avoid canned and fast foods. ○ Use spices other than salt in cooking. ○ Avoid lying in one position for longer than 2 h. ○ Raise head of bed or sit in chair if having difficulty breathing. ○ Restrict fluid intake as necessary (e.g., usual in kidney and liver disease) ○ Weigh at the same time every day wearing the same clothes and using the same scale	Knowledge and support provide motivation for change and increases potential for positive outcome.
• Teach purposes and side effects of medication, e.g., diuretics or cardiac medications.	Appropriate use of medication and reduction of side effects.

Fluid-Volume Excess

FLOWCHART EVALUATION: EXPECTED OUTCOME 1

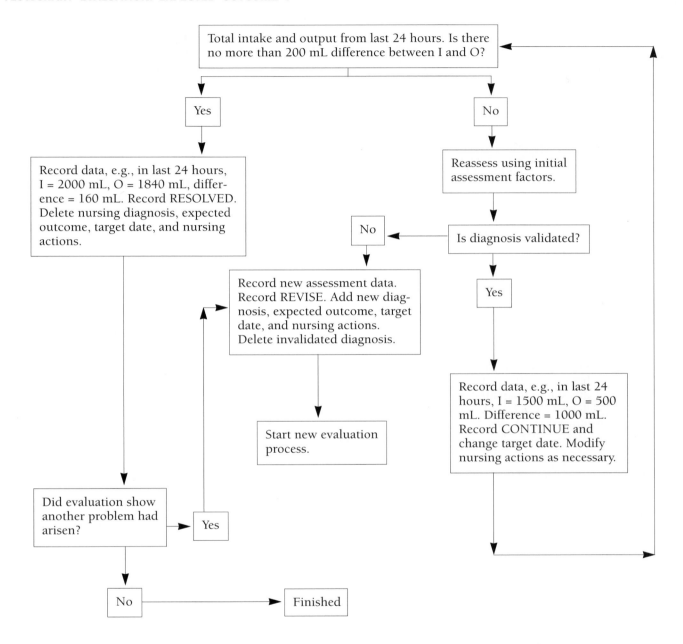

Fluid-Volume Excess

FLOWCHART EVALUATION: EXPECTED OUTCOME 2

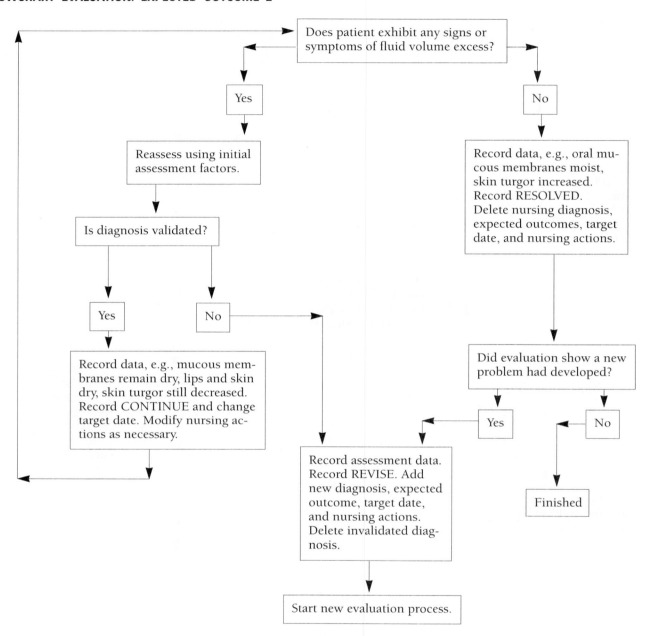

Hyperthermia

DEFINITION

A state in which an individual's body temperature is elevated above his or her normal range.[23]

NANDA TAXONOMY: EXCHANGING 1.2.2.3

DEFINING CHARACTERISTICS[23]

1. Major defining characteristics
   a. Increase in body temperature above normal range
2. Minor defining characteristics
   a. Flushed skin
   b. Warm to touch
   c. Increased respiratory rate
   d. Tachycardia
   e. Seizures or convulsions

RELATED FACTORS[23]

1. Exposure to hot environment
2. Vigorous activity
3. Medications or anesthesia
4. Inappropriate clothing
5. Increased metabolic rate
6. Illness or trauma
7. Dehydration
8. Inability or decreased ability to perspire

RELATED CLINICAL CONCERNS

1. Any infectious process
2. Septicemia
3. Hyperthyroidism
4. Any disease leading to dehydration, for example, diarrhea, vomiting, hemorrhage
5. Any condition causing pressure on the brain stem
6. Heat stroke

HAVE YOU SELECTED THE CORRECT DIAGNOSIS?

Risk for Altered Body Temperature   This diagnosis indicates that the person is potentially unable to regulate heat production and dissipation within a normal range. In Hyperthermia, the patient's ability to produce heat is not impaired. Heat dissipation is impaired to the degree that Hyperthermia results.

Ineffective Thermoregulation   Ineffective Thermoregulation indicates that the patient's body temperature is fluctuating between being elevated and being subnormal. In Hyperthermia the temperature does not fluctuate; it remains elevated until the underlying cause of the elevation is negated or until administration of medications such as Tylenol and aspirin.

Hypothermia   Hypothermia means the patient's body temperature is subnormal. This indicates the exact opposite measurement from Hyperthermia.

EXPECTED OUTCOMES

1. Will return to normal body temperature (range between 97.3 and 98.8°F) by (date) and/or
2. Will identify at least (number) measures to use in correcting hyperthermia.

TARGET DATES

Because hyperthermia can be life-threatening, initial target dates should be in terms of hours. After the patient has demonstrated some stability toward a normal range, the target date can be increased to 2 to 4 days.

NURSING ACTIONS/INTERVENTIONS WITH RATIONALES

Adult Health

ACTIONS/INTERVENTIONS	RATIONALES
• Monitor temperature every hour on the (hour/half hour) while awake and temperature remains elevated. Measure temperature every 2 h during night (note times here). After temperature begins to decrease, lengthen time between temperature measurements.	Hyperthermia is incompatible with cellular life.
• Sponge patient with cool water or rubbing alcohol, or apply continuous cold packs, or place patient in a tub of tepid water until temperature is lowered to at least 102°F. (Be careful to not overchill the patient.) Dry patient well and keep dry and clean.	Basic measures to assist in temperature reduction via heat dissipation. Overchilling could cause shivering, which increases heat production.

Continued

ACTIONS/INTERVENTIONS	RATIONALES
• Use a fan or place in front of an air conditioner. Cool environment to no more than 70°F.	Promotes cooling via heat dissipation.
• Monitor and use equipment according to manufacturer's guidelines and policies of unit, e.g., cooling blanket.	
• Give antipyretic drugs as ordered. Closely monitor effects, and document effects within 30 min after medications given.	Antipyretics assist in temperature reduction. Monitoring ensures that patient is not changed to a condition of hypothermia; it allows the health care team to assess the effectiveness of the antipyretic. Ineffectiveness would require changing to a different antipyretic.
• Maintain seizure precautions until temperature stabilizes.	Hyperthermia can lead to febrile seizures due to overstimulation of the nervous system.
• Give sips of salt water every 30 min if conscious and not vomiting.	Assists in maintaining fluid and electrolyte balance.
• Encourage fluids up to 3000 mL every 24 h.	Helps maintain fluid and electrolyte balance and assists in replacing fluid lost through perspiration.
• Give skin, mouth, and nasal care at least every 4 h while awake (note times here). Change bed linens and pajamas as often as necessary.	Hyperthermia promotes mouth breathing in an effort to dissipate heat. Mouth breathing dries the oral mucous membrane. Keeping bed linens and pajamas dry helps prevent shivering.
• Do not give stimulants.	Stimulants cause vasoconstriction which could increase hyperthermia.
• Gather data relevant to underlying contributing factors at least once per shift.	Control of underlying factors helps prevent occurrence of hyperthermia.
• Provide health care teaching, beginning on admission, regarding: ○ Need for frequent temperature checks ○ Related medical or nursing care ○ Safety when using ice packs or electric cooling blanket ○ How family can assist in care ○ Importance of hydration ○ Possible fear or altered comfort of patient with fever due to discomfort, fast heart rate, dizziness, and general feeling of illness ○ Possible seizure activity	Relieves anxiety and allows patient and family to participate in care. Initiates home care planning.
• Carry out appropriate infection control in the event or potential event of infectious disease process according to actual or suspected organisms.	Prevents spread of infection.
• Assist in promoting a quiet environment.	Allows for essential sleep and rest. Hyperthermia causes increased metabolic rate.

Child Health

ACTIONS/INTERVENTIONS	RATIONALES
• Monitor temperature every 30 min until temperature stabilizes.	Frequent assessment per tympanic (aural) thermometer or as specified will provide cues to evaluate efficacy of treatment and monitors underlying pathology.
• Administer antipyretics, antiseizure, or antibiotic medications as ordered with precaution for: ○ Maintenance of IV line ○ Drug safe range for child's age and weight ○ Potential untoward response ○ IV compatibility ○ Infant's or child's renal, hepatic, and GI status	Unique components for each individual patient must be considered within usual treatment modalities to help bring safe and timely return of temperature while avoiding iatrogenic complications.

- Provide padding to siderails of crib or bed to prevent injury in event of possible seizures.

- Ensure that airway maintenance is addressed by appropriate suctioning and airway equipment according to age.

Protection from injury in likelihood of uncontrolled sudden bodily movement serves to protect patient from further problems. Uses universal seizure precautions. As a part of seizure activity, there is always the potential of loss of consciousness with respiratory involvement.

Women's Health

Newborn (Newborn is included with Women's Health because newborn care is administered by nurses on either a maternity, obstetrical, or mother-baby unit.)

ACTIONS/INTERVENTIONS	RATIONALES
• When under heat source or bililights, monitor the infant every hour for increased redness and sweating. Check heat source at least every 30 min (overhead, isolettes, or bililights).	Provides safe environment for infant.
• Monitor infant's temperature, skin turgor, and fontanel (bulging or sunken) for signs and symptoms of dehydration every 30 min while under heat source. First temperature measurement should be rectal; thereafter can be axillary.	Provides essential information as to infant's current status and promotes a safe environment for infant.
• Check for urination; infant should wet at least 6 diapers every 24 h.	Basic monitoring of infant's physiologic functioning.
• Replace lost fluids by offering the infant breast, water, or formula at least every 2 h on the (odd/even) hour.	Decreases insensible fluid loss and maintains body temperature within normal range. This action will decrease the infant's needs for IV glucose.

• Pregnancy:
  ○ Teach patient to avoid use of hot tubs or saunas.
    (1) During first trimester: Concerns about possible CNS defects in fetus and failure of neural tube closure.[42]
    (2) During second and third trimesters: Concerns about cardiac load for mother.[42]
  ○ Provide cooling fans for mothers during labor and for patients on $MgSO_4$ therapy.
  ○ Keep labor room cool for mother's comfort.
	Provides safe environment for mother and prevents injury to fetus.

Psychiatric Health

ACTIONS/INTERVENTIONS	RATIONALES

• Monitor clients receiving neuroleptic drugs for decreased ability to sweat by observing for decreased perspiration and an increase in body temperature with activity, especially in warm weather. Monitor these clients for hyperpyrexia (up to 107°F). Notify physician of alterations in temperature. Note alteration in the client's plan of care and initiate the following actions:
  ○ Client should not go outside in the warmest part of the day during warm weather.
  ○ Maintain client's fluid intake up to 3000 mL every 24 h by (this is especially important for clients who are also receiving lithium carbonate; lithium levels should be carefully evaluated):
    (1) Having client's favorite fluids on the unit.
	Clients who are receiving neuroleptic medications are at risk for developing neuroleptic malignant syndrome, which can be life-threatening.[32]

Continued

ACTIONS/INTERVENTIONS	RATIONALES

(2) Having client drink 240 mL (an 8-oz glass) of fluids every hour while awake and 240 mL with each meal. If necessary, the nurse will sit with the client while the fluid is consumed.
     (3) Maintaining record of client's intake and output.
   ○ Dress client in light, loose clothing.
   ○ If client is disoriented or confused, provide one-on-one observation.
 • Decrease client's activity level by:
   ○ Decreasing stimuli
   ○ Sitting with client and talking quietly or involving client in a table game or activity that requires little large muscle movement (note activities that client enjoys here)
   ○ Assigning room near nurse's station and dayroom areas
 • Monitor client's mental status every hour.
 • Do not provide clients with alteration in mental status with small electrical cooling devices unless they receive constant supervision.
 • Give client as much information as possible about his or her condition and measures that are implemented to decrease temperature.
 • Teach client and family measures to decrease or eliminate risk for hyperthermia (see Home Health for teaching information).
 • Consult with appropriate assistive resources as indicated.
	High fevers can alter mental status and thus decrease the client's ability to make proper judgments.
	 Increased physical activity increases body temperature, and the decreased ability to sweat, secondary to medications, inhibits the body's normal adaptive response.[38]

Gerontic Health

Nursing actions for the gerontic patient with this diagnosis are the same as those for Adult Health and Home Health.

Home Health

ACTIONS/INTERVENTIONS	RATIONALES

• Monitor for factors contributing to hyperthermia (see Defining Characteristics).
 • Teach client and family the signs and symptoms of hyperthermia.
   ○ Flushed skin
   ○ Increased respiratory rate
   ○ Increased heart rate
   ○ Increase in body temperature
   ○ Seizure precautions and care
 • Teach measures to decrease or eliminate the risk of hyperthermia:
   ○ Wearing appropriate clothing
   ○ Taking appropriate care of underlying disease
   ○ Avoiding exposure to hot environments
   ○ Preventing dehydration
   ○ Using antipyretics
   ○ Performing early intervention with gradual cooling
 • Involve client and family in planning, implementing, and promoting reduction or elimination of the risk for hyperthermia.
	Identification of risk factors provides for intervention to reduce or prevent negative outcomes.
	 Provides data for early intervention.
	
	 Provides basic knowledge that increases the probability of successful self-care.
	
	 Involvement provides opportunity for increased motivation and ability to appropriately intervene.

- Assist client and family to identify lifestyle changes that may be required:
  - Measure temperature using appropriate method for developmental age of person.
  - Learn survival techniques if client works or plays outdoors.
  - Ensure proper hydration.
  - Transport to health care facility.
  - Use emergency transport system.

Knowledge and support provide motivation for change and increase potential for a positive outcome.

Hyperthermia

FLOWCHART EVALUATION: EXPECTED OUTCOME 1

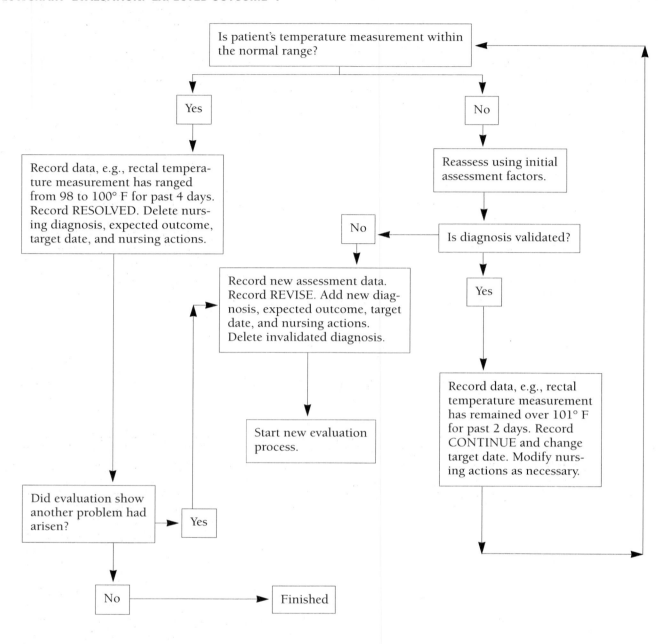

Hyperthermia

FLOWCHART EVALUATION: EXPECTED OUTCOME 2

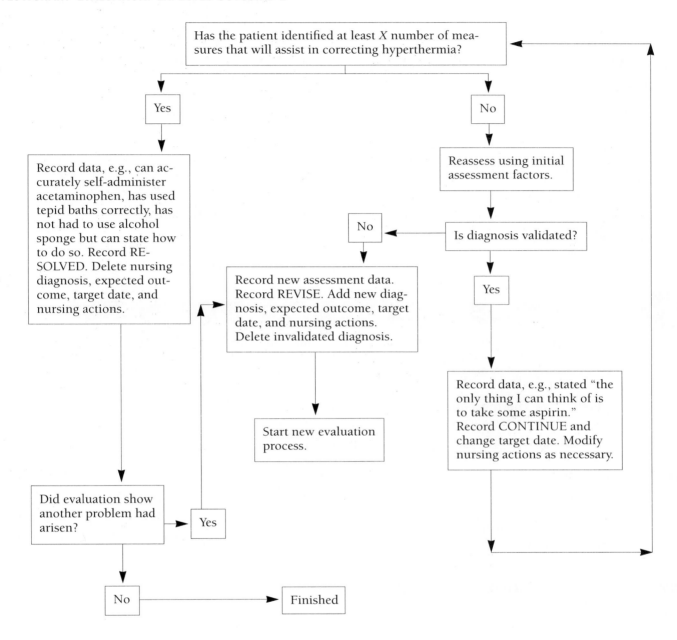

Has the patient identified at least *X* number of measures that will assist in correcting hyperthermia?

Yes

Record data, e.g., can accurately self-administer acetaminophen, has used tepid baths correctly, has not had to use alcohol sponge but can state how to do so. Record RESOLVED. Delete nursing diagnosis, expected outcome, target date, and nursing actions.

Did evaluation show another problem had arisen?

Yes

No → Finished

Record new assessment data. Record REVISE. Add new diagnosis, expected outcome, target date, and nursing actions. Delete invalidated diagnosis.

Start new evaluation process.

No

Reassess using initial assessment factors.

Is diagnosis validated?

No

Yes

Record data, e.g., stated "the only thing I can think of is to take some aspirin." Record CONTINUE and change target date. Modify nursing actions as necessary.

Hypothermia

DEFINITION

The state in which an individual's body temperature is reduced below normal range.[23]

NANDA TAXONOMY: EXCHANGING 1.2.2.2

DEFINING CHARACTERISTICS[23]

1. Major defining characteristics
   a. Reduction in body temperature below normal range
   b. Shivering (mild)
   c. Cool skin
   d. Pallor (moderate)
2. Minor defining characteristics
   a. Slow capillary refill
   b. Tachycardia
   c. Cyanotic nail beds
   d. Hypertension
   e. Piloerection

RELATED FACTORS[23]

1. Exposure to cool or cold environment
2. Illness or trauma
3. Damage to hypothalamus
4. Inability or decreased ability to shiver
5. Malnutrition
6. Inadequate clothing
7. Consumption of alcohol
8. Medications causing vasodilation
9. Evaporation from skin in cool environment
10. Decreased metabolic rate
11. Inactivity
12. Aging

RELATED CLINICAL CONCERNS

1. Hypothyroidism
2. Anorexia nervosa
3. Any injury to the brain stem

HAVE YOU SELECTED THE CORRECT DIAGNOSIS?

Risk for Altered Body Temperature This diagnosis indicates that the person is potentially unable to regulate heat production and heat dissipation within a normal range. In Hypothermia, the patient's ability to dissipate heat is not impaired. Heat production is impaired to the degree that Hypothermia results.

Ineffective Thermoregulation The body temperature fluctuates between being too high and too low. In Hypothermia, the temperature does not fluctuate; it remains low.

Hyperthermia The patient's temperature is above normal, not below normal.

EXPECTED OUTCOMES

1. Will return to normal body temperature range (between 97.3 and 98.8°F) by (date) and/or
2. Will identify at least (number) measures to use in correcting hypothermia

TARGET DATES

Hypothermia can be life-threatening; therefore, initial target dates should be in terms of hours. After the patient has demonstrated some stability toward a normal range, target dates can be increased to 2 to 4 days.

NURSING ACTIONS/INTERVENTIONS WITH RATIONALES

Adult Health

ACTIONS/INTERVENTIONS	RATIONALES
• Warm the patient quickly. Use blankets, warming blankets, warm water (102–105°F), extra clothing, warm drinks, and warm room. Do not use a heat lamp or hot-water bottles. Prevent air drafts in room. Monitor safe functioning of equipment used in thermoregulation.	Basic measures that assist in increasing core temperature and prevent excess heat dissipation. Heat lamps and hot-water bottles warm only a limited area and increase the likelihood of local tissue damage.
• Monitor temperature measurement every hour until temperature returns to normal levels and stabilizes.	Assesses effectiveness of therapy.
• Prevent injury. Gently massage body; however, do not rub a body part if frostbite is evident.	Massage helps stimulate circulation; however, massage of a frostbitten area will promote tissue death and gangrene. In frostbite, circulation has to be gradually reestablished through warming.

- Address skin protective needs by frequent monitoring for breakdown or altered circulation.
- Give fluids such as salt and soda solution. Have patient sip slowly (if conscious and not vomiting). Do not give alcohol.
- Monitor respiratory rate and depth and breath sounds every hour. Provide for airway suctioning and positioning as needed.
- Bathe with appropriate protection and covering.
- Devote appropriate attention to prevention of major complications such as shock, cardiac failure, tissue necrosis, infection, fluid and electrolyte imbalance, convulsions or loss of consciousness, respiratory failure, and renal failure.
- Administer medications as ordered.
- Monitor effects, and record within 30 min after administration.
- Obtain a detailed history regarding:
  ○ Onset
  ○ Related trauma and causative factors
  ○ Duration of hypothermia
- Provide opportunities for patient and family to ask questions and relay concerns by including 30 min for this every shift. (Note times here.)
- Allow for appropriate attention to resolution of psychological trauma, especially in instances of severe exposure to cold, at least once per shift. (Note times here.)
- Teach patient and family measures to decrease or eliminate the risk for hypothermia, to include:
  ○ Wearing appropriate clothing when outdoors
  ○ Maintaining room temperature at minimum of 65°F
  ○ Wearing clothing in layers
  ○ Covering the head, hands, and feet when outdoors (especially the head)
  ○ Removing wet clothing
- Teach patient about the kinds of behavior that increase the risk for hypothermia:
  ○ Drug and alcohol abuse
  ○ Working, living, or playing outdoors
  ○ Poor nutrition, especially when body fat is reduced below normal levels as in anorexia nervosa
- Teach patient and family signs and symptoms of early hypothermia:
  ○ Confusion, disorientation
  ○ Slurred speech
  ○ Low blood pressure
  ○ Difficulty in awakening
  ○ Weak pulse
  ○ Cold stomach
  ○ Impaired coordination
- Make appropriate arrangements for follow-up after discharge from hospital. Identify support groups in the community for the patient and family.
- Consult with appropriate assistive resources as indicated:
  ○ Obtain an energy audit by public service company to identify possible sources of heat loss.
  ○ Refer patient to social services to provide information on emergency shelters, clothing, and food banks.
  ○ Recommend financial counseling if heating the home is financially difficult.

Hypothermia causes peripheral vasoconstriction, which leads to a high risk for impaired skin integrity.
Assists in maintaining fluid and electrolyte balance.
Alcohol would promote vasoconstriction.

Hypothermia and its related factors promote the development of respiratory complications.

Prevents heat loss.
Awareness of the complications of hypothermia will help prevent the complication.

Assists in monitoring effectiveness of therapy.

Decreases anxiety and facilitates home care teaching.

Helps in reducing patient's anxiety and facilitates patient's resolving of the lingering effects of trauma.

Permits patient to participate in self-care and promotes compliance to prevent future episodes.

Foster resources for long-term management in terms of adequate housing, financial resources, and social habits.

Promotes effective long-term management and prevention of future episode.

Child Health

ACTIONS/INTERVENTIONS	RATIONALES
• Provide for maintenance of body temperature by hat (stockinette for infant) and using an open radiant warmer, isolette, or heating blanket.	Heat loss is greatest via the head in young infants as well as by convection and evaporation. Suitable maintenance of temperature by appropriate equipment will help to maintain neutral body core temperature.
• Incorporate other health care team members to address collaborative needs.	Provision of support for long-term follow-up will place value on the need for care and the importance of compliance. Assists in reducing anxiety.
• Provide teaching to address unknown and necessary information for child and family in terms they can relate to (e.g., temperature measurement).	Serves to establish foundation of trust and provides essential basis for follow-up care.
• Anticipate safety needs according to patient's age and development status.	Each opportunity for reinforcing the importance of safety as a part of well-child follow-up should not be overlooked. Emphasize caution with rectal thermometer to prevent trauma to anal sphincter and tissue, and caution family regarding the use of mercury-glass thermometer and breakage. In the event of the use of electronic equipment, emphasize the importance of protection of skin, constant surveillance, and unique safety needs per manufacturer.

Women's Health

NOTE: This nursing diagnosis will pertain to the woman the same as to any other adult. The reader is referred to the other sections for specific nursing actions pertaining to women and hypothermia. Infants control their body temperature with nonshivering thermogenesis; this process is accompanied by an increase in oxygen and calorie consumption. Therefore, use of a radiant warmer or prewarmed mattress for initial care provides environmental heat giving rather than heat losing. However, it is important to note that hypothermia and cold stress in the neonate are related to the amount of oxygen needed by the infant to control apnea and acid-base balance. It is estimated that to replace a heat loss during a temperature drop of 3.5°C (6.3°F), the infant will require a 100 percent increase in oxygen consumption for more than 1½ h. Metabolic acidosis can occur quickly if the infant becomes hypothermic.[26]

Newborn

ACTIONS/INTERVENTIONS	RATIONALES

• To prevent hypothermia in the newborn:
  ○ Dry new infant thoroughly.
  ○ Cover with blanket.
  ○ Lay next to mother's body (cover mother and infant by placing blanket over them).
  ○ Place infant under radiant heat source.
  ○ Keep out of drafts.
• Observe infant for hypoglycemia. Check temperature every hour until stable, then every 4 h for 24 h. May be taken rectally, by axilla, or by skin (continuous probe).
	Prevention of heat loss in the infant will reduce oxygen and calorie consumption and prevent metabolic acidosis.

Psychiatric Health

ACTIONS/INTERVENTIONS	RATIONALES
• Monitor client's mental status every 2 h (note times here); report alterations to physician. • If client is receiving antipsychotics or antidepressants, report this fact to the physician when temperature alteration is first noted. • Protect client from contact with uncontrolled hot objects such as space heaters and radiators by teaching clients and family to remove them from the environment. • Allow client to use heating pads and electric blankets only with supervision. • Teach client the potential for medication to affect body temperature regulation, especially in the elderly.	Antipsychotic and antidepressant medications can alter thermoregulation, which results in hypothermia.[38] Basic safety measures.

Gerontic Health

Nursing actions for the gerontic health patient with this diagnosis are the same as those given for Adult Health and Mental Health.

Home Health

ACTIONS/INTERVENTIONS	RATIONALES

• Involve client and family in planning, implementing, and promoting reduction or elimination of the risk for hypothermia.
• Assist client and family to identify lifestyle changes that may be required:
  ○ Avoiding drug and alcohol abuse
  ○ Learning survival techniques if client works or plays outdoors (e.g., camping, hiking, or skiing)
  ○ Keeping person dry
  ○ Transporting to health care facility
  ○ Using emergency transport system
	Involvement provides likelihood of increased motivation and ability to appropriately intervene.
	
	Knowledge and support provide motivation for change and increase the potential for a positive outcome.

Hypothermia

FLOWCHART EVALUATION: EXPECTED OUTCOME 1

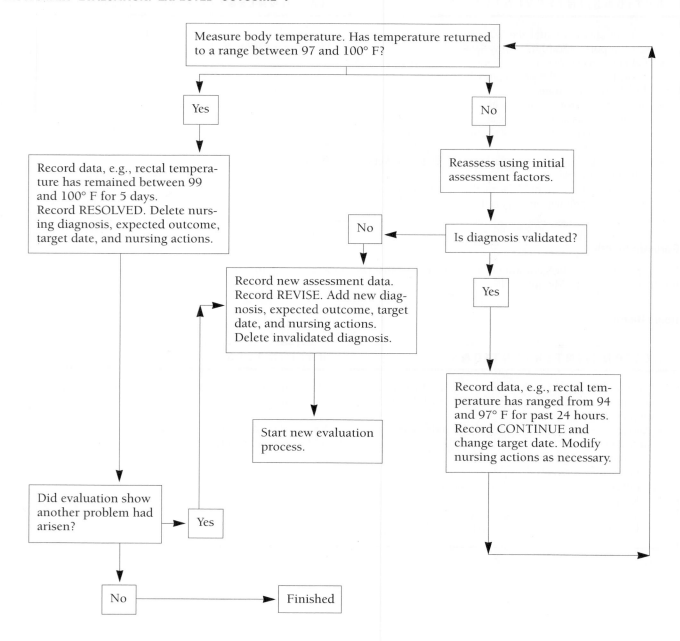

Measure body temperature. Has temperature returned to a range between 97 and 100° F?

Yes

No

Record data, e.g., rectal temperature has remained between 99 and 100° F for 5 days. Record RESOLVED. Delete nursing diagnosis, expected outcome, target date, and nursing actions.

Reassess using initial assessment factors.

No

Is diagnosis validated?

Yes

Record new assessment data. Record REVISE. Add new diagnosis, expected outcome, target date, and nursing actions. Delete invalidated diagnosis.

Start new evaluation process.

Record data, e.g., rectal temperature has ranged from 94 and 97° F for past 24 hours. Record CONTINUE and change target date. Modify nursing actions as necessary.

Did evaluation show another problem had arisen?

Yes

No

Finished

Hypothermia

FLOWCHART EVALUATION: EXPECTED OUTCOME 2

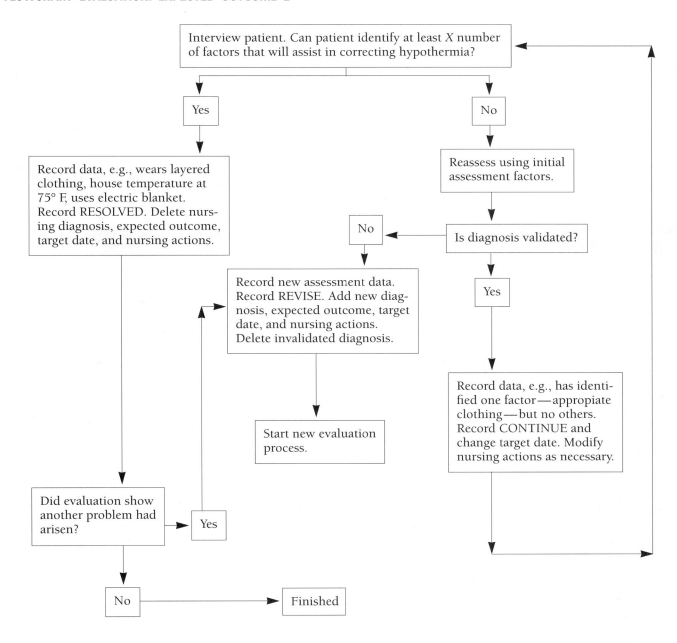

Infant Feeding Pattern, Ineffective

DEFINITION

A state in which an infant demonstrates an impaired ability to suck or coordinate the suck-swallow response.[23]

NANDA TAXONOMY: MOVING 6.5.1.4

DEFINING CHARACTERISTICS[23]

1. Major defining characteristics
   a. Inability to initiate or sustain an effective suck
   b. Inability to coordinate sucking, swallowing, and breathing
2. Minor defining characteristics
   None given.

RELATED FACTORS[23]

1. Prematurity
2. Neurologic impairment or delay
3. Oral hypersensitivity
4. Prolonged NPO
5. Anatomic abnormality

RELATED CLINICAL CONCERNS

1. Prematurity
2. Cerebral palsy
3. Thrush
4. Hydrocephalus
5. Any condition that would require major surgery immediately after birth

HAVE YOU SELECTED THE CORRECT DIAGNOSIS?

Ineffective Breast-Feeding   With this diagnosis the infant is able to suckle and swallow but there is dissatisfaction or difficulty with the breast-feeding process. The key difference would be based on the defining characteristics of Ineffective Breast-Feeding versus Ineffective Infant Feeding Pattern. If the infant demonstrates problems with initiating, sustaining, or coordinating sucking, swallowing, and breathing, then Ineffective Infant Feeding Pattern is the most appropriate diagnosis.

Altered Nutrition, Less Than Body Requirements   Certainly this diagnosis could be the result of Ineffective Infant Feeding Pattern if the feeding problem is not remedied. However, correction of the primary problems would prevent the development of this diagnosis.

EXPECTED OUTCOMES

1. Will demonstrate normal ability to suck-swallow by (date) and/or
2. Will gain at least (number) ounces by (date)

TARGET DATES

This diagnosis would be life-threatening; therefore, progress should initially be evaluated every few hours. After the infant has begun to exhibit at least some sucking-swallowing, then the target date can be moved to every 2 days.

NURSING ACTIONS/INTERVENTIONS WITH RATIONALES

Adult Health

For this diagnosis, Child Health and Women's Health (Newborn) serve as the generic actions. This diagnosis would not be used in adult health.

Child Health

ACTIONS/INTERVENTIONS	RATIONALES

• Monitor for all possible contributory factors:
  ○ Actual physiologic sucking potential
  ○ Other objective concerns, e.g., swallowing or respiratory
  ○ Objective history data, e.g., prematurity or congenital anomalies
  ○ Maternal or infant reciprocity
  ○ Subjective data from caregivers or parents
	A thorough assessment and monitoring will serve as the critical basis for appropriate individualizing and prioritizing a plan of health care.

• Provide anticipatory support to infant for respiratory difficulties that could increase the probability of aspiration.	Airway maintenance is a basic safety precaution for this infant. Airway and suctioning equipment will be standard (see nursing actions for Risk for Aspiration).

- Ascertain the most appropriate feeding protocol for the infant with attention to:
  - Nutritional needs according to desired weight gain
  - Actual feeding mode, e.g., modified nipple, larger hole nipple, syringe adapted for feeding, position for feeding, or gastric tube
  - Health status and prognosis
  - Compliance factors
  - Socioeconomic factors
  - Maternal-infant concerns
- Explore the feelings caregivers or parents have related to the Ineffective Feeding Pattern.

- Strictly monitor and calculate intake, output, and caloric count on each shift, and total each 24 h.

- Weigh infant daily or more often as indicated.

- Collaborate with other health care professionals to better meet the infant's needs.
- Allow for appropriate time to prepare infant for feeding, and provide a calm, smoothing milieu.

- Encourage family to participate in feeding and plans for feeding.
- Provide teaching based on an assessment of parental knowledge needs and/or deficits.

- Allow for time to clarify feeding protocols, questions, and discharge planning.

A realistic yet holistic approach will provide a foundation for multidisciplinary management with best likelihood for success. Specific criteria will provide measurable progress parameters.

Often the expression of feelings will reduce anxiety and may allow further potential alterations to be minimized by early intervention.
Caloric intake and hydration status are indirectly and directly used to monitor the infant's progress in tolerance of feeding and feeding efficacy.
Weight gain would serve as a major indicator of effective feeding and assist in assessment of hydration.
A multidisciplinary approach is most effective in level and cost of care.
A nonhurried, nonstressful milieu will promote the infant's relaxation and allow the infant to perceive feeding as a pleasant experience.
Inclusion of family empowers the family and augments their self-confidence and coping.
Knowledge provides a means of decreasing anxiety. When based on assessed needs, it will reflect the individualized needs and more likely meet the parent's learning needs.
Appropriate attention to questions and concerns parents may have will assist in reducing anxiety, thereby allowing for learning and a greater likelihood of adherence to the therapeutic regimen.

Women's Health

ACTIONS/INTERVENTIONS	RATIONALES
• Provide support and information to mother and significant other. Explain the infant's inability to suck, and provide suggestions and options (based on etiology of sucking problem) to correct or reduce problem.[30,44,45]	The basic rationale for all the nursing actions in this diagnosis is to provide nutrition to the infant in the most appropriate, cost-effective, and successful manner.
• Describe the anatomy and physiology of sucking to the mother.	Assists in decreasing anxiety, provides a base for teaching, and permits long-range planning.
• Explain importance of positioning for both bottle- and breast-feeding.[45-47]	Encourages proper suckling by the infant.
• Provide support and supervision to assist mother in encouraging infant to suck properly.	
• Assist mother and family to assess appropriate intake by observing the infant for at least 6–8 wet diapers in 24 h (after milk has come in).	Assures that infant is getting enough nutrition and is not becoming dehydrated.[34,35,44]
• If necessary, provide supplemental nutrition system while teaching infant to suck, e.g., dropper, syringe, spoon, cup, or supplementation device.[48,49]	Pays attention to basic nutrition while also attending to problem with sucking.
• Refer patient's mother to lactation consultant or clinical nurse specialist for assistance and support in teaching infant to suck.	
• Assist mother and significant others to choose feeding system for infant (breast, bottle, or tube) that will supply best nutrition.	Provides basic support to encourage essential nutrition.

Psychiatric Health

This diagnosis would not be used in mental health.

Gerontic Health

This diagnosis is not appropriate for the gerontic patient.

Home Health

The nursing actions for Home Health would be the same as for Women's Health.

Infant Feeding Pattern, Ineffective

FLOWCHART EVALUATION: EXPECTED OUTCOME 1

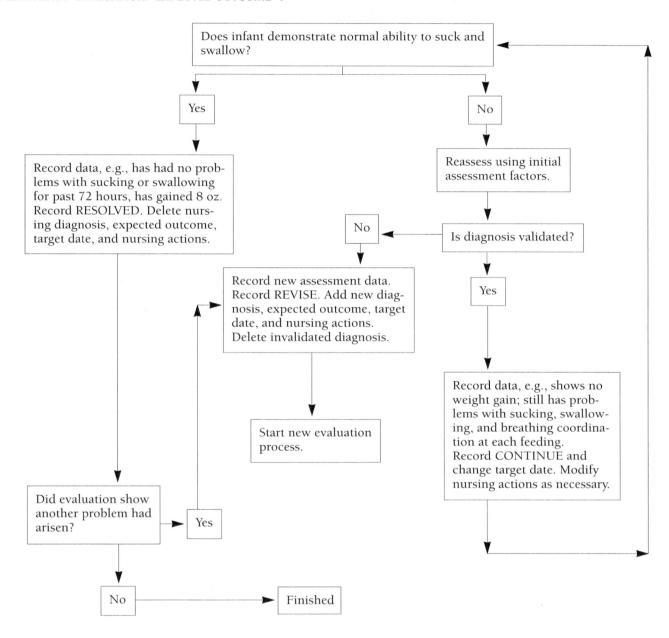

Infant Feeding Pattern, Ineffective

FLOWCHART EVALUATION: EXPECTED OUTCOME 2

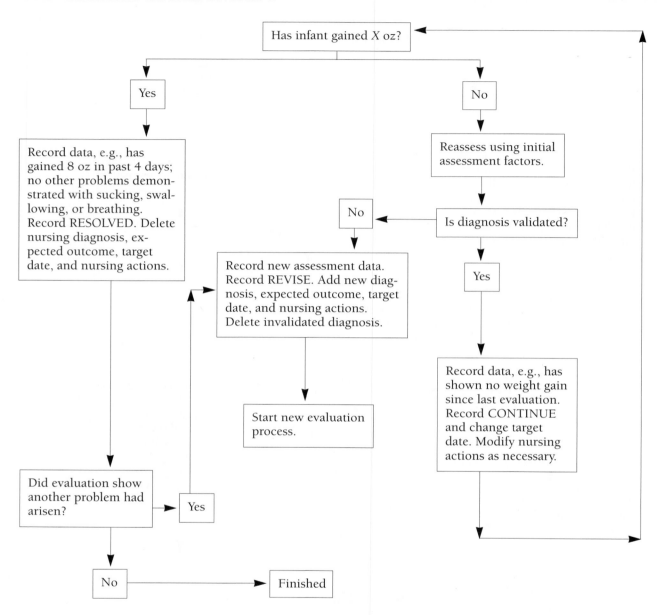

Has infant gained *X* oz?

Yes

No

Record data, e.g., has gained 8 oz in past 4 days; no other problems demonstrated with sucking, swallowing, or breathing. Record RESOLVED. Delete nursing diagnosis, expected outcome, target date, and nursing actions.

Reassess using initial assessment factors.

No

Is diagnosis validated?

Record new assessment data. Record REVISE. Add new diagnosis, expected outcome, target date, and nursing actions. Delete invalidated diagnosis.

Yes

Start new evaluation process.

Record data, e.g., has shown no weight gain since last evaluation. Record CONTINUE and change target date. Modify nursing actions as necessary.

Did evaluation show another problem had arisen?

Yes

No

Finished

Nutrition, Altered, Less Than Body Requirements

DEFINITION

The state in which an individual experiences an intake of nutrients insufficient to meet metabolic needs.[23]

NANDA TAXONOMY: EXCHANGING 1.1.2.2

DEFINING CHARACTERISTICS[23]

1. Major defining characteristics
   a. Loss of weight with adequate food intake
   b. Body weight 20 percent or more under ideal
   c. Reported inadequate food intake less than RDA (recommended daily allowance)
   d. Weakness of muscles required for swallowing or mastication
   e. Reported or evidence of lack of food
   f. Aversion to eating
   g. Reported altered taste sensation
   h. Satiety immediately after ingesting food
   i. Abdominal pain with or without pathology
   j. Sore, inflamed buccal cavity
   k. Capillary fragility
   l. Abdominal cramping
   m. Diarrhea and/or steatorrhea
   n. Hyperactive bowel sounds
   o. Lack of interest in food
   p. Perceived inability to ingest food
   q. Pale conjunctival and mucous membranes
   r. Poor muscle tone
   s. Excessive loss of hair
   t. Lack of information; misinformation
   u. Misconception
2. Minor defining characteristics
   None given.

RELATED FACTORS[23]

Inability to ingest or digest food or absorb nutrients due to biologic, psychologic, or economic factors.

RELATED CLINICAL CONCERNS

1. Anorexia nervosa or bulimia
2. Cancer
3. AIDS
4. Alzheimer's disease
5. Anemia
6. Ostomies
7. Schizophrenia, paranoid

STOP

HAVE YOU SELECTED THE CORRECT DIAGNOSIS?

Altered Oral Mucous Membrane   If the oral mucous membranes are severely inflamed or damaged, food intake could be so painful that the person ceases intake to avoid the pain. While the end result might be Altered Nutrition, Less Than Body Requirements, initial intervention would have to be aimed at handling the oral mucosal problem.

Altered Bowel Elimination, Diarrhea   In this instance the body cannot absorb the necessary nutrients because the food material passes through the gastrointestinal tract too rapidly.

Altered Tissue Perfusion   Once the food has been ingested, digested, and absorbed, its components must get to the cells. If there is Altered Tissue Perfusion, the nutrients may not be able to get to the cells in sufficient quantities to do any good.

Self-Care Deficit, Feeding, or Altered Sensory Perception, Visual, Olfactory, and/or Gustatory, or Altered Health Maintenance   One of these diagnoses may be the primary problem. If the person does not sense hunger through the usual means—seeing, smelling, or tasting—or if the person thinks he or she has already eaten, then the desire to eat may not exist. Even if the person senses hunger, the inability to feed oneself, to shop for food, or to prepare food could result in less than adequate nutrition.

Altered Comfort, Pain   If the preparation or actual eating of food increases pain level, then the patient might elect to avoid eating to assist in pain control.

Fear, Dysfunctional Grieving, Social Isolation, Body Image Disturbance, Alteration in Self-Esteem, and Spiritual Distress   These diagnoses are psychosocial problems that can impact nutrition. Each of these may create a decreased desire to eat, or even if food is eaten, the person may vomit because the stomach will not accept the food. Additionally, if the person eats, he or she may only pick at the food and not ingest enough to maintain the body's need for nutrients.

Knowledge Deficit   The person may not really know how much or what kind of food is more beneficial to his or her body.

EXPECTED OUTCOMES

1. Will gain (number) of pounds by (date) and/or
2. Will design and implement a personal nutritional improvement plan by (date) that is accurate, achievable, and realistic.

TARGET DATES

This diagnosis reflects a long-term-care problem; therefore, a target date of 5 days or more, from the date of admission, would be acceptable.

NURSING ACTIONS/INTERVENTIONS WITH RATIONALES

Adult Health

ACTIONS/INTERVENTIONS	RATIONALES
• Increase food and fluid intake at each meal or feeding via: 　○ Reducing noxious stimuli 　○ Opening all food containers and releasing odors outside patient's room 　○ According to individual needs, either providing privacy for eating or providing communal dining 　○ Administering appropriate medications 30 min before meals (e.g., analgesics or antiemetics); recording effects of medications within 30 min of administration 　○ If patient requires suctioning, doing so at least 15 min before mealtime (keep suctioning equipment available but out of immediate eating site)	Basic methods and procedures that enhance appetite. Suctioning removes secretions that may cause nausea. Timing of activities promotes rest prior to meals.
• Provide a rest period of at least 30 min prior to meal. • Give oral hygiene 30 min before meals and as required.	Conserves energy for feeding self and digestion. Moistens and cleanses oral mucous membranes, which promotes eating.
• Assist patient to eat or feed patient: 　○ Raise the head of bed. 　○ Help patient wash hands. 　○ Open cartons and packages. 　○ Cut food into small, bite-size pieces. 　○ Provide assistive devices (e.g., large-handled spoon or fork, all-in-one utensil, or plate guard).	
• Offer small, frequent feedings every 2–3 h rather than just 3 meals per day. Allow patient to assist with food choices and feeding schedules.	Three large meals a day give a sense of fullness, and the size of servings may be overwhelming to patient. Smaller meals facilitate gastric emptying, thus promoting a larger food intake overall.
• Force fluid intake between meals: 　○ Limit fluid intake at meals. 　○ Offer wine at meals or immediately prior to meals.	Alcohol stimulates gastric secretions and stimulates the appetite.
• Encourage patient to eat slowly.	Allows the patient to savor the taste of food. Facilitates the digestion process. Stimulates salivation.
• Have patient chew gum before meals or have patient visualize lemons or sour pickles. • Offer between-meal supplements. Focus on high-protein diet and liquids. • Avoid gas-producing foods and carbonated beverages.	Provides additional caloric intake. Providing high-protein foods and fluids helps prevent muscle-tissue loss. Gas-producing foods promote nausea and a feeling of fullness.
• Avoid very hot or very cold foods.	Extremes in temperature lead to a decrease in appetite and promote irritation of oral mucous membranes.
• Encourage significant others to bring special food from home.	Familiar food promotes appetite and empowers patient and family in regard to the diet. Allows an opportunity for teaching diet.
• Allow rest periods of at least 30 min after feeding. • Measure and total intake and output every 8 h. Total every 24 h.	Facilitates digestion and reduces stress.

- Make sure intake and output are balancing at least every 72 h.
- Weigh daily at (state time) and in same-weight clothing. Have patient empty bladder before weighing. Teach patient this routine for continued weighing at home.
- Encourage exercise at least twice per shift to the extent possible without tiring. If exercise capacity is limited, do passive and active ROM every 4 h at (state times here) while awake.
- Monitor:
  - Vital signs every 4 h while awake at (state times here) and as required based on measurement results
  - Airway, sensorium, chest sounds, bowel sounds, skin turgor, mucous membranes, bowel function, urine specific gravity, and glucose level at least once per shift
  - Laboratory values (e.g., electrolyte levels, hematocrit, hemoglobin, blood glucose, serum albumin, and total protein)
- Provide frequent positive reinforcement for:
  - Weight gain
  - Increased intake
  - Ignoring weight loss
  - Using consistent approach
- Teach patient and significant others:
  - Balanced diet based on the basic four food groups
  - Role of diet in health (e.g., healing, energy, and normal body functioning)
  - How to keep food diary with calorie count
  - Adding spices to food to improve taste and aroma
  - Use of exchange lists
  - Relaxation techniques
- Refer, as necessary, to other health care providers.

Allows monitoring of renal function and ensures weight gain is not due to fluid retention.
Assesses effectiveness of therapy and interventions.
Promotes patient's control of weight after discharge.

Stimulates appetite and prevents complications from immobility.

Allows early detection of complications and assists in monitoring effectiveness of therapy.

Provides essential information needed to prevent future episodes.

Provides ongoing support for long-term care.

ADDITIONAL INFORMATION

There will be situations in which the patient's nutritional condition has progressed to the point that tube feedings, intravenous therapy, or total parenteral nutrition will become necessary. In addition to the nursing actions for the overall nursing diagnosis of Altered Nutrition, Less Than Body Requirements, the following actions should be added.

Tube Feedings

ACTIONS/INTERVENTIONS	RATIONALES
• Check placement and patency prior to each feeding. Initial placement should be checked using radiographic verification since auscultatory methods are not always accurate. Check gastric aspiration for acidic pH.[50,51]	Prevents aspiration and monitors for complication of stress ulcer.
• Aspirate tube prior to each feeding. Measure amount of residual from previous feeding. If 150 mL or more, delay feeding and notify physician.	Prevents overloading of stomach and initiates assessment for reason stomach is not emptying.
• Check temperature of feeding before administering. Temperature should be slightly below room temperature.	Prevents abdominal cramping and reflux.
• Measure amount of feeding exactly. Flush tube with water immediately after feeding.	Avoid overloading stomach. Flushing ensures that all feeding has entered stomach and prevents clogging of tube.
• Crush medications in water or dissolve in water before giving. Flush tube with water immediately after administering medication.	Permits maintenance of therapeutic regimen and prevents clogging of tube by medication.

Continued

ACTIONS/INTERVENTIONS	RATIONALES
• Keep patient in semi-Fowler's position for at least 30 min following feeding.	Prevents reflux and aspiration of feeding.
• Cleanse and lubricate nares after each feeding.	Helps prevent breakdown of nasal mucosa. Promotes comfort.
• Check taping of tube following each feeding.	Ensures security of tube and promotes comfort.
• If feeding is to be administered by gravity method (preferred), make sure all air is out of tubing.	Air in stomach is uncomfortable, creates feeling of fullness, promotes nausea, and displaces space needed for nutritional feeding.

Continuous Tube Feeding

In certain situations, such as severe dysphagia, clients may be placed on continuous feeding via a pump. When continuous feeding is in effect, the following additional actions should be implemented:

ACTIONS/INTERVENTIONS	RATIONALES
• Maintain the head of the bed at a 30-degree angle at all times.	Decreases the risk of aspiration and lets gravity assist in fluid flow through stomach.
• Monitor infusion rate at least every 4 h around the clock at (times).	Ensures that correct flow rate is being maintained.
• Monitor respiratory rate, effort, and lung sounds at least every 4 h around the clock at (times).	Allows monitoring for possible aspiration.
• Request medication in liquid form whenever possible.	Decreases the potential blocking off of feeding tube with particulate matter.
• Check for security of tube placement at least every 4 h around the clock at (times).	Guards against tube displacement.
• Provide oral care every 4 h while awake at (times). Oral care is especially important when the nasogastric route is used.	An increase in mouth breathing leads to drying of the oral cavity and accumulation of debris in the mouth.

Intravenous

ACTIONS/INTERVENTIONS	RATIONALES
• Check insertion site for warmth, redness, swelling, leakage, and pain at least every 4 h at (state times here).	Basic monitoring for infiltration and venous irritation.
• Check flow rate at a maximum of every hour on the (hour/half-hour).	Prevents fluid overload.
• Check for signs and symptoms of circulatory overload at least every 2 h (state times here) (e.g., headache, neck vein distention, tachycardia, increased blood pressure, or respiratory changes).	
• Change tubing according to agency's stated standard or policy.	Implementation of CDC guidelines; prevention of complications from tubing.

Total Parenteral Nutrition

ACTIONS/INTERVENTIONS	RATIONALES
• Do not administer without pump.	The pump allows for accurate flow rate.
• Change tubing and filter daily at (state time here).	Ensures proper flow of parenteral nutrition and avoids complications.

• Change dressing every other day beginning (date):
  ○ Use aseptic technique.
  ○ Gently cleanse area around catheter (state specifically how here—most agencies have specific policy).
  ○ Use a bacteriostatic, not antibiotic, ointment.
  ○ Apply a dry, airtight dressing
	Basic infection-preventive measures.

• Check insertion site for warmth, redness, swelling, leakage, and pain at least every 4 h at (state times here).	Basic monitoring for infiltration and venous irritation.

Child Health

NOTE: This diagnosis represents a long-term-care issue. Therefore, a series of subgoals of smaller amounts of weight to be gained in a lesser period of time may be necessary. Long-term goals are still to be formulated and revised as the patient's status demands. Also, there will undoubtedly be instances in which overlap may exist for other nursing diagnoses. Specifically, as an example, in the instance of an alteration in nutrition related to actual failure to thrive, one must refer to appropriate role performance on the part of the mother with consideration for holistic nursing management. It would be most critical to include a few specific nursing process components to reflect the critical needs for the mother-infant dyad.

ACTIONS/INTERVENTIONS	RATIONALES
• Feed the infant on a regular schedule which offers nutrients appropriate to metabolic needs. For example, an infant of less than 5 lb will eat more often, but in lesser amounts (2–3 oz every 2–3 h) than an infant of 15 lb (4–5 oz every 3–4 h).	The stomach capacity and digestive concerns for each patient must be considered to realistically plan for weight gain over a slow, steady, incremental time frame.

• Assist or feed patient:
  ○ Elevate head of bed or place infant in infant seat, and older infant or toddler in highchair with safety belt in place. If necessary, hold infant. (This will be dictated in part by patient's status and presence of various tubes and equipment.)
  ○ Help patient wash hands. For infants and toddlers, administer diaper change as needed.
  ○ Warm foods and formula as needed, and test on wrist before feeding infant or child.
  ○ Provide aids appropriate for age and physical capacity as needed, such as two-handed cups for toddlers, favorite spoon, or Velcro strap for utensils for child with cerebral palsy.
  ○ Offer small, age-appropriate feedings with input from family members regarding child's preferences.
  ○ Encourage patient to eat slowly and to chew food thoroughly. For infant, bubble before, during, and after feeding.
	Appropriate attention to aesthetic, physical, and emotional details related to feeding will help to provide the optimal potential for pleasant, long-lasting eating patterns. The limitation of psychologic, emotional duress cannot be overemphasized and must be considered in each parent-child unit.

• Provide role-modeling opportunities in a nonthreatening, nonjudgmental manner to assist parents in learning about feeding an infant or child.	Nonthreatening role-modeling and personal encouragement fosters compliance and lessens anxiety.
• Weigh patient on same scale and at same time (state time here) daily. Weigh infants without clothes, older children in underwear.	Weight gain serves as a critical indicator of efficacy of treatment. Maintaining consistency in weighing lessens the number of potential intervening variables that would result in an accurate weight.

Continued

ACTIONS/INTERVENTIONS	RATIONALES

• Teach patient and family:
   ○ Balanced diet appropriate for age using basic four food groups.
   ○ Role of diet in health (e.g., healing, energy, and normal body functioning). If infant is medically diagnosed as Failure to Thrive, offer appropriate emotional support and allow at least 30 min 3 times a day (state times here) for exploring dyad relationships.
   ○ How to use spices and child-oriented approach in encouraging child to eat (e.g., peach fruit salad with peach as a face, garnished with cherries and raisins for eyes and nose, half of a pineapple round for mouth).
   ○ Monitoring for possible food allergies, especially in toddlers with history of allergies.
   ○ How to weigh self appropriately if applicable, or for parents to weigh child.
 • Provide positive reinforcement as often as appropriate for parents and child demonstrating critical behavior.
	Reinforcement of desired behaviors fosters long-term compliance, thereby empowering the family with satisfaction and confidence for ultimate self-care management with minimal intervention by others.

Women's Health

NOTE: Poverty and substance abuse are often associated with nutritional deficits. Remember that underweight women who are pregnant will exhibit a different pattern of weight gain than normal-weight women. This difference is exhibited in a rapid weight gain at the beginning of the first trimester of about 1 lb per week by 20 weeks. In the underweight woman, weight gain can be as much as 18 to 20 lb. Remember to teach the parents signs and symptoms of weight loss in the neonate.[26]

ACTIONS/INTERVENTIONS	RATIONALES

• Collaborate with dietitian in planning and teaching diet:
   ○ Emphasize high-quality calories (cottage cheese, lean meats, fish, tofu, whole grains, fruits, and vegetables).
   ○ Avoid excess intake of fats and sugar.
   ○ Assist patient in identifying methods to keep caloric intake within the recommended limit.
 • Verify prepregnant weight.
 	
 • Determine if weight loss during first trimester is due to nausea and vomiting.
 • Check activity level against daily dietary intake.
 • Check for food intolerances.
 • Check environmental influences:
   ○ Hot weather
   ○ Cultural practices
   ○ Pica eating
   ○ Economic situation
   ○ Ascertain economic status and ability to buy food
   ○ Monitor woman's emotional response to the pregnancy and to additional weight gain
	Gives baseline from which to plan better nutrition.
	
	 Assist in planning realistic diet changes within the patient's means and according to the patient's particular needs and habits.

NOTE: Dieting is never recommended during pregnancy because it deprives mother and fetus of nutrients needed for tissue growth and because weight loss is accompanied by maternal ketosis, a direct threat to fetal well-being.[5,42]

- Identify additional caloric needs and sources of those calories for the nursing mother[52,53]:
  - Additional 500 cal/day above normal dietary intake is needed to produce adequate milk (depending on the individual, a total of 2500–3000 cal/day).
  - Additional fluids are necessary to produce adequate milk.
- Collaborate with nutritionist to provide a healthy dietary pattern for the lactating mother.

Provides basis for ensuring good nutrition and assists in successful breast-feeding.

- Monitor mother's energy levels and health maintenance:
  - Does she complain of fatigue?
  - Does she have sufficient energy to complete her daily activities?
  - Does the dietary assessment show irregular dietary intake?
  - Is she more than 10 percent below the ideal weight for her body stature?
- For breast-feeding the newborn or neonate during the first 6 mo, teach mother:
  - The major source of nourishment is human milk.
  - Vitamin supplements can be used as recommended by physician:
    (1) Vitamin D
    (2) Fluoride
    (3) If indicated, iron
- Infants should be taking in approximately 420 mL daily soon after birth and building to 1200 mL daily at the end of 3 mo.

Provides for good nutritional status of the newborn.

- Monitor for fluid deficit at least daily:
  - "Fussy baby," especially if immediately after feeding
  - Constipation (remember that breast-fed babies have fewer stools than formula-fed babies)

Allows early intervention for this problem.

- Weight loss or slow weight gain: Closely monitor baby, mother, and nursing routine:
  - Is baby getting empty calories (e.g., a lot of water between feedings)?
  - Avoid nipple confusion, which results from switching baby from breast to bottle and vice versa many times.
  - Instruct mother in "cup feeding" of nursing infant to assure adequate fluid intake and avoid nipple confusion.[34,35]

Provides infant with nutrition, while supporting the breast-feeding mother.[44]

  - Count number of diapers per day (should have 6–8 really wet diapers per day).
  - Is there intolerance to mother's milk or bottle formula?
  - Is there illness or lactose intolerance?
  - Infrequent nursing can cause slow weight gain.

Psychiatric Health

NOTE: Due to long-term-care requirements for these clients, target dates should be determined in weeks or months, not hours or days.

ACTIONS/INTERVENTIONS	RATIONALES
• Do not attempt teaching or long-term goal setting with client until concentration has improved (symptom of starvation).	Starvation can impact cognitive functioning.[54]
• Establish contract with client to remain on prescribed diet and not to perform maladaptive behavior (i.e., vomiting or use of laxatives). State specific behavior for client here.	Provides client with sense of control and clearly establishes the consequences and rewards for behavior.
• Place client on 24-h constant observation (this will be discontinued when client ends maladaptive behavior or at specific times that nursing staff assess are low risk).	Provides consistency and structure during the stressful early period of treatment.
• Place client on constant observation during meals and at high-risk times for maladaptive behavior (such as 1 h after meals or while using the bathroom). This action will take effect when the preceding one is discontinued.	Provides support for client during stressful period.
• Do not allow client to discuss weight or calories. Excessive discussion of food is also discouraged.	Decreases client's abnormal focus on food and promotes normal eating patterns. This behavior is more indicative of starvation than an eating disorder.[54]
• Require client to eat prescribed diet (all food on tray each meal except for those 3 or 4 foods client was allowed to omit in the admission contract). List client's omitted food here.	Promotes client's sense of control and participation in decision making within appropriate limits.
• Sit with client during meals, and provide positive support and encouragement for the feelings and concerns the client may have.	Provides a positive supportive context for client.[54]
• Do not threaten client with punishment (tube feeding or IVs).	
• Report all maladaptive behavior to the client's primary nurse or physician for confrontation in individual therapy sessions.	
• Spend (number) minutes with client every (number) minutes to establish relationship.	
• Respond to queries related to fears of being required to gain too much weight with reassurance that the goal of treatment is to return client to health and that he or she will not be allowed to become overweight.	
• If client vomits, have him or her assist with the clean-up and require him or her to drink an equal amount of a nutritional replacement drink.	Provides natural consequences for behavior.
• Encourage client to attend group therapy (specific encouraging behavior should be listed here such as assisting client to complete morning care on time or other interventions that are useful for this client).	Provides support from peers and a source of honest feedback.[54]
• Encourage client's family by (list specific encouraging behaviors for this family) to attend family therapy sessions.	Provides support for the family and an opportunity for the family to work through their concerns together.[54]
• Assist client with clothing selection. Clothes should not be too loose, hiding weight loss, or too tight, assisting client to feel overweight even though appropriate weight is achieved.	Altered body image makes it difficult for clients to make appropriate choices; honest feedback and support from the nursing staff makes the transition to "healthy" choices easier.
• When maintenance weight is achieved, assist client with selection of appropriate foods from hospital menu.	As symptoms of starvation are resolved, clients are better able to make appropriate choices, and gradual returning of control prepares the client to accept responsibility at discharge.[54]
• When maintenance weight is achieved, refer client to dietitian for teaching about balanced diet and home maintenance.	
• When maintenance weight is achieved, refer to occupational therapist for practice with menu planning, trips to grocery stores to purchase food, and meal preparation.	

- When maintenance weight is achieved, plan passes with client for trips to restaurants for meals.

- Allow client to exercise (number) minutes (number) times per day while supervised (this will be altered as client reaches maintenance weight).
- Allow client to do the following exercises during the exercise period. (These are graded to the client's physical condition. Consultation with the occupational therapist is useful.)
- Allow client (number) of (number) minute walks on hospital grounds with a staff member each day.

Provides further information to client to assist in maintaining desired weight. Provides visible reward for weight maintenance.

Assists client in developing realistic goals for exercise according to age and ability.

Gerontic Health

Nursing actions for the gerontic patient with this diagnosis are the same as those in Adult Health.

Home Health

NOTE: Due to long-term-care requirements for these clients, target dates should be determined in weeks or months, not hours or days.

ACTIONS/INTERVENTIONS	RATIONALES

• Reduce associated factors, for example:
  ○ Minimize noxious odors by using foods that require minimal cooking; or if someone else is cooking for client, arrange for client to be away from cooking area.
  ○ Provide social atmosphere desired by client.
  ○ Plan medications to decrease pain and nausea around mealtime.
  ○ Plan meals away from area where treatments are performed.
  ○ Maintain oral hygiene before and after meals. Instruct client and family in proper brushing, flossing, and use of water pick.
  ○ Encourage client to prepare favorite foods.
  ○ Avoid foods that contribute to noxious symptoms such as gas, nausea, or GI distress.
  ○ Discourage fasting. Teach stress-reduction exercises.
  ○ Maintain exercise program as tolerated.
	Provides positive environment to promote nutritional intake.

• Teach client to add high-calorie, high-protein, and high-fat items to meal preparation activities; e.g., use milk in soups, add cheese to food, and use butter or margarine in soups and vegetables.	Promotes weight gain and prevents loss of muscle mass.
• Teach or provide assistance to rest before meals. If client is doing the meal preparation, teach to cook large quantities and freeze several meals at a time and to seek assistance in meal preparation when fatigued.	Provides optimal conditions to avoid overfatigue.

Nutrition, Altered, Less Than Body Requirements

FLOWCHART EVALUATION: EXPECTED OUTCOME 1

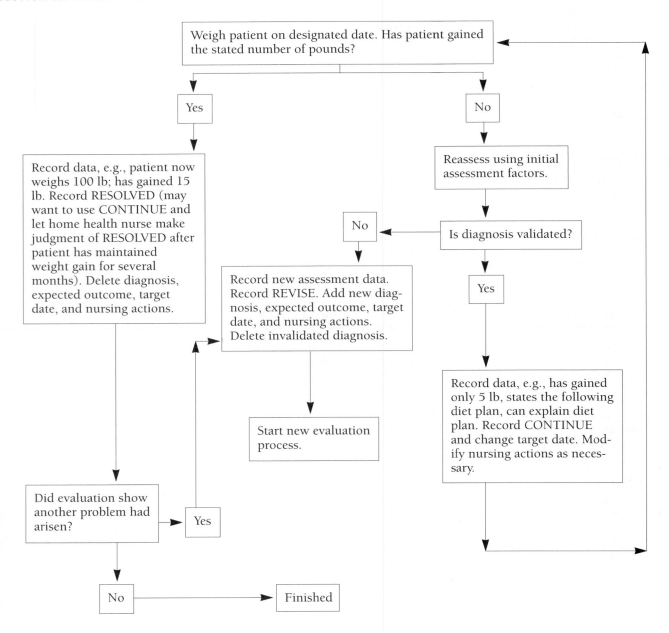

Nutrition, Altered, Less Than Body Requirements

FLOWCHART EVALUATION: EXPECTED OUTCOME 2

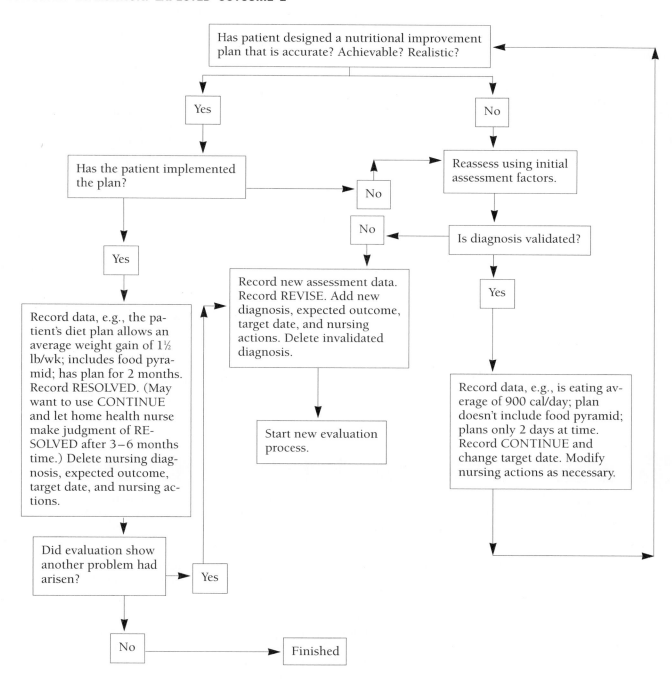

Nutrition, Altered, Risk for or More Than Body Requirements

DEFINITION

The state in which an individual is at risk of experiencing an intake of nutrients which exceeds metabolic needs.[23]

ACTUAL The state in which an individual is experiencing an intake of nutrients which exceeds metabolic needs.[23]

NANDA TAXONOMY: EXCHANGING 1.1.2.1 AND 1.1.2.3

DEFINING CHARACTERISTICS[23]

1. Major defining characteristics
   A. Risk for: Presence of risk factors such as:
      (1) Reported or observed obesity in one or both parents*
      (2) Rapid transition across growth percentiles in infants or children*
      (3) Reported use of solid food as major food source before 5 months of age
      (4) Observed use of food as reward or comfort measure
      (5) Reported or observed higher baseline weight at beginning of each pregnancy
      (6) Dysfunctional eating patterns:
         (a) Pairing food with other activities
         (b) Concentrating food intake at end of day
         (c) Eating in response to external cues such as time of day or social situation
         (d) Eating in response to internal cues other than hunger such as anxiety
   B. More than body requirements:
      (1) Weight 10 percent over ideal for height and frame
      (2) Weight 20 percent over ideal for height and frame*
      (3) Triceps skin fold greater than 15 mm in men or 25 mm in women*
      (4) Sedentary activity level
      (5) Reported or observed dysfunctional eating pattern:
         (a) Pairing food with other activities
         (b) Concentrating food intake at end of day
         (c) Eating in response to external cues such as time of day or social situation
         (d) Eating in response to internal cues other than hunger, for example, anxiety
2. Minor defining characteristics
   None given.

RELATED FACTORS[23]

1. Risk for: The risk factors also serve as the related factors.
2. More Than body requirements: Excessive intake in relation to metabolic needs.

RELATED CLINICAL CONCERNS

1. Alzheimer's disease
2. Morbid obesity
3. Hypothyroidism
4. Disorders requiring medicating with corticosteroids
5. Any disorder resulting in prolonged immobility

HAVE YOU SELECTED THE CORRECT DIAGNOSIS?

Knowledge Deficit The patient, because of cultural background, may not know the appropriate foods groups and the nutritional value of the foods. Additionally, the cultural beliefs held by a patient may not value thinness. Therefore, the people of a particular culture may actually promote obesity.

Altered Health Maintenance Due to other problems, the patient may not be able or willing to modify nutritional intake even though he or she has information about good nutritional patterns.

Other Possible Diagnoses Several diagnoses from the psychosocial realm may be the underlying problem that has resulted in Risk for or More Than Body Requirements. Powerlessness, Self-Esteem Disturbance, Social Isolation, Body Image Disturbance, or Ineffective Individual Coping may also need to be dealt with in the patient who is at Risk for or actually has Altered Nutrition, More Than Body Requirements.

EXPECTED OUTCOMES

1. Will lose (number) of pounds by (date) and/or
2. Will have (percentage) decrease in body fat by (date)

NOTE: Goal is 22 percent fat for women and 15 percent fat for men.[43]

TARGET DATES

Because this diagnosis reflects long-term care in terms of both cause and correction, a target date of 5 days or over would not be unreasonable.

---

* Critical.

NURSING ACTIONS/INTERVENTIONS WITH RATIONALES
Adult Health

ACTIONS/INTERVENTIONS	RATIONALES

• Assist patient to identify dysfunctional eating habits, during first day of hospitalization, by:
  ◦ Reviewing 1 week's dietary intake
  ◦ Associating times of eating and types of food with corresponding events, e.g., in response to internal cues or in response to external cues
  ◦ Reviewing 1 week's exercise pattern
• Check activity level against daily dietary intake.
	Provides basic information needed to plan changes in dysfunctional habits to begin weight-loss program.

• Discuss with patient potential or real motivation for desiring to lose weight at this time. • Discuss with patient past attempts at weight loss and factors that contributed to his or her success or failure.	Assists in understanding the patient's rewards for goals and assists in establishment of goals and rewards. Provides increased individualization and continuity of care, which facilitates the development of a therapeutic relationship.[55]
• Limit patient's intake to number of calories recommended by physician and/or nutritionist.	Reduces calories to promote weight loss yet maintains body's nutritional status.
• Weigh patient daily at (state time). Teach patient to weigh self at the same time each morning in same clothing. Help patient to establish a graphic to allow visualization of progress, e.g., bar chart, chart with gold star for each weight-loss day.	Provides a visible means of ascertaining weight-loss progress.
• Provide good skin care and monitor skin daily, especially skin folds and areas where skin meets skin.	These areas are especially prone to impaired skin integrity due to the collection of moisture and continuous friction.
• Measure total intake and output every 8 h. Encourage intake of low-calorie, caffeine-free drinks.	Ensures renal functioning and maintenance of fluid balance. A significant amount of weight loss in the first few days is due to fluid excretion. Low-calorie, caffeine-free drinks help offset "hunger pains."
• Collaborate with physical therapist in establishing an exercise program.	Exercise burns calories and tones muscles.
• Assist patient in selecting an exercise program by providing patient with a broad range of options, and have client select one he or she will enjoy.	Will assist in narrowing the range between calories consumed and calories burned. Facilitates development of adaptive coping behaviors.
• Develop a schedule and goals for implementing the exercise plan. (Set goals that are achievable; usually this is 50 percent of what the patient estimates is achievable.) Develop a reward schedule for achievement of exercise goals, and record this plan here.	Promotes patient self-esteem when goals can be accomplished and provides motivation for continued efforts.
• Teach stress reduction techniques, and have patient return-demonstrate for at least 30 min at least twice a day at (times), e.g., progressive relaxation, scheduled quiet time, or time management.	Helps to alleviate eating associated with stress. Facilitates patient's development of alternative coping behaviors.

• Assist patient to establish a food diary, during first day of hospitalization, which should be maintained until weight has stabilized within normal limits:
  ◦ What eating: Caloric intake
  ◦ Where eating: All actual sites
  ◦ When eating: Time of day, length of time spent eating, or circumstances leading to deciding to eat
  ◦ Activity during this time
  ◦ Feelings and emotions before, during, and after eating
  ◦ Provide space for listing of all physical activity, e.g., walked 1½ blocks from car to office.
• Review diary with patient on a daily basis, and list those factors that will assist with a weight-loss plan and those that will hinder a weight-loss plan.
	Helps patient to identify real intake and to identify behavorial and emotional antecedents to dysfunctional eating behavior.[56–58]

Continued

ACTIONS/INTERVENTIONS	RATIONALES
• Teach patient principles of balanced diet, or refer him or her to dietitian for instructions at least 3 days prior to discharge: ○ Food guide pyramid ○ Recommended daily allowances ○ Weighing and measuring foods ○ Exchange lists • Instruct patient to grocery shop from a list and soon after eating. • Discuss with patient those foods that provide the greatest risk of decreasing self-control, and develop a plan for eliminating them from the diet. • Use visual aids to increase effectiveness of diet teaching. • Schedule adequate time for teaching. Convey positive attitude, and reinforce information about food groups.	Provides basic knowledge needed to control weight at home. Promotes self-care. Promotes patient's perception of control.
• Spend 30 min at least twice a day at (times) with the patient reviewing the benefits of weight loss and the progress made to this point. Do not focus on the concept of loss when talking with the patient; use terms such as *reduction* and *gains in self-concept* to provide positive ideas.	Promotes a positive orientation and sense of control for the patient.[55]
• Discuss with the patient other life achievements and strategies that assisted with attaining these achievements. Focus on the concept of perseverance in attaining the achievement, or discuss with the patient the last long trip taken and apply the concept of persevering and planning that allowed the trip to be taken. Relate the ideas of persevering and planning to the task of weight loss.	Promotes positive orientation and focuses on strengths patient already possesses.
• Present the concept of approaching goals one day at a time rather than attempting or reflecting on all of the task.	Promotes positive orientation by setting readily achievable goals.
• Review pros and cons of alternate weight-loss options with patient: ○ Fad diets ○ Diet pills ○ Liquid diet preparations ○ Surgery ○ Diuretics ○ Laxatives ○ Bingeing and purging	Promotes safety in weight-loss plan. Avoids serious complications such as heart failure due to questionable weight-loss ideas.
• Demonstrate adaptations in eating that could promote weight loss: ○ Smaller plate ○ One-half of usual serving ○ No second servings ○ Laying fork down between bites ○ Chewing each bite at least *X* number of times	Assists in behavior modification needed to lose weight.
• Teach alternative food preparation habits that will reduce calories while increasing nutritional content of diet: ○ Boil or broil instead of frying food. ○ Use nonstick spray for pans instead of butter, margarine, or fat. ○ Use fruits and vegetables. ○ Increase use of fish or poultry over beef or pork.	Reduction of fat in meal preparation assists in calorie reduction and weight loss. Often excess food is consumed for water content when water would satisfy the need. Facilitates development of adaptive eating behaviors.

- Drink water or herbal tea for thirst; do not confuse thirst for hunger.
- Reduce or eliminate fat and sugar from recipes.
- Reduce or eliminate fat and sugar from recipes.
- Use fresh ingredients whenever possible for increased flavor.
- Use fresh fruit canned in its own juice for sweetening instead of sugar.
- Use plain yogurt or blended and seasoned tofu as substitutes for sour cream.

- Provide patient with a calorie list of fast-food items, and plan for maintaining desired goals by:
  - Developing a list of those fast-food items that provide the best food value for the calories
  - Assisting the patient with developing recipes to use at home that are calorie-wise and easily prepared to decrease the temptation to use fast food
  - Developing a list of those restaurants that provide options for reducing calorie intake such as those with salad bars or the option to eliminate certain items from a serving such as high-calorie condiments

Promotes patient's perception of control. Provides planned strategies for coping before entering potentially difficult situations.

- Have patient design own weight-loss plan at least 3 days prior to discharge to allow practice and revision as necessary:
  - Caloric intake
  - Activity
  - Behavioral or lifestyle changes, i.e., those behaviors that will replace factor that inhibits weight loss

Allows patient to assume control for long-term therapy. The more the patient is involved in planning care, the higher the probability he or she will maintain compliance.

- Encourage patient to increase activity by:
  - Walking up stairs instead of riding elevators at work
  - Taking walks in the evening before retiring

- Consult with family and visitors regarding importance of patient's adhering to diet. Caution against bringing food, etc., from home.

Involves others in supporting patient in weight-loss effort.

- Discuss with patient and significant others the necessary alterations in eating behavior, and develop a list of ways the significant others can be supportive of these alterations.

- Use appropriate behavior modification techniques to reinforce teaching. Refer patient and family to psychiatric nurse practitioner for appropriate techniques to use at home as well as assistance with guilt, anxiety, etc., over being obese.

Reinforcement supports change.

- Plan for times when patient will indulge in high-calorie meals or snacks, such as holidays, by developing an attitude of nonfailure and regained control or coping. Time may be planned for the patient to "break" the diet.

Promotes patient's perception of control.

- If bingeing has been a problem and other techniques have not effectively eliminated it, then assist the patient in planning the next binge to the final detail.

The patient's *not* following through with the planned binge will demonstrate his or her control over binges, and his or her strength can be promoted. The patient following through with the planned binge can also demonstrate control; the patient regains power and can then proceed to schedule and plan binges, altering the frequency and amount consumed gradually. Either option should be positively received by the nurse with appropriate follow-up to promote the patient's positive orientation.[55,58]

- Suggest patient contract with a significant other or home health nurse prior to discharge.

Provides added reinforcement and support for continued weight loss.

Continued

ACTIONS/INTERVENTIONS	RATIONALES
• Develop a list of rewards for positive changes. These rewards should be ones the patient will give himself or herself or that can be given by the health care team or patient support system and should not be related to food. The patient's reward schedule should be listed here.	Many patients will have difficulty identifying nonfood rewards, and a great deal of support may be needed. Rewards should initially be scheduled on a daily basis for successful achievement of behavior related to weight loss and can then be gradually expanded to weekly or monthly rewards that promote the patient's self-esteem and provide motivation for continued efforts.
• Instruct patient to postpone desire to eat between meals by doing 5 min of slow deep breathing and reviewing 3 of the identified positive motivating factors for weight loss for this patient. If the desire to eat remains, have the patient drink a glass of water or cup of herb tea and spend 10 min engaged in an activity such as writing a letter, working on a hobby, reading, sewing, or playing with children or spouse or significant other—anything but watching television (this activity generally contains too many food cues).	Provides patient time to substitute positive coping behavior for dysfunctional eating behavior.[56]
• Refer patient to community resources at least 3 days prior to discharge from hospital.	Provides long-range support for continued success with weight loss.

Child Health

Orders are the same as for the adult. Make actions specific to the child according to the child's developmental level.

Women's Health

ACTIONS/INTERVENTIONS	RATIONALES
• Verify the prepregnancy weight. • Obtain a 24-h diet history. Ask patient to select a typical day. • Calculate the woman's calorie and protein intake. • Rule out excessive edema and hypertension. Measure ankles and abdominal girth and record. Remeasure each day. Measure BP every 4 h while awake at (state times here).	Provides basis for planning diet with patient.

• Encourage client to increase her activity by:
  ○ Joining exercise groups for pregnancy (usually found in childbirth classes in community)
  ○ Joining swim exercise groups for pregnancy (usually found at YWCAs or community centers)
• Refer patient to appropriate support groups for assistance in exercise programs for the pregnant woman (e.g., physical therapist, local groups who have swimming classes for pregnant women, and childbirth classes).
	Assists in maintaining desired weight gain; improves muscle tone and circulation.

• If recommended intake is 2400 cal/day but 24-h diet recall reveals a higher caloric intake:
  ○ Recommend reduction of fat in diet (e.g., decrease amount of cooking oil used, use less salad dressing and margarine, cut excess fat off meat, and take skin off chicken before preparing).
  ○ Monitor size of food portions.
  ○ Stress that appetite can be controlled with high-quality sources of energy and protein.
	Basic measures and teaching factors to assist in weight control.

- Assist mothers with cultural or economic restrictions to introduce more variety into their diets.
- Stress that weight gain is the only way the fetus can be supplied with nourishment.
- Point out that added body fat will be burned and will provide necessary energy during lactation (breast-feeding).
- Assist pregnant adolescents within 3 yr of menarche to plan diets that have needed additional nutrients.
- Discourage any attempts at weight reduction or dieting.

Diet has to be planned to meet the growth needs of the adolescent as well as those of the fetus.

NOTE: Dieting is never recommended during pregnancy because it deprives mother and fetus of nutrients for tissue growth and because weight loss is accompanied by maternal ketosis, a direct threat to fetal well-being.[22,40]

Additional Information

A satisfactory pattern of weight gain for the average woman is[5]:

10 wk gestation	650 g (approximately 1.5 lb)
20 wk gestation	4000 g (approximately 9.0 lb)
30 wk gestation	8500 g (approximately 19.0 lb)
40 wk gestation	12,500 g (approximately 27.5 lb)

Over the course of the pregnancy, a total weight gain of 25 to 35 lb is recommended for both nonobese and obese pregnant women. During the second and third trimesters, a gain of about 1 lb/wk is considered desirable.

Psychiatric Health

Nursing actions for the mental health client with this diagnosis are the same as those actions for Adult Health.

Gerontic Health

Nursing actions for the gerontic patient with this diagnosis are the same as those actions in Adult Health and Home Health.

Home Health

ACTIONS/INTERVENTIONS	RATIONALES

- Assist client in identifying lifestyle changes that may be required:
  ○ Regular exercise at least 3 times per week that includes stretching and flexibility exercises and aerobic activity (20 min) at target training rate
  ○ Nutritional habits that include decreasing fat and simple carbohydrates and increasing complex carbohydrates
	Knowledge and support provide motivation for change and increase the potential for positive outcomes.

- Assist client and family in identifying cues other than focus on weight and calories, such as feeling of well-being, percent of body fat, increased exercise endurance, and better-fitting clothes.	Excess focus on the weight as measured by the scale and on calorie counting may increase the probability of failure and encourage the pattern of repeated weight loss followed by weight gain. This pattern results in increased percentage of body fat.

- Have client and family design personalized plan:
  ○ Menu planning
  ○ Decreased fats and simple carbohydrates and increased complex carbohydrates
  ○ Regular, balanced exercise
  ○ Lifestyle changes
	A personalized plan improves the probability of adherence to the plan.

Nutrition, Altered, Risk for or More Than Body Requirements

FLOWCHART EVALUATION: EXPECTED OUTCOME 1

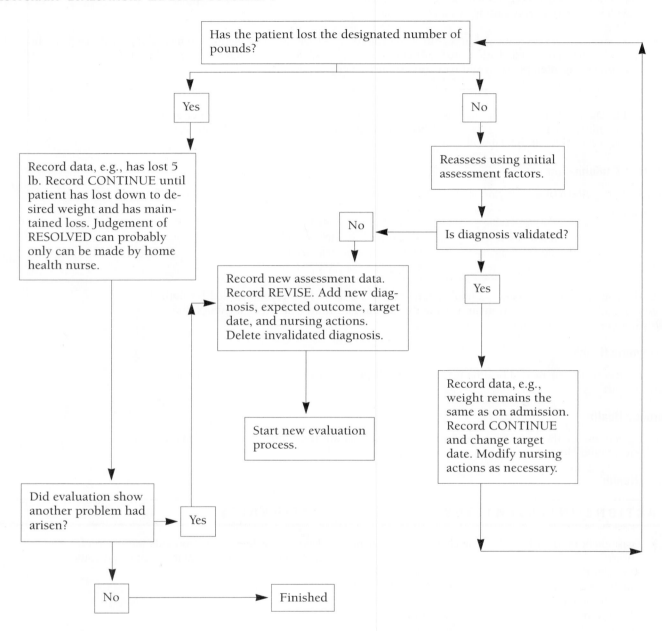

Nutrition, Altered, Risk for or More Than Body Requirements

FLOWCHART EVALUATION: EXPECTED OUTCOME 2

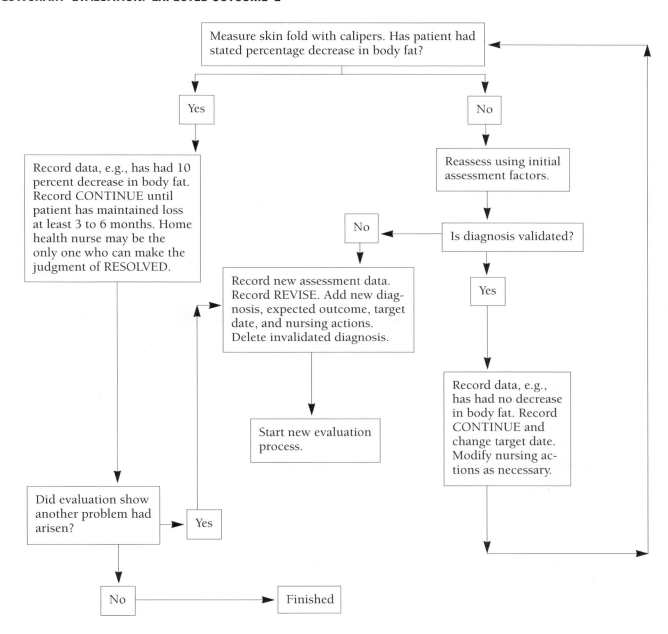

Swallowing, Impaired

DEFINITION

The state in which an individual has decreased ability to voluntarily pass fluids and/or solids from the mouth to the stomach.[23]

NANDA TAXONOMY: MOVING 6.5.1.1

DEFINING CHARACTERISTICS[23]

1. Major defining characteristics
   a. Observed evidence of difficulty in swallowing, for example, stasis of food in oral cavity
   b. Coughing or choking
   c. Evidence of aspiration
2. Minor defining characteristics
   None given.

RELATED FACTORS[23]

1. Neuromuscular impairment (e.g., decreased or absent gag reflex, decreased strength or excursion of muscles involved in mastication, perceptual impairment, or facial paralysis)
2. Mechanical obstruction (e.g., edema, tracheostomy tube, or tumor)
3. Fatigue
4. Limited awareness
5. Reddened, irritated oropharyngeal cavity

RELATED CLINICAL CONCERNS

1. Cerebrovascular accident
2. Any neuromuscular diagnosis, for example, myasthenia gravis, muscular dystrophy, cerebral palsy, Parkinson's disease, Alzheimer's disease, poliomyelitis
3. Hyperthyroidism
4. Any medical diagnosis related to decreased level of consciousness, for example, seizures, concussions, or increased intracranial pressure
5. Tracheoesophageal problems, for example, fistula, tumor, edema, or presence of tracheostomy tube
6. Anxiety

HAVE YOU SELECTED THE CORRECT DIAGNOSIS?

Altered Oral Mucous Membrane   Impaired Swallowing implies that there is a mechanical or physiologic obstruction between the oropharynx and the esophagus. An Altered Oral Mucous Membrane indicates that only the oral cavity is involved. Structures below the oral cavity, per se, are not affected. If liquids or solids are able to pass through the oral cavity, even though pain or difficulty might be present, there will be nothing obstructing its passage through the esophagus to the stomach. Therefore, if solids or liquids are able to pass into the stomach without crowing, coughing, or choking, the appropriate nursing diagnosis is **not** Impaired Swallowing.

Altered Nutrition, Less Than Body Requirements   Certainly Altered Nutrition, Less Than Body Requirements, would be a consideration and probably a secondary problem to Impaired Swallowing. Choosing between the two diagnoses would be based on the related factors, with Impaired Swallowing taking priority over the Altered Nutrition initially.

EXPECTED OUTCOMES

1. Will be able to freely swallow (solids) (liquids) by (date) and/or
2. Will not have any aspiration problems by (date)

TARGET DATES

Since Impaired Swallowing can be life-threatening, the patient should be checked for progress daily. After the condition has improved, progress could be checked at 3-day intervals.

NURSING ACTIONS/INTERVENTIONS WITH RATIONALES

Adult Health

ACTIONS/INTERVENTIONS	RATIONALES
• Monitor for lesions or infectious processes of the mouth and oropharynx at least once per shift.	Lesions or ulcers in the mouth promote difficulty in swallowing.
• Test, prior to every offering of food, fluid, etc., for presence of gag reflex.	Prevents choking and aspiration.

- Test swallowing capacity with clear, sterile water **only**, prior to offering food or fluids. Have suctioning equipment and tracheostomy tray on standby in patient's room.

- Support hydration and caloric intake. Collaborate with physician regarding the need for IVs, hyperalimentation, etc.

- Maintain appropriate upright position during feeding.
- Warm fluids before offering to patient.

- Stay with the patient while he or she tries to eat.

- Be supportive to patient during swallowing efforts.
- Consult with nutritionist about patient's preferred food list and about enhancing the nutritional value of those foods that are easier for the patient to swallow (e.g., adding vitamins to warm liquids).
- Provide for rest periods before and after eating.

- Measure and document intake and output each shift. Total each 24 h.
- Weigh patient each day at the same time (note time here) and in same-weight clothing.
- Advance diet as tolerated.
- Teach the patient who has had supraglottic surgery an alternate method of swallowing:
  - Have the patient clear his or her throat by coughing and expectorating. If patient unable to expectorate, suction the secretions.
  - Have the patient inhale as the food is put in the mouth.
  - Have the patient then perform a Valsalva maneuver as he or she is swallowing.
  - Have the patient cough, swallow again, and exhale deeply.
  - Start with soft, nonacidic, noncrumbly foods rather than liquids. Liquids are more difficult to control.
  - Provide privacy for the patient as he or she learns alternate swallowing.
  - Teach at least one other family member or significant other how to support patient in alternate swallowing, suctioning, Heimlich maneuver, etc.
- Refer patient as needed to other health care team members.

Provides equipment needed in case of aspiration or respiratory obstruction emergency.

Maintains fluid and electrolytes even though patient may not be able to swallow.

Gravity assists in facilitation of swallowing.
Warm fluids assist swallowing through mild relaxation of esophageal muscles.
Basic safety measure for patient who has difficulty swallowing.
Swallowing difficulty is very frustrating for the patient.

Coughing episodes are frequent with impaired swallowing, and coughing is very tiring.
Basic monitoring of patient's condition. Permits a consistent and more accurate comparison.

Facilitates active swallowing and support for patient as he or she begins to adapt to impaired swallowing.

Collaboration supports a holistic approach to patient care.

Child Health

ACTIONS/INTERVENTIONS	RATIONALES
- Monitor for contributory factors, especially palate formation, possible tracheoesophageal fistula, or other congenital anomalies.	A thorough assessment will best identify those patients who have greater-than-usual likelihood of swallowing difficulties due to structural, acquired, or circumstantial conditions.
- Maintain infant in upright position after feedings for at least 1½ h.	An upright position will favor, by gravity, the digestion and absorption of nutrients, thereby decreasing the likelihood of reflux and resultant potential for choking.

Continued

ACTIONS/INTERVENTIONS	RATIONALES
• Address anticipatory safety needs for possible choking: 　○ Have appropriate suctioning equipment available. 　○ Teach parents CPR. 　○ Provide parenting support for CPR and suctioning. 　○ Assist family to identify ways to cope with swallowing disorder, e.g., the need for extra help in feeding. • Administer medications as ordered. Avoid powder or pill forms. Use elixirs or mix as needed.	Usual anticipatory airway management is appropriate in long-term patient management while education and teaching concerns can be addressed in a supportive environment, thereby reducing anxiety in event of cardiopulmonary arrest secondary to impaired swallowing. Pills or powders may increase the likelihood of impaired swallowing in young children and/or infants. Appropriate mixing with fruit syrups or using manufacturer's elixir or suspension form of the drug lessens the likelihood of impaired swallowing.

Women's Health

The nursing actions for a woman with the nursing diagnosis of Impaired Swallowing are the same as those for Adult Health.

Psychiatric Health

NOTE: The following nursing actions are specific considerations for the mental health client who has Impaired Swallowing that is caused or increased by anxiety. Refer to Psychiatric Health nursing actions for the diagnosis of Anxiety for interventions related to decreasing and resolving the client's anxiety. If swallowing problems are related to an eating disorder, refer to Psychiatric Health nursing actions for Altered Nutrition, Less Than Body Requirements, for additional nursing actions.

ACTIONS/INTERVENTIONS	RATIONALES
• Provide a quiet, relaxed environment during meals by discussing with client the situations that increase anxiety and excluding those factors from the situation. Provide things such as favorite music and friends or family that increase relaxation. (Note information provided by client here, especially those things that need to be provided by the nursing staff.)	Promotes client's control and facilitates relaxation response, thus inhibiting the sympathetic nervous system response.[55,57]
• Provide medications in liquid or injectable form. (Note any special preference client may have in presentation of medications here.)	Liquids are easier to swallow than tablets. Providing medications by injection would prevent any swallowing problems.
• Teach client deep muscle relaxation. (Refer to the mental health nursing actions for Anxiety for actions related to decreasing anxiety.)	Promotes client control and inhibits the sympathetic nervous system response.
• Discuss with client foods that are the easiest and the most difficult to swallow. Note information from this discussion here. (Note time and person responsible for this discussion here.)	Promotes client control.
• Plan client's most nutritious meals for the time of day he or she is most relaxed, and note that time here.	
• Provide client with high-energy snacks several times during the day. (Note snacks preferred by client and time they are to be offered here.)	Provides additional calories in frequent small amounts.

- Assign primary nurse to sit with client 30 min (this can be increased to an hour as client tolerates interaction time better) 2 times a day to discuss concerns related to swallowing. (This can be included in the time described under the nursing actions for Anxiety.) As the nurse-client relationship moves to a working phase, discussion can include those factors that precipitated client's focus on swallowing. These factors could be a trauma directly related to swallowing, such as an attack in which the client was choked or in which oral sex was forced.

  Provides increased individuation and continuity of care, facilitating the development of a therapeutic relationship. The nursing process requires that a trusting and functional relationship exist between nurse and client.[55]

- Teach client and client's support system nutrition factors that will improve swallowing and maintain adequate nutrition. Note here the names of those persons client would like included in this teaching. Note here the time arranged and person responsible for this teaching.

  Promotes long-term support for assistance with problem.

Gerontic Health

Nursing actions for the gerontic patient with this diagnosis are the same as those for Adult Health and Psychiatric Health.

Home Health

ACTIONS/INTERVENTIONS	RATIONALES
Teach measures to decrease or eliminate Impaired Swallowing: ○ Principles of oral hygiene ○ Small pieces of food or pureed food as necessary ○ Aspiration precautions, e.g., eat and drink sitting up, do not force-feed or fill mouth too full, and CPR ○ Proper nutrition and hydration ○ Use of adaptive equipment as required Teach patient to monitor for factors contributing to Impaired Swallowing, e.g., fatigue, obstruction, neuromuscular impairment, or irritated oropharyngeal cavity, on at least a daily basis.	Prevents or diminishes problems. Promotes self-care and provides database for early intervention.
Involve client and family in planning, implementing, and promoting reduction or elimination of Impaired Swallowing by establishing regular family conferences to provide for mutual goal setting and to improve communication.	Goal setting and communication promote positive outcomes.
Assist client and family in lifestyle changes that may be required. ○ Client may need to be fed. ○ Mealtimes should be quiet, uninterrupted, and at consistent times on a daily basis. ○ Client may require special diet and special utensils.	Knowledge and support provide motivation for change and increase the potential for a positive outcome.

Swallowing, Impaired

FLOWCHART EVALUATION: EXPECTED OUTCOME 1

Swallowing, Impaired

FLOWCHART EVALUATION: EXPECTED OUTCOME 2

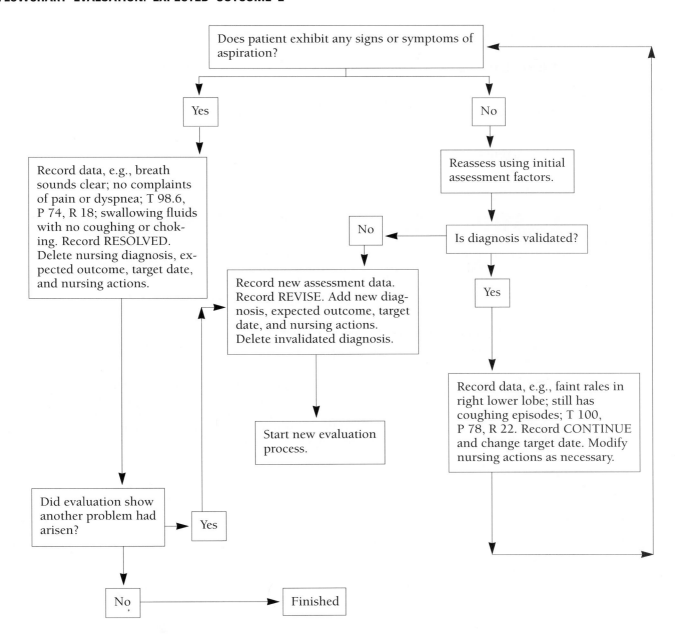

Does patient exhibit any signs or symptoms of aspiration?

Yes

No

Record data, e.g., breath sounds clear; no complaints of pain or dyspnea; T 98.6, P 74, R 18; swallowing fluids with no coughing or choking. Record RESOLVED. Delete nursing diagnosis, expected outcome, target date, and nursing actions.

Reassess using initial assessment factors.

No

Is diagnosis validated?

Record new assessment data. Record REVISE. Add new diagnosis, expected outcome, target date, and nursing actions. Delete invalidated diagnosis.

Yes

Start new evaluation process.

Record data, e.g., faint rales in right lower lobe; still has coughing episodes; T 100, P 78, R 22. Record CONTINUE and change target date. Modify nursing actions as necessary.

Did evaluation show another problem had arisen?

Yes

No

Finished

Thermoregulation, Ineffective

DEFINITION

The state in which the individual's temperature fluctuates between hypothermia and hyperthermia.[23]

NANDA TAXONOMY: EXCHANGING 1.2.2.4

DEFINING CHARACTERISTIC[23]

1. Major defining characteristics
   a. Fluctuations in body temperature above or below the normal range.
2. Minor defining characteristics
   None given.

RELATED FACTORS[23]

1. Trauma or illness
2. Immaturity
3. Aging
4. Fluctuating environmental temperature

RELATED CLINICAL CONCERNS

1. Any infection
2. Any surgery
3. Septicemia

HAVE YOU SELECTED THE CORRECT DIAGNOSIS?

Hyperthermia   Hyperthermia means that a person maintains a body temperature greater than normal for himself or herself. In Ineffective Thermoregulation, the client's temperature is changing between Hyperthermia and Hypothermia. If the temperature measurement is remaining above normal, the correct diagnosis is Hyperthermia, not Ineffective Thermoregulation.

Hypothermia   Hypothermia means that a person maintains a body temperature below normal for himself or herself. If the temperature is consistently remaining below normal, the correct diagnosis is Hypothermia, not Ineffective Thermoregulation.

Risk for Altered Body Temperature   With this diagnosis the patient has a potential inability to regulate heat production and heat dissipation within a normal range. The key point to remember is that a temperature abnormality does not exist yet but the risk factors present indicate that such a problem could develop. If the temperature measurements are fluctuating between hypothermia and hyperthermia, the correct diagnosis is Ineffective Thermoregulation.

EXPECTED OUTCOMES

1. Will maintain a body temperature between 97 and 99°F by (date) and/or
2. Will identify at least (number) of measures to use in correcting Ineffective Thermoregulation by (date)

TARGET DATES

Initial target dates will be stated in terms of hours. After stabilization, an appropriate target date would be 3 days.

NURSING ACTIONS/INTERVENTIONS WITH RATIONALES
Adult Health

ACTIONS/INTERVENTIONS	RATIONALES
• Monitor vital signs at least every hour on the (hour/half-hour). • Maintain room temperature at all times at 72°F. Provide warmth or cooling as needed to maintain temperature in desired range; avoid drafts and chilling for the patient.	Tracks basic trends in temperature fluctuations. Permits early recognition of ineffective thermoregulation. Offsets environmental impact on thermoregulation.

- Reduce stress for patient. Provide quiet, nonstimulating environment.

- If the patient is hypothermic, see nursing actions for hypothermia on page 152.
- If patient is hyperthermic, see nursing actions for hyperthermia on page 145.
- Make referrals for appropriate follow-up before dismissal from hospital.

Assists body to maintain homeostasis. Stress could contribute to problems with thermoregulation due to increased basal metabolic rate.
Thermoregulation problems may vary from hypothermia to hyperthermia.

Provides long-range, cost-effective support.

Child Health

ACTIONS/INTERVENTIONS	RATIONALES
• Protect child from excessive chilling during bathing or procedures. • Assist in answering parent's or child's questions regarding temperature-monitoring procedures or administration of medications. • Assist parents in dealing with anxiety in times of unknown causes or prognosis by allowing 30 min per shift for venting anxiety (state times here). Interview parents specifically to ascertain anxiety. • Involve parents and family in child's care whenever appropriate, especially for comforting child.	Evaporation and significant change of temperature for even short periods of time will contribute to heat loss for the young child or infant, especially during illness. Appropriate teaching fosters compliance and reduces anxiety. Because the emphasis on monitoring and treating altered thermoregulation is so great, it can be easy to overlook the parents and their concerns. Specific attention must be given to ascertaining how the patient and family are feeling about all the many concerns generated. Parental involvement fosters empowerment and regaining of self-care, thereby reestablishing the likelihood for effective family coping.

Women's Health

This nursing diagnosis will pertain to women the same as it would for any other adult. The reader is referred to the Adult Health and Home Health nursing actions for this diagnosis.

Psychiatric Health

The nursing actions for this diagnosis in the mental health client are the same as those for Adult Health.

Gerontic Health

Nursing actions for the gerontic patient with this diagnosis are the same as those actions for Adult Health and Home Health.

Home Health

ACTIONS/INTERVENTIONS	RATIONALES
• Monitor for factors contributing to Ineffective Thermoregulation (illness, trauma, immaturity, aging, or fluctuating environmental temperature).	Allows early recognition and early implementation of therapy.
• Involve client and family in planning, implementing, and promoting reduction or elimination of Ineffective Thermoregulation.	Personal involvement and input increase likelihood of maintenance of plan.
• Teach client and family early signs and symptoms of Ineffective Thermoregulation (see Hyperthermia and Hypothermia).	
• Teach client and family measures to decrease or eliminate Ineffective Thermoregulation (see Hyperthermia and Hypothermia).	
• Assist client and family to identify lifestyle changes that may be required (see Hyperthermia and Hypothermia).	Provides basic information and planning to successfully manage condition at home.

Thermoregulation, Ineffective

FLOWCHART EVALUATION: EXPECTED OUTCOME 1

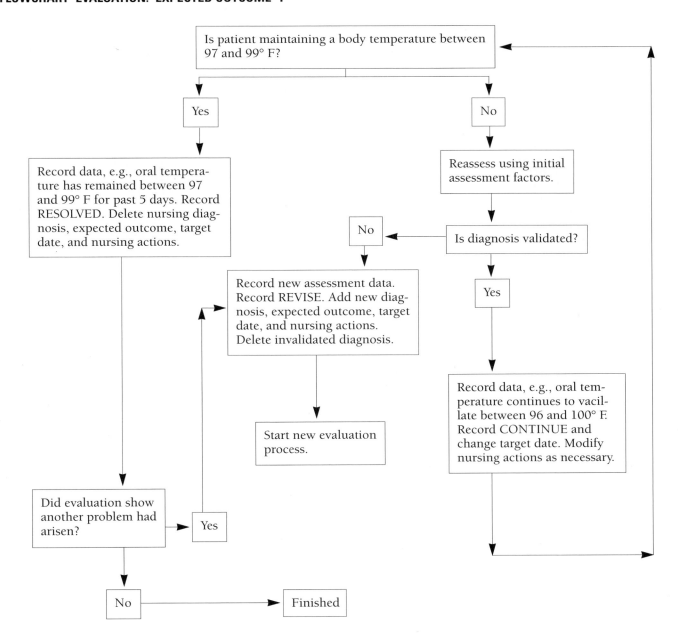

Thermoregulation, Ineffective

FLOWCHART EVALUATION: EXPECTED OUTCOME 2

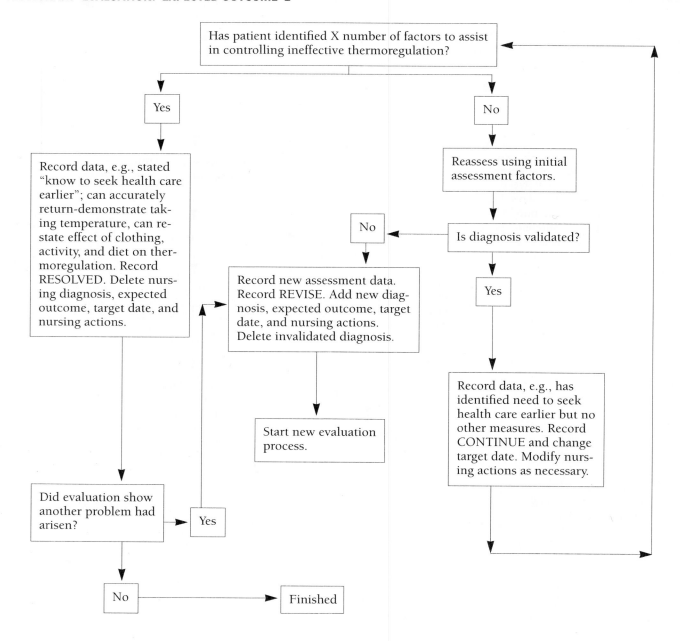

Tissue Integrity, Impaired

DEFINITION[23]

TISSUE INTEGRITY, IMPAIRED A state in which an individual experiences damage to mucous membrane, corneal, integumentary, or subcutaneous tissue.

RISK FOR IMPAIRED SKIN INTEGRITY A state in which the individual's skin is at risk of being adversely altered.

IMPAIRED SKIN INTEGRITY A state in which the individual's skin is adversely altered.

ALTERED ORAL MUCOUS MEMBRANE The state in which an individual experiences disruptions in the tissue layers of the oral cavity.

NANDA TAXONOMY: EXCHANGING 1.6.2.1, 1.6.2.1.2.2, 1.6.2.1.2.1, AND 1.6.2.1.1

DEFINING CHARACTERISTICS[23]

1. Major defining characteristics
   A. Impaired Tissue Integrity
      (1) Damaged or destroyed tissue (cornea, mucous membrane, integumentary, or subcutaneous)
   B. Risk factors for Impaired Skin Integrity
      (1) External (environmental)
         (a) Hypo- or hyperthermia
         (b) Chemical substance
         (c) Mechanical factors
            (1) Shearing forces
            (2) Pressure
            (3) Restraint
         (d) Radiation
         (e) Physical immobilization
         (f) Excretions or secretions
         (g) Humidity
      (2) Internal (somatic)
         (a) Medication
         (b) Alterations in nutritional state
            (1) Obesity
            (2) Emaciation
         (c) Altered metabolic state
         (d) Altered circulation
         (e) Altered sensation
         (f) Altered pigmentation
         (g) Skeletal prominence
         (h) Developmental factors
         (i) Alterations in skin turgor (change in elasticity)
         (j) Psychogenic
         (k) Immunologic
   C. Impaired Skin Integrity
      (1) Disruption of skin surfaces
      (2) Destruction of skin layers
      (3) Invasion of body structures
   D. Altered Oral Mucous Membrane
      (1) Oral pain or discomfort
      (2) Coated tongue
      (3) Xerostomia (dry mouth)
      (4) Stomatitis
      (5) Oral lesions or ulcers
      (6) Lack of or decreased salivation
      (7) Leukoplakia
      (8) Edema
      (9) Hyperemia
      (10) Oral plaque
      (11) Desquamation
      (12) Vesicles
      (13) Hemorrhagic gingivitis
      (14) Carious teeth
      (15) Halitosis
2. Minor defining characteristics
   None given.

RELATED FACTORS[23]

1. Impaired Tissue Integrity
   a. Altered circulation
   b. Nutritional deficit or excess
   c. Fluid deficit or excess
   d. Knowledge deficit
   e. Impaired physical mobility
   f. Irritants
      (1) Chemical (including body excretions, secretions, and medications)
      (2) Thermal (temperature extremes)
      (3) Mechanical (pressure, shear, and friction)
      (4) Radiation (including therapeutic radiation)
2. Risk for Impaired Skin Integrity
   The risk factors also serve as the related factors.
3. Impaired Skin Integrity
   a. External (environmental)
      (1) Hypo- or hyperthermia
      (2) Chemical substance
      (3) Mechanical factors
         (a) Shearing forces
         (b) Pressure
         (c) Restraint
      (4) Radiation
      (5) Physical immobilization
      (6) Humidity
   b. Internal (somatic)
      (1) Medication
      (2) Alterations in nutritional state
         (a) Obesity
         (b) Emaciation
      (3) Altered metabolic state
      (4) Altered circulation
      (5) Altered sensation
      (6) Altered pigmentation
      (7) Skeletal prominence
      (8) Developmental factors
      (9) Immunologic deficit
      (10) Alterations in skin turgor (change in elasticity)
4. Altered Oral Mucous Membrane
   a. Pathologic conditions: Oral cavity (radiation to head or neck)
   b. Dehydration
   c. Trauma
      (1) Chemical, for example, acidic foods, drugs, noxious agents, and alcohol
      (2) Mechanical, for example, ill-fitting dentures, braces, tubes (endotracheal or nasogastric), and surgery in oral cavity

d. NPO for more than 24 hours
e. Ineffective oral hygiene
f. Mouth breathing
g. Malnutrition
h. Infection
i. Lack of or decreased salivation
j. Medication

RELATED CLINICAL CONCERNS

1. Any condition requiring immobilization of patient
2. Burns: Chemical, thermal, or radiation
3. Accidents: Motor vehicle, farm equipment, motorcycles, and so on
4. AIDS
5. Congestive heart failure
6. Diabetes mellitus

HAVE YOU SELECTED THE CORRECT DIAGNOSIS?

Impaired Skin Integrity   If the tissue damage involves only the skin and its subcutaneous tissues, then the most correct diagnosis is Impaired Skin Integrity. Risk for Impaired Skin Integrity would be the most appropriate diagnosis if the patient was presenting a majority of risk factors for a skin integrity problem but the problem has not yet developed.

Altered Oral Mucous Membrane   If the tissue damage involves only the oral mucous membranes, then the best diagnosis is Altered Oral Mucous Membrane. Impaired Tissue Integrity is a higher-level diagnosis and would cover a wider range of tissue types. Altered Oral Mucous Membranes and the two diagnoses related to Skin Integrity are more specific and exact diagnoses and should be used before Impaired Tissue Integrity if the problem can be definitively isolated to either the oral mucous membrane or the skin.

EXPECTED OUTCOMES

1. Will exhibit no signs or symptoms of increased tissue integrity problems (e.g., increased size or infection) by (date) and/or
2. Will implement plan to avoid future episodes of Impaired Tissue Integrity by (date)

TARGET DATES

Tissue integrity problems can begin developing within hours of a patient's admission if caution is not taken regarding turning, cleaning, and so on. Therefore, an initial target date of 2 days after admission would be most appropriate.

NURSING ACTIONS/INTERVENTIONS WITH RATIONALES
Adult Health

ACTIONS/INTERVENTIONS	RATIONALES
• Perform active or passive ROM exercises at least once per shift at (state times here).	Stimulates circulation, which provides nourishment and carries away waste, thus reducing the likelihood of tissue breakdown.
• Ambulate to extent possible.	
• Change position at least hourly, and teach patient to change position at least every 30 min. Do not position on affected area.	
• If patient is unable to turn self, have several persons available to help lift, then turn.	
• Gently massage pressure points and bony prominences following each position change.	
• Teach patient and significant others how to turn patient without shearing force being involved. Be sure bed has siderails and a trapeze (overhead) bar for assistance with turning. Move slowly.	
• Use soft, wrinkle-free linen only.	
• Place cornstarch or powder on linens.	

- Make sure footboard is in place for patient to use for bracing.
- Avoid use of rubber or plastic in direct contact with patient.
- Reduce pressure on affected skin surface by using: Pressure predisposes tissue breakdown.
  - Egg crate
  - Alternating air mattress
  - Sheepskin
  - Commercial wafer barriers
  - Thick dressing used as pad on bony prominences
  - Bed cradle
- Collaborate with dietitian regarding well-balanced diet. Assist patient to eat as necessary.   Prevents tissue breakdown due to negative nitrogen balance.
- Monitor dietary intake, and avoid irritant food and fluid intake (e.g., highly spiced food or extremes of temperature).   These factors would increase probability of oral mucous membrane problems.
- Encourage fluid intake to at least 2000 mL per 24 h.   Maintains fluid and electrolyte balance, which is necessary for tissue repair and normal functioning.

- Measure and total intake and output every 8 h.
- Cleanse perineal area carefully after each urination or bowel movement. Monitor closely for any urinary or fecal incontinence.   Allowing body wastes to remain on skin promotes tissue breakdown. Incontinence would increase probability of such an event.
- Teach patient principles of good skin hygiene.   Promotes self-care and self-management to prevent problem.

- Have patient cough and deep breathe every 2 h on the (odd/even) hour.   Basic care measures to offset other complications that develop in tandem with impaired tissue integrity.
- Administer oral hygiene at least 3 times a day after each meal and PRN: Basic care measures to maintain oral mucosa.
  - Brush teeth, gums, and tongue with soft-bristled brush, sponge stick, or gauze-wrapped finger.
  - Floss teeth
  - Rinse mouth thoroughly after brushing. Avoid commercial mouthwashes and preparations with alcohol, lemon, or glycerin. Use normal saline or oxidizing agent (mild hydrogen peroxide solution, Gly-oxide, sodium bicarbonate solution).
  - If patient is unable to rinse, turn on side and do oral irrigation.
  - Teach patient how to use water pick.
  - Teach patient and significant others proper oral hygiene.
  - If patient has dentures, cleanse with equal parts of hydrogen peroxide and water.
  - Apply lubricant to lips at least every 2 h on the (odd/even) hour.
- Maintain good body hygiene. Be sure patient has at least a sponge bath every day **unless** skin is too dry.
- Monitor for signs of infection at least daily.   Infection, through production of toxins, wastes, and so on, increases the probability of tissue damage.

- Keep room temperature and humidity constant. Room temperature should be keep close to 72°F and humidity at a low level unless otherwise ordered.   Keeps skin cool and dry to prevent perspiration.
- Darken room, as necessary, to protect eyes.
- Encourage patient to chew sugar-free gum to stimulate salivation.
- Administer medications as ordered and record response (e.g., topical oral antibiotics, or analgesic mouthwashes). Record response within 30 min of administration.
- Encourage patient to avoid smoking.   Highly irritating to mucous membranes.
- Provide between-meal food or fluids that patient has identified as soothing, e.g., warm or cool.

Continued

ACTIONS/INTERVENTIONS	RATIONALES
• If lesions develop, cleanse area daily at (time) according to prescribed regimen.	
• Protect open surface with such products as:	
○ Karaya powder	
○ Skin gel	
○ Wafer barrier	
○ Other commercial skin preparations	
• Collaborate with an enterostomal therapist and the physician regarding care specific to the patient (list individualized care procedures here).	
• Change dressings when needed using aseptic techniques. Collaborate with physician regarding dressing type and use of topical agents.	
• Teach patient and significant others care of wound prior to discharge.	Basic care measures for impaired skin integrity.
• Avoid use of adhesive tape. If tape must be applied, use nonallergic tape.	
• Avoid use of doughnut ring.	
• Use mild, unscented soap (or soap substitute) and cool or lukewarm water.	
• Avoid vigorous rubbing, but do massage gently using a lanolin-based unscented lotion.	
• Pat area dry. Be sure area is thoroughly dry.	
• Expose to air, sunlight, or heat lamp at least 4 times a day at (state times here). Check patient at least every 5 min if using heat lamp.	
• Monitor:	These measures would allow early detection of any complications.
○ Skin surface and pressure areas at least every 4 h at (state times here) for blanching, erythema, temperature difference (e.g., increased warmth), or moisture	
○ Size and color of lesion at least every 4 h at (state times here)	
○ Fluid and electrolyte balance	
• Particularly watch for signs or symptoms of edema. Collaborate with physician regarding frequency of measurement of electrolyte levels.	
• Caution patient and assist to avoid scratching irritated areas:	Avoids further irritation of already damaged tissue.
○ Trim and file nails.	
○ Apply cool compresses.	
• Collaborate with physician regarding medicated baths (e.g., oatmeal) and topical ointments.	
• Teach patient to press rather than scratch area that is itching.	
• Refer to community health agencies and other health care providers as appropriate.	Provides ongoing support and cost-effective use of available resources.

Child Health

ACTIONS/INTERVENTIONS	RATIONALES
• Handle infant gently; especially caution paramedical personnel regarding need for gentle handling.	The epidermis of infants and young children is thin and lacking in subcutaneous depth. Others, such as x-ray technicians, may not realize the fragile nature of skin as they carry out necessary procedures.
• Place patient on sheepskin or flotation pad, or if parents choose, allow infant or child to be held frequently.	Alternating surface contact and position favors circulatory return to central venous system.

- Caution patient and parents to avoid scratching irritated area:
  - Trim nails with appropriate scissors; receive parental permission if necessary.
  - Make small mitts if necessary from cotton stockinette used for precasting.
- Monitor perineal area for possible allergy to diapers.

Anticipate potential injury of delicate epidermis, especially when irritation may prompt itching.

Various synthetics in diapers may evoke allergenic responses and either cause or worsen existent skin irritation.

- Encourage fluids:
  - Infants: 250–300 mL/24 h
  - Toddler: 1150–1300 mL/24 h
  - Preschooler: 1600 mL/24 h
  (These are approximate ranges. The physician may order specific amounts according to the child's age and condition.)

Adequate hydration will assist in normal homeostatic mechanisms which will affect the skin's integrity.

- Provide protection such as bandage or padding to tissue site involved.
- Monitor and document circulation to affected tissue via:
  - Peripheral arterial pulses
  - Blanching or capillary refill
  - Tissue color
  - Sensation to touch or temperature
  - Tissue general condition, e.g., bruising or lacerations
  - Drainage, e.g., amount, odor, or color
  - ROM limitations

Anticipation and protection from injury serves to limit the depth and/or degree of altered skin integrity.
These factors represent basic appropriate criteria for circulatory checks. They may be added to in instances of specific concerns such as compartment syndrome associated with hand trauma.

- Administer oral hygiene according to needs and status:
  - Glycerin and lemon swabs for NPO infant
  - Special orders for postoperative cleft palate or cleft lip repair

Appropriate oral hygiene will decrease the likelihood of altered integrity of surrounding tissues and is critical for care of altered associated oral disorders.

- Teach parents to limit time infant sucks bottle in reclining position to best prevent bottle syndrome and decayed teeth.

Evidence suggests that bottle syndrome is prevented by not having infant go to sleep with bottle. Completion of feeding and removal of bottle are suggested before placing infant in crib.

- Protect the altered tissue site as needed during movement by providing support to the limb.

Provision of support and usual use of body parts will favor adequate circulation and prevent further injury.

- Provide ROM and ambulation as permitted to encourage vascular return.
- Position patient while in bed so that the head of the bed is elevated slightly and involved limb is elevated approximately 20 degrees.

Appropriate venous return is favored by resultant gravity with limb higher than heart.

- Address altered thermoregulation, and especially protect patient from chilling or shock due to dehydration or sepsis.

In severe instances of altered thermoregulation or related pathology, there may not be the usual manifestations of derivations from normals. It may also be difficult to assess sensation in the young infant due to the infant's inability to provide verbal feedback.

- Use restraints judiciously for involved limb or body site.

Any undue constriction or threat to circulation must be weighed appropriately in making decisions as to whether or not to restrain the child.

- Monitor intravenous infusion and administration of medications carefully. Avoid use of sites in close proximity to area of altered tissue integrity.
- Allow patient and family time to express concerns by providing at least 30 min per shift for family counseling (state times here).

This is usual protocol for IV therapy and must be considered paramount as IV meds or solutions pose serious threats to the veins and surrounding tissues.
Reduces anxiety since the family's concerns can be made known and their feelings valued.

Continued

ACTIONS/INTERVENTIONS	RATIONALES
• Teach patient and family: 　◦ Need for follow-up care 　◦ Signs and symptoms to be reported: 　　(1) Increased temperature (101°F or above) 　　(2) Foul odors or drainage 　　(3) Delayed healing or increase in damage site size 　　(4) Loss of sensation or pulsation in limb or site 　　(5) Any increase in pain 　◦ Prosthetic device if indicated 　◦ Aids in mobility, such as crutches or walker 　◦ Need to avoid constrictive clothing 　◦ Appropriate dietary restrictions or needs	Appropriate education serves to build self-confidence and effects long-term compliance with treatment and health management.

Women's Health

ACTIONS/INTERVENTIONS	RATIONALES
• Monitor perineum and rectum after childbirth for injury or healing at least once per shift at (state times here). Monitor episiotomy site for redness, edema, or hematomas each 15 min immediately after delivery for 1 h, then once each shift thereafter.	Assesses basic physical condition as a basis for providing care and preventing complications.
• Collaborate with physician regarding: 　◦ Applying ice packs or cold pads to perineum for the first 8–12 h after delivery to reduce edema and increase comfort 　◦ Sitz baths twice a day at (state times here) and as necessary for pain and discomfort 　◦ Analgesics and topical anesthetics as necessary for pain and discomfort	Provides comfort and promotes healing.
• Teach good perineal hygiene and self-care: 　◦ Rinse perineal area with warm water after each voiding. 　◦ Pat dry gently from front to back to prevent contamination. 　◦ Apply perineal pad from front to back to prevent contamination. 　◦ Change pads frequently to prevent infection and irritation.	Promotes healing and encourages self-care.
• Provide factual information on resumption of sexual activities after childbirth: 　◦ First intercourse should be after adequate healing period (usually 3–4 wk). 　◦ Intercourse should be slow and easy (woman on top can better control angle, depth, and penetration).	Provides basic information to promote safe self-care.
• Teach postmenopausal women the signs and symptoms of atrophic vaginitis: 　◦ Watery discharge 　◦ Burning and itching of vagina or vulva • Encourage examinations (Pap smears) for estrogen levels at least annually. • In collaboration with physician, encourage use as needed of: 　◦ Estrogen replacement creams or vaginal suppositories 　◦ Extra lubrication during intercourse	Provides basic information that promotes self-care and health maintenance.

- Teach breast-feeding mothers about breast care:
  - Inspect nipples for cracks or fissures.
  - Wear supportive bra (breast binder to relieve engorgement).
  - Shower daily, do not use soap on breast, and allow to air dry.
  - Use lanolin-based cream (vitamin E cream, Masse, or A&D cream) to prevent drying and cracking of nipples.
- Enhance let-down reflex:
  - Nurse early and frequently. Ten minutes on each side is easier on sore nipples than nursing for longer periods less frequently.
  - Nurse at both breasts each feeding. Switch sides to begin nursing each time, e.g., if baby nursed first on left side at last feeding, begin on right side this time. A safety pin or small ribbon on bra strap will remind mother which side she used first last time.
  - Change positions from one feeding to next (distributes sucking pressure).
  - Check baby's position on breast. Be certain areola is in mouth, not just nipple.
  - Begin nursing on least sore side first, if possible; then switch baby to other side.
  - Apply ice to nipple just before nursing to decrease pain (fold squares and put them in the freezer to apply as needed).
- Collaborate with physician regarding use of analgesics. Caution patient to not take over-the-counter medication since some medications are passed to the baby via breast milk.

NOTE: Between the third and sixth months of pregnancy, the process of tooth calcification (hardening) begins in the fetus. What the mother consumes in her diet will affect the development of the unborn child's teeth. A well-balanced diet will usually provide correct amounts of nutrients for both mother and child.

- Teach patient to practice good oral hygiene at least twice a day as well as PRN:
  - Each time patient eats or, if nauseated and vomiting, vomits, patient should clean gums and teeth.
  - If the smell of toothpaste or mouthrinse makes patient nauseated, patient should use baking soda.
- Reduce the number of times sugar-rich foods are eaten between meals.
- Teach patient to snack on fruits, vegetables, cheese, cottage cheese, whole grains, or milk.

- Have patient increase daily calcium intake to at least a total of 1.2 g of calcium per day.
- Collaborate with obstetrician and dentist to plan needed dental care during pregnancy.
- Assist in planning best time in pregnancy for dental visits:
  - Not during the first 3 mo if:
    (1) Previous obstetric history of miscarriage
    (2) Threatened miscarriage
    (3) Other medical indications
    (4) Hypersensitive to gagging (will increase nausea and vomiting)

Provides basic information that assists in preventing skin breakdown and promotes self-care and successful lactation.

Promotes let-down reflex and successful breast-feeding.

Promotes sense of mother's well-being. Assists in promoting proper growth and development of fetus and encourages health maintenance.

Provides basic information to patient that promotes health maintenance and increases awareness of need for self-care.

Continued

ACTIONS/INTERVENTIONS	RATIONALES

○ Not during the last 3 mo if:
  (1) Not able to sit in dental chair for long periods of time
  (2) Obstetric history of premature labor
- Instruct patient to have x-rays only when it is absolutely necessary. Caution patient to request a lead apron when having x-rays.

Prevents x-ray exposure to fetus.

ADDITIONAL INFORMATION

Nursing actions for newborn health immediately follow the women's health nursing actions. As previously mentioned, newborn actions are inclined in this section because newborn care is most often administered by nurses in the obstetrical or women's health area. Focus needs to be made on the newborn simply because the newborn's oral mucous membrane problems can be easily overlooked.

- In collaboration with dentist, teach parents the oral and dental needs of the neonate:
  ○ Use of fluoride
  ○ Proper use of pacifiers
  ○ Not using homemade pacifiers
  ○ Use of pacifiers as recommended by dentist
  ○ Allowing infant who is teething to chew on soft toothbrush (will encourage later brushing of teeth since allows infant to become familiar with toothbrush in mouth)
  ○ Holding on to brush
  ○ Giving brush to infant only when adult is present
- Teach parents how to administer oral hygiene:
  ○ Massage and rub infant's gums with finger daily.
  ○ Inspect oral cavity daily for hygiene and problems.
- Take infant for first dental visit between 18 mo and 2 yr.
- Dental caries (decay) can be a result of prolonged nursing or delayed weaning:
  ○ Do not allow infant to nurse at breast or bottle beyond required feeding time.
  ○ Do not allow infant to sleep habitually at the breast or with a bottle in the mouth.
  ○ Teach the neonate's parents to:
    (1) Avoid giving sweet liquids (soft drinks) or fruit juices in bottle.
    (2) Wean child from bottle to cup soon after first birthday.
    (3) When continuing to nurse infant, give water in cup soon after first birthday.
    (4) Use good handwashing techniques to prevent infection with or reinfection of thrush.
    (5) Do not place infant on sheets where mother has been sitting.
    (6) Thoroughly clean breast or bottle-feeding equipment.

Promotes good health and provides information as a basis for parental care of infant. Assists in preventing infection.

Psychiatric Health

ACTIONS/INTERVENTIONS	RATIONALES
• Refer to Chapter 8 for stress reduction measures and interventions for the stressors that produce psychogenic skin reactions.	
• If client is placed in restraints:	
○ Monitor the integrity of skin under restraints every hour.	
• Apply lanolin-based lotion and cornstarch or powder to area under restraint at least every 2 h on the (odd/even) hour and PRN.	Lubricates skin and decreases risk for breakdown.
○ Pad restraints with nonabrasive materials such as sheepskin.	Decreases mechanical friction against the skin and decreases risk for breakdown.
○ Keep area of restraint next to the skin clean and dry.	
○ Release restraints one at a time every 2 h on (odd/even) hour and PRN. Remove restraints as soon as the client will tolerate one-to-one care without risk to self or others.	
○ Maintain proper movement and alignment of affected body parts.	Decreases mechanical friction on specific areas for long periods of time, thus decreasing risk for breakdown.
○ Change client's position every 2 h on (odd/even) hour.	
○ Offer client fluids every 15 min. List preferred fluids here.	Hydration improves skin condition.
○ While client is very agitated and physically active, provide constant one-to-one observation.	
○ While limb is out of restraints, have client move limb through ROM.	Promotes circulation and assists in preventing the consequences of immobility.
○ If client is in four-point restraints, place him or her on side or stomach and change this position every 2 h on (odd/even) hour.	Client safety is of primary importance. This positioning prevents aspiration by facilitating drainage of fluids away from the airway.
○ Monitor skin condition of pressure areas.	
○ If client is in four-point restraint, provide one-on-one observation.	Provides supportive environment to client.
○ Continually remind client of reason for restraint and conditions for having the restraints removed.	
○ Talk with client in calm, quiet voice, and use client's name.	
○ Use restraints that are wide and have padding. Make sure padding is kept clean and dry and free of wrinkles.	
• If Impaired Tissue Integrity is the result of self-harm, place client on one-on-one observation until the risk of future harm has diminished.	Client safety is of primary importance. Provides ongoing supervision to inhibit impulsive behavior and encourages use of alternative coping behaviors.
• Monitor self-inflicted injuries hourly for the first 24 h for signs of infection and further damage. Note information on a flow sheet. After the first 24 h, monitor on a daily basis.	Early identification and treatment of infection can prevent more serious damage.
• Provide equipment and time for the client to practice oral hygiene at least after each meal.	Removes debris and food particles, thus reducing the risk of tissue injury.
• Discuss with client lifestyle changes to improve condition of mucous membranes, including nutritional habits, use of tobacco product, use of alcohol, maintenance of proper hydration, and effects of frequent vomiting.	Alerts client to lifestyle patterns that increase risk for injury to oral mucous membranes. If risk factors are present, frequent assessment and increased attention to oral hygiene can decrease the risk of membrane breakdown.
• Discuss with client side effects of medications that contribute to alterations in oral mucous membranes such as antibiotics, antihistamines, phenytoin, antidepressants, and antipsychotics.	

Continued

ACTIONS/INTERVENTIONS	RATIONALES
• Teach client to use nonsucrose candy or gum to stimulate flow of saliva. • Teach client to avoid excessive wind and sun exposure, especially with antipsychotic drugs. • If client is taking antipsychotic drugs, suggest the use of a sunscreen containing PABA.	Maintains hydration of membranes and decreases chance of breakdown. These medications can cause photosensitivity.[25]

Gerontic Health

ACTIONS/INTERVENTIONS	RATIONALES
• Nursing actions for this diagnosis in the gerontic patient are essentially the same as those for adult health and home health with the following special notations: Use only superfatted, nonperfumed, mild, nondetergent and hexachlorophene-free soap in bathing the patient.[59] • When drying the skin after bathing, pat the skin dry rather than rubbing, and apply lubricating lotion while the skin is still damp.	The incidence of dry skin in the older adult is increased due to decreased production of natural skin oils. Increases the moisture level of the patient's skin. Careful attention to dry skin conditions in the older adult will assist in maintaining tissue integrity for the older adult.

Home Health

ACTIONS/INTERVENTIONS	RATIONALES

• Teach self-monitoring techniques to prevent tissue breakdown and to initiate early treatment:
  ○ Inspect the skin at least daily. Change positions at least every 2 h.
  ○ Massage pressure points and bony prominences gently at least 3 times a day.
  ○ Avoid rubber or plastic mattress covers or sheets.
  ○ Use proper body alignment and padding to reduce pressure on affected areas.
  ○ At least once per day engage in physical activity (active or passive) which will develop a full ROM of all joints and relieve pressure on risk area.
  ○ Consult health care provider for treatment of actual skin lesions.
  ○ Avoid scratching lesions.
• Teach signs and symptoms of tissue breakdown, e.g., redness over bony prominences, pain or discomfort in localized area, skin lesions, or itching.
• Teach measures to promote tissue integrity:
  ○ Keep skin clean and dry. Wash urine and feces off skin immediately.
  ○ Maintain adequate hydration, e.g., oral fluids, mild soap for bathing, and use of nonscented lotion or petroleum jelly on skin after bathing.
  ○ Maintain adequate protein intake.
  ○ Use mild laundry detergent on clothes. Double-rinse clothes, linens, and diapers if skin is sensitive.
	Promotes self-care.
	
	Provides data for early intervention.
	
	Provides knowledge and skills that will prevent or minimize skin breakdown.

- Change position at least every 2 h on (odd/even) hour. Avoid prolonged sitting, standing, or lying in one position.
- Use sunscreen to prevent sun damage.
- Avoid excessive wind and sun exposure.
- Wear properly fitting shoes.
- Avoid shearing force when moving in bed or chair.

Tissue Integrity, Impaired

FLOWCHART EVALUATION: EXPECTED OUTCOME 1

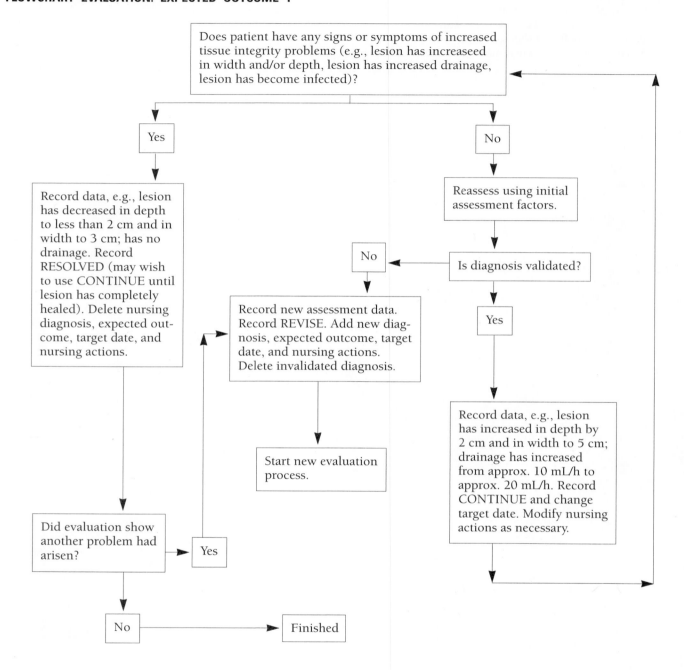

Does patient have any signs or symptoms of increased tissue integrity problems (e.g., lesion has increaseed in width and/or depth, lesion has increased drainage, lesion has become infected)?

Yes

No

Record data, e.g., lesion has decreased in depth to less than 2 cm and in width to 3 cm; has no drainage. Record RESOLVED (may wish to use CONTINUE until lesion has completely healed). Delete nursing diagnosis, expected outcome, target date, and nursing actions.

Reassess using initial assessment factors.

No

Is diagnosis validated?

Yes

Record new assessment data. Record REVISE. Add new diagnosis, expected outcome, target date, and nursing actions. Delete invalidated diagnosis.

Start new evaluation process.

Record data, e.g., lesion has increased in depth by 2 cm and in width to 5 cm; drainage has increased from approx. 10 mL/h to approx. 20 mL/h. Record CONTINUE and change target date. Modify nursing actions as necessary.

Did evaluation show another problem had arisen?

Yes

No

Finished

Tissue Integrity, Impaired

FLOWCHART EVALUATION: EXPECTED OUTCOME 2

Elimination Pattern

Pattern Description

The elimination pattern focuses on bowel and bladder functioning. While excretion also occurs through the skin and the lungs, the primary mechanisms of waste excretion are the bowel and bladder.

A problem within the elimination pattern may be the primary reason for seeking health care or may arise secondary to another health problem such as impaired mobility. Very few of the other patterns or nursing diagnoses will not have an ultimate impact on the elimination pattern from either a physiologic, psychologic, or sociologic direction.

Included in the elimination pattern are the individual's habits in terms of excretory regularity as well as aids the individual uses to maintain regularity or any devices used to control either bowel or bladder incontinence.

Pattern Assessment

1. Is there stool leakage when patient coughs, sneezes, or laughs?
   a. Yes (Bowel Incontinence)
   b. No
2. Is there involuntary passage of stool?
   a. Yes (Bowel Incontinence)
   b. No
3. Does patient take laxative on a routine basis?
   a. Yes (Colonic Constipation; Perceived Constipation)
   b. No
4. Has the number of bowel movements decreased?
   a. Yes (Constipation; Colonic Constipation)
   b. No
5. Are stools hard formed?
   a. Yes (Constipation; Colonic Constipation)
   b. No
6. Does patient have to strain to have bowel movement?
   a. Yes (Constipation; Colonic Constipation)
   b. No
7. Does patient believe he or she is frequently constipated?
   a. Yes (Perceived Constipation)
   b. No
8. Does patient expect to have a bowel movement at the same time each day?
   a. Yes (Perceived Constipation)
   b. No
9. Are bowel sounds increased?
   a. Yes (Diarrhea)
   b. No
10. Has the number of bowel movements increased?
    a. Yes (Diarrhea)
    b. No
11. Does the patient complain of loose, liquid stools?
    a. Yes (Diarrhea)
    b. No
12. Is there increased frequency of voiding?
    a. Yes (Altered Urinary Elimination; Stress Incontinence; Urge Incontinence)
    b. No

13. Is there dribbling of urine when the patient laughs, coughs, or sneezes?
    a. Yes (Stress Incontinence)
    b. No
14. Once the need to void is felt, is the patient able to reach toilet in time?
    a. Yes
    b. No (Urge Incontinence; Functional Incontinence)
15. Does the patient complain of bladder spasms?
    a. Yes (Reflex Incontinence; Urge Incontinence)
    b. No
16. Is there a decreased awareness of the need to void?
    a. Yes (Reflex Incontinence; Total Incontinence)
    b. No
17. Is there a decreased urge to void?
    a. Yes (Reflex Incontinence)
    b. No
18. Does the patient void in small amounts?
    a. Yes (Urge Incontinence; Urinary Retention)
    b. No
19. Is there urine flow without bladder distention?
    a. Yes (Total Incontinence)
    b. No
20. Is the bladder distended?
    a. Yes (Urinary Retention)
    b. No
21. Is there decreased urine output?
    a. Yes (Urinary Retention)
    b. No

Conceptual Information

Elimination, simply defined, refers to the excretion of waste and nondigested products of the metabolic process. Elimination is essential in maintaining the fluid, electrolyte, and nutritional balance of the body. A disruption in an individual's usual elimination pattern can be life-threatening since a person cannot live long without the ability to rid his or her body of waste products.[1,2]

Elimination depends on the interrelated functioning of the gastrointestinal system, urinary system, nervous system, and skin. This chapter will include only the lower urinary tract and gastrointestinal tract since the skin and nervous system are related to nursing diagnoses in other chapters. Also, since the nursing diagnoses related to elimination refer only to elimination and not the collection and formation of the waste materials, inclusion of other conceptual information would be confusing.

Our society has a dichotomous attitude toward elimination. A great deal of time, effort, and money is expended in designing and advertising bathrooms and aids to elimination, but to discuss elimination is considered rude.[1] Therefore, obtaining a reliable, complete elimination pattern assessment may be difficult. Added to this difficulty is the fact that each person has his or her own normal elimination habit.

Elimination is highly individualized and can be influenced by age, circadian rhythms, culture, diet, activity, stress, and a number of other factors. Elimination has elements of both involuntary and voluntary control. The mechanisms that control the production of waste materials and the neural signals that the bladder or bowel needs to be emptied are primarily involuntary. However, each person can usually control both the timing of bowel and bladder evacuation and the use of abdominal and perineal muscles to assist in evacuation.

Food and fluid intake are extremely important in elimination. A fluid intake of 2000 mL/day and a food intake of high-fiber foods would, in the majority of instances, ensure an adequate elimination pattern.[3,4] Alteration in elimination may cause psychosocial problems, such as social isolation due to embarrassment, as well as physiologic problems, such as fluid and/or electrolyte imbalance.

BOWEL ELIMINATION

The lower gastrointestinal tract includes the small and large intestines. The small bowel includes the duodenum, jejunum, and ileum and is about 20 feet in length and 1 inch in diameter. The large bowel includes the cecum, colon, and rectum and terminates at the anus. The large bowel is about 5 feet long and about 2½ inches in diameter. The small bowel and large bowel connect at the ileocecal valve.[2]

The intestines receive partially digested food from the stomach and move the food element through the lower tract, thus assisting in proper absorption of water, nutrients, and electrolytes. The intestines also provide secretory and storage functions. They secrete mucus, potassium, bicarbonate, and enzymes.

The chyme (small intestine contents) is moved by peristalsis, and the feces (large intestine contents) are propelled by mass movements that are stimulated by the gastrocolic reflex. The gastrocolic reflex occurs in response to food entering the stomach and causing distention, so mass movement occurs only a few times a day. The gastrocolic reflex occurs within 30 minutes after eating and is most predominant after the first meal of the day. Therefore, after the first meal of the day is the most frequent time for bowel elimination. Other reflexes involved in elimination are the duodenocolic reflex and the defecation reflex. The duodenocolic reflex is stimulated by the distention of the duodenum as food passes from the stomach to the duodenum. The gastrocolic and duodenocolic reflexes stimulate rectal contraction and, usually, a desire to defecate. The defecation reflex occurs in response to feces entering the rectum. This reflex promotes relaxation of the internal anal sphincter, thus also promoting a desire to defecate. Extra fluids upon morning waking potentiate the gastrocolic reflex. If the fluids are warm or contain caffeine, they will also stimulate peristalsis.[1,2]

The secretions of the gastrointestinal tract assist with food passage and further digestion. The passage rate of the contents through the intestines helps determine the absorption amount. The small intestine is responsible for about 90 percent of the absorption of amino acids, sodium, calcium chloride, fatty acids, bile salts, and water. Potassium and bicarbonate are excreted. The usual amount of time for chyme to move from the stomach to the ileocecal valve varies from 3 to 10 hours. It takes about 12 hours for feces to travel from the ileocecal valve to the rectum. One bowel movement may be the result of meals eaten over the past 3 to 4 days, but most of the food residue from any particular meal will have been excreted within 4 days. Passage of contents is primarily influenced by the amount of residue and the motility rate. Feces are normally evacuated on a moderately regular schedule, but the schedule will vary from three times daily to once per week depending on the individual.

When proper absorption does not occur, necessary nutrients and electrolytes are lost for subsequent body use. Small bowel loss can cause metabolic acidosis and hypokalemia. Large bowel loss can lead to dehydration and hyponatremia.

The squatting, leaning forward position is the most supportive position for defecation because it increases intra-abdominal pressure and promotes easier abdominal and perineal muscle contraction and relaxation. Beside positioning, diet, and fluid intake, other aids to elimination include enemas and laxatives.

Enemas assist in evacuation through either promotion of peristalsis, chemical irritation, or lubrication. Volume enemas, 500 to 1000 mL of fluid, cause distention, which increases peristalsis. The addition of heat and soapsuds, for example, adds chemical irritation and increases peristalsis. Straight tap-water enemas should be used cautiously since they are hypotonic and may disturb electrolyte balance. Electrolyte enemas are usually prepackaged and are hypertonic. Hypertonic enemas increase fluid amounts in the bowel through osmosis, thus slightly increasing distention and providing a relatively mild chemical irritation. Both the distention and irritation also result in increased peristalsis. Oil enemas are usually small-volume enemas (100 to 200 mL) and provide lubrication as well as stool softening.[1,5]

Laxatives assist elimination through producing bulk, providing lubrication, causing chemical irritation, or softening stool. The action of laxatives ranges from harsh to mild.

Both laxatives and enemas can be abused. Persistent use of either will diminish normal reflexes so that the individual will begin to require more and more aid. The individual then establishes an aid-dependent habit just as a drug abuser does.

While constipation and diarrhea are the two most common problems with bowel elimination, flatulence may be an associated problem. Flatus (intestinal gas) is normal. A problem arises when the individual cannot pass the gas or when abnormally large amounts of gas are produced. Flatus is produced by swallowed air, diffusion of gases from the bloodstream to the gastrointestinal tract, from carbon dioxide formed by the action of bicarbonate with hydrochloric acid or fatty acids, and from bacterial decomposition of food residue. Common causes of gas problems include gas-producing foods (beans, for example), highly irritating foods (pizza, for example), constipating medications (codeine, for example), and inactivity. The problems relate directly to the amount of gas produced and decreased motility. Increased flatus causes distention, which, in turn, can cause pain, respiratory difficulty, and further problems with intestinal motility.[1]

As previously mentioned, any bowel elimination problem can ultimately be life-threatening. Any bowel elimination problem, whether it be constipation, diarrhea, or flatulence, that lasts over 1 to 2 weeks in an adult or over 2 to 3 days for an infant or elderly person requires immediate health care intervention.

URINARY ELIMINATION

The lower urinary tract is composed of the ureters, bladder, and urethra. These anatomic structures serve as storage and excretory pathways for the waste secreted by the kidneys. The ureters extend from the kidney pelvis to the trigone area in the bladder. The ureters are small tubes composed of smooth muscle, which propels urine by peristalsis from the kidney to the bladder. The bladder stores the urine until it is excreted through the urethra. Between the base of the bladder and the top of the urethra is the urethral sphincter. The sphincter opens under learned voluntary control. Opening the urethral sphincter allows the urine to pass through the urethra and meatus for elimination. The female urethra is about 3 to 5 cm long, and the male urethra is about 20 cm long.[2]

The desire to void occurs when the bladder (adult) has reached a capacity of 250 to 450 mL of urine. As urine collects to the bladder capacity, the stretch receptors in the bladder muscle are activated. This stretching stimulates the voiding reflex center in the spinal cord (sacral levels 2, 3, and 4), which sends signals to the midbrain and the pons. These stimuli result in inhibition of the spinal reflex center and pudendal nerve, which allows relaxation of the external sphincter and contraction of the bladder, and voiding occurs. The bladder is under parasympathetic control with the learned voluntary control being guided by the cortex, midbrain, and medulla.[1,2]

The anatomically correct positions for voiding are sitting for the female and standing for the male. It is important to note that in some cultural groups the correct voiding position for the male is squatting. Either standing or squatting is anatomically correct. Difficulties arise if the male is lying down, for example, in traction or a body cast. An individual generally voids 200 to 450 mL each voiding time, and it is within normal limits to void 5 to 10 times per day. Common times for urination are upon arising and before retiring. Other times will vary with habits and correspond with work breaks and availability of toilet facilities.[1,2]

Urine volume will vary according to the individual. Urine volume depends on normal kidney functioning, amount of fluid and food intake, environmental temperature, fluid requirements of other organs, presence of open wounds, output by other areas (skin, bowel, or respiration), and medications such as diuretics. The amount of solutes in the urine, an intact neuromuscular system, and the actions of the antidiuretic hormone also influence output. A significant impact on urinary output is the opportunity to void at socially acceptable times in private.[1]

Inadequate urinary output may arise from either the kidney not producing urine (suppression) or blockage of urine flow (retention) somewhere between the kidney and external urinary meatus. Suppression may result from disease of the kidneys or other body structures and inadequate fluid intake. Retention may be either mechanical or functional in nature. Mechanical retention is due to anatomic blockage such as a stricture or a calculus. *Functional retention* actually refers to any retention that is not mechanical and includes such areas as neurogenic problems.[2]

Urinary control relates to the integrity and strength of the urinary sphincters and perineal musculature. Inability to control urinary output will soon lead to social isolation due to embarrassment over control and odor. Urinary incontinence is more common than most health care professionals realize. Studies[6,7] have indicated that urinary incontinence is quite common among healthy premenopausal middle-aged women. These studies found no relationship between continence status, number of children, history of gynecologic surgery, smoking, physical activity, or intake of alcohol and caffeine. The studies found also that very few of these women sought treatment for this incontinence.

Bladder-retraining programs may vary according to individual hospitals and physicians. Consultation with a rehabilitation nurse clinician will provide the most current and reliable information regarding a successful bladder-retraining program.[8] Two measures that may assist with incontinence are Crede's maneuver and the Valsalva maneuver. Crede's maneuver involves placing the fingertips together at the midline of the pelvic crest, then massaging deeply and smoothly down to the pubic bone. Check with the physician first since there are contraindications such as ureteral reflux.[5] The Valsalva maneuver involves asking the patient to simulate having a bowel movement. Have the patient take a deep breath, hold it, and then bear down as if expelling a bowel movement. Check with the physician first since there are contraindications such as glaucoma, eye surgery, and impaired circulation.[5]

Urine is a waste product formed as a part of body metabolism. Urine is normally produced at a rate of 30 to 50 mL/h. Under normal circumstances output will balance with intake about every 72 hours. An hourly output of less than 30 mL, a 24-hour output of 500 mL or less, or an intake-output imbalance lasting over 72 hours requires immediate intervention.[1,4]

Developmental Considerations

Elimination depends on the interrelatedness of fluid intake, muscle tone, regularity of habits, culture, state of health, and adequate nutrition.[9]

INFANT

Kidney function does not reach adult levels until 6 months to 1 year of life. Nervous system control is inadequate, and renal function does not reach a mature status until approximately 1 year of life.[9] Voiding is stimulated by cold air. The infant usually voids 15 to 60 mL at each voiding during the first 24 hours of life and may void reflexively at birth. If the infant has not voided by 12 hours after birth, there is cause for concern. By the third day, the infant may void 8 to 10 times during each 24 hours, equaling about 100 to 400 mL. Urinary output is affected by the amount of fluid consumed, the amount of activity (increased activity equals less urine), and the environmental temperature (increased temperature equals less urine).[10] Uric acid crystals may be found in concentrated urine, causing a rusty discoloration to the diaper.[10]

The muscles and elastic tissues of the infant's intestines are poorly developed, and nervous system control is adequate. Water and electrolyte absorption is functional but immature. The intestines are proportionately longer than in the adult. While some digestive enzymes are present, they can break down only simple foods. These digestive enzymes are unable to break down complex carbohydrates or protein.

Meconium is the first waste material that is eliminated by the bowel. This usually occurs during the first 24 hours. After 24 hours, the characteristics of the bowel movement change as it mixes with milk. The characteristics of the stool will depend on whether the infant is breast-fed or bottle-fed. The breast-fed infant will have soft, semiliquid stools that are yellow or golden in color. The bottle-fed infant will have a more formed stool which is light yellow to brown in color.

The infant may have 4 to 8 soft bowel movements a day during the first 4 weeks of life. Flatus often accompanies the passage of stool, and there may be a sour odor to the bowel movement. By the fourth week of life, the number of bowel movements has decreased to 2 to 4 a day. By 4 months, there is a predictable interval between bowel movements.

It is common for the infant to push or strain at stool. However, if the stools are very hard or dry, the infant should be assessed for constipation. The bottle-fed infant is more prone to constipation than the breast-fed infant.

Infants sometimes suffer from what is known as *colic*. Colic is described as daily periods of distress caused by rapid, violent peristaltic waves and increased gas pressure in the rectum.[10] The cause is unknown but may have to do with the simple (rather than the complex) digestive enzymes of the infant or a decreased amount of vitamin A, K, or E. Most authorities agree that colic disappears as digestive enzymes become more complex and when normal bacterial flora accumulate.[10]

TODDLER AND PRESCHOOLER

By 2 years of age, the kidneys are able to conserve water and to concentrate urine almost on an adult level, except under stress. The bladder increases in size and is able to hold about 88 mL of urine.

Nervous system and gastrointestinal maturation has occurred during infancy and the beginning of the toddler years. By the time children are 2 to 3 years of age, they are ready to control bowel and bladder functioning. Bowel elimination control is usually attained first; daytime bladder control is second, and nighttime bladder control is third. The child must be able to walk a few steps, control the sphincter, recognize and interpret that the bladder is full, and be able to indicate that he or she wants to go to the bathroom. The child must also value dryness. He or she must recognize that it is more socially acceptable to be dry than to be wet.

Parents should not attempt toilet training, even if the child is ready, if there are family or environmental stressors. Regression is normal during toilet training and, coupled with undue stress, could cause physical or psychosocial problems.

Bladder training takes time to accomplish. Both the parent and the child must have patience and not get unduly upset when accidents occur. In fact, nighttime bladder control may not be attained until 5 to 8 years of life. Doctors and researchers disagree on the age at which nighttime bedwetting (enuresis) becomes a problem.[10] Parents should limit fluids at night, have the child void before going to bed, and get the child up at least once during the night to assist in attaining nighttime control.

In order to toilet train, the parent should watch for patterns of defecation. Eating stimulates peristaltic activity and

evacuation. The child can then be taken to the toilet at the expected time after eating. The child should be told what is expected while on the toilet. Give the child enough time to evacuate the bowel, but do not have the child sit on the toilet too long. The child (and the parent) may then become frustrated.

Children at this age like to please their parents. Evacuation of the bowel is a natural process and should not be approached as if it is a dirty or unnatural process. The children should be rewarded when able to defecate, but they should not be punished if unable to have a bowel movement. Children should be encouraged to feel proud of their accomplishment; children should never be punished or made to feel ashamed for not giving what is expected.

Children usually do not need enemas or laxatives to make them regular. In fact, those artificial aids may be dangerous. Lack of parental understanding of the elimination process and child development, coupled with harsh punishment for "accidents," may lead a child to an obsessive, meticulous, and rigid personality.

Accidents can and do occur even after a child has been completely toilet trained. These accidents usually occur because the child ignores the defecation urge when he or she is engrossed in an activity and does not want to take the time to go to the bathroom or when other stressors have a higher priority at the moment.

SCHOOL-AGE CHILD

The urinary system is functioning maturely by this age. The normal output is 500 mL/day. Urinary tract infections are common because of careless hygiene practices in females. The gastrointestinal system attains adult functional maturity during the school years.

ADOLESCENT

There are no noticeable differences in patterns of urinary elimination in this age group. The intestines grow in length and width. The muscles of the intestines become thicker and stronger.

This developmental stage is important in developing bowel habits. The teenager is engaged in developing sexuality. This group may ignore warning signals for elimination because they do not want to leave their activities or because of the close association of the anus to the teenager's developing sexual organs. Additionally, if a problem arises with elimination, adolescents are reluctant to talk about it with either their peers or an adult.

YOUNG ADULT

There is no noticeable difference in patterns of elimination during this developmental period. Total urinary output for 24 hours is 1000 to 2000 mL. The rate of passage of feces is influenced by the nature of the foods consumed and the physical health of the individual. Hemorrhoids are possible in this developmental group, especially females.

ADULT

Adequate daily fluid intake helps to maintain proper elimination functions. There is a gradual decrease in the number of nephrons and therefore decreased renal functioning with age. Additionally, bladder tone diminishes; thus, the adult may urinate more frequently.

Digestive enzymes (gastric acid, pepsin, ptyalin, and pancreatic enzymes) begin to decrease. This may lead to an increasing incidence of intestinal disorders, cancer, and gastrointestinal complaints.

OLDER ADULT

Renal function is slowed by both the structural and functional aging changes, mainly because of decreases in the number of nephrons. Vascular sclerosing also occurs in the renal system, and this, combined with fewer nephrons, decreases available blood so that the GFR (glomerular filtration rate) becomes markedly reduced. While the GFR reduction is still sufficient to handle normal demands, stress or illness can significantly alter the older adult's renal status.[11] Decreased concentrations and dilution ability of the kidneys occur as a result of changes in the renal tubules. Waste products are effectively processed by the kidneys, but over a longer period of time. The decreased efficiency of the kidneys helps make older adults especially vulnerable to medication side effects and problems regarding drug excretion.[12]

The older male adult may have an enlarged prostate gland. Prostatic enlargement can lead to urethritis, incomplete bladder emptying, and difficulty in starting the stream of urine. Bladder changes, resulting from loss of smooth-muscle elasticity, can result in a decreased bladder capacity. Uninhibited bladder contractions may interrupt bladder filling and lead to a premature urge to void. Increased residual urine and incomplete emptying of the bladder result in a higher incidence of urinary tract infections in older adults of both sexes.

Changes in the gastrointestinal tract include a continued decrease in digestive enzymes and questionable changes in absorption in the small intestines. The large intestine may have reduced blood flow secondary to vascular twisting, and there is debate regarding decreased motility in the colon. Problems related to constipation may occur due to increased tolerance for rectal distention rather than decreased motility.[12]

Major factors that affect GI and GU function in older adults include immobility and medications. Immobility can lead to kidney stones, UTIs secondary to stasis, and alterations in food intake, digestion, and elimination.[13] Medications such as anticholinergics and opiates can result in delayed motility in the GI tract. Diuretics, hypnotics, and antipsychotics must be considered in light of their effect on GU function.[14]

APPLICABLE NURSING DIAGNOSES

Bowel Incontinence

DEFINITION

A state in which an individual experiences a change in normal bowel habits characterized by involuntary passage of stool.[15]

NANDA TAXONOMY: EXCHANGING 1.3.1.3

DEFINING CHARACTERISTICS[15]

1. Major defining characteristics
   a. Involuntary passage of stool
2. Minor defining characteristics
   None given

RELATED FACTORS[15]

1. Gastrointestinal disorders
2. Neuromuscular disorders
3. Colostomy
4. Loss of rectal sphincter control
5. Impaired cognition

RELATED CLINICAL CONCERNS

1. Alzheimer's disease
2. Guillain-Barré syndrome
3. Spinal cord injury
4. Intestinal surgery
5. Gynecologic surgery

HAVE YOU SELECTED THE CORRECT DIAGNOSIS?

Constipation The problem may really be due to constipation with impaction. Incontinence may occur because some feces are leaking around the impaction site and the individual is unable to control its passage and thus appears incontinent.

Self-Care Deficit, Toileting If the individual is unable to appropriately care for his or her evacuation needs, incontinence may result.

Diarrhea Diarrhea relates to frequent bowel movements, but the patient is aware of rectal filling and can control the feces until reaching the toilet. With incontinence the patient may not be aware of rectal filling, and the stool passage is involuntary.

EXPECTED OUTCOMES

1. Will have no more than one soft, formed stool per day by (date) and/or
2. Will return to usual bowel elimination habits by (date)

TARGET DATES

Target dates should be based on the individual's usual bowel elimination pattern. Incontinence may require additional retraining time and effort. Therefore, a target date 5 days from admission would be most realistic. Also remember that there must be a realistic potential that bowel continence can be regained by the patient.

NURSING ACTIONS/INTERVENTIONS WITH RATIONALES

Adult Health

ACTIONS/INTERVENTIONS	RATIONALES
• Check for fecal impaction on admission, and implement nursing actions for constipation if impaction is noted.	Impaction may lead to leakage of bowel contents around impacted area.
• Record each incontinent episode when it occurs as well as the amount, color, and consistency of each stool.	Assists in determining pattern of incontinence.
• Record events associated with incontinent episode, including events both before and after the episode (i.e., activity, stress, location, people present, etc).	Assists in determining pattern of incontinence.
• Monitor anal skin integrity at least once per shift at (times).	Allows early detection of any tissue integrity problems.
• Keep anal area clean and dry.	Bowel contents are damaging to the skin and promote tissue integrity problems.
• Provide room deodorizer and chlorophyll tablets for patient.	Decreases embarrassment due to odors.
• Provide emotional support for patient through teaching, providing time for listening, etc.	Patient may find incontinence embarrassing and may try to isolate self.
• Initiate bowel training at least 4 days prior to discharge: ○ Administer suppository half-hour after eating. ○ Toilet half-hour after suppository insertion. ○ Toilet prior to activity. ○ Stimulate defecation reflex with circular movement in rectum using gloved, lubricated finger.	Establishes consistent pattern and conditions control of elimination.
• Teach patient, beginning as soon after admission as possible: ○ Pelvic floor strengthening exercises (see Constipation) ○ Diet, i.e., the role of fiber and fluids ○ Use of assistive devices such as Velcro closings on clothes and pads ○ Perineal hygiene ○ Appropriate use of suppositories and antidiarrheal medications ○ Refer patient for home health care assistance.	Basic knowledge promotes understanding of condition and assists patient to change behavior as well as empowering the patient for self-care.

Child Health

Nursing actions for Incontinence in the child are the same as those for Adult Health. Modifications would be made for child's age and size, for example, medication dosages and fluid amounts.

Women's Health

Bowel incontinence in women caused by uterine prolapse and pelvic relaxation with displacement of pelvic organs (particularly the rectum) is relieved only by surgical repair.[16] Otherwise, nursing actions for bowel incontinence in Women's Health are the same as in Adult Health.

Psychiatric Health

ACTIONS/INTERVENTIONS	RATIONALES

• If a pattern forms around specific events, develop plan to:
  ○ Encourage person to use bathroom before the event.
  ○ Alter the manner in which specific task is performed to prevent stress (note alterations here).
  ○ Discuss with client alternative ways of coping with stress. (Refer to Chap. 8 for specific nursing actions related to reduction of anxiety and Chap. 11 for specific nursing actions related to Ineffective Coping.)
	Promotes client's perceived control and increases potential for client's involvement in treatment plan.

• If assessment suggests secondary gains associated with episodes, decrease these by:
  ○ Withdrawing social contact after an episode
  ○ Having client clean himself or herself
  ○ Providing social contact or interactions with the client at times when no incontinence is experienced
	Provides negative consequences for inappropriate coping behavior.

• If not related to secondary gain, spend (number) minutes with client after each episode to allow expression of feelings. • Discuss with client effects this problem has on lifestyle.	Verbalization of feelings in a nonthreatening environment models acceptance of feelings and positive coping behavior. Increases client's awareness of impact inappropriate coping behaviors have on lifestyle. Provides data for development of alternative coping, promoting client's perceived control.

Gerontic Health

ACTIONS/INTERVENTIONS	RATIONALES
• Record events associated with incontinent episode. • Monitor medication intake for potential to result in bowel incontinence. • Teach toileting skills to caregivers of cognitively impaired older adults. In early dementia, labeling the bathroom and reminding the individual to toilet may result in continence.	Assists in determining pattern of incontinence. Older adult may have difficulty in reaching commode or bathroom easily. Medications with a sedative effect may decrease the ability of the patient to reach toilet facilities in a timely manner. Depending on the stage of the disease, a person with dementia may forget to toilet or have difficulty finding a bathroom that is not readily identified.

Home Health

ACTIONS/INTERVENTIONS	RATIONALES

• Teach patient and family:
  ○ To use appropriately all prescribed and over-the-counter medications
  ○ To monitor color, frequency, consistency, and pattern of symptoms
  ○ To ensure adequate bowel elimination:
  (1) Proper diet
  (2) Fluid and electrolyte balance
  (3) Pelvic floor and abdominal exercises
  ○ To monitor skin integrity
  ○ To keep bed linens and clothing clean and dry
	These activities assist in preventing constipation and provide data for early recognition of problem.
	
	These measures prevent secondary problems from occurring due to the existing problem.

Bowel Incontinence

FLOWCHART EVALUATION: EXPECTED OUTCOME 1

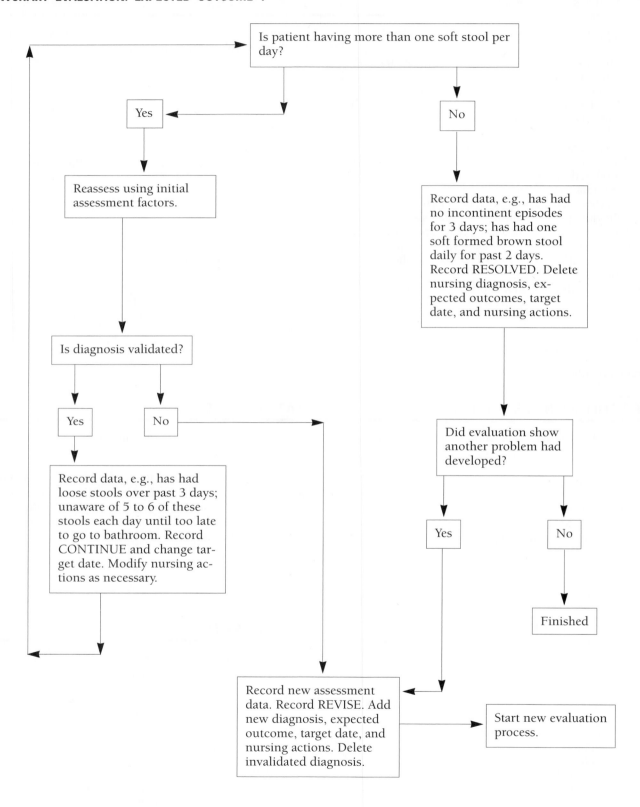

Is patient having more than one soft stool per day?

Yes

No

Reassess using initial assessment factors.

Record data, e.g., has had no incontinent episodes for 3 days; has had one soft formed brown stool daily for past 2 days. Record RESOLVED. Delete nursing diagnosis, expected outcomes, target date, and nursing actions.

Is diagnosis validated?

Yes

No

Record data, e.g., has had loose stools over past 3 days; unaware of 5 to 6 of these stools each day until too late to go to bathroom. Record CONTINUE and change target date. Modify nursing actions as necessary.

Did evaluation show another problem had developed?

Yes

No

Finished

Record new assessment data. Record REVISE. Add new diagnosis, expected outcome, target date, and nursing actions. Delete invalidated diagnosis.

Start new evaluation process.

Bowel Incontinence

FLOWCHART EVALUATION: EXPECTED OUTCOME 2

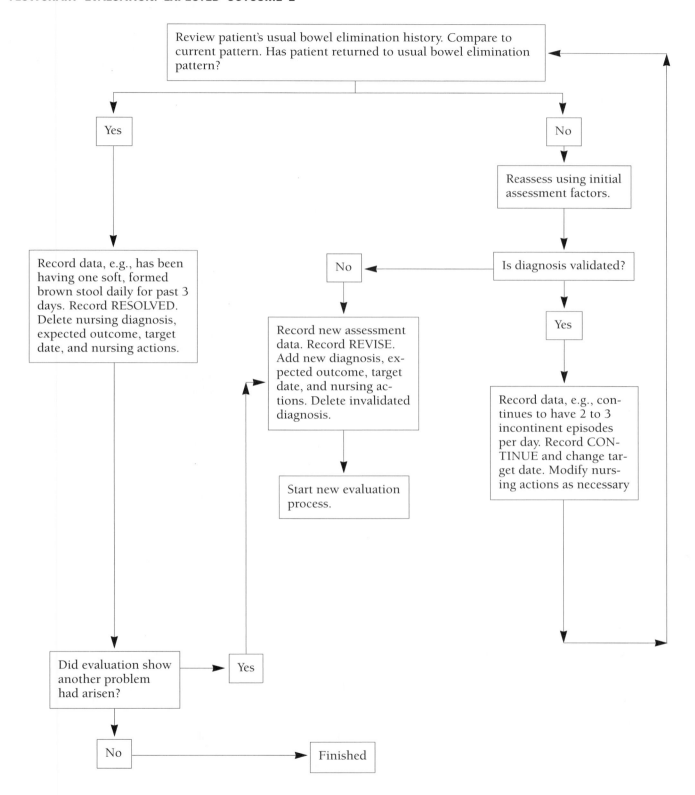

Constipation

DEFINITION

CONSTIPATION A state in which an individual experiences a change in normal bowel habits characterized by a decrease in frequency and/or passage of hard dry stools.[15]

COLONIC CONSTIPATION The state in which an individual's pattern of elimination is characterized by hard, dry stool, which results from a delay in passage of food residue.[15]

PERCEIVED CONSTIPATION The state in which an individual makes a self-diagnosis of constipation. A person with this diagnosis may try to ensure a daily bowel movement through abuse of laxatives, enemas, and suppositories.[15]

NANDA TAXONOMY: EXCHANGING 1.3.1.1, 1.3.1.1.1, AND 1.3.1.1.2

DEFINING CHARACTERISTICS[15]

1. Constipation
   a. Major defining characteristics
      (1) Decreased activity level
      (2) Frequency less than usual pattern
      (3) Hard-formed stools
      (4) Palpable mass
      (5) Reported feeling of pressure in rectum
      (6) Reported feeling of rectal fullness
      (7) Straining at stool
   b. Other Possible Characteristics
      (1) Abdominal pain
      (2) Appetite impairment
      (3) Back pain
      (4) Headache
      (5) Interference with daily living
      (6) Use of laxative
2. Colonic Constipation
   a. Major Defining Characteristics
      (1) Decreased frequency
      (2) Hard, dry stool
      (3) Straining at stool
      (4) Painful defecation
      (5) Abdominal distention
      (6) Palpable mass
   b. Minor
      (1) Rectal pressure
      (2) Headache
      (3) Appetite impairment
      (4) Abdominal pain
3. Perceived Constipation
   a. Major defining characteristics
      (1) Expectation of a daily bowel movement with the resulting overuse of laxatives, enemas, and suppositories
      (2) Expected passage of stool at same time each day
   b. Minor defining characteristics
      None given.

RELATED FACTORS[15]

1. Constipation
   a. To be developed
2. Colonic Constipation
   a. Less than adequate fluid intake
   b. Less than adequate dietary intake
   c. Less than adequate fiber
   d. Less than adequate physical activity
   e. Immobility
   f. Lack of privacy
   g. Emotional disturbances
   h. Chronic use of medication and enemas
   i. Stress
   j. Change in daily routines
   k. Metabolic problems, for example, hypothyroidism, hypocalcemia, or hypokalemia
3. Perceived Constipation
   a. Cultural or family health belief
   b. Faulty appraisal
   c. Impaired thought processes

RELATED CLINICAL CONCERNS

1. Anemias
2. Hypothyroidism
3. Hemorrhoids
4. Renal dialysis
5. Abdominal surgery

HAVE YOU SELECTED THE CORRECT DIAGNOSIS?

Altered Nutrition, Less or More Than Body Requirements This might be the primary nursing diagnosis. Either of these diagnoses influences the amount and consistency of the feces.

Fluid-Volume Deficit This diagnosis might also be the primary problem. The feces need adequate lubrication to pass through the gastrointestinal tract. If there is a Fluid-Volume Deficit, the feces are harder, more solid, and unable to move through the system.

Diarrhea or Bowel Incontinence Constipation can be misdiagnosed as Diarrhea or Bowel Incontinence. Diarrhea or incontinence may be a secondary condition to constipation as semiliquid feces may pass around the area of constipation.

Impaired Physical Mobility This diagnosis could be the underlying cause of constipation. Decrease in physical mobility affects every body system. In the GI tract, peristalsis is slowed, which may lead to a backlog of feces and to constipation.

Self-Care Deficit, Toileting This diagnosis may also be the primary diagnosis. Difficulty in reaching appropriate toileting facilities and difficulty in cleansing oneself after toileting could lead to a decision to delay bowel movement with a result of constipation.

Ineffective Individual Coping and Anxiety These diagnoses are two psychosocial nursing diagnoses from which Constipation needs to be differentiated. Both of these psychosocial diagnoses initiate stress as an autonomic response, and the parasympathetic system stimuli (which control motility of the GI tract) are reduced. This reduced motility may lead to constipation.

EXPECTED OUTCOMES

1. Will return, as nearly as possible, to usual bowel elimination habits by (date) and/or
2. Will design and carry out a plan to avoid constipation by (date)

TARGET DATES

Target dates should be based on the individual's usual bowel elimination habits. A target date 3 to 5 days from admission would be reasonable for the majority of patients.

NURSING ACTIONS/INTERVENTIONS WITH RATIONALES

Adult Health

ACTIONS/INTERVENTIONS	RATIONALES
• Record amount, color, and consistency of bowel movement following each bowel movement. Question patient regarding bowel movements at least once per shift. Also record if patient has had no bowel movement on a shift.	Basic assessment of problem severity as well as monitoring effectiveness of therapy.
• Monitor and record symptoms associated with passage of bowel movement: ○ Any straining, pain, or headache ○ Any rectal bleeding or fissures	Allows early detection of additional problems.
• If fecal impaction: ○ Attempt digital removal using gloves and lubrication. ○ Administer oil retention enema of small volume. Have the patient retain for at least 1 h. ○ Use small-volume saline enema if oil retention does not relieve impaction.	Prioritization of methods used to break up and remove impaction.
• Collaborate with physician regarding use of glycerin or other types of suppositories.	
• Measure and total intake and output every shift. Be sure to include estimation of loss by perspiration.	Allows monitoring of fluid balance.
• Force fluids, of patient's choice, to at least 2000 mL daily. Encourage 8 oz of fluid every 2 h on the (odd/even) hour beginning at awakening each morning.	Increases moisture and water content of feces for easier movement through intestines and anus.
• Increase patient's activity to extent possible through ambulation at least 3 times per shift while awake.	Activity promotes stimulation of bowel and will assist in elimination.
• Assist patient with exercises every 4 h while awake. Have patient repeat each exercise at least 5 times: ○ Bent-knee sit-ups ○ Straight- or bent-leg lifts ○ Alternating contraction and relaxation of perineal muscles while sitting in a chair and with feet placed apart on floor	Strengthens pelvic floor and abdominal muscles.

Continued

ACTIONS/INTERVENTIONS	RATIONALES
• Assist patient with implementation of stress reduction techniques at least once per shift.	Promotes relaxation and can increase feces passage through the intestines.
• Digitally stimulate anal sphincter at scheduled times (usually after meals—state times here).	Stimulates defecation reflex and urge.
• Provide privacy and sufficient time for bowel elimination.	Decreases stress and promotes relaxation, which increases likelihood of bowel movement.
• Help patient assume anatomically correct position for bowel movements.	Promotes effective use of abdominal muscles and allows gravity to assist in defecation.
• Use rectal tube, heat, activity, and change of position, every 2 h on the (odd/even) hour, for problems with flatulence.	Promotes passage of flatus.
• Monitor anal skin integrity at least once per shift.	Straining at stool can cause splits and tears of the anal tissue.
• Provide room deodorizer for patient as needed.	Helps to eliminate odors, which decreases patient's embarrassment.
• Use cool compresses to anus every 2 h as needed.	Alleviates anal itching.
• Teach patient, starting as soon after admission as possible:	Promotes understanding of self-care needs prior to discharge.[17]
○ The importance of a bowel routine and the need to respond to the urge to defecate as soon as possible	
○ To stimulate gastrocolic reflex through drinking prune juice or hot liquid upon arising	
○ To allow sufficient time for bowel movement and plan time for elimination	
○ To include high-fiber foods and extra liquid in daily diet	
○ To avoid prolonged use of elimination aids such as laxatives and enemas	
○ To avoid straining	
○ To use proper perineal hygiene	
○ To describe the relationship of diet and activity to bowel elimination	
• Collaborate, as soon as possible after admission:	Provides basic resources and information needed; promotes holistic approach to treatment.
○ With dietitian regarding a high-fiber, high-roughage diet (the more food a patient eats, the fewer laxatives the patient will require)	
○ With physical therapist regarding exercise program	
○ With physician regarding mild analgesics and ointments for control of pain associated with bowel movement	
○ With physician regarding use of stool softeners, laxatives, suppositories, and enemas	
○ With enterostomal therapist regarding ostomy care (i.e., irrigations, stoma and skin care, and appliances)	
○ With psychiatric nurse clinician regarding counseling for patient and family regarding possible underlying emotional components	
○ With home health nurse regarding follow-up planning for home and usual daily activities of living with emphasis on stress, etc.	

Child Health

Nursing actions for Constipation in the child are the same as those for Adult Health. Modifications would be made for child's age and size, for example, medication dosages and fluid amounts.

Women's Health

ACTIONS/INTERVENTIONS	RATIONALES
• Assist patient in identifying lifestyle adjustments that may be needed due to changes in physiologic function or needs during experiential phases of life (e.g., pregnancy, postpartum, and after gynecologic surgery).	Provides information needed as basis for planning care and health maintenance.
• Teach client changes that occur during pregnancy that contribute to decreased gastric motility and potential constipation, e.g., fluid intake may decrease due to nausea and vomiting of early pregnancy; increased use of mother's body fluid intake to produce lactation can lead to decrease in fluid intake overall; supplemental iron during pregnancy can lead to severe constipation; and fear of injury or pain upon defecation after birth can lead to constipation.	Provides basic information for self-care during pregnancy, birthing process, and postpartum.

• Teach anatomic shifting of abdominal contents due to fetal growth.
• Teach hormonal influences (e.g., increased progesterone) on bodily functions:
  ○ Decreased stomach emptying time
  ○ Decreased peristalsis
  ○ Increase in water reabsorption
  ○ Decrease in exercise
  ○ Relaxation of abdominal muscles
  ○ Increase in flatulence
	Provides information as a basis for nutrition plan during pregnancy. Promotes self-care.

• Teach the effects of the increase in oral iron or calcium supplements on the gastrointestinal tract, e.g., constipation. Describe the physical changes present in the immediate postpartum period that affect the gastrointestinal tract:
  ○ Lax abdominal muscles
  ○ Fluid loss (perspiration, urine, lochia, or dehydration during labor and delivery)
  ○ Hunger
	Provides basis for teaching patient plan of self-care at home and promotes healing process.

• Assist patient in planning diet that will promote healing, replace lost fluids, and help with return to normal bowel evacuation.
• Instruct in the use of ointments, anesthetic sprays, sitz baths, and witch hazel compresses to relieve episiotomy pain and reduce hemorrhoids.
• Instruct in pelvic floor exercises (Kegel exercises) to assist healing and reduction of pain.
• Teach nursing mothers alternate methods of assistance with bowel evacuation other than cathartics (cathartics are expressed in breast milk):
  ○ Prune juice
  ○ Hot liquids
  ○ High-fiber, high-roughage diet
  ○ Daily exercise
	Promotes successful lactation, good self-care, and good nutrition and provides basis for teaching care.

• Describe the physical changes present in the immediate postoperative period (C-section and gynecologic surgery) that affect the gastrointestinal tract:
  ○ Fluid loss (blood loss or dehydration as a result of being NPO and surgery)
  ○ Decreased peristalsis
  ○ Bowel manipulation during surgery
  ○ Increased use of analgesics and anesthesia
	Provides basis for teaching and planning of care. Promotes and encourages self-care.

Psychiatric Health

The nursing actions for this diagnosis in Psychiatric Health are the same as those for Adult Health. Please refer to those recommended actions.

Gerontic Health

ACTIONS/INTERVENTIONS	RATIONALES
• Review medication record for drugs that may have constipation as a side effect.	Older adults receiving antidepressants, anticholinergics, tranquilizers, or certain antacids may experience constipation due to the drug-delayed motility of waste matter through the intestine. Older adults are more likely to be on multiple medications that can result in constipation.
• Collaborate with physician regarding changes in medication to avoid the side effect of constipation.	

Home Health

NOTE: Adult Health actions are appropriate for Home Health. The locus of control shifts from the nurse to the client, family, or caregiver.

ACTIONS/INTERVENTIONS	RATIONALES
• The nurse will teach others to complete activities.	Client and members of family may have different ideas regarding appropriate elimination patterns.
• Teach client and family the definition of *constipation*. Determine if problem is perceived by client and family as being due to incorrect definition or is based on physiologic dysfunction.	Nursing interventions for physiologic definition are outlined in the Adult Health nursing actions. Nursing interventions for varying definitions will require family involvement.
• Assist client and family in identifying lifestyle changes that may be required: 　○ Establishment of a regular elimination routine based on cultural and individual variations 　○ Stress management techniques 　○ Decrease in concentrated, refined foods 　○ Identification of any food intolerances or allergies and avoidance of those foods 　○ Appropriate use and frequency of use of prescribed and over-the-counter medications 　○ Physiologic parameters of constipation	Home-based care requires involvement of family. Bowel elimination problems may require adjustments in family activities.

Constipation

FLOWCHART EVALUATION: EXPECTED OUTCOME 1

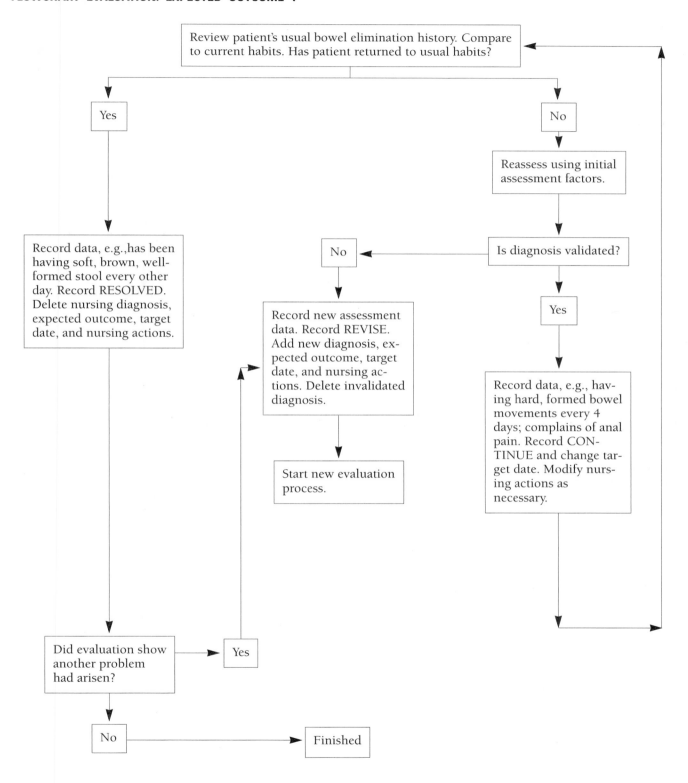

Constipation

FLOWCHART EVALUATION: EXPECTED OUTCOME 2

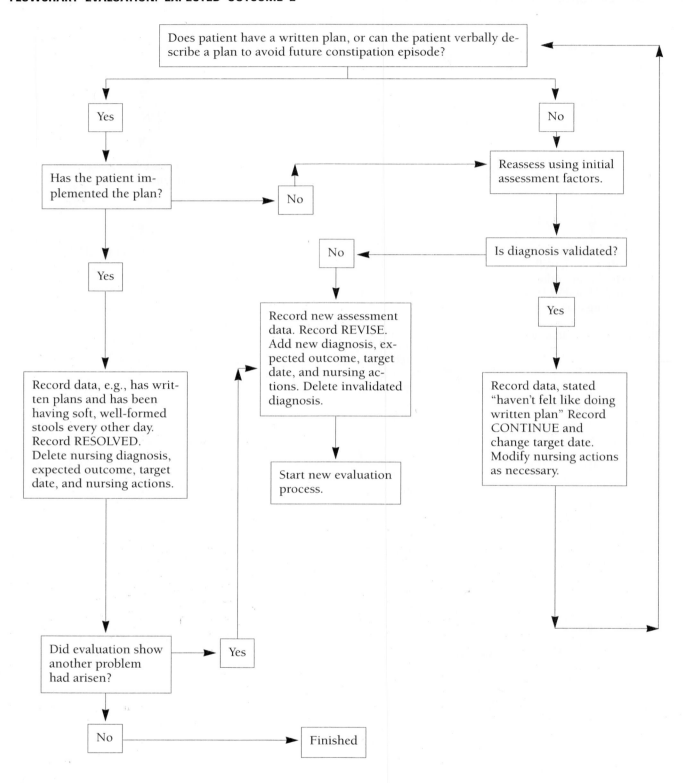

Diarrhea

DEFINITION

A state in which an individual experiences a change in normal bowel habits characterized by the frequent passage of loose, fluid, unformed stools.[15]

NANDA TAXONOMY: EXCHANGING 1.3.1.2

DEFINING CHARACTERISTICS[15]

1. Major defining characteristics
   a. Abdominal pain
   b. Cramping
   c. Increased frequency of bowel sounds
   d. Loose liquid stools
   e. Urgency
2. Other possible characteristics
   a. Change in color

RELATED FACTORS[15]

1. Gastrointestinal disorders
2. Metabolic disorders
3. Nutritional disorders
4. Endocrine disorders
5. Infectious process
6. Tube feedings
7. Fecal impaction
8. Change in dietary intake
9. Adverse effects of medication
10. High stress levels

RELATED CLINICAL CONCERNS

1. Inflammatory bowel disease (ulcerative colitis, Crohn's disease, enteritis)
2. Anemias
3. Gastric bypass or gastric partitioning surgery
4. Gastritis

HAVE YOU SELECTED THE CORRECT DIAGNOSIS?

Constipation   Diarrhea may be secondary to constipation. In instances of severe constipation or impaction, semiliquid feces can leak around the areas of impaction and will appear to be diarrhea.

Altered Nutrition, Less Than Body Requirements   If the individual is not ingesting enough food or sufficient bulk to allow feces to be well formed, diarrhea may well result.

Fluid-Volume Deficit or Fluid-Volume Excess   While research has not definitely supported the impact of fluid volume on bowel elimination, it is a common practice to pay attention to these diagnoses when either constipation or diarrhea is present. The basic idea appears to be that the amount of fluid ingested or absorbed by the body can affect the consistency of the fecal material.

Anxiety, Self-Esteem Disturbance, or Ineffective Individual Coping   Any of these psychosocial diagnoses precipitates a stress response. Indices of stress include gastrointestinal signs and symptoms, including diarrhea, vomiting, and "butterflies" in the stomach.

Sleep Pattern Disturbance   If a person's biologic clock is changed because of altered sleep-wake patterns, body responses attuned to the biologic clock will also be altered. This includes usual elimination patterns, and diarrhea may result.

EXPECTED OUTCOMES

1. Will have no more than one soft, formed bowel movement per day by (date) and/or
2. Will return to usual bowel elimination habits by (date)

TARGET DATES

Target dates should be based on the individual's usual bowel elimination habits. Thus, a target date 3 days from the day of admission would be reasonable for the majority of patients. Since diarrhea can be particularly life-threatening for infants and older adults, a target date of 2 days would not be too soon.

NURSING ACTIONS/INTERVENTIONS WITH RATIONALES
Adult Health

ACTIONS/INTERVENTIONS	RATIONALES
• Record amount, color, consistency, and odor following each bowel movement.	Basic monitoring of conditioning as well as monitoring of effectiveness of therapy.
• Monitor weight and electrolytes at least every 2 days while diarrhea persists (state dates here).	Monitors hydration status.
• Measure and total intake and output every shift.	Monitors hydration status.
• Decrease bowel stimulation through placing patient on NPO status or clear liquid diet and intravenous hydration. Slowly reintroduce solid foods.	Rests the bowel while maintaining fluid and electrolyte balance.
• Place on enteric precautions until cause of diarrhea is determined.	Some types of diarrhea are infectious and are communicable.
• Make sure bathroom facilities are readily available.	Helps to prevent accidents and prevent embarrassment for patient.
• Administer antidiarrheal medications as ordered, and document results within 1 h after administration, e.g., Diarrhea decreased from 1 stool every 30 min to 1 stool every 2 h.	Documents effectiveness of medication.
• Increase fluid intake to at least 2500 mL per day.	Maintains hydration status.
• Offer fluids high in potassium and sodium at least once per hour, e.g., Gatorade, Pedialyte.	
• Serve fluids at tepid temperature (avoid temperature extremes such as very hot or very cold).	
• List patient's fluid likes and dislikes here.	
• Provide perineal skin care after each bowel movement. Monitor anal skin integrity at least once each shift.	Dries moisture, prevents skin breakdown, and prevents perineal infection.
• If tube feedings are causal factor, collaborate with physician regarding:	Modifying any of the listed items may decrease incidence of diarrhea.
◦ Infusion rate	
◦ Temperature of feeding	
◦ Dilution of feeding	
◦ Following feeding with water	
◦ Administration of Hydrocil at onset of tube feeding (increases stool consistency)[18]	
• Provide room deodorizer, chlorophyll tablets, and fresh parsley for patient's use.	Assists in elimination of odor; promotes pleasant environment.
• Assist patient with stress reduction exercises at least once per shift; provide quiet, restful atmosphere.	Promotes relaxation and decreases stimulation of bowel.
• Collaborate with dietitian regarding low-fiber, low-residue, soft diet.	Helps to identify foods that stimulate bowel and exacerbate diarrhea.
• List here those foods that patient has described as being irritating.	
• Teach patient:	Increases patient's knowledge of causes, treatment, and complications of diarrhea. Promotes self-care.
◦ Diet: Avoiding irritating foods, including basic food pyramid groups, influence of high-fiber foods, and influence of fruits.	
◦ Fluids: Maintaining intake and output balance, influence of environmental temperature, influence of activity, and influence of caffeine and milk	
◦ Medications: Caution with over-the-counter medications, those that are antidiarrheal, and those that promote diarrhea, e.g., antacids.	

Child Health

ACTIONS/INTERVENTIONS	RATIONALES
• Weigh diapers for urine and stools; assess specific gravity after each voiding.	A strict assessment of intake and output serves as a basis for monitoring the efficiency of the treatment and may provide a database for treatment protocol. Hydration is monitored via specific gravity as an indication of the renal ability to adjust to fluid and electrolyte imbalance. Dehydration is extremely dangerous for the infant and requires close monitoring to offset the effects of dehydration.

• Monitor for signs and symptoms of dehydration:
  ◦ Depressed anterior fontanel in infants
  ◦ Poor skin turgor
  ◦ Decreased urinary output
• Monitor signs and symptoms associated with bowel movement, including cramping, flatus, and crying.
 	
• Provide prompt and gentle cleansing after each diaper change. For older children offer warm soaks after each diarrheal episode.
• Collaborate with physician regarding:
  ◦ Frequent stooling (more than 3 times per shift)
  ◦ Excessive vomiting
  ◦ Possible dietary alterations for specific formula or diet
  ◦ Monitoring electrolytes and renal function
  ◦ Maintenance of IV fluids
  ◦ Antidiarrheal medications
	Associated signs and symptoms serve as supportive data to follow the altered bowel function with an emphasis on related pain or discomfort.
	Skin breakdown occurs in a short period of time due to frequent bowel movements and the resultant skin irritation.
	These nursing measures constitute routine measures to monitor diarrhea and its related problems. Prompt reporting and intervention decrease the likelihood of more serious complications.

Women's Health

NOTE: Some women experience diarrhea 1 or 2 days before labor begins. It is not certain why this occurs, but it is thought to be due to the irritation of the bowel by the contracting uterus and the decrease in hormonal level (estrogen and progesterone) in late pregnancy. For diarrhea that is a precursor to labor, the following action applies.

ACTIONS/INTERVENTIONS	RATIONALES

• Offer oral electrolyte solutions such as:
  ◦ Gatorade
  ◦ Classic Coca-Cola
  ◦ Jello
  ◦ 10-K
  ◦ Pedialyte
	Provides nutrition, electrolytes, and minerals that support a successful labor process.

Psychiatric Health

ACTIONS/INTERVENTIONS	RATIONALES
• Discuss with client the role stress and anxiety play in this problem. • Develop with client stress reduction plan and practice specific interventions 3 times a day at (list times here). • Refer to Chapter 8 for specific nursing actions related to the diagnosis of Anxiety.	Diarrhea can be related to autonomic nervous system response to emotions.[19] Promotes client's adaptive response to stress and promotes client's sense of control.

Gerontic Health

ACTIONS/INTERVENTIONS	RATIONALES
• Monitor medication intake to assess for potential side effect of diarrhea. • Collaborate with physician regarding possible alterations in medications to decrease the problem of diarrhea.	The older adult may be having diarrhea as a result of antibiotic therapy, use of drugs with a laxative effect such as magnesium-based antacids, or as a sign of drug toxicity secondary to antiarrhythmics such as digitalis, quinidine, or propranolol.

Home Health

ACTIONS/INTERVENTIONS	RATIONALES

• Teach client and family:
  ○ How to monitor perianal skin integrity
  ○ Techniques of perianal hygiene
  ○ Techniques of maintaining fluid and electrolyte balance (see Adult Health)
  ○ Administering antidiarrheal medications
• Assist client and family to set criteria to help them to determine when a physician or other intervention is required, e.g., child's having over 3 stools in 1 day.
• Assist client and family in identifying lifestyle changes that may be required:
  ○ Avoid drinking local water when traveling in areas where water supply may be contaminated (foreign countries or streams and lakes when camping).
  ○ Practice stress management.
  ○ Avoid laxative or enema abuse.
  ○ Avoid foods that cause symptoms.
  ○ Avoid bingeing behavior.
• Refer patient to appropriate assistive resources as indicated.
	Similar to Adult Health. For Home Health the locus of control is now the client and family, not the nurse.
	
	Provides client and family background knowledge to seek appropriate assistance as need arises.
	
	Behaviors to prevent recurrence of or continuation of the problem.
	
	Additional assistance may be required to maintain health. Use of readily available resources is cost-effective.

Diarrhea

FLOWCHART EVALUATION: EXPECTED OUTCOME 1

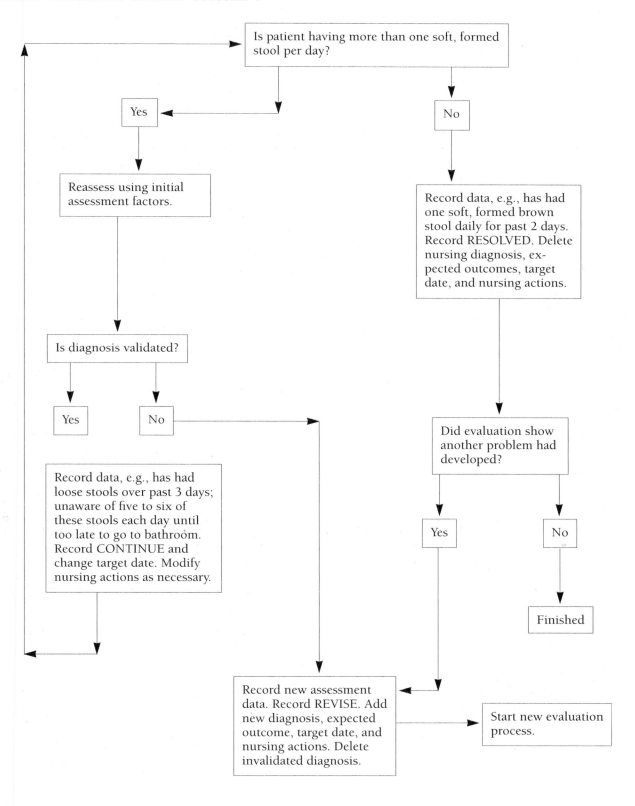

Is patient having more than one soft, formed stool per day?

Yes

Reassess using initial assessment factors.

Is diagnosis validated?

Yes

No

Record data, e.g., has had loose stools over past 3 days; unaware of five to six of these stools each day until too late to go to bathroom. Record CONTINUE and change target date. Modify nursing actions as necessary.

No

Record data, e.g., has had one soft, formed brown stool daily for past 2 days. Record RESOLVED. Delete nursing diagnosis, expected outcomes, target date, and nursing actions.

Did evaluation show another problem had developed?

Yes

No

Finished

Record new assessment data. Record REVISE. Add new diagnosis, expected outcome, target date, and nursing actions. Delete invalidated diagnosis.

Start new evaluation process.

Diarrhea

FLOWCHART EVALUATION: EXPECTED OUTCOME 2

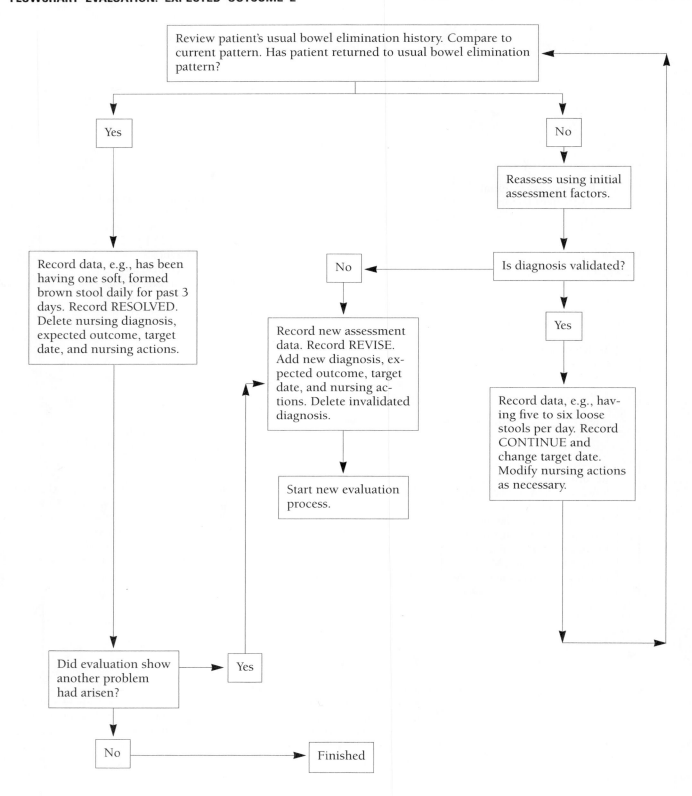

Urinary Elimination, Altered, Incontinence

DEFINITIONS

ALTERED URINARY ELIMINATION The state in which the individual experiences a disturbance in urine elimination.[15]

FUNCTIONAL INCONTINENCE The state in which an individual experiences an involuntary, unpredictable passage of urine.[15]

REFLEX INCONTINENCE The state in which an individual experiences an involuntary loss of urine, occurring at somewhat predictable intervals when a specific bladder volume is reached.[15]

STRESS INCONTINENCE The state in which an individual experiences a loss of urine of less than 50 mL occurring with increased abdominal pressure.[15]

TOTAL INCONTINENCE The state in which the individual experiences a continuous and unpredictable loss of urine.[15]

URGE INCONTINENCE The state in which the individual experiences involuntary passage of urine occurring soon after a strong sense of urgency to void.[15]

NANDA TAXONOMY: EXCHANGING 1.3.2, 1.3.2.1.1, 1.3.2.1.2, 1.3.2.1.3, 1.3.2.1.4, AND 1.3.2.1.5

DEFINING CHARACTERISTICS[15]

1. Altered Urinary Elimination
   a. Major defining characteristics
      (1) Dysuria
      (2) Frequency
      (3) Hesitancy
      (4) Incontinence
      (5) Nocturia
      (6) Retention
      (7) Urgency
   b. Minor defining characteristics
      None given
2. Functional Incontinence
   a. Major defining characteristics
      (1) Urge to void or bladder contractions sufficiently strong to result in loss of urine before reaching an appropriate receptacle
   b. Minor defining characteristics
      None given
3. Reflex Incontinence
   a. Major defining characteristics
      (1) No awareness of bladder filling
      (2) No urge to void or feelings of bladder fullness
      (3) Uninhibited bladder contraction or spasm at regular intervals
   b. Minor defining characteristics
      None given
4. Stress Incontinence
   a. Major defining characteristics
      (1) Reported or observed dribbling with increased abdominal pressure
   b. Minor defining characteristics

      (1) Urinary urgency
      (2) Urinary frequency (more often than every 2 hours)
5. Total Incontinence
   a. Major defining characteristics
      (1) Constant flow of urine occurring at unpredictable times without distention, or uninhibited bladder contractions or spasms
      (2) Unsuccessful incontinence refractory treatments
      (3) Nocturia
   b. Minor defining characteristics
      (1) Lack of perineal or bladder filling awareness
      (2) Unawareness of incontinence
6. Urge Incontinence
   a. Major defining characteristics
      (1) Urinary urgency
      (2) Frequency (voiding more often than every 2 hours)
      (3) Bladder contracture or spasm
   b. Minor defining characteristics
      (1) Nocturia (more than 2 times per night)
      (2) Voiding in small amounts (less than 100 mL) or in large amounts (more than 550 mL)
      (3) Inability to reach toilet in time

RELATED FACTORS[15]

1. Altered Urinary Elimination
   a. Multiple causality including:
      (1) Anatomic obstruction
      (2) Sensorimotor impairment
      (3) Urinary tract infection
2. Functional Incontinence
   a. Altered environment
   b. Sensory, cognitive, or mobility deficits
3. Reflex Incontinence
   a. Neurologic impairment (e.g., spinal cord lesion that interferes with conduction of cerebral messages above the level of the reflex arc)
4. Stress Incontinence
   a. Degenerative changes in pelvic muscles and structural supports associated with increased age
   b. High intra-abdominal pressure (e.g., obesity or gravid uterus)
   c. Incompetent bladder outlet
   d. Overdistention between voidings
   e. Weak pelvic muscles and structural supports
5. Total Incontinence
   a. Neuropathy preventing transmission of reflex indicating bladder fullness
   b. Neurologic dysfunction causing triggering of micturition at unpredictable times
   c. Independent contraction of detrusor reflex due to surgery
   d. Trauma or disease affecting spinal cord nerves
   e. Anatomic (fistula)
6. Urge Incontinence
   a. Decreased bladder capacity (e.g., history of PID, abdominal surgeries, or indwelling urinary catheter)

b. Irritation of bladder stretch receptors causing spasm (e.g., bladder infections)
c. Alcohol
d. Caffeine
e. Increased fluids
f. Increased urine concentration
g. Overdistention of bladder

RELATED CLINICAL CONCERNS

1. Spinal cord injury
2. Urinary tract infection
3. Alzheimer's disease
4. Pregnancy
5. Abdominal surgery
6. Prostate surgery

HAVE YOU SELECTED THE CORRECT DIAGNOSIS?

Constipation Anything in the body that creates additional pressure on the bladder or bladder sphincter may precipitate voiding. Constipation can create this additional pressure because of the increased amount of fecal material in the sigmoid colon and rectum. Incontinence may then be a direct result of constipation or fecal impaction.

Fluid-Volume Excess or Fluid-Volume Deficit Since urination depends on input of the stimulus that the bladder is full and since one of the ways the body responds to excess fluid volume is by increasing urinary output, the very fact that there is excess volume may result in the bladder's inability to keep up with the kidney's production of urine. Thus, incontinence may occur. Conversely, Fluid-Volume Deficit can result in incontinence by eliminating the sensation of a full bladder and by decreasing the person's awareness of the sensation.

Impaired Physical Mobility As previously stated, the individual must be able to control the sphincter, walk a few steps, recognize and interpret that the bladder is full, and be able to indicate that he or she wants to go to the bathroom. Even if the person has some control of the sphincter and has correctly recognized and interpreted the cues of a full bladder, if he or she is unable to get to the bathroom or get there in time because of mobility problems, incontinence may result. This may happen especially in a hospital.

Impaired Verbal Communication The ability to verbally communicate the need to urinate is important. If the person is unable to tell someone or have someone understand that he or she wants to go to the bathroom, incontinence may occur.

EXPECTED OUTCOMES

1. Will remain continent at least 90 percent of the time by (date) and/or
2. Will design and carry out a personal continence plan by (date)

TARGET DATES

Incontinence will require training time and effort; therefore, a target date 5 days from the date of admission would be reasonable to evaluate the patient's progress toward meeting the expected outcome. Additionally, there must be a realistic potential that urinary continence may never be regained by the patient. For this reason, it would need to be qualified for use with handicapped or neurologically deficient clients according to the exact level of continence hoped for.

NURSING ACTIONS/INTERVENTIONS WITH RATIONALES

Adult Health

ACTIONS/INTERVENTIONS	RATIONALES

• Record:
  ○ Time and amount of each voiding
  ○ Whether voiding was continent or incontinent
  ○ Patient's activity before and after incontinent incidence
	Monitors voiding pattern and effectiveness of treatment.

• Monitor, at least every 2 h on the (odd/even) hour, for continence.	Basic methods to monitor hydration, prevent tissue integrity problems, prevent infection, and promote comfort.

- Monitor:
  - Weight at least every 3 days
  - Lab values (e.g., electrolytes, WBC, or urinalyses)
  - For dependent edema
  - Perineal skin integrity at least once per shift
  - Intake and output, each shift
  - For bladder distention at least every 2 h on the (odd/even) hour
- Apply medicated ointment as ordered.
- Use heat lamp as ordered.
- Consult with enterostomal therapist regarding any stoma care.
- Give sitz bath.
- Respond **immediately** to patient's request for voiding.
- Schedule toileting:
  - Schedule at least 30 min before recorded incontinence times.
  - Awaken patient once during night for voiding.
  - Encourage patient to consciously hold urine to stretch bladder.
  - Teach biofeedback techniques.
- Stimulate voiding at scheduled time by:
  - Assisting patient to maintain normal anatomic position for voiding
  - Having patient lightly brush inner thighs or lower abdomen
  - Running warm water over perineum (measure amount first)
  - Having patient listen to dripping water
  - Placing patient's hands in warm water
  - Using Crede's or Valsalva maneuver
  - Gently tapping over bladder
  - Drinking water while trying to void
  - Providing privacy
  - Providing night light and clear path to bathroom
  - Sitting on firm towel roll when incontinence threatens
  - Gradually increasing length of time, by 15 min, between voidings
- Schedule fluid intake:
  - Avoid fluids containing caffeine and other fluids that produce a diuretic effect (e.g., coffee, grapefruit juice, and alcohol).
  - Encourage 8 oz of fluid every 2 h on the (odd/even) hour during the day.
  - Limit fluids after 6 p.m.
- Maintain bowel elimination. Monitor bowel movements, and record at least once each shift.
- Beginning on day of admission, teach and have patient return-demonstrate perineal skin care.
- Beginning on day of admission, guard and teach patient to guard against nosocomial infection.
- Assist patient with stress reduction and relaxation techniques at least once per shift.
- Collaborate with physician regarding:
  - Intermittent catheterization
  - Medications (e.g., urinary antiseptics, analgesics, or anticholinergics)
- Collaborate with dietitian regarding foods and fluids to acidify urine, e.g., cranberry juice or citrus fruits.
- Collaborate with rehabilitation nurse clinician to establish a bladder retraining program.

Immediate response may prevent an incontinent episode.

Voiding at scheduled intervals prevents overdistention and helps to establish a voiding pattern.

Assists in predicting times of voiding. Decreases urge to void at unscheduled times.

Fullness in bowel may exert pressure on bladder causing bladder incontinence.
Prevents skin irritation, infection, and odor.

Promotes relaxation and self-control of voiding.

Prevents complications related to bladder overdistention.

Decreases the probability of bladder infections.

Allows establishment of a program that is current in content and procedures.

Continued

ACTIONS/INTERVENTIONS	RATIONALES
• Teach patient exercises to strengthen pelvic floor muscles (10 times each at least 4 times per day—state times here): 　○ Contracting posterior perineal muscles as if trying to stop a bowel movement 　○ Contracting anterior perineal muscles as if trying to stop voiding 　○ Starting and stopping urine stream 　○ Bent-knee sit-ups 　○ Bent-leg lifts	Strengthens pelvic floor muscles to better control voiding.
• Teach the patient the importance of maintaining a daily routine: 　○ Voiding upon arising 　○ Awakening self once during the night 　○ Voiding immediately before retiring 　○ Not postponing voiding unnecessarily	Helps to establish urinary elimination pattern and prevents overdistention of bladder.
• Encourage patient that he or she can be continent again and encourage to avoid social isolation: 　○ Wearing street clothes with protective pads in undergarments 　○ Maintaining bladder-retraining program 　○ Responding as soon as possible to voiding urge 　○ Taking oral chlorophyll tablets 　○ Losing weight if necessary	Helps preserve self-concept and body image. Promotes compliance.
• Refer patient to home health care agency for follow-up.	Provides continuity of care and support system for ongoing care at home.

Child Health

Nursing actions for the child with incontinence are the same as for Adult Health with appropriate modifications for child's age and weight.

Women's Health

ACTIONS/INTERVENTIONS	RATIONALES
• Assist patient in identifying lifestyle adjustments that may be needed to accommodate changing bladder capacity due to anatomic changes of pregnancy. • Teach patient: 　○ To recognize symptoms of urinary tract infection (urgency, burning, or dysuria) 　○ How to take temperature (make sure patient knows how to read thermometer) 　○ To seek immediate medical care if symptoms of urinary tract infection appear	Bladder capacity is reduced due to enlarging uterus, displacement of abdominal contents by enlarged uterus, and pressure on bladder by enlarged uterus.

Psychiatric Health

　　NOTE: Clients on hypnotics, antidepressants, and antipsychotics are at risk for this diagnosis. If alteration is related to psychosocial issues and has no physiologic component, initiate the following nursing actions (refer to Adult Health for physiologically produced problems).

ACTIONS/INTERVENTIONS	RATIONALES
• Monitor times, places, persons present, and emotional climate around inappropriate voiding episodes.	Identifies target behaviors and establishes a baseline measurement of behavior with possible reinforcers for inappropriate behavior.[20]
• Remind client to void before a high-risk situation or remove secondary-gain process from situation.	Removes positive reinforcement for inappropriate behavior.[21]
• Provide the client with supplies necessary to facilitate appropriate voiding behavior (e.g., urinal for client in locked seclusion area).	Appropriate behavior cannot be implemented without the appropriate equipment.
• Inform client of acceptable times and places for voiding and of consequences for inappropriate voiding (note consequences here).	Negative reinforcement eliminates or decreases behavior.[21]
• Have client assist with cleaning up any voiding that has occurred in an inappropriate place.	Provides a negative consequence for inappropriate behavior.[21]
• Provide as little interaction with client as possible during cleanup.	Lack of social response acts as negative reinforcements.[20,21]
• Provide client with positive reinforcement for voiding in appropriate place and time (list specific reinforcers for this client here).	Positive reinforcement encourages appropriate behavior.[21]
• Spend (number) minutes with client every hour in an activity the client has identified as enjoyable; do not provide this time or discontinue time if client inappropriately voids during the specified time (list identified activities here).	Interaction with the nurse can provide positive reinforcement. Withdrawing attention for inappropriate behavior provides negative reinforcement.[21]
• If client voids inappropriately (number) times during a shift, he or she will spend (number) minutes (no more than 30) in time-out. Each inappropriate voiding in time-out adds 5 min to this time.	Negative consequences decrease or eliminate undesirable behavior.[21]
• As behavior improves, add rewards for accumulated times of appropriate voiding (e.g., on 2-h pass for 1 day of appropriate voiding). Record these rewards here.	Intermittent reinforcement can render a response more resistant to extinction once it has been established.[22]

Refer to Chapters 8 and 11 for interventions related to the specific alterations that would promote this coping pattern.

Gerontic Health

ACTIONS/INTERVENTIONS	RATIONALES
• Review medication record for drugs such as sedatives, hypnotics, or diuretics that may contribute to urinary incontinence.	Sedatives and hypnotics may result in a delayed response to the urge to void. Diuretic therapy, depending on dosage and time of administration, may result in an inability to reach the bathroom in a timely manner.

Home Health

NOTE: If this nursing diagnosis is made, it is imperative that a physician referral be made. If referred to home care under a physician's care, it is important to maintain and evaluate response to prescribed treatments.

ACTIONS/INTERVENTIONS	RATIONALES

• Assist client and family in identifying lifestyle changes that may be required:
  ◦ Using proper perineal hygiene
  ◦ Taking showers instead of tub baths
  ◦ Drinking fluids to cause voiding every 2–3 h to flush out bacteria
  ◦ Scheduling fluid intake
  ◦ Voiding after intercourse
  ◦ Avoiding perfumed soaps, toilet paper, or feminine hygiene sprays
  ◦ Wearing cotton underwear
  ◦ Using proper handwashing techniques
  ◦ Following a daily routine of voiding (see Adult Health actions)
  ◦ Establishing a bladder-retraining program
  ◦ Doing exercises to strengthen pelvic floor muscles
  ◦ Providing an environment conducive to continence
  ◦ Street clothes and protective underwear
  ◦ Air purifier
  ◦ Activities as tolerated
  ◦ Unobstructed access to bathroom
  ◦ Avoiding fluids that produce diuretic effect, e.g., caffeine, alcohol, or teas
	Basic measures to prevent recurrence.

• Teach client and family to dilute and acidify the urine:
  ◦ Increasing fluids
  ◦ Introducing cranberry juice, poultry, etc., to increase acid ash
	Bacteria multiply rapidly in alkaline urine.

• Teach client and family to monitor and maintain skin integrity:
  ◦ Keep skin clean and dry.
  ◦ Keep bed linens and clothing clean and dry.
  ◦ Use proper perineal hygiene.
	Prevents or minimizes problems secondary to incontinence.

• Assist client and family to set criteria to help them to determine when a physician or other intervention is required, e.g., hematuria, fever, or skin breakdown. • Monitor and teach importance of appropriate medications and treatments ordered by physician. • Refer patient to appropriate assistive resources as indicated.	Assists in preventing or minimizing further physiologic damage.

Urinary Elimination, Altered, Incontinence

FLOWCHART EVALUATION: EXPECTED OUTCOME 1

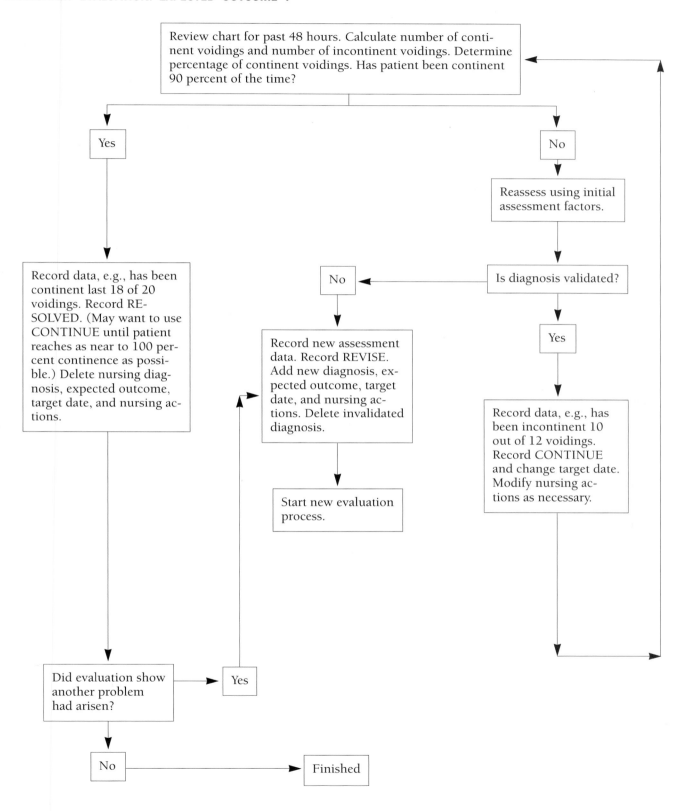

Urinary Elimination, Altered, Incontinence

FLOWCHART EVALUATION: EXPECTED OUTCOME 2

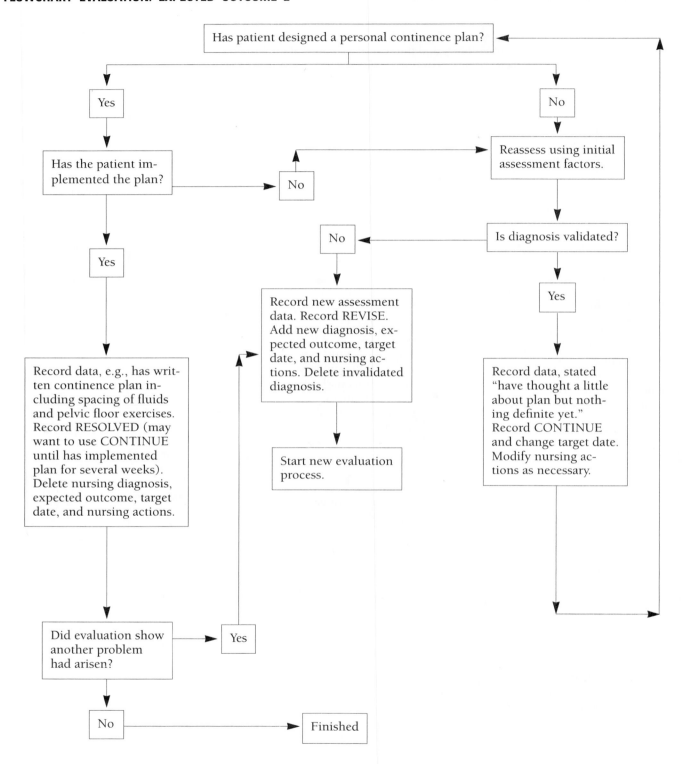

Urinary Retention

DEFINITION

The state in which the individual experiences incomplete emptying of the bladder.[15]

NANDA TAXONOMY: EXCHANGING 1.3.2.2

DEFINING CHARACTERISTICS[15]

1. Major defining characteristics
   a. Bladder distention
   b. Small, frequent voiding or absence of urine output
2. Minor defining characteristics
   a. Sensation of bladder fullness
   b. Dribbling

   c. Residual urine
   d. Dysuria
   e. Overflow incontinence

RELATED FACTORS[15]

1. High urethral pressure caused by weak detrusor
2. Inhibition of reflex arc
3. Strong sphincter
4. Blockage

RELATED CLINICAL CONCERNS

1. Benign prostatic hyperplasia
2. Hysterectomy
3. Urinary tract infection
4. Cancer

HAVE YOU SELECTED THE CORRECT DIAGNOSIS?

Incontinence Overflow incontinence frequently occurs in patients whose primary problem is really retention. The bladder is overdistended in retention, and some urine is passed involuntarily because of the pressure of the retained urine on the bladder sphincter.

Self-Care Deficit, Toileting In neurogenic bladder conditions, the bladder is chronically overdistended, resulting in urinary retention.

EXPECTED OUTCOMES

1. Will void under voluntary control and empty bladder at least every 4 hours by (date) and/or
2. Will demonstrate no signs or symptoms of urinary retention by (date)

TARGET DATES

Urinary retention poses many dangers to the patient. An acceptable target date to evaluate for lessening of retention would be within 24 to 48 hours after admission.

NURSING ACTIONS/INTERVENTIONS WITH RATIONALES

Adult Health

ACTIONS/INTERVENTIONS	RATIONALES
• Monitor bladder for distention at least every 2 h on the (odd/even) hour.	Monitors pattern and determines effectiveness of treatment; helps prevent complications.
• Measure and record intake and output each shift.	Monitors fluid balance.
• Maintain fluid intake:	Assures sufficient fluid intake, but restricts fluid when
○ Encourage fluids to at least 2000 mL per day.	activity decreases. Assists in preventing nocturia.
○ Limit fluids after 6 p.m.	
• Monitor:	Constipation may block bladder opening and lead to
○ Bowel elimination at least once per shift	retention. Empty bowel will facilitate free passage of
○ Urinalyses, electrolytes, and weight at least every 3 days	urine.
• Increase patient activity:	Strengthens muscles and promotes kidney and bladder
○ Ambulate at least twice per shift while awake at (times).	functioning.
○ Collaborate with physical therapist, soon after admission, regarding an exercise program.	

Continued

ACTIONS/INTERVENTIONS	RATIONALES
• Collaborate with rehabilitation nurse clinician to initiate bladder-retraining program.	Allows establishment of a program that is current in content and procedures.
• Stimulate micturition reflex every 4 h while awake at (times):	Helps relax sphincter and strengthens voiding reflex.
○ Assist patient to assume anatomically correct position for voiding.	
○ Remind patient to consciously be aware of need-to-void sensations.	
• Teach patient to assist bladder contraction:	
○ Crede's maneuver	
○ Valsalva maneuver	
○ Abdominal muscle contraction	
• Beginning on day of admission, teach patient the following exercises:	Strengthens pelvic floor muscles.
○ Bent-knee sit-ups	
○ Bent-leg lifts	
○ Contracting posterior perineal muscles as if trying to stop a bowel movement	
○ Contracting anterior perineal muscles as if trying to stop voiding	
○ Starting and stopping urine stream	
• Collaborate with physician regarding:	Relieves bladder distention, assists to schedule voiding, and prevents infection.
○ Intermittent catheterization	
○ Medications (e.g., urinary antiseptics or analgesics)	
• Refer to home health agency at least 2 days prior to discharge for continued monitoring.	Provides continuity of care and a support system for ongoing home care.

Child Health

NOTE: For infants and children who weigh less than 20 lb, it is necessary to calculate exact intake and output and fluid requisites according to the etiologic factors present. Attention must be paid to the child's physiologic developmental level regarding urinary control.

ACTIONS/INTERVENTIONS	RATIONALES
• Provide opportunities for child and parents to verbalize concerns or views related to body image disturbances related to urinary control and retention. Spend at least 30 min per shift in privacy with child and parents to permit this verbalization.	Assists in reducing anxiety and attaches value to the patient's and parent's feelings. Promotes the development of a therapeutic relationship.
• Monitor parental (patient as applicable) knowledge of preventive health care for patient:	Parental knowledge will assist in the reduction of anxiety and will provide a greater likelihood for compliance with desired plan of care.
○ Teaching and observation of urinary catheterization	
○ Maintenance of catheters and supplies	
○ How to obtain supplies	
○ How to obtain a sterile culture specimen	
○ Appropriate restraint of infant	
○ Potential regarding urinary control	
• Provide opportunities for parental participation in the care of the infant or child:	Appropriate parental involvement provides opportunities for trial care and allows parents to practice care in a safe, supportive environment prior to time of more total self-care.
○ Feedings	
○ Bathing	
○ Monitoring intake and output	
○ Planning for care to include individual preferences when possible	
○ Assisting with procedures when appropriate	
○ Provision of safety needs	
○ Cautious handwashing to prevent infection	
○ Appropriate emotional support	

- ○ Appropriate diversional activity and relaxation
- ○ Need for pain medication
- Collaborate with other health care professionals as needed.
- Assist family to identify support groups represented in the community for future needs.

Identification of support for the family will best assist them to comply with the desired plan of care while reducing anxiety and promoting self-care.

Women's Health

ACTIONS/INTERVENTIONS	RATIONALES
• Collaborate with physician regarding intermittent catheterization.	It is not easy to catheterize a woman postpartum nor is it desirable to introduce an added risk of infection, so every effort and support should be directed toward helping the woman to void on her own. If, however, she is unable to void or to empty her bladder, an indwelling catheter may be placed for 24–48 h to rest the bladder and allow it to heal, edema to subside, and bladder and urethral tone to return.[23]

Psychiatric Health

NOTE: Clients receiving antipsychotic and antidepressant drugs are at increased risk for this diagnosis. Refer to Adult Health for general actions related to this diagnosis.

ACTIONS/INTERVENTIONS	RATIONALES
• Place clients receiving antipsychotic or antidepressant medication on daily assessment for this diagnosis. Elderly clients should be evaluated more frequently if their physical status indicates.	Early intervention and treatment assures better outcome.
• Monitor bladder for distention at least every 4 h at (times) if verbal reports are unreliable or if they indicate a voiding frequency greater than every 4 h.	
• Increase client's activity by: ○ Walking with client (number) minutes 3 times a day at (list times here) ○ Collaborating with physical therapist regarding an exercise program ○ Placing client in a room distant from the day area, nursing stations, and other activity if condition does not contraindicate this ○ Providing physical activities that client indicates are of interest (list those here with the time for each)	Activity maintains muscle strength necessary for maintenance of normal voiding patterns (see Adult Health for specific exercises to strengthen pelvic floor muscles).
• Teach deep muscle relaxation, and spend 30 minutes twice a day at (list times here) practicing this with client. Associate relaxation with breathing so that client can eventually relax with deep breathing while attempting to void.	Anxiety can increase muscle tension and therefore contribute to urinary retention.[23]

Gerontic Health

ACTIONS/INTERVENTIONS	RATIONALES
• Review medication record for use of antidepressant and antipsychotic medications.	The use of antidepressant and antipsychotic medications can result in urinary retention as a side effect.

Home Health

NOTE: If this nursing diagnosis is made, it is imperative that physician referral be made. Vigorous intervention is required to prevent damage or systemic infection. If patient is referred to home care under physician's care, it is important to maintain and evaluate response to prescribed treatments.

ACTIONS/INTERVENTIONS	RATIONALES
• Assist client and family in lifestyle changes that may be required: ○ Monitor bladder for distention. ○ Record intake and output. ○ Stimulate micturition reflex (see Adult Health). ○ Institute bladder retraining program (see Additional Information). ○ Perform exercises to strengthen pelvic floor muscles. ○ Use proper position for voiding. ○ Maintain fluid intake. ○ Maintain physical activity as tolerated. ○ Use straight catheterization.	Similar to Adult Health. Locus of control now is with family and client.
• Assist client and family to set criteria to help them to determine when a physician or other intervention is required, e.g., specified intake and output limit, pain, or bladder distention.	Knowledge will assist client and family to seek timely interventions.
• Monitor and teach importance of appropriate medications and treatment ordered by physician.	Provides client and family with knowledge to care for problem.
• Refer to appropriate assistive resources as indicated.	Additional support may be required to help the client and family maintain care at home.

Urinary Retention

FLOWCHART EVALUATION: EXPECTED OUTCOME 1

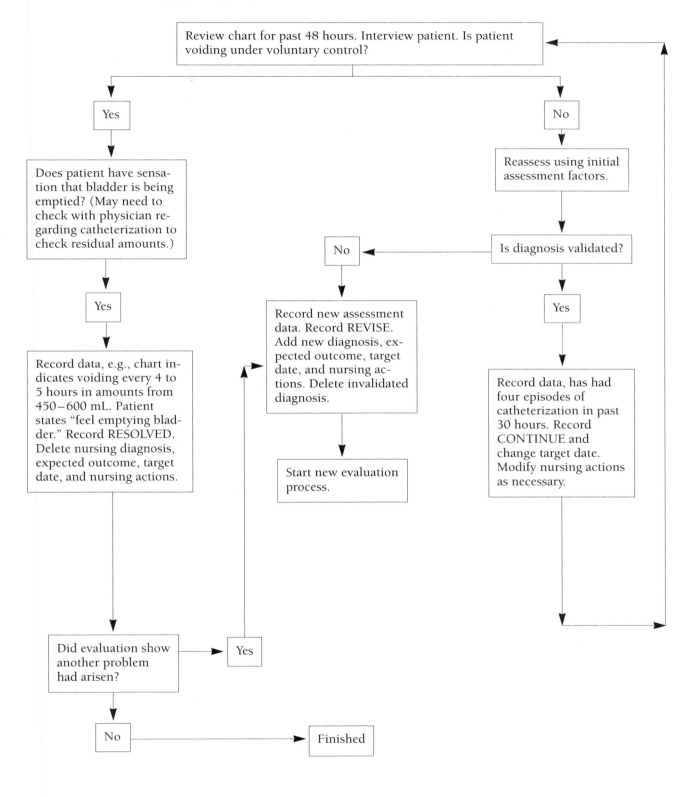

Urinary Retention

FLOWCHART EVALUATION: EXPECTED OUTCOME 2

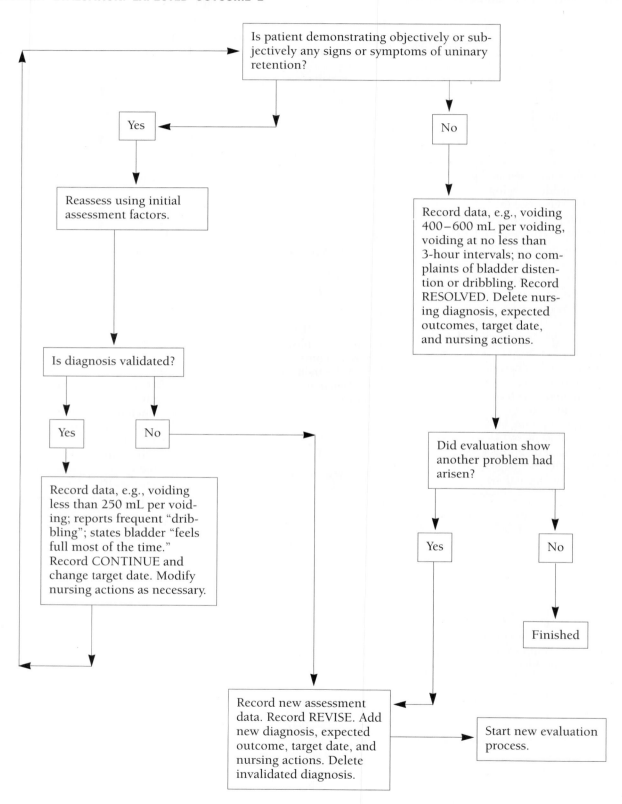

Is patient demonstrating objectively or subjectively any signs or symptoms of urinary retention?

Yes

No

Reassess using initial assessment factors.

Record data, e.g., voiding 400–600 mL per voiding, voiding at no less than 3-hour intervals; no complaints of bladder distention or dribbling. Record RESOLVED. Delete nursing diagnosis, expected outcomes, target date, and nursing actions.

Is diagnosis validated?

Yes

No

Record data, e.g., voiding less than 250 mL per voiding; reports frequent "dribbling"; states bladder "feels full most of the time." Record CONTINUE and change target date. Modify nursing actions as necessary.

Did evaluation show another problem had arisen?

Yes

No

Finished

Record new assessment data. Record REVISE. Add new diagnosis, expected outcome, target date, and nursing actions. Delete invalidated diagnosis.

Start new evaluation process.

Activity-Exercise Pattern

Pattern Description

This pattern focuses on the activities of daily living (ADL) and the amount of energy an individual has available to support these activities. The ADL include all aspects of maintaining self-care and incorporate leisure time as well. Because the individual's energy level and mobility for ADL are affected by the proper functioning of the neuromuscular, cardiovascular, and respiratory systems, nursing diagnoses related to dysfunctions in these systems are included.

As with the other patterns, a problem in the activity-exercise pattern may be the primary reason for the patient's entering the health care system or may arise secondary to problems in another functional pattern. Any admission to a hospital may promote the development of problems in this area because of the therapeutics required for the medical diagnosis (e.g., bedrest) or because of agency rules and regulations (e.g., limited visiting hours).

Pattern Assessment

1. Does the patient's heart rate or BP increase abnormally in response to activity?
   a. Yes (Activity Intolerance)
   b. No
2. Does the patient have dyspnea after activity?
   a. Yes (Activity Intolerance)
   b. No
3. Does the patient have a medical diagnosis related to the cardiovascular or respiratory system?
   a. Yes (High Risk for Activity Intolerance)
   b. No
4. Does the patient have a history of Activity Intolerance?
   a. Yes (High Risk for Activity Intolerance)
   b. No
5. Does the patient complain of fatigue, weakness, or lack of energy?
   a. Yes (Activity Intolerance or Fatigue)
   b. No
6. Is the patient unable to maintain usual routines?
   a. Yes (Fatigue or Self-Care Deficit)
   b. No
7. Does the patient report difficulty in concentrating?
   a. Yes (Fatigue)
   b. No
8. Review self-care chart. Does the patient have any self-care deficits?
   a. Yes (Self-Care Deficit [Specify which area])
   b. No
9. Can the patient engage in usual hobby while in hospital?
   a. Yes
   b. No (Diversional Activity Deficit)
10. Does the family need help with home maintenance after patient goes home?
    a. Yes (Impaired Home Maintenance Management)
    b. No
11. Does the patient have insurance?
    a. Yes
    b. No (Impaired Home Maintenance Management)

12. Is the patient within height and weight norm for age?
    a. Yes
    b. No (Altered Growth and Development)
13. Can the patient perform developmental skills appropriate for age level?
    a. Yes
    b. No (Altered Growth and Development)
14. Are there any abnormal movements?
    a. Yes (Disorganized Infant Behavior)
    b. No
15. Does the infant respond appropriately to stimuli?
    a. Yes
    b. No (Disorganized Infant Behavior)
16. Does the patient's cardiogram indicate arrhythmias?
    a. Yes (Decreased Cardiac Output)
    b. No
17. Is the patient's jugular vein distended?
    a. Yes (Decreased Cardiac Output)
    b. No
18. Are the patient's peripheral pulses within normal limits?
    a. Yes
    b. No (Decreased Cardiac Output, Altered Tissue Perfusion, High Risk for, or Peripheral Neurovascular Dysfunction)
19. Are the patient's extremities cold?
    a. Yes (Altered Tissue Perfusion or High Risk for Peripheral Neurovascular Dysfunction)
    b. No
20. Does the patient have claudication?
    a. Yes (Altered Tissue Perfusion or High Risk for Peripheral Neurovascular Dysfunction)
    b. No
21. Does the patient have full range of motion?
    a. Yes
    b. No (Impaired Physical Mobility)
22. Does the patient have problems moving self in bed or in ambulating?
    a. Yes (Impaired Physical Mobility)
    b. No
23. Is the patient paralyzed?
    a. Yes (High Risk for Disuse Syndrome)
    b. No
24. Is the patient immobilized by casts or traction?
    a. Yes (High Risk for Disuse Syndrome or High Risk for Peripheral Neurovascular Dysfunction)
    b. No
25. Does the patient have a spinal cord injury at T7 or above and paroxysmal hypertension?
    a. Yes (Dysreflexia)
    b. No
26. Does the patient have a spinal cord injury at T7 or above and bradycardia or tachycardia?
    a. Yes (Dysreflexia)
    b. No
27. Review mental status examination. Is the patient exhibiting confusion or drowsiness?
    a. Yes (Impaired Gas Exchange)
    b. No
28. Review blood gases. Does the patient demonstrate hypercapnia?

a. Yes (Impaired Gas Exchange or Inability to Sustain Spontaneous Ventilation)
b. No

29. Were rales (crackles) or rhonchi (wheezes) present on chest auscultation?
    a. Yes (Ineffective Airway Clearance)
    b. No

30. Is respiratory rate increased above normal range?
    a. Yes (Ineffective Airway Clearance or Ineffective Breathing Pattern)
    b. No

31. Is the patient on a ventilator? If yes, does the patient have restlessness or an increase from baseline of BP, P, or R when attempts at weaning are tried?
    a. Yes (Dysfunctional ventilatory weaning response)
    b. No

32. Does the patient have dyspnea and shortness of breath?
    a. Yes (Ineffective Breathing Pattern or Inability to Sustain Spontaneous Ventilation or Activity Intolerance)
    b. No

33. Is the patient exhibiting pursed-lip breathing?
    a. Yes (Ineffective Breathing Pattern)
    b. No

Conceptual Information

There are several nursing diagnoses included in this pattern that, at first glance, seem to have little relationship to each other. However, closer investigation demonstrates that there is one concept common to all of the diagnoses: immobility. Immobility or the impulses that control and coordinate mobility can contribute to the development of any of these diagnoses, or any of these diagnoses can ultimately lead to the development of immobility.

Mobility and immobility are end points on a continuum with many degrees of impaired mobility or partial mobility between the two points.[1] Immobility is usually distinguished from impaired mobility by the permanence of the limitation. A person who is quadriplegic has immobility because it is permanent; a person with a long cast on the left leg has impaired mobility because it is temporary.[2]

Mobility is defined as the ability to move freely, and it is one of the major means by which we define and express ourselves. The central nervous system integrates the stimuli from sensory receptor nerves of the peripheral nervous system and projection tracts of the central nervous system to respond to the internal or external environment of the individual. This integration allows for movements and expressions. A problem with mobility can be a measure of the degree of illness or health problem an individual has.[3]

Patients with self-care deficits are most often those who are experiencing some type of mobility problem.[2] The problem with mobility requires greater energy expenditure, which leads to activity intolerance, diversional activity deficit, and impaired home maintenance simply due to the lack of energy or nervous system response to engage in these activities.

Problems with mobility and nervous system response also lead to other physical problems. When a person has impaired mobility or immobility, bedrest is quite often prescribed or is voluntarily sought in an effort to conserve energy. Several authors[3-5] describe the physical problems that can occur secondary to prolonged bedrest:

1. **Respiratory:** Decreased chest and lung expansion causes slower and more shallow respiration. Pooling of secretions occurs secondary to decreased respiratory effort and the effects of gravity. The cough reflex is decreased due to decreased respiratory effort, gravity, and decreased muscle strength. Acid-base balance is shifted, causing a retention of carbon dioxide. Respiratory acidosis causes changes in mentation: vasodilation of cerebrovascular blood vessels and increased cerebral blood flow, headache, mental cloudiness, disorientation, dizziness, generalized weakness, convulsions, and unconsciousness. Additionally, because of the buildup of carbon dioxide in the lungs, adequate oxygen cannot be inspired, leading to tissue hypoxia.

2. **Cardiovascular:** Circulatory stasis is caused by vasodilation and impaired venous return. Muscular inactivity leads to vein dilation in dependent parts. Gravity effects also occur. Decreased respiratory effort and gravity lead to decreased changes in thoracic and abdominal pressures that usually assist in promoting blood return to the heart. Quite often patients have increased use of the Valsalva maneuver, which leads to increases in preload and afterload of cardiac output and ultimately a decreased cardiac output. Continued limitation of activity leads to decreased cardiac rate, circulatory volume, and arterial pressure due to redistribution of body fluids. Venous stasis contributes to the potential for deep venous thrombosis and pulmonary embolus. After prolonged bedrest, the normal neurovascular mechanism of the cardiovascular system that prevents large shifts in blood volume does not adequately function. When the individual who has experienced extended bedrest attempts to assume an upright position, gravity pulls an excessive amount of blood volume to the feet and legs, depriving the brain of adequate oxygen. As a result, the individual experiences orthostatic hypotension.[4]

3. **Musculoskeletal:** Inactivity causes decreased bone stress and decreased muscle tension. Osteoblastic and osteoclastic activities become imbalanced, leading to calcium and phosphorus loss. Decreased muscle use leads to decreased muscle mass and strength due to infrequent muscle contractions and protein loss.

4. **Metabolic:** Basal metabolic rate and oxygen consumption decrease, leading to decreased efficiency in using nutrients to build new tissues. Normally, body tissues break down nitrogen, but apparently muscle mass loss with accompanying protein loss leads to nitrogen loss and a negative nitrogen balance. Changes in tissue metabolism lead to increased potassium and calcium excretion. Decreased energy use and decreased basal metabolic rate (BMR) lead to appetite loss, which leads to decreased nutrient intake necessary to offset losses.

5. **Skin:** The negative nitrogen balance previously discussed, coupled with continuous pressure on bony prominences, leads to a greatly increased potential for skin breakdown.

Immobility is not the sole causative factor of the nursing diagnoses in this pattern. Many of the diagnoses can be related to specific medical diagnoses such as congestive heart failure or may occur as a result of diagnoses in this pattern, for example, Altered Growth and Development. However, the concept of immobility does serve to point out the interrelatedness of the diagnoses.

Since fatigue plays a major role in determining the quality and amount of musculoskeletal activity undertaken, consideration of the factors that influence fatigue is an essential part of nursing assessment for the activity-exercise pattern. Fatigue might be considered in two general categories: experiential and muscular. The degree to which the individual participates in activity is significant in determining the fatigue experienced. Activities that the individual enjoys are less likely to produce fatigue than are those not enjoyed. Preferences should be considered within the framework of capacity and needs. Obviously other factors that must be considered include the physical and medical condition of the person and his or her emotional state, level of growth and development, and state of health in general. Oxygenation needs and extrinsic factors would also need to be addressed. If there is overstimulation as with noise, extremes of temperature, or interruption of routines, a greater amount of fatigue or disorganized behavior can be expected. Sensory understimulation with resultant boredom can also contribute to fatigue.

Fatigue can develop as a result of too much waste material accumulating and too little nourishment going to the muscles. Muscle fatigue usually is attributed to the accumulation of too much lactic acid in the muscles. Certain metabolic conditions, such as congestive heart failure, place a person at greater risk for fatigue.

Developmental Considerations

Activity is influenced by diet, musculoskeletal factors, and respiratory and cardiovascular mechanisms. Developmental considerations for diet are addressed in Chapter 3. The developmental considerations discussed below specifically relate to musculoskeletal, respiratory, and cardiovascular factors.

INFANT

Physical and motor abilities are influenced by many things, including genetic, biologic, and cultural factors. Nutrition, maturation of the central nervous system, skeletal formation, overall physical health status, amount of stimulation, environmental conditions, and consistent loving care also play a part in physical and motor abilities.[6] Girls usually develop more rapidly than boys, although the activity level is higher in boys.[6]

All muscular tissue is formed at birth, but growth occurs as the infant uses the various muscle groups. This use stimulates increased strength and function.

The infant engages in various types of play activity at various times in infancy because of developing skills and changing needs. The infant needs the stimulation of parents in this play activity to fully develop. However, parents should be aware of the dangers in overstimulation. Fatigue, inattention, and injury to the infant may result.[6]

Interruptions in the normal developmental sequence of play activities due to illness or hospitalization, for example, can have a detrimental effect on the future development of the infant or child. An understanding of the normal sequence of play development is important to have so that therapeutic interventions can be designed to approximate the developmental needs of the individual.

The structural description of play development focuses on the Piagetian concepts of the increasing cognitive complexity of play activities. Elementary sensorimotor-based games emerge first, with the gradual development of advanced social games in adulthood.[7]

Play activities assist in the child's development of psychomotor skills and cognitive development. Socialization skills are learned and practiced via the interaction with others during play. As the child begins to learn more about his or her body during play, he or she will incorporate more complicated gross and fine motor skills. Play is extremely valuable in the development of language and other communication skills. Play helps the individual to establish control over self and the environment and provides a sense of accomplishment. Through play activities, the infant learns to trust the environment. Play also affords the child the opportunity to express emotions that would be unacceptable in other normal social situations.

Practice games begin during the sensorimotor level of cognitive development at 1 to 4 months of age and continue with increasing complexity throughout childhood. These games include skills that are performed for the pleasure of functioning, that is, for the pleasure of practice.

Symbolic games appear later during the sensorimotor period than do practice games—about age 12 to 18 months. Make-believe is now added to the practice game. Elements of absent objects or persons are represented by other objects. As previously stated, activity is influenced by respiratory and cardiovascular mechanisms.

The respiratory mechanisms or air-conducting passages (the nose, pharynx, larynx, trachea, bronchi, bronchioles, and alveoli) and lungs of the infant are small, delicate, and immature. The air that enters the nose is cool, dry, and unfiltered. The nose is unable to filter the air, and the mucous membranes of the upper respiratory tract are unable to produce enough mucus to humidify or warm the inhaled air. Therefore, the infant is more susceptible to respiratory tract infections.[7]

Additionally, the infant is a nose breather. When upper respiratory tract infections do occur, the infant is unable to appropriately clear the airways and may get into some difficulty until he or she learns to breathe through his or her mouth (at about 3 to 4 months of age). The cough of the infant is not very effective, and the infant quickly becomes fatigued with the effort.[7]

In the lungs, the alveoli are functioning, but not all alveoli may be expanded. Therefore, there is a large amount of dead space in the lungs. The infant has to work harder to exchange enough oxygen and carbon dioxide to meet body demands. The elevated respiratory rate of the infant (30 to 60 per minute) reflects this increased work. Additionally, arterial blood gases of the infant may show an acid-base imbalance. The rate and rhythm of respiration in the infant are somewhat irregular, and it is not unusual for the infant to use accessory muscles of respiration. Retractions with respiration are common.

The alveoli of the infant increase in number and complexity very rapidly. By 1 year of age, the alveoli and the lining of the air passages have matured considerably.

Respiratory tract obstructions are common in this age group because of the short trachea and the almost straight-line position of the right main stem bronchus. Additionally, the epiglottis does not effectively close over the trachea during swallowing. Thus, foreign objects are aspirated into the lungs.

In terms of cardiovascular development, the foramen ovale closes during the first 24 hours, and the ductus arteriosus closes after several days. The neonate can survive mild oxygen deprivation longer than an adult. The Apgar scoring system is used to measure the physical status of the newborn and includes heart rate, color, and respiration. There is no day-night rhythm to the neonate's heart rate, but from the sixth week on the rate will be lower at night than during the day. Axillary temperature and age-sized blood pressure cuffs should be used to assess vital signs. The pulse is 120 to 150 beats per minute, respiration ranges from 35 to 50 per minute, and BP ranges from 40 to 90 mm Hg systolic and 6 to 20 mm Hg diastolic. Vital signs become more stable over the first year. Listening for murmurs should be done over the base of the heart rather than at the apex. Breath sounds are bronchovesicular. The neonate has limited ability to respond to environmental temperature changes and will lose heat rapidly. This leads to an increased basal metabolic rate (BMR) and an increased workload on the heart. Until age 7, the apex is palpated at the fourth interspace just to the left of the midclavicular line.

TODDLER AND PRESCHOOLER

By this age, the child is walking, running, climbing, and jumping. The toddler is very active and very curious. He or she gets into everything. This helps the toddler organize his or her world and develop spatial and sensory perception.[6] It is during this period that the child begins to see himself or herself as a person separate from his or her parents and the environment. This increasing level of autonomy also presents a challenge for the caregivers. The child alternates between the security of the parents and the exciting exploration of the environment.

The toddler is fairly clumsy, but gross and fine motor coordination is improving. Neuromuscular maturation and repetition of movements help the child further develop skills.[6] Muscles grow faster than bones during these years. Safety is a major concern for children of this age. The toddler, especially, wants to do many things for himself or herself, thus testing control of self and the environment.

Bathing and Hygiene

By the age of 3, the child can wash and dry his or her hands with some wetting of clothes and can brush his or her teeth with assistance to perform the task adequately. By the fourth birthday the child may bathe himself or herself with assistance. The child will be able to bathe himself or herself without assistance by the age of 5. Both parents and nurses must keep in mind the safety issues involved in bathing; the child requires supervision in selection of water temperature and in the prevention of drowning.

Dressing and Grooming

At age 18 to 20 months the child has the fine motor skills required to unzip a large zipper. By 24 to 48 months the child can unbutton large buttons. The child can put on a coat with assistance by age 2; the child can undress himself or herself in most situations and can put on his or her own coat without assistance by age 3. At $3\frac{1}{2}$ years the child can unbutton small buttons, and by 4 years he or she can button small buttons. Dressing without assistance and beginning ability to lace shoes are accomplishments of the 5-year-old. The development of fine motor skills is required for most of the tasks of dressing. It is important that the child's clothing have fasteners that are appropriate for the motor skill development. The child will require assistance with deciding the appropriateness of clothing selected; seasonal variations in weather and culturally accepted norms regarding dressing and grooming are learned by the child with assistance.

Feeding

The child can drink from a cup without much spilling by 18 months. The child will have frequent spills while trying to get the contents of a spoon into his or her mouth at this age. By 2 years of age the child can drink from a cup; use of the spoon has improved at this age, but the child will still spill liquids (soup) from a spoon when eating. The child can eat from a spoon without spilling by $3\frac{1}{2}$ years. Accomplished use of the fork occurs at 5 years.

Toileting

By age 3 the child can go to the toilet without assistance; the child can pull pants up and down for toileting without assistance at this stage as well. The development of food preferences, preferred eating schedules and environment, and toileting behavior are imparted to the child by learning. Toileting, food, and the eating experiences may also include pleasures, control issues, and learning tasks in addition to the development of the motor skills required to accomplish the task. Delays or regressions in the tasks of self-feeding may reflect issues other than a self-care deficit, for example, discipline, family coping, and role relationships.

During the preschool years, the child seems to have an unlimited supply of energy. However, he or she does not know when to stop and may continue activities past the point of exhaustion. Parents should provide a variety of activities for the age group, as the attention span is short.

The lung size and volume of the toddler have now increased, and thus the oxygen capacity of the toddler has increased. The toddler is still susceptible to respiratory tract infections but not to the extent of the infant. The rate and rhythm of respiration have decreased, and respirations average 25 to 35 per minute. Accessory muscles of respiration are infrequently used now, and respirations are primarily diaphragmatic.

The respiratory structures (trachea and bronchi) are positioned farther down in the chest now, and the epiglottis is effective in closing off the trachea during swallowing. Thus, aspiration and airway obstruction are reduced in this age group.

The respiratory rate of the preschooler is about 30 per

minute. The preschooler is still susceptible to upper respiratory tract infections. The lymphatic tissues of the tonsils and adenoids are involved in these respiratory tract infections. Tonsillectomies and adenoidectomies are not performed "routinely" any more. These tissues serve to protect the respiratory tract, and valid reasons must exist to warrant their removal.

The temperature of the toddler ranges around 99°F ± 1° (orally); pulse ranges around 105 beats per minute ±35; respirations range from 20 to 35 per minute; and blood pressure ranges from 80 to 100 mm Hg systolic and 60 to 64 mm Hg diastolic. The size of the vascular bed increases in the toddler, thus reducing resistance to flow. The capillary bed has increased ability to respond to environmental temperature changes. Lung volume increases. Breath sounds are more intense and more bronchial, and expiration is more pronounced. The toddler's chest should be examined with the child in an erect position, then recumbent, and then turned to the left side. Arrhythmias and extrasystoles are not uncommon but should be recorded.

The temperature of the preschooler is 98.6°F ± 1° (orally); pulse ranges from 80 to 100 beats per minute; respiration is 30 per minute ±5; and BP is 90/60 mm Hg ±15. There is continued increase of the vascular bed, lung volume, and so on, in keeping with physical growth.

SCHOOL-AGE CHILD

Whereas the muscles were growing faster than the bones during the toddler and preschool years, the skeletal system is growing rapidly during these years—faster than the muscles are growing. Children may experience "growing pains" because of the growth of the long bones. There is a gradual increase in muscle mass and strength, and the body takes on a leaner appearance. The child loses his or her baby fat, muscle tone increases, and loose movements disappear. Adequate exercise is needed to maintain strength, flexibility, and balance and to encourage muscular development.[7] Males have a greater number of muscle cells than females. Posture becomes more upright and straighter but is not necessarily influenced by exercise. Posture is a function of the strength of the back muscles and the general state of health of the child. Poor posture may be reflective of fatigue as well as skeletal defects[7] with fatigue being exhibited by such behaviors as quarrelsomeness, crying, or lack of interest in eating. Skeletal defects such as scoliosis begin to appear during this period.

Neuromuscular coordination is sufficient to permit the schoolchild to learn most skills[6]; however, care should be taken to prevent muscle injuries. Hands and fingers manipulate things well. Although children, age 7, have a high energy level, they also have an increased attention span and cognitive skills. Therefore, they tend to engage in quiet games as well as active ones. Seven-year-olds tend to be more directed in their range of activities. Games with rules develop as the child engages in more social contacts. These games characteristically emerge during the operational phase of cognitive development in the school-age child. These rule games may also be practice or symbolic in nature, but now the child attaches social significance and order to the play by imposing the structure of rules.

Eight-year-olds have grace and balance. Nine-year-olds move with less restlessness; their strength and endurance increase, and their hand-eye coordination is good.[6] Competition among peers is important to test out their strength, agility, and coordination. While 10- to 12-year-old children are better able to control and direct their high energy level, they do have energetic, active, restless movements with tension release through finger drumming, foot tapping, or leg swinging.

The respiratory rate of the school-age child slows to 18 to 22 per minute. The respiratory tissues reach adult maturity, lung volume increases, and the lung capacity is proportionate to body size. The school-age child is still susceptible to respiratory tract infections. The frontal sinuses are fairly well developed by this age, and all the mucous membranes are very vulnerable to congestion and inflammation. The temperature, pulse, and respiration of the school-age child are gradually approaching adult norms, with temperature ranging from 98 to 98.6°F, pulse (resting) 60 to 70 beats per minute, and respiration from 18 to 20 per minute. Systolic BP ranges from 94 to 112 mm Hg, and diastolic from 56 to 60 mm Hg. The heart grows more slowly during this period and is smaller in relation to the rest of the body. Since the heart must continue to supply the metabolic needs, the child should be advised against sustained physical activity and be watched for tiring. After age 7 the apex of the heart lies at the interspace of the fifth rib at the midclavicular line. Circulatory functions reach adult capacity. The child will still have some vasomotor instability with rapid vasodilation. A third heart sound and sinus arrhythmias are fairly common but, again, should be recorded.

ADOLESCENT

Growth in skeletal size, muscle mass, adipose tissue, and skin are significant in adolescence. The skeletal system grows faster than the muscles; thus stress fractures may result. The large muscles grow faster than the smaller muscles with the occasional result of poor posture and decreased coordination. Males are clumsier than females. Muscle growth continues in males during late adolescence because of androgen production.[6]

Physical activities provide a way for adolescents to enjoy the stimulation of conflict in a socially acceptable way. Some form of physical activity should be encouraged to promote physical development, prevent overweight, formulate a realistic body image, and promote peer acceptance.

The respiratory rate of the adolescent is 16 to 20 per minute. Parts of the body grow at various rates, but the respiratory system does not grow proportionately. Therefore, the adolescent may have inadequate oxygenation and become more fatigued. The lung capacity correlates with the adolescent's structural form. Males have a larger lung capacity than females due to greater shoulder width and chest size. Males have greater respiratory volume, greater vital capacity, and a slower respiratory rate. The male's lung capacity matures later than the female's. The female's lungs mature at age 17 or 18.

The heart continues to grow during adolescence but more slowly than the rest of the body, so inadequate oxygenation and fatigue are common. The heart continues to enlarge until age 17 or 18. Systolic pulse pressure increases, and the temperature is the same as in an adult. The pulse ranges from 50 to 68 beats per minute, respiration ranges from 18 to 20 per minute, and BP is 100 to 120/50 to 70 mm Hg. Females have slightly higher pulse rates and basal body temperature and lower systolic pressures than males. Hypertension incidence increases. Essential hypertension incidence is approximately equal between races for this age group.

Athletes have slower pulse rates than peers. Heart sounds are heard readily at the fifth left intercostal space. Functional murmurs should be outgrown by this time. Chest pain may arise from musculoskeletal changes, but cardiovascular pain should always be investigated. Cardiovascular problems are the fifth leading cause of death in adolescents.

More rest and sleep are needed now than earlier. The teenager is expending large amounts of energy and functioning with an inadequate oxygen supply; both of these factors contribute to fatigue and cause the need for additional rest. Parents may need to set limits. Rest does not necessarily mean sleep and can also include quiet activities.[6]

There is a correlation between the maturation of the skeletal system and the reproductive system. Because of the very rapid growth during this period, the adolescent may not have sufficient energy left for strenuous activities. He or she tires easily and may frequently complain of needing to sit down. Gradually the adolescent is able to increase both speed and stamina during exercise. An increase in muscular and skeletal strength, as well as the increased ability of the lungs and heart to provide adequate oxygen to the tissue, facilitate maintenance of hemodynamics and rate of recovery after exercise. The body reaches its peak of physiologic resilience during late adolescence and young adulthood. Both strength and tolerance to strenuous activity can be increased by regular physical training and an individualized conditioning program.

Faulty nutrition is another major cause of fatigue in the adolescent. Poor eating habits established during school-age years, combined with the typical quick-service, quick-energy food consumption patterns of adolescents, frequently lead to anemia, which in itself can lead to activity intolerance.[7]

The adolescent may be given responsibility for assisting with the maintenance of the family home, or may be responsible for his or her own home if living independently from the family of origin. The role exploration characteristic of adolescence may lead to temporary changes in hygiene practices.

Recreational activities in adolescence often take the form of organized sports and other competitive activities. Social relationships are developed and enhanced, specific motor and cognitive skills related to a specific sport are refined, and a sense of mastery can be developed. Group activities and peer approval and acceptance are important. The adolescent responds to peer activities and experiments with different roles and lifestyles. The nurse must distinguish self-care practices that are acceptable to the peer group from those that indicate a self-care deficit.

YOUNG ADULT

Growth of the skeletal system is essentially complete by age 25. Muscular efficiency is at its peak between 20 and 30. Energy level and control of energy are high. Thereafter, muscular strength declines with the rate of muscle aging depending on the specific muscle group, the activity of the person, and the adequacy of his or her diet.

Regular exercise is helpful in controlling weight and maintaining a state of high-level wellness. Muscle tone, strength, and circulation are enhanced by exercise. Problems arise especially when sedentary lifestyles decrease the amount of exercise available with daily activities. Caloric intake and exercise should be balanced.

Adequate sleep is important for good physical and mental health. Lack of sleep results in progressive sluggishness of both physical and cognitive functions. This age group gets the majority of its activity from work and leisure activities. The young adult should learn to balance his or her work with leisure-time activities. Getting started in a career can be very stressful and can lead to burnout if an appropriate balance is not found. Physical fitness reflects ability to work for a sustained period with vigor and pleasure, without undue fatigue, with energy left over for enjoying hobbies and recreational activities and for meeting emergencies.[6]

Basic to fitness are regular physical exercise, proper nutrition, adequate rest and relaxation, conscientious health practices, and good medical and dental care. Regular physical fitness is a natural tranquilizer releasing the body's own endorphins, which reduce anxiety and muscular tension.

The respiratory system of the young adult has completely matured. Oxygen demand is based on exercise and activity now but gradually decreases between age 20 and 40. The body's ability to use oxygen efficiently is dependent on the cardiovascular system and the needs of the skeletal muscles.

The respiratory system and cardiovascular systems change gradually with age, but the rate of change is highly dependent on the individual's diet and exercise pattern. Generally, contraction of the myocardium decreases. The maximum cardiac output is reached between the ages of 20 and 30. The arteries become less elastic. The maximum breathing capacity decreases between ages 20 and 40. Cardiac and respiratory function can be improved with regular exercise. Hypertension (BP 140/90 mm Hg or higher) and mitral valve prolapse syndrome are the most common cardiovascular medical diagnoses of the young adult.

ADULT

The basal metabolism rate gradually decreases. Although there is a general and gradual decline in quickness and level of activity, people who were most active among their age group during adolescence and young adulthood tend to be the most active during middle and old age. In women, there is frequently a menopausal rise in energy and activity.[8] Judicious exercise balanced with rest and sleep modify and retard the aging process. Exercise stimulates circulation to all parts of the body, thereby improving body functions. Exercise can also be an outlet for emotional tension. If the person is beginning exercises after being sedentary, certain precautions should be taken, such as gradually increasing exercise to a moderate level, exercising consistently, and avoiding overexertion. Recent research indicates that cardiovascular risk factors can be reduced in women by low-intensity walking.[9]

The adult is beginning to have a decrease in bone mass and a loss of skeletal height. Muscle strength and mass are directly related to active muscle use. The adult needs to maintain the patterns of activity and exercise of young adulthood and not become sedentary. Otherwise, muscles lose mass structure and strength more rapidly.

Temperature for the adult ranges from 97 to 99.6°F, pulse ranges from 50 to 100 beats per minute, respiration ranges from 16 to 20 per minute; and BP 120/80 mm Hg ± 15. Cardiac output gradually decreases, and the decreasing elasticity of the blood vessels causes more susceptibility to hypertension and cardiovascular diseases. Females become as prone to coronary disease after menopause as males, so estrogen appears to be a protective agent. The BMR generally decreases. Essential and secondary hypertension and angina occur more frequently in this age group.

The lung tissue becomes thicker and less elastic with age. The lungs cannot expand as they once did, and breathing capacity is reduced. The respiratory rate may increase to compensate for the reduced breathing capacity.

The normal adult should be able to perform activities of daily living without assistance. The needs for close relationships and intimacy of adulthood can be initiated by leisure activities with identified partners or a small group of close friends (e.g., hiking, tennis, golf, or attending concerts or theaters). The middle-aged adult is often interested in the personal satisfaction of diversional activities.

The adult will most likely be responsible for home maintenance as well as outside employment. Role strain or overtaxation of the adult is possible. Illness or injury to the adults in the household will significantly affect the ability of the family unit to maintain the home.

OLDER ADULT

The older adult faces gradual decline in function through the years. A decrease in skeletal mass affects all the bones of the skeleton. Decrease in skeletal mass leads to decreased strength. The tissues of the joints and bones stiffen due to increased collagen; thus, movement and range of motion markedly decrease. The oxygen supply to the muscles may also be decreased as a result of the reduced cardiac output. Mobility is lessened, and the older adult moves more slowly. The older adult should be encouraged to maintain optimum range of motion through planned exercise and activity.

There is a decline in exercise tolerance and work capacity as one ages. Cardiovascular changes, decreased pulmonary function, disuse of muscle groups, poor nutrition, and debilitating diseases may all contribute to less-than-optimum functioning and decreased mobility. With a decreased oxygen supply, the muscles may function, but cardiac output may be so poor that normal activity is impossible. Decreased sensory and motor abilities and muscle weakness may occur more frequently in the older adult. Lung tissue continues to lose elasticity and becomes thicker. Alveolar sacs collapse, and thus there are fewer functional units exposed to gas exchange. Additionally, the muscles of respiration have become rigid so lung expansion is not as great. The blood flow through the lungs is decreased because of reduced cardiac output. All these changes result in a reduced breathing capacity, a decreased amount of oxygen in the blood (decreased P_{O_2}), an increase in air trapped in the lungs (increased P_{CO_2}), and changes in respiratory rate, rhythm, and depth. The work of breathing is increased by a decrease in adequate functioning. The ability and effectiveness of the cough are also decreased due to diminished muscle tone and decreased sensitivity to stimuli.[6]

Physiologic cell and tissue changes (increased connective and collagen tissues, disappearance of some cellular elements, reduction in the number of normally functioning cells, increased amount of fat, decreased oxygen utilization, decreased cardiac output, or decreased muscle strength) require the heart to work harder to provide adequate oxygenation. Exercise or stress raises heart rate and BP more in the older adult than in younger adults, and it takes longer for these rates to return to normal. Heart valves become more rigid and thick. This may give rise to the development of murmurs. Inelasticity of vessels, loss of cell integrity, and decrease in cardiac output and stroke volume combine to produce hypoxia. Blood flow through the coronary arteries decreases. Maximum breathing capacity, vital capacity, and inspiratory reserve volume decrease. The area of alveolar contact decreases as does the diffusing capacity; hence, there is a decrease in the oxygen content of the blood. Congestive heart failure, chronic occlusive arterial disease, and stasis ulcers rise in incidence with this age group. The BP usually measures 140/80 to 150/90 mm Hg, but the rest of the vital signs remain in the same range as for the middle-aged adult. Downward dislocation of the cardiac apex and increased kyphosis may alter isolation of the apical pulse and usual chest landmarks.

Cardiovascular diseases are the highest cause of death in the older adult group, with the most common medical diagnosis being atherosclerosis.

Since there is decreased physical reserve and muscle strength, the older adult should view exercise and activity as a means of promoting and maintaining health and well-being. Activity and exercise can help keep an individual in shape and maintain an optimal functioning level. The older adult should pace exercise and activity and recognize that it will take longer to do things than it once did.[6]

Time available for leisure activities may dramatically increase for the individual at retirement or for the couple who has accomplished child-rearing or career-establishing tasks. Diversional activities provide physical activity as well as reestablish social contacts and form new friendships.

The older adult is more likely to experience the impairments discussed in the physiologic section, thereby altering his or her ability to maintain his or her own homes. Impaired elderly may live with their adult children, thereby placing additional responsibilities on the adult children for adequate home maintenance.

While changes do occur, the older population is a diverse group, and so individual assessment is of highest priority. The above-cited changes associated with aging may not apply to all older adults. There are many very independent older persons in our society, and the number is increasing.

APPLICABLE NURSING DIAGNOSES

Activity Intolerance, Risk for or Actual

DEFINITION

RISK FOR A state in which an individual is at risk of experiencing insufficient physiological or psychological energy to endure or complete required or desired daily activities.[10]

ACTUAL A state in which an individual has insufficient physiological or psychological energy to endure or complete required or desired daily activities.[10]

NANDA TAXONOMY: MOVING 6.1.1.2 AND 6.1.1.3

DEFINING CHARACTERISTICS[10]

1. Risk for Activity Intolerance
   a. Major defining characteristics (risk factors)
      (1) History of previous intolerance
      (2) Deconditioned status
      (3) Presence of circulatory or respiratory problems
      (4) Inexperience with the activity
   b. Minor defining characteristics
      None given
2. Activity Intolerance
   a. Major defining characteristics
      (1) Verbal report of fatigue or weakness (**critical**)
      (2) Abnormal heart rate or blood pressure response to activity
      (3) Exertional discomfort or dyspnea
      (4) Electrocardiographic changes reflecting arrhythmias or ischemia
   b. Minor defining characteristics
      None given

RELATED FACTORS[10]

1. Risk for Activity Intolerance
   The risk factors also serve as the related factors for this diagnosis.
2. Activity Intolerance
   a. Bedrest or immobility
   b. Generalized weakness
   c. Sedentary lifestyle
   d. Imbalance between oxygen supply and demand

RELATED CLINICAL CONCERNS

1. Anemias
2. Congestive heart failure
3. Valvular heart disease
4. Cardiac arrhythmia
5. Chronic obstructive pulmonary disease (COPD)
6. Metabolic disorder
7. Musculoskeletal disorders

HAVE YOU SELECTED THE CORRECT DIAGNOSIS?

Impaired Physical Mobility This diagnosis implies that an individual would be able to move independently if something were not limiting the motion. Activity Intolerance implies that the individual is freely able to move but cannot endure or adapt to the increased energy or oxygen demands made by the movement or activity.

Self-Care Deficit Self-Care Deficit indicates that the patient has some dependence on another person. Activity Intolerance implies that the patient is independent but is unable to perform activities because the body is unable to adapt to the increased energy and oxygen demands made. A person may have a self-care deficit due to activity intolerance.

Ineffective Individual Coping Persons with the diagnosis of Ineffective Individual Coping may be unable to participate in their usual roles or in their usual self-care because they feel they lack control or the motivation to do so. Activity Intolerance, on the other hand, implies that the person is willing and able to participate in activities but is unable to endure or adapt to the increased energy or oxygen demands made by the movement or activity.

EXPECTED OUTCOMES

1. Will verbalize less fatigue and weakness by (date) and/or
2. Will participate in increased self-care activities by (date). Specify which self-care activities, that is, bathing, feeding, dressing, or ambulation, and the frequency, duration, or intensity of the activity.

EXAMPLE
Will increase walking by at least 1 block each week for 8 weeks.

TARGET DATES

Appropriate target dates will have to be very individualized according to the degree of activity intolerance. An appropriate range would be 3 to 5 days.

NURSING ACTIONS/INTERVENTIONS WITH RATIONALES

Adult Health

ACTIONS/INTERVENTIONS	RATIONALES
• Monitor current potential for desired activities including: ○ Physical limitations related to illness or surgery ○ Factors that relate to desired activities ○ Realistic expectations for actualizing potential for desired activities ○ Objective criteria by which specific progress may be measured, e.g., distance, time, and observable signs or symptoms such as apical pulse, respiration ○ Previous level of activities patient enjoyed	Provides baseline for planning activities and increase in activities.
• Assist patient with self-care activities as needed. Let patient determine how much assistance is needed.	Allows patient to have some control and choice in plan; helps patient to gradually decrease the amount of activity intolerance.
• Monitor and record blood pressure, pulse, and respiration before and after activities.	Vital signs increase with activity and should return to baseline within 5–7 min postactivity. Maximal effort should be greater than or equal to 60–80% over the baseline.
• Encourage progressive activity and increased self-care as tolerated. Schedule moderate increase in activities on a daily basis, e.g., will walk 10 ft farther each day.	Gradually increases tolerance for activities.
• Collaborate with physician regarding oxygen therapy.	Promotes teamwork. Oxygen may be needed for shortness of breath associated with increased activity.
• Collaborate with a physical therapist in establishing an appropriate exercise plan.	Provides most appropriate activities for patient.
• Collaborate with an occupational therapist for appropriate diversional activity schedule.	
• Teach client appropriate exercise methods to prevent injury, e.g., no straight-leg sit-ups; proper muscle stretching and warm-up before aerobic exercise; reaching target heart rate; stopping exercise if experiencing pain, excessive fatigue, nausea, or breathlessness.	Basic safety measures to avoid complicating condition.
• Encourage rest as needed between activities. Assist patient in planning a balanced rest-activity program.	Planned rest assists in maintaining and increasing activity tolerance.
• Provide for a quiet, nonstimulating environment. Limit number of visitors and length of their stay. Teach relaxation and alternate pain relief measures. Assess internal and external motivators for activities, and record here.	Determine various methods to motivate behavior.
• Encourage adequate dietary input by ascertaining patient's food preferences and consulting with dietitian.	Provides adequate nutrition to meet metabolic demands.
• Assist the patient in weight reduction as required.	Decreased weight requires less energy and oxygen use.
• Teach patient relationship between nutrition and exercise tolerance, and assist in developing a diet that is appropriate for nutritional and metabolic needs (see Chap. 3 for further information). Assist patient in acquiring equipment to perform desired exercise (list needed equipment here; this could include proper shoes, eyeglasses, or weights).	Assists patient to learn alternate methods to conserve energy in activities of daily living.
• Instruct patient in energy-saving techniques of daily care, e.g., preparing meals sitting on a high stool rather than standing.	
• Provide opportunities of 15–30 min per shift for allowing patient and family to verbalize concerns regarding activity.	

- Introduce necessary teaching according to the readiness of patient and family with appropriate modifications to best meet patient's needs.
- Provide patient and family opportunities to contribute to plans for activity as appropriate. Allow for individual preference and suggestions on an ongoing basis.
- Provide opportunities for success in meeting expected goals by using subgoals or increments that lead to desired activity.

Assists in reducing anxiety, promotes long-range planning, and provides a teaching opportunity. Ensures that teaching meets patient's level of understanding and need. The more the patient and family participate in planning, the more likely they are to implement the desired regimen.

Achieving success motivates the patient to continue the activity.

Child Health

ACTIONS/INTERVENTIONS	RATIONALES
• Provide learning modules and practice sessions with materials suitable for child's age and developmental capacity, e.g., dolls, videos, or pictures.	Developmentally appropriate materials will enhance learning and will maintain child's attention.
• Provide for continuity in care by assigning same nurses for care during critical times for teaching and implementation.	Continuity of caregivers fosters trust in the nurse-patient relationship, which enhances learning.
• Modify expected behavior to incorporate appropriate developmental needs, e.g., allow for shared cards, messages, or visitors to lobby if possible for adolescent patients.	Valuing of patient's developmental needs fosters self-esteem and serves as a reward for efforts.
• Reinforce adherence to regimen with stickers or other appropriate measures to document progress.	Extrinsic rewards may help to symbolize concrete progress and reinforce appropriate behaviors for achieving goals.

Women's Health

ACTIONS/INTERVENTIONS	RATIONALES
PREMATURE RUPTURE OF MEMBRANES[11,12] **NOTE:** Approach to treatment is controversial and depends upon practice in your particular area.	
• Carefully monitor fetal heart rate to detect cord compression and/or cord prolapse.	
• Carefully monitor for signs and symptoms of amnionitis.	
◦ Check maternal temperature every 4 h.	
◦ Evaluate for uterine tenderness at least twice a day.	
◦ Check daily leukocyte counts.	
◦ Avoid vaginal exams.	
• Keep patient and partner informed, and encourage their participation in management decisions.	
• Explain and provide answers to questions regarding:	Assists in reducing fears of expectant parents and increasing the likelihood of a good outcome for the pregnancy.
◦ Possible preterm delivery	
◦ Fetal lung maturity and possible use of corticosteriods to accelerate fetal lung maturity	
• Provide comfort measures to decrease intolerance of bedrest:	
◦ Back or body massage	
◦ Diversional activities, such as TV, reading, or handicrafts	
◦ Bedside commode (if acceptable to treatment plan)	

Continued

ACTIONS/INTERVENTIONS	RATIONALES

PRETERM LABOR[13-15]

NOTE: Although there is disagreement on the definition, the most widely used definition of preterm labor is 6 to 8 contractions per hour or 4 contractions in 20 min *associated with* cervical change.[13]

- Thoroughly explain to patient and partner the process of preterm labor.
- Discuss options of activity allowed. (**NOTE:** This varies, and there is controversy in the literature on the value of bedrest for preterm labor; therefore, look at practice in your area.)
- Discuss various treatment possibilities:
  - Prolonged bedrest or at least a marked reduction in activity
  - Intravenous volume expansion (IV therapy)
  - Tocolytic therapy (IV, oral, or pump)
  - Use of magnesium sulfate
  - Use of prostaglandin synthesis inhibitors such as indomethacin
  - Use of calcium channel blockers
- Carefully monitor those patients on tocolytic therapy for:
  - Pulmonary edema
  - Hypokalemia
  - Hyperglycemia
  - Shortness of breath
  - Chest pain
  - Cardiac dysrhythmia
  - ECG "ischemia" changes
  - Hypotension
- Carefully monitor uterine contractions (strength, quality, frequency, and duration).
- Monitor fetal heart rate in association with contractions.
- Provide diversional activities for those patients on bedrest.
- Refer patient for home monitoring and evaluation if appropriate:
  - Assess patient's ability to identify contractions.
  - Evaluate patient's support system at home.
  - Assess patient's access to health care provider.

Provides parents with information, increases motivation to continue with reduced activity, and allows informed choices.

Increases compliance, decreases cost, and decreases maternal stress when she can achieve treatment at home instead of in an acute care setting.

PREGNANCY-INDUCED HYPERTENSION (PIH)[16,17]

- Explain the various screening procedures for PIH to patient and partner:
  - Blood pressure measurement
  - Urine checked for protein
  - Assessment of total and interval weight gain
  - Signs and symptoms of sudden edema of hands and face, sudden 5-lb weight gain in 24–48 h, epigastric pain, or spots before eyes or blurred vision
- Discuss treatment plan with patient and partner:
  - Bedrest on either side (right or left)
  - Magnesium sulfate therapy
  - Reduction in noise, visual stimuli, and stress
  - Careful monitoring of fetal heart rate
  - Possible sonogram to determine IUGR
  - Good nutrition with a maximum RDA sodium intake of 110 to 3300 mg/day

- Assess patient's support system to determine if patient can be treated at home.[18,19]
- Assist family plan for needed caretaking and housekeeping activities if patient is at home.[18,19]
- Consult with perinatologist and visiting nurse to implement collaborative care plan.
- Ensure that family knows procedure for obtaining emergency service.

UNCOMPLICATED PREGNANCY

NOTE: Even though there are often no complications in pregnancy, it is not unusual, particularly during the last 4 to 6 weeks, to have activities restricted because of edema, bouts with false labor, and fatigue. This fatigue continues after the birth, when the mother and father become responsible for the care of a newborn infant 24 h a day.

- Discuss with the expectant parents methods of conserving energy while continuing their daily activities during the last weeks of pregnancy.
- Assist expectant mother in developing a plan whereby she can take frequent (2 in the morning, 2 in the afternoon), short breaks during the workday to:
  - Retain energy and reduce fatigue
  - Reduce the incidence of false labor
  - Increase circulation and thus reduce dependent lower limb edema and increase oxygen to the placenta and fetus

Provides opportunity to rest throughout the day and therefore the ability to maintain as many routine activities as possible. Increases oxygen flow to the uterus and the fetus, thereby reducing the possibility of preterm labor and severe fatigue.

- Assist expectant parents to plan for the possibility of reducing the number of hours the woman works during the week. Look at work schedule and talk with employer about:
  - Working every other day
  - Working only half-day each day
  - Working 3 days in the middle of the week, i.e., Tuesday, Wednesday, and Thursday, or having a 4-day weekend to rest
  - Job sharing

AFTER DELIVERY

- Instruct patient in energy-saving activities of daily care:
  - Take care of self and baby only
  - Let partner and others take care of housework and other children.
  - Let partner and others take care of baby for a prearranged time during the day so mother can spend quality time with other children.
  - Learn to sleep when baby sleeps.
  - Turn off phone or turn on answering machine.
  - Have specific times set for visiting of friends or relatives.
  - If breast-feeding, partner can change infant and bring infant to mother at night. (Mother does not always have to get up and go to infant.)
- Consider taking baby to bed with parent.

A common problem with a new baby is overwhelming fatigue for the mother. These measures will assist in decreasing the fatigue.

Newest research shows that taking the baby to bed with mother and father at night for the first few weeks:
  - Allows the mother, father, and infant to get more rest
  - Allows baby to nurse longer and sleep for longer periods faster
  - Possibly reduces the incidence of SIDS as the baby mimics the breathing patterns of the mother and father
Promotes positive learning and acquaintance activities for the new parents. Allows infant to feel more secure and therefore increases infant-to-parent attachment.

Continued

Psychiatric Health

ACTIONS/INTERVENTIONS	RATIONALES
• Discuss with client his or her perceptions of activity appropriate to his or her current capabilities.	Provides an understanding of the client's worldview so that care can be individualized and interventions developed that are acceptable to both the nurse and the client.[20]
• If the client estimates a routine that far exceeds current capabilities (as with eating disorder clients or clients experiencing elated mood):	
◦ Establish appropriate limits on exercise. (The limits and consequences for not maintaining limits established should be listed here. If the excessive exercise pattern is related to an elated mood, set limits in a manner that allows client some activity while not greatly exceeding metabolic needs until psychologic status is improved.)	Negative reinforcement eliminates or decreases behavior.[21] Because of their high energy level, elated clients need some large motor activity that will discharge energy but not present a risk for physical harm.[22]
◦ Begin client slowly, i.e., with stretching exercise for 15 min twice a day.	Goals need to be achievable to promote the sense of accomplishment and positive self feelings, which will in turn increase motivation.[20]
◦ As physical condition improves, gradually increase exercise to 30 min of aerobic exercise once per day.	A regimen that provides positive cardiovascular fitness without risk of overexertion.[22]
◦ Discuss with client appropriate levels of exercise considering his or her age and metabolic pattern.	Overexertion can decrease benefits of exercise by increasing risk for injury.[23]
◦ Discuss with client the hazards of overexercise.	
◦ Establish a reward system for clients who maintain the established exercise schedule (the schedule for the client should be listed here with those reinforcers that are to be used).	Positive reinforcement encourages appropriate behavior.[21]
◦ Stay with client while he or she is engaged in appropriate exercise.	Interaction with the nurse can provide positive reinforcement.[21]
◦ Develop a schedule for the client to be involved in an occupational therapy program to assist client in identifying alternative forms of activity other than aerobic exercise.	Promotes accurate perception of body size, nutrition, and exercise needs.
◦ Limit number of walks off the unit to accommodate client's weight, level of exercise on the unit, and physiology (the frequency and length of the walk should be listed here).	
• For further information related to eating disorder clients, see Altered Nutrition, Less Than Body Requirements.	
• If client's expectations are much less than current capabilities (as with depressed or poorly motivated client), implement the following actions:	Goals need to be achievable to promote sense of accomplishment and positive self feelings, which will in turn increase motivation.[20]
◦ Establish very limited goals that client can accomplish, e.g., a 5-min walk in a hallway once a day or walking in the client's room for 5 min. The goal established should be listed here.	
◦ Establish a reward system for achievement of goals (the reward program should be listed here with a list of items the client finds rewarding).	Positive reinforcement encourages appropriate behavior.[21]
◦ Develop a schedule for the client to be involved in an occupational therapy program (note schedule here).	Provides client with opportunity to improve self-help skills while engaged in a variety of activities.
◦ Establish limits on the amount of time the client can spend in bed or in his or her room during waking hours (establish limits the client can achieve, and note limits here).	Exercise raises levels of endorphins in the brain, which has a positive effect on depression and general feeling of well-being.[22,24]
◦ Stay with client during exercise periods and time out of the room until the client is performing these tasks without prompting.	Interaction with the nurse can provide positive reinforcement.[21]

- Provide the client with firm support for initiating the activity.

- Place a record of goal achievement where client can see and mark each step toward the goal with a reward marker.
- Provide positive verbal reinforcement for goal achievement and progress.
- For further information about clients with depressed mood, refer to Ineffective Individual Coping (Chap. 11).
- Monitor effect current medications may have on activity tolerance, and teach client necessary adjustments.

- Schedule time to discuss plans and special concerns with client and client's support system. This could include teaching and answering questions. Schedule daily during initial days of hospitalization and one longer time just before discharge. Note schedule times and person responsible for this.

Attention from the nurse can provide positive reinforcement and increase client's motivation to accomplish goal.
Provides concrete evidence of goal attainment and motivation to continue these activities that will promote well-being.

Psychotropic medications may cause postural hypotension, and the client should be instructed to change position slowly.
Recognizes the reciprocity between the client's illness and the family context.[25]

Gerontic Health

NOTE: Research on activity intolerance in older adults is very minimal. The few studies that do address activity and exercise are usually done on "healthy elders."[26]

ACTIONS/INTERVENTIONS	RATIONALES
- Determine, with the assistance of the patient, particular time periods of highest energy and plan care accordingly.	Maximizes potential to successfully participate in or complete care requirements.
- Teach patient to monitor pulse before, during, and after activity.	Promotes self-monitoring and provides means of determining progress across care settings.
- Refer patient to occupational therapy and physical therapy for determination of a progressive activity program.	Collaboration ensures a plan that will result in activity for maximum effect.
- Provide positive feedback for incremental successes. Focus on measurable increases in activity levels.	Provides motivation to continue program.

Home Health

ACTIONS/INTERVENTIONS	RATIONALES

- Teach client and family appropriate monitoring of causes, signs, and symptoms of high risk for or actual activity intolerance:
  - Prolonged bedrest
  - Circulatory or respiratory problems
  - New activity
  - Fatigue
  - Dyspnea
  - Paint
  - Vital signs (before and after activity)
  - Malnutrition
  - Previous inactivity
  - Weakness
  - Confusion
	Provides baseline for prevention and/or early intervention.

Continued

ACTIONS/INTERVENTIONS	RATIONALES

• Assist client and family in identifying lifestyle changes that may be required:
  ○ Progressive exercise to increase endurance
  ○ ROM and flexibility exercises
  ○ Treatments for underlying conditions (cardiac, respiratory, musculoskeletal, circulatory, etc.)
  ○ Motivation
  ○ Assistive devices as required (walkers, canes, crutches, wheelchairs, exercise equipment, etc.)
  ○ Adequate nutrition
  ○ Adequate fluids
  ○ Stress management
  ○ Pain relief
  ○ Prevention of hazards of immobility
  ○ Changes in occupations, family, or social roles
  ○ Changes in living conditions
  ○ Economic concerns
	Lifestyle changes require sufficient support to achieve.

• Teach client and family purposes and side effects of medications and proper administration techniques.	Changes locus of control to client and family and supports self-care.
• Assist client and family to set criteria to help them to determine when physician or other intervention is required.	Provides additional support for client.
• Consult with or refer to appropriate assistive resources as indicated.	

Activity Intolerance, Risk for or Actual

FLOWCHART EVALUATION: EXPECTED OUTCOME 1

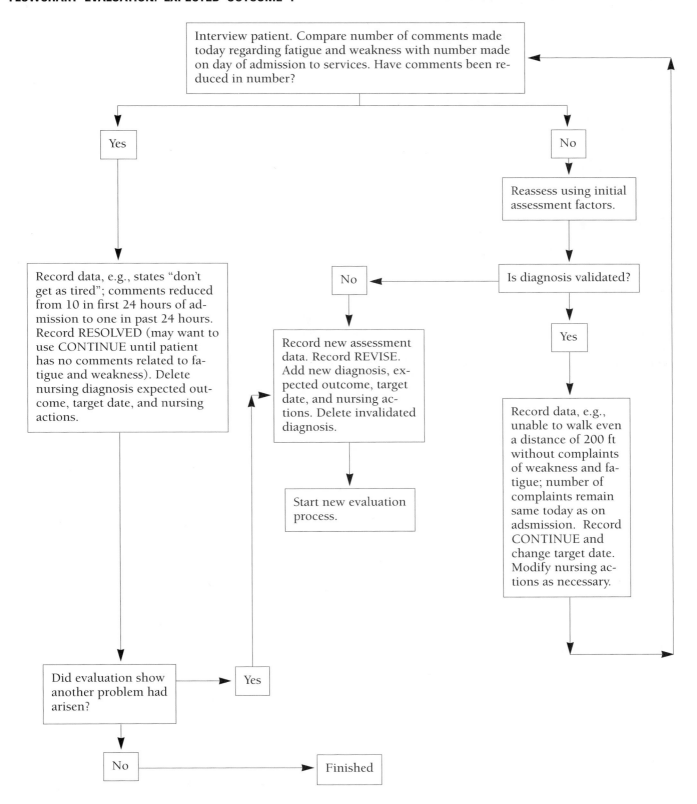

Activity Intolerance, Risk for or Actual

FLOWCHART EVALUATION: EXPECTED OUTCOME 2

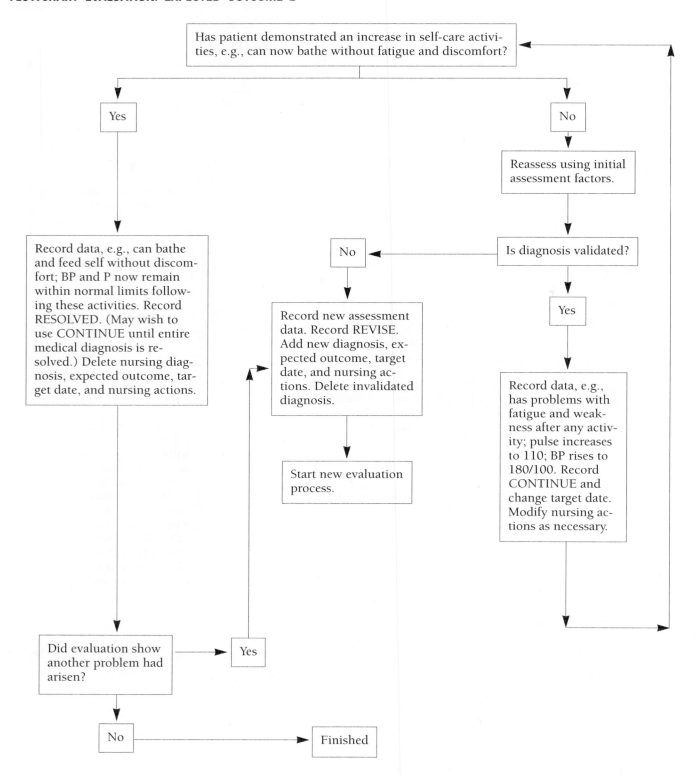

Has patient demonstrated an increase in self-care activities, e.g., can now bathe without fatigue and discomfort?

Yes

No

Reassess using initial assessment factors.

Record data, e.g., can bathe and feed self without discomfort; BP and P now remain within normal limits following these activities. Record RESOLVED. (May wish to use CONTINUE until entire medical diagnosis is resolved.) Delete nursing diagnosis, expected outcome, target date, and nursing actions.

No

Is diagnosis validated?

Record new assessment data. Record REVISE. Add new diagnosis, expected outcome, target date, and nursing actions. Delete invalidated diagnosis.

Yes

Record data, e.g., has problems with fatigue and weakness after any activity; pulse increases to 110; BP rises to 180/100. Record CONTINUE and change target date. Modify nursing actions as necessary.

Start new evaluation process.

Did evaluation show another problem had arisen?

Yes

No

Finished

Airway Clearance, Ineffective

DEFINITION

A state in which an individual is unable to clear secretions or obstructions from the respiratory tract.[10]

NANDA TAXONOMY: EXCHANGING 1.5.1.2

DEFINING CHARACTERISTICS[10]

1. Major defining characteristics
   a. Abnormal breath sounds: crackles, gurgles, wheezes
   b. Cough, ineffective or absent
   c. Communicates verbally, difficulty with sputum
   d. Communicates chest congestion
2. Minor defining characteristics
   None given

RELATED FACTORS[10]

1. Decreased energy; fatigue
2. Tracheobronchial infection, obstruction, secretion, sputum, tenacious and copious
3. Perceptual or cognitive impairment
4. Trauma

RELATED CLINICAL CONCERNS

1. Adult respiratory distress syndrome (ARDS)
2. Pneumonia
3. Cancer of the lung
4. Chronic obstructive pulmonary disease (COPD)
5. Congestive heart failure
6. Cystic fibrosis
7. Inhalation injuries
8. Neuromuscular diseases

HAVE YOU SELECTED THE CORRECT DIAGNOSIS?

Ineffective Breathing Pattern   This diagnosis implies an alteration in the rate, rhythm, depth, or type of respiration such as hyperventilation or hypoventilation. These patterns are not effective in supplying oxygen to the cells of body or in removing the products of respiration. However, air is able to move freely through the air passages. In Ineffective Airway Clearance, the air passages are obstructed in some way.

Impaired Gas Exchange   This diagnosis means that air has been inhaled through the air passages but that oxygen and carbon dioxide are not appropriately exchanged in the alveolar-capillary level. Air has been able to pass through clear air passages, but a problem arises at the cellular level.

Fluid-Volume Deficit   When fluid volume is insufficient to assist in liquefying thick, tenacious respiratory tract secretions, Fluid-Volume Deficit then becomes the primary diagnosis. In this instance, the patient would be unable to effectively expectorate the secretions no matter how hard he or she tried, and Ineffective Airway Clearance would result.

Pain   If pain is sufficient to prevent the patient from coughing to clear the airway, then Ineffective Airway Clearance will result secondary to the pain.

EXPECTED OUTCOMES

1. Will have an open, clear airway by (date) and/or
2. Will easily expectorate secretions from airway by (date)

TARGET DATES

Ineffective airway clearance is life-threatening; therefore, progress toward meeting the expected outcome should be evaluated at least on a daily basis.

ADDITIONAL INFORMATION

The various ways of measuring lung volume and capacity are summarized and defined in Table 5–1.

Table 5–1 LUNG CAPACITIES AND VOLUMES

Measurement	Average Value, Adult Make, mL (resting)	Definition
Tidal volume (TV)	500	Amount of air inhaled or exhaled with each breath
Inspiratory reserve volume (IRV)	3100	Amount of air that can be forcefully inhaled after a normal tidal volume inhalation
Expiratory reserve volume (ERV)	1200	Amount of air that can be forcefully exhaled after a normal tidal volume exhalation
Residual volume (RV)	1200	Amount of air left in the lungs after a forced exhalation
Total lung capacity (TLC)	6000	Maximum amount of air that can be contained in the lungs after a maximum inspiration: $$TLC = TV + IRV + ERV + RV$$
Vital capacity (VC)	4800	Maximum amount of air that can be expired after a maximum inspiration: $$VC = TV + IRV + ERV$$ Should be 80% of TLC
Inspiratory capacity (IC)	3600	Maximum amount of air that can be inspired after a normal expiration: $$IC = TV + IRV$$
Functional residual capacity (FRC)	2400	Volume of air remaining in the lungs after a normal tidal volume expiration: $$FRC = ERV + RV$$

NURSING ACTIONS/INTERVENTIONS WITH RATIONALES

Adult Health

ACTIONS/INTERVENTIONS	RATIONALES
• Maintain appropriate emergency equipment as dictated by situation (e.g., tracheostomy sterile setup, or suctioning apparatus).	Basic safety precautions.
• Monitor respiratory rate, depth, and breath sounds at least every 4 h.	Basic indicators of airway patency.
• Collaborate with physician regarding frequency of blood gas measurements.	Assists in determining changes in ventilatory status, promotes teamwork.
• Give mucolytic agents via nebulizer or intermittent positive-pressure breathing (IPPB) treatments or continuous positive airway pressure (CPAP) as ordered.	Helps thin and loosen secretion; expands airways.
• Monitor effects and side effects of medications used to open patient's airways (bronchodilators, corticosteroids), e.g., for an aminophylline IV drip, ensure appropriate dilution, note incompatibility factor, monitor for nausea, increased heart rate, irritability, etc. Document effect within 30 min after administration.	Assists in determining if airflow or lung volume is improved via medication.
• Maintain adequate fluid intake to liquefy secretions. Encourage intake up to 3000 mL per day (unless contraindicated). Measure output each 8 h.	Assists in liquefaction of secretions and provides moisture to the pulmonary mucosa.

• Have patient's favorite fluids available:
   ○ Remind patient to drink fluids at least every hour while awake.
   ○ Provide warm or hot drinks instead of cold fluids.	

• Assist patient in coughing, huffing, and breathing efforts to make them more productive:
   ○ Sit in upright position.
   ○ Take a deep, slow breath while expanding abdomen, allowing diaphragm to expand.
   ○ Hold breath for 3–5 s.
   ○ Exhale the breath slowly through the mouth while abdomen moves inward.
   ○ Pause briefly before next breath in.
	Deep breathing and diaphragmatic breathing allow for greater lung expansion and ventilation as well as a more effective cough.

○ Cough with the second breath inward; cough forcefully from chest (these should be two short, forceful coughs).

○ Place hands on upper abdomen and exert inward, upward pressure during cough (splint incision or painful areas during procedure).

○ Maintain adequate humidity in environment (80%).

• Observe patient practicing proper breathing techniques 30 min twice a day (note time of practice sessions here).

• Assist with cupping and clapping activities every 4 h while awake at (times). Teach family these procedures.

Cupping and clapping loosen secretions and assist expectoration. Teaching family allows them to participate in care under supervision and promotes continuation of the procedure after discharge.

Removes tenacious secretions from airways.

• Assist patient with clearing secretions from mouth or nose by:

○ Providing tissues

○ Using gentle suctioning if necessary

• Assist patient with oral hygiene at least every 4 h while awake at (times):

○ Lubricate lips with a moisturizing agent.

○ Do not allow the use of oil-based products around the nose.

Oral hygiene clears away dried secretions and freshens the mouth. Oil-based products may obstruct breathing passages.

• Discuss with patient importance of maintaining proper position to include:

○ Side-lying position while in bed

○ Sitting or standing position with shoulders back and back as straight as possible to facilitate expansion of the diaphragm

Facilitates expansion of the diaphragm; decreases probability of aspiration.

• Remind patient of proper positioning as required.

• Promote rest and relaxation by scheduling treatments, and activities with appropriate rest periods.

Avoids overexertion and worsening of condition.

• Instruct patient to avoid irritating substances, large crowds, and persons with upper respiratory infections.

Prevents infection or airway spasms.

• Discuss with patient factors contributing in ineffective airway clearance, e.g., cigarettes or alcohol. Refer patient, prior to discharge, to a stop smoking program at a community agency such as:

○ American Cancer Society

○ American Heart Association

○ American Lung Association

Smoking increases production of mucus and paralyzes or causes loss of cilia.

• Refer patient for appropriate consultations as needed, e.g., respiratory therapy or physical therapy.

• Provide for appropriate follow-up by scheduling appointments before dismissal.

Promotes cost-effective use of resources and follow-up care.

Child Health

ACTIONS/INTERVENTIONS	RATIONALES
• Monitor patient factors that relate to ineffective airway clearance, including: ○ Feeding tolerance or intolerance ○ Allergens ○ Emotional aspects ○ Stressors of recent or past activities ○ Congenital anomalies ○ Parental anxieties ○ Infant or child temperament ○ Abdominal distention ○ Related vital signs, especially heart rate	Provides an individualized data baseline that facilitates individualized care planning.

Continued

ACTIONS/INTERVENTIONS	RATIONALES
○ Diaphragmatic excursion ○ Retraction in respiratory effort ○ Choking, coughing ○ Flaring of nares ○ Appropriate functioning of respiratory equipment • Provide appropriate attention to suctioning and related respiratory maintenance: ○ Appropriate size for catheter as needed ○ Appropriate administration of humidified oxygen as ordered by physician if applicable ○ Appropriate follow-up of blood gases ○ Documentation of oxygen administration, characteristics of secretion obtained by suctioning, vital signs during suctioning, reporting apical pulse below 70 or above 149 beats per minute for infant, below 90 or above 120 beats per minute for young child. • Encourage patient's input in planning care for patient with attention to individual preferences when possible. • Provide health teaching as needed based on assessment and child's situation. • Plan for appropriate follow-up with health team members. • Reduce apprehension by providing comforting behavior and meeting developmental needs of patient and family. • Allow for diversional activities to approximate tolerance of child. • Encourage family members to assist in care of patient with use of return-demonstration opportunities for teaching required skills. • Provide for appropriate safety maintenance, especially with oxygen administration (no smoking) and appropriate precautions for age and developmental level. • Allow ample time for parental mastery of skills identified in care of child.	Assures basic maintenance of airway and respiratory function. Gives priority attention to child's status and developmental level. Promotes family empowerment and thus promotes the likelihood of more effective management of therapeutic regimen after discharge. Allows for timely home care planning, family time for asking questions, practicing of techniques, etc., before discharge. Assists in reducing anxiety and promotes continuance of therapeutic regimen. Provides for long-term support and effective management of therapeutic regimen. Sensitivity to individual feelings and needs builds trust in the nurse-patient-family relationship. Realistic opportunities for diversion will be chosen according to what the patient is capable of doing and will leave the patient feeling refreshed and renewed for having participated. Return-demonstration provides feedback to evaluate skills and reinforcement in a supportive environment. Involvement of parents also satisfies emotional needs of both parent and child. Appropriate safety measures must be taken with the use of combustible potentials whose use out of prescribed parameters may be toxic. Greater success in compliance and confidence is afforded by providing ample time for skills that require mastery.

Women's Health

NOTE: The following nursing actions pertain to the newborn infant in the delivery room, immediately following delivery. See Adult Health and Home Health for actions related to the mother.

ACTIONS/INTERVENTIONS	RATIONALES
• Evaluate and record the respiratory status of the newborn infant: ○ Suction and clear mouth and pharynx with bulb syringe. ○ Avoid deep suctioning if possible.	Basic measures to clear newborn's airway. Deep suctioning would stimulate reflexes that could result in aspiration.

- Continue to evaluate infant's respiratory status and act if necessary to resuscitate. Depending on infant's response, the following nursing measures can be taken:
  - Administer warm, humid oxygen with face mask.
  - If no improvement, administer oxygen with bag and mask.
  - If no improvement, be prepared for:
    (1) Endotracheal intubation
    (2) Ventilation with positive pressure
    (3) Cardiac massage
    (4) Transport to neonatal intensive care unit

Basic protocol for infant who has difficulty immediately after birth.

Psychiatric Health

ACTIONS/INTERVENTIONS	RATIONALES
• Collaborate with physician for possible use of saline gargles or anesthetic lozenge for sore throats (report all sore throats to physician, especially if client is receiving antipsychotic drugs and in the absence of other flu or cold symptoms).	These medications can cause blood dyscrasias, which present with the symptoms of sore throat, fever, malaise, unusual bleeding, and easy bruising. Early intervention is important for patient safety.[27]
• Remind client to chew food well, and sit with client during mealtime if cognitive functioning indicates a need for close observation. Note any special adaptations here (i.e., soft foods, observation during meals, etc.).	Provides safety for client with alterations of mental status.

Gerontic Health

ACTIONS/INTERVENTIONS	RATIONALES
• Encourage coughing and deep-breathing exercises every 2 h on the (odd/even) hour.	Provides exercise in techniques that assist in clearing the airway.
• Provide small, frequent feedings during periods of dyspnea.	Conserves energy and promotes ventilation efforts.
• Instruct patient regarding early signs of respiratory infections, e.g., increased amount or thickness of secretions, increased cough, or changes in color of sputum produced.	Early recognition of signs of infection promotes early intervention and avoidance of severe infection.
• Encourage increased mobility, as tolerated, on a daily basis.	Mobility helps to increase rate and depth of respiration as well as decreasing pooling of secretions.
• Teach patient to complete prescribed course of antibiotic therapy.	Due to economic factors, patients commonly stop therapy before the designated time frame, "saving" the medication for possible future episodes.
• Monitor for the use of sedative medications that can decrease the level of alertness and respiratory effort.	These medications can decrease the level of alertness and respiratory effort.
• Collaborate with physician regarding the use of cough suppressants.	Decreases episodes of persistent, nonproductive coughing.

Home Health

ACTIONS/INTERVENTIONS	RATIONALES

• Teach client and family appropriate monitoring of signs and symptoms of ineffective airway clearance:
  ○ Cough (effective or ineffective)
  ○ Sputum
  ○ Respiratory status (cyanosis, dyspnea, and rate)
  ○ Abnormal breath sounds (noisy respirations)
  ○ Nasal flaring
  ○ Intercostal, substernal retraction
  ○ Choking, gagging
  ○ Diaphoresis
  ○ Restlessness, anxiety
  ○ Impaired speech
  ○ Collection of mucus in mouth
	Provides for early recognition and intervention for problem.

• Assist client and family in identifying lifestyle changes that may be required:
  ○ Eliminating smoking
  ○ Treating fear or anxiety
  ○ Treating pain
  ○ Performing pulmonary hygiene:
    (1) Clearing the bronchial tree by controlled coughing
    (2) Decreasing viscosity of secretions via humidity and fluid balance
    (3) Postural drainage
  ○ Learning stress management
  ○ Ensuring adequate nutritional intake
  ○ Learning diaphragmatic breathing
  ○ Administering pain relief
  ○ Beginning progressive ambulation (avoiding fatigue)
  ○ Maintaining position so that danger of aspiration is decreased
  ○ Maintaining body position to minimize work of breathing and cleaning airway
  ○ Ensuring adequate oral hygiene
  ○ Clearing secretions from throat
  ○ Suctioning as needed
  ○ Keeping area free of dust and potential allergens or irritants
  ○ Ensuring adequate hydration (monitoring intake and output)
	Provides basic information for client and family that promotes necessary lifestyle changes.

• Teach client and family purposes, side effects, and proper administration techniques of medications.	
• Assist client and family to set criteria to help them to determine when physician or other intervention is required.	Locus of control shifts from nurse to client and family, thus promoting self-care.
• Teach family basic CPR.	
• Consult with or refer to appropriate assistive resources as indicated.	Provides additional support for client and family and uses already available resources in a cost-effective manner.

Airway Clearance, Ineffective

FLOWCHART EVALUATION: EXPECTED OUTCOME 1

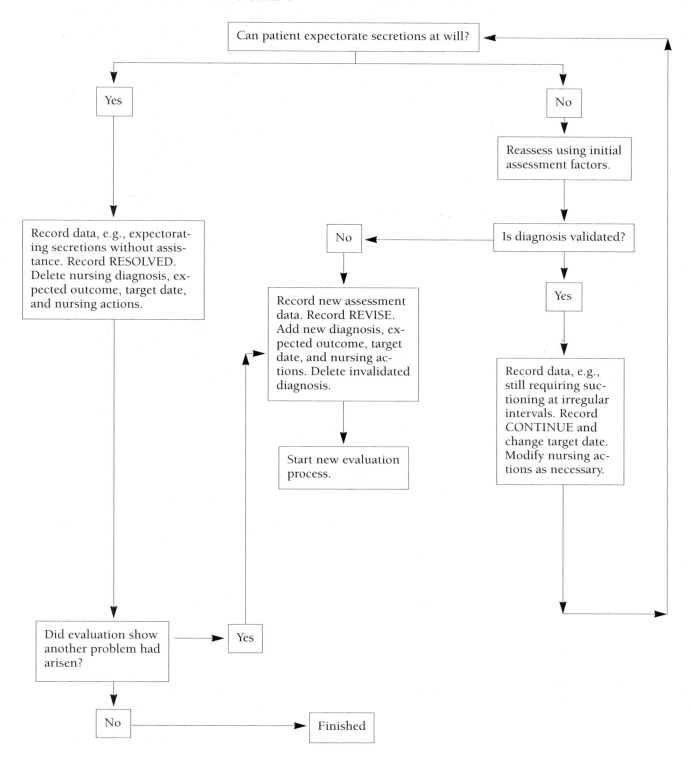

Airway Clearance, Ineffective

FLOWCHART EVALUATION: EXPECTED OUTCOME 2

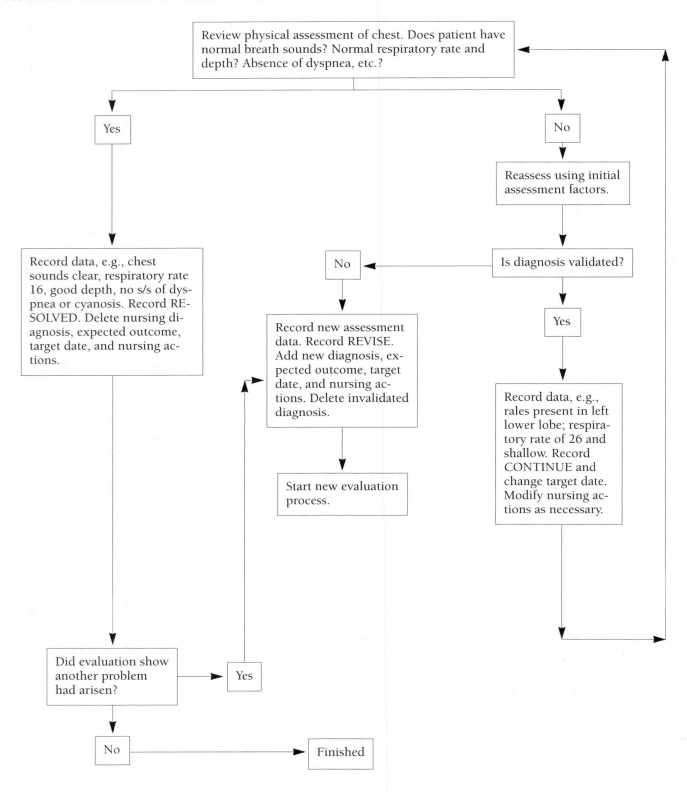

Breathing Pattern, Ineffective

DEFINITION

A state in which the rate, depth, timing, rhythm, or chest or abdominal wall excursion during inspiration, expiration, or both does not maintain optimum ventilation for the individual.[10]

NANDA TAXONOMY: EXCHANGING 1.5.1.3

DEFINING CHARACTERISTICS[10]

1. Major defining characteristics
   a. Dyspnea (shortness of breath)
   b. Respiratory rate:
   Adults (age 14 or greater): <11 or >24
   Infants: <25 or >60
   Ages 1 to 4: <20 or >30
   Ages 5 to 14: <15 or >25
   c. Depth of breathing
   Adults VT: <200 or >500 mL at rest
   Infants: 6 to 8 mL/kg
   d. Timing ratio of inspiration and expiration (if measured):
   Inspiratory time: <1:2 or >2:4
   Fractional inspiratory time: <0.36 or >0.47
   Inspiration longer than expiration
   e. Irregular breathing rhythm (e.g., apnea, frequent signs, use of accessory muscles of breathing inappropriate to level of activity, asynchronous thoracoabdominal motion)
   f. Grunting
   g. Nasal flaring (infants)
   h. Paradoxical breathing patterns
   i. Use of accessory muscles
   j. Altered chest excursion
2. Minor defining characteristics
   None given

RELATED FACTORS[10]

1. Neuromuscular impairment
2. Pain
3. Musculoskeletal impairment
4. Perception or cognition impairment
5. Anxiety
6. Decreased energy; fatigue

RELATED CLINICAL CONCERNS

1. Chronic obstructive or restrictive pulmonary disease
2. Pneumonia
3. Asthma
4. Acute alcoholism (intoxication or overdose)
5. Congestive heart failure
6. Chest trauma
7. Myasthenia gravis

STOP

HAVE YOU SELECTED THE CORRECT DIAGNOSIS?

Ineffective Airway Clearance Ineffective Airway Clearance means that something is blocking the air passage, but when air gets to the alveoli, there is adequate gas exchange. In Ineffective Breathing Pattern, the ventilatory effort is insufficient to bring in enough oxygen or to get rid of sufficient amounts of carbon dioxide. However, air is able to freely move through the air passages.

Impaired Gas Exchange This diagnosis indicates that enough oxygen is brought into the respiratory system and the carbon dioxide that is produced is exhaled, but there is insufficient exchange of oxygen and carbon dioxide at the alveolar-capillary level. There is no problem with either the ventilatory effort or the air passageways. The problem exists at the cellular level.

EXPECTED OUTCOMES

1. Will demonstrate an effective breathing pattern by (date) as evidenced by (specify criteria here, for example, normal breath sounds, arterial blood gases within normal limits, no evidence of cyanosis) and/or
2. Will return-demonstrate methods necessary to improve breathing patterns by (date)

TARGET DATES

Evaluation should be made on an hourly basis since this diagnosis has the potential to be life-threatening. After the patient has stabilized, target dates can be spaced farther apart.

NURSING ACTIONS/INTERVENTIONS WITH RATIONALES

Adult Health

ACTIONS/INTERVENTIONS	RATIONALES
• Administer oxygen as ordered.	Maintains or improves arterial blood gases (ABGs); reduces anxiety.

• Monitor baseline respiratory data:
  ○ Respiratory rate and pattern
  ○ Use of intercostal and accessory muscles
  ○ Position of comfort
  ○ Nares for flaring
  ○ Grunting or related noises such as stridor
  ○ Coughing; nature of secretions
  ○ Breath sounds
  ○ Related vital signs, especially apical pulse and blood pressure
  ○ Aids required for respiration and airway maintenance
  ○ Skin color, hydration, and elimination
  ○ Arterial blood gases as ordered
  ○ Appropriate related equipment such as arterial line or IV
  ○ Oxygen administration per order
  ○ Documentation of all of the above
	Basic monitoring of overall condition and its related progress or lack of progress.

• Collaborate with physician on monitoring of blood gases; report abnormal results immediately.	ABGs are important indicators of ventilatory effectiveness. Promotes team approach to planning.
• Perform nursing actions to maintain airway clearance (see Ineffective Airway Clearance—enter those orders here).	Maintains a patient airway for gas exchange.
• Reduce chest pain using noninvasive techniques and analgesics.	Promotes chest expansion.
• Maintain appropriate attention to relief of pain and anxiety via positioning, suctioning, and administration of medications as ordered.	
• Maintain appropriate caution for possible side effects of respiratory depression for specific medications such as morphine or Valium.	
• Raise head of bed 30 degrees or more if not contraindicated.	Allows gravity to assist in lowering the diaphragm and provides greater chest expansion.
• Instruct in diaphragmatic deep breathing and pursed-lip breathing. Have patient return-demonstrate, and perform these activities at least every hour.	Promotes lung expansion and slightly increases pressure in the airways, allowing them to remain open longer; increases oxygenation and exhalation of carbon dioxide.
• Reduce fear and anxiety by spending at least 15 min every 2 h on the (odd/even) hour with patient.	Reduces tension and stress; reduces oxygen demand and work of breathing.
• Administer or assist with IPPB or CPAP as ordered. Remain with patient during treatment.	Promotes expansion of airways and exchange of gases; staying with the patient reduces anxiety.
• Turn every 2 h on the (odd/even) hour.	Promotes mobility of any secretions and promotes lung expansion.
• Encourage patient's mobility as tolerated (see Impaired Physical Mobility).	Promotes tolerance for activities and helps with lung expansion and ventilation.
• Instruct patient in effects of smoking, air pollution, etc., prior to discharge, on breathing pattern.	Knowledge will assist patient to avoid harmful environments and to protect himself or herself from the effects of such activities.

• Provide teaching based on needs of patient and family regarding:
  ○ Illness
  ○ Procedures and related nursing care
  ○ Implications for rest and relief of anxiety secondary to respiratory failure
  ○ Advocacy role
	Reduces anxiety; starts appropriate home care planning; assists family in dealing with health care system.

Child Health

ACTIONS/INTERVENTIONS	RATIONALES
• Maintain appropriate emergency equipment in an accessible place. (Specify actual size of endotracheal tube for infant, child, or adolescent, trach set size, and suctioning catheters or chest tube for size of patient.)	Standard accountability for emergency equipment and treatment is basic to patient care and especially so when risk factors are increased.
• Allow at least 5–15 min per shift for parents and child to verbalize concerns related to illness.	Appropriate time for ventilation may be hard to determine, but efforts to do so demonstrate valuing of patient and family needs and serve to reduce anxiety.
• Determine perception of illness by patient and parents.	How the parents and child see (perceive) the patient's problem will provide meaningful data that serve to ensure sensitivity in care and will provide information regarding teaching needs. Provides cues to questions regarding continued implementation of therapeutic regimen.
• Include parents in care of child as appropriate, to include comfort measures, assisting with feeding, and the like.	Parental involvement is critical in maintaining emotional bonds with the child. Also augments sense of contributing to child's care with opportunities for mastering the skills in a supportive environment.
• Collaborate with appropriate related health team members as needed.	Appropriate coordination of services will best meet the patient's needs with attention to the patient's individuality.

Women's Health

ACTIONS/INTERVENTIONS	RATIONALES
• Assist patient and significant other in identifying lifestyle changes that may be required to prevent Ineffective Breathing Pattern during pregnancy, e.g., stopping smoking or avoiding crowds during influenza epidemics.	Increased cardiovascular fitness supports increased respiratory effectiveness.
• Develop exercise plan for cardiovascular fitness during pregnancy.	
• Teach patient to avoid wearing constrictive clothing during pregnancy.	Any constriction will contribute to further breathing difficulties, which will become more difficult as the expanding uterus contributes to abdominal contents pressing against the diaphragm.[28]
• Teach and encourage patient to practice correct breathing techniques for labor.	Assists in preventing hyperventilation.
• During the latter stages of pregnancy, encourage patient to: ◦ Walk up stairs slowly ◦ Lie on left or right side, to get more oxygen to fetus ◦ Position herself in bed with pillows for optimum comfort and adequate air exchange ◦ Take frequent rest breaks during the workday	During this stage the chest cavity has less room to expand because of the enlarging uterus.[29] Often edema of the latter stage of pregnancy causes "stuffy" noses and full sinuses.
• Carefully monitor maternal respiration during the laboring process.	Analgesics and anesthesia can cause maternal hypoxia and reduce fetal oxygen.
• If prolonged decrease in FHT immediately prior to delivery, administer pure oxygen (10–12 L/min) to mother before delivery and until cessation of pulsation in cord.	
• Evaluate and record the respiratory status of the newborn infant: ◦ Determine the 1-min Apgar score. ◦ Suction and clear mouth and pharynx with bulb syringe. ◦ Avoid deep suctioning if possible.	Basic care measures to ensure effective respiration in the newborn infant.

Continued

ACTIONS/INTERVENTIONS	RATIONALES
• Dry excess moisture off infant with towel or blanket.	Helps stimulate infant; prevents evaporative heat loss.

• Stimulate (if necessary), using firm but gentle tactile stimulation:
  ∘ Slapping sole of foot
  ∘ Rubbing up and down spine
  ∘ Flicking heel
• Place infant in warm environment:
  ∘ Under radiant heat warmer
  ∘ Next to mother's skin
• Cover infant's head with stocking cap.
• Cover both mother and infant with warm blanket.
• Determine and record the 5-min Apgar score.	

• Continue to evaluate infant's respiratory status and be prepared to act if necessary to resuscitate. Depending on infant's response, the following nursing measures can be taken:
  ∘ Administer warm, humid oxygen with face mask.
  ∘ If no improvement, administer oxygen with bag and mask.
  ∘ If no improvement, be prepared for:
   (1) Endotracheal intubation
   (2) Ventilation with positive pressure
   (3) Cardiac massage
   (4) Transporting to neonatal intensive care unit
	Basic protocol to care for the newborn who has respiratory problems.

Psychiatric Health

NOTE: The following orders are for Ineffective Breathing Pattern Related to Anxiety. For those problems related to physiologic problems, refer to Adult Health nursing actions.

ACTIONS/INTERVENTIONS	RATIONALES
• Monitor causative factors.	Provides information on client's current status so interventions can be adapted appropriately.
• Place client in a calm, supportive environment.	Anxiety is contagious, as is calm. A calm reassuring environment can communicate indirectly to the client that the situation is safe and that the nurse can assist him or her in mobilizing their internal resources, thus facilitating client's sense of control.
• Maintain a calm, supportive attitude, reassuring client that you will assist him or her in maintaining control. • Give client clear, concise directions.	Anxiety can decrease client's ability to focus on and understand a complex presentation of information.
• Have client maintain direct eye contact with nurse. Modulate based on client's ability to tolerate eye contact. This should not be done in a manner that appears to "stare client down."	Communicates interest in the client and assists client in tuning out extraneous stimuli.
• Instruct client to take slow, deep breaths. Demonstrate breaths to client, and practice with client. Provide client with constant, positive reinforcement for appropriate breathing patterns.	Helps to stimulate relaxation response.
• Remain with client until episode is resolved. • If client does not respond to the attempts to control breathing, have client breathe into a paper bag. • Distract client from focus on breathing by beginning a deep muscle relaxation exercise that begins at client's feet.	Reassures client of safety and security. Rebreathing air with a higher CO_2 content will slow the respiratory rate. Interrupts pattern of thought that reinforces anxiety and therefore increases breathing difficulties.

- Use successful resolution of a problematic breathing episode as an opportunity to teach client that he or she can gain conscious control over breathing and that these episodes are not out of his or her control.
- Teach client and significant others proper breathing techniques to include:
  ○ Maintaining proper body alignment
  ○ Using diaphragmatic breathing (See Ineffective Airway Clearance for information on this technique.)
  ○ Use of deep muscle relaxation before the onset of ineffective breathing pattern begins
- Practice with client diaphragmatic breathing twice a day for 30 min. Note practice times here.
- Develop a plan with client for initiating slow, deep breathing when an ineffective breathing pattern begins.

- Identify with client those situations that are most frequently associated with the development of ineffective breathing patterns, and assist him or her in practicing relaxation in response to these situations 1 time a day for 30 min. Note times of practice sessions here.

Promotes client's self-esteem and perceived control; also provides positive reinforcement for adaptive coping behaviors.

Promotes perceived control and adaptive coping behaviors. Provides information that will facilitate positive reinforcement from the support system increasing the probability for the success of the behavior change.[30]

Enhances relaxation response.

Early recognition of problematic situations facilitates client's ability to gain control and utilize adaptive coping behaviors.
Positive imagery promotes positive psychophysiologic responses and enhances self-esteem, which improves possibility of positive outcome.[23]

Gerontic Health

ACTIONS/INTERVENTIONS	RATIONALES
• Monitor respiratory rate, depth, effort, and lung sounds every 4 h around the clock.	Minimum database needed for this diagnosis.
• Due to age-related "air trapping," have patient focus on improving expiratory effort. Instruct patient to inhale to the count of 1 and exhale for 3 counts.[31]	Decreased alveoli and decreased elasticity leads to air trapping, which results in hyperinflation of lungs.
• Collaborate with occupational therapist and respiratory therapist regarding other measures to enhance respiratory function.	Occupational therapist can teach patient less energy-expending means to complete activities of daily living. Respiratory therapist can assist patient and family in learning how to perform pulmonary toileting at home.
• In the event of a chronic Ineffective Breathing Pattern, refer the patient to a support group such as those sponsored by the American Lung Association.	Provides long-term support for coping with problems; provides updated information; provides role modeling from other group members.
• Instruct in relaxation techniques, e.g., guided imagery or progressive muscle relaxation, to reduce stress.	May assist in decreasing the episodes of acute breathing problems in those with chronic ineffective breathing pattern.
• Where applicabale, monitor for knowledge of proper medication use, especially if inhalers are a part of the therapy.	Maximum benefit may be derived from proper drug administration and usage. Inhalers may be difficult to operate due to physical problems and lack of information regarding proper usage.

Home Health

NOTE: If this diagnosis is suspected when caring for a patient in the home, it is imperative that a physician referral be obtained immediately. If the patient has been referred to home health care by a physician, the nurse will collaborate with the physician in the treatment of the patient.

ACTIONS/INTERVENTIONS	RATIONALES

• Teach client and family appropriate monitoring of signs and symptoms of ineffective breathing pattern:
  ○ Cough
  ○ Sputum production
  ○ Fatigue
  ○ Respiratory status: Cyanosis, dyspnea, rate
  ○ Lack of diaphragmatic breathing
  ○ Nasal flaring
  ○ Anxiety or restlessness
  ○ Impaired speech
	Provides for early recognition and intervention for problem.

• Assist client and family in identifying lifestyle changes that may be required to prevent ineffective breathing pattern:
  ○ Stopping smoking
  ○ Prevention and early treatment of lung infections
  ○ Avoidance of known irritants and allergens
  ○ Practicing pulmonary hygiene:
    (1) Clearing bronchial tree by controlled coughing
    (2) Decreasing viscosity of secretions via humidity and fluid balance
    (3) Clearing postural drainage
  ○ Treatment of fear, anxiety, anger, depression, thorax trauma, or narcotic overdoses
  ○ Adequate nutritional intake
  ○ Stress management
  ○ Adequate hydration
  ○ Breathing techniques (diaphragmatic, pursed lips)
  ○ Progressive ambulation
  ○ Pain relief
  ○ Preventing hazards of immobility
  ○ Appropriate use of oxygen (dosage, route, and safety factors)
	Provides basic information for client and family that promotes necessary lifestyle changes,

• Teach patient and family purposes, side effects, and proper administration techniques of medication.	
• Assist client and family to set criteria to help them to determine when physician or other intervention is required.	Locus of control shifts from nurse to family, thus promoting self-care.
• Teach family basic CPR.	

Breathing Pattern, Ineffective

FLOWCHART EVALUATION: EXPECTED OUTCOME 1

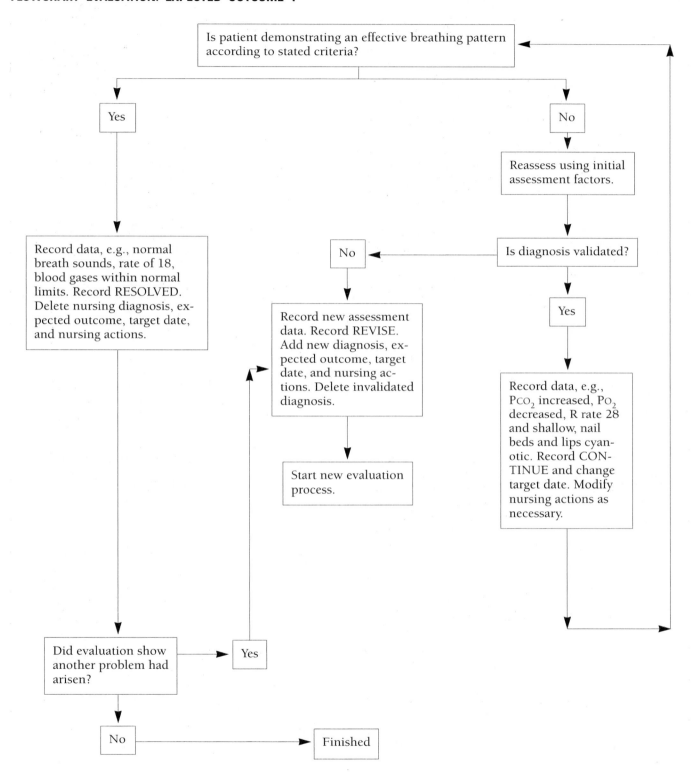

Breathing Pattern, Ineffective

FLOWCHART EVALUATION: EXPECTED OUTCOME 2

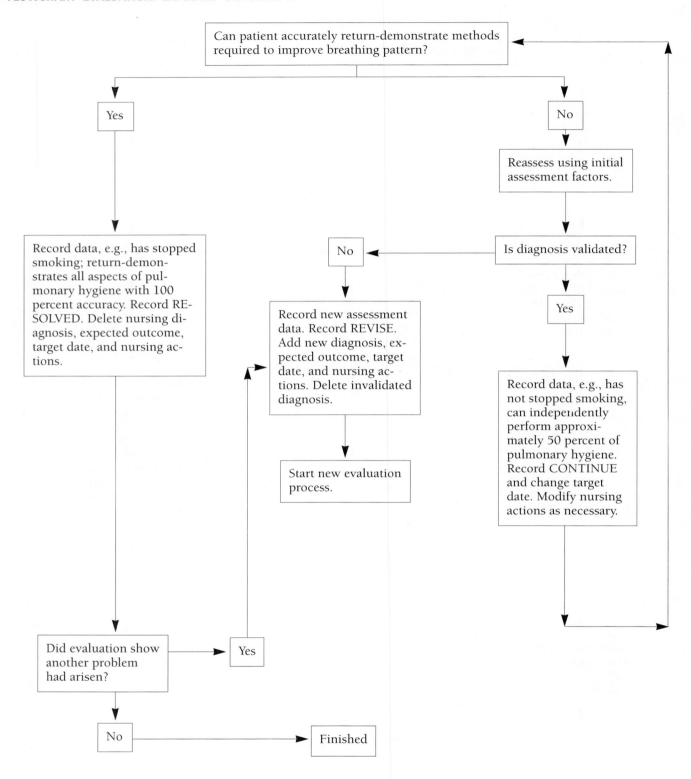

Cardiac Output, Decreased

DEFINITION

A state in which the blood pumped by the heart is inadequate to meet the metabolic demands of the body.[10]

NANDA TAXONOMY: EXCHANGING 1.4.2.1

DEFINING CHARACTERISTICS[10]

1. Major defining characteristics
   a. Variations in blood pressure readings
   b. Arrhythmias
   c. Fatigue
   d. Jugular vein distention
   e. Skin color changes
   f. Rales
   g. Oliguria
   h. Decreased peripheral pulses
   i. Cold, clammy skin
   j. Dyspnea
   k. Orthopnea and/or PND
   l. Restlessness
   m. Chest pain
   n. Weight gain
   o. Wheezing
   p. Edema
   q. Elevated PA pressures
   r. Increased respiratory rate
   s. Use of accessory muscles
   t. ECG changes
   u. Ejection factor <40 percent
   v. Abnormal chest x-ray (pulmonary vascular congestion)
   w. Abnormal cardiac enzymes
   x. Altered mental status
2. Minor defining characteristics
   None given

RELATED FACTORS[10]

To be developed.

RELATED CLINICAL CONCERNS

1. Congestive heart failure
2. Myocardial infarction
3. Valvular heart disease
4. Inflammatory heart disease, for example, pericarditis
5. Hypertension
6. Shock
7. Chronic obstructive pulmonary disease

HAVE YOU SELECTED THE CORRECT DIAGNOSIS?

Altered Tissue Perfusion Decreased cardiac output relates specifically to a heart malfunction while Altered Tissue Perfusion relates to deficits in the peripheral circulation that will have cellular-level impact. Tissue perfusion problems may develop secondary to decreased cardiac output but can also exist without cardiac output problems.[32] In either diagnosis, close collaboration will be needed with medical practitioners to ensure the best possible interventions for the patient.

EXPECTED OUTCOMES

1. Will exhibit no signs or symptoms of decreased cardiac output by (date) and/or
2. Will implement a self-designed plan to lessen the likelihood of future decreased cardiac output episodes by (date)

TARGET DATES

Because the nursing diagnosis Decreased Cardiac Output is life-threatening, progress toward meeting the expected outcomes should be evaluated at least daily for 3 to 5 days. If significant progress is demonstrated, then the target date can be increased to 3-day intervals. Patients who develop this diagnosis should be referred to a medical practitioner immediately and transferred to a critical care unit.

ADDITIONAL INFORMATION

Cardiac output (CO) refers to the amount of blood ejected from the left ventricle into the aorta per minute. Cardiac output is equivalent to the stroke volume (SV), which is the amount of blood ejected from the left ventricle with each contraction times the heart rate (HR) or the number of beats per minute:

$$CO = SV \times HR$$

The average amount of cardiac output is 5.6 L per minute. This amount will vary according to the individual's amount of exercise and body size.

Cardiac output is dependent on the relationship between stroke volume and the heart rate. Cardiac output is maintained by compensatory adjustment of these two variables. If the rate slows, the time for ventricular filling (diastole) increases. This allows for an increase in the preload and a subsequent increase in stroke volume. If the stroke volume falls, the heart rate increases to compensate. Stroke volume is affected by preload, contractility, and afterload.

Preload refers to the amount of stretching of the myocardial fibers. The fibers stretch due to the increase in the volume of blood delivered to the ventricles during diastole. The degree of myocardial stretch before contraction is preload. Preload is determined by the venous return and ejection frac-tion (amount of blood left in the ventricle at the end of systole). Prolonged excessive stretching will lead to a decrease in cardiac output.

Contractility is a function of the intensity of the actinomycin linkages. Increased contractility increases ventricular emptying and results in increased stroke volume. Contractility can be increased by sympathetic stimulation or by the administration of such drugs as calcium and epinephrine. *Afterload* is the amount of tension developed by the ventricle during contraction. The amount of peripheral resistance will predominantly determine the amount of tension. Excessive increases in the afterload will reduce stroke volume and cardiac output.

The heart rate is predominantly influenced by the autonomic nervous system through both the sympathetic and parasympathetic nervous systems. The sympathetic fibers can increase both rate and force, while the parasympathetic fibers act in an opposite direction. Other factors such as the central nervous system pressoreceptor reflexes, cerebral cortex impulses, body temperature, electrolytes, and hormones also affect the heart rate, but the autonomic nervous system keeps the entire system in balance.[33]

NURSING ACTIONS/INTERVENTIONS WITH RATIONALES

Adult Health

ACTIONS/INTERVENTIONS	RATIONALES
• Place on cardiac monitor and continuously monitor cardiac rhythm and rate.	Myocardial perfusion can be more accurately assessed.
• Monitor, at least every 2 h on the (odd/even) hour: ○ Vital signs ○ Chest and heart sounds ○ Apical-radial pulse deficit; pedal pulses ○ Pulse pressure ○ Other hemodynamic readings (e.g., wedge pressures, PAP, PCWP, central venous pressure [CVP]) ○ Neck vein filling ○ Peripheral edema (extremities, eyelids, sacral areas) ○ Level of consciousness ○ Activity intolerance ○ Mental status ○ Skin changes ○ Peripheral pulses ○ Liver position	Establishes baseline and allows for accurate monitoring of changes from baselines.
• Collaborate with physician regarding frequency of measurement of the following and closely monitor results: ○ Arterial blood gases ○ Electrolytes ○ Cardiac enzymes ○ Complete blood cell count ○ Electrolyte balance	Additional baseline data needed for accurate monitoring of condition.
• Explain reasons for tests and monitoring to patient as well as the role he or she plays in ensuring accurate results.	Decreases anxiety and promotes more accurate monitoring results.
• Administer oxygen and medications as ordered, and monitor effects.	Enhances myocardial perfusion and decreases workload.
• Monitor flow rate of oxygen.	
• Measure urinary output hourly.	Fluid overload or underload can compromise cardiac output.
• Measure and record intake and total at least every 8 h. Collaborate with physician regarding limitation of intake.	
• Monitor pain, and institute immediate relief measures.	Pain can increase cardiac output; relief measures also decrease anxiety.
• Keep siderails up and bed in low position particularly during periods of altered mental status.	Basic patient safety.
• Weigh daily at (time) and in same-weight clothing.	Helps to determine changes in fluid volume.

ACTIONS/INTERVENTIONS	RATIONALES

• Provide skin care at least every 2 h on the (odd/even) hour:
  ○ Change position and support in anatomic alignment.
  ○ Elevate edematous extremities, and use measures such as a bed cradle to keep pressure off edematous parts.
  ○ Use sheepskin, egg crate mattress, or alternating air mattress under patient.
  ○ Keep linens free of wrinkles.
  ○ Keep skin clean and dry.
  ○ Avoid shearing forces when moving patient.
  ○ Use cornstarch on bed and skin to facilitate patient's movement.
	Promotes tissue perfusion; decreases pressure area thus decreasing the likelihood of impaired tissue integrity.

• Do ROM exercises at least once per shift, and position patient carefully.	Promotes circulation; reduces consequences of impaired mobility. Careful positioning assists breathing and avoids pressure.

• Monitor intravenous therapy:
  ○ Flow rate
  ○ Insertion site
	Prevents fluid overload or underload. Monitor IV site for patency of veins and for presence of infection.

• Provide adequate rest periods:
  ○ Schedule at least one 5-min rest after any activity.
  ○ Schedule 30- to 60-min rest period after each meal.
	Decreases stress on already stressed circulatory system.

• Limit visitors and visiting time. Explain need for restriction to patient and significant others. If presence of significant other promotes rest, allow to stay beyond time limits.	
• Monitor bowel elimination, abdominal distention, and bowel sounds at least once per shift during waking hours. Collaborate with physician regarding stool softener.	Avoids straining and Valsalva maneuver, which comprise cardiac output.
• Assist patient with stress management and relaxation techniques every 4 h while awake (state times here). Support patients in usual coping mechanisms.	Decreases anxiety and promotes cardiac output.
• Plan to spend at least 15 min every 4 h providing emotional support to patient and significant others.	Decreases anxiety.
• Collaborate with dietitian regarding dietary restrictions when developing plan of care, and reinforce prior to discharge (e.g., sodium, fluids, calories, and cholesterol).	These dietary factors can compromise cardiac output.

• Collaborate with occupational therapist and family regarding diversional activities. Refer patient to:
  ○ Physical therapist for home exercise program
  ○ Visiting nurse service
	Promotes collaboration and holistic care.

Child Health

ACTIONS/INTERVENTIONS	RATIONALES

• Provide in-depth monitoring and documentation related to the following:
  ○ Ventilator if applicable:
    (1) If continuous positive airway pressure (CPAP), adjust setting according to physician's order
    (2) Peak pressure as ordered
    (3) O_2 percentage desired as ordered
  ○ Intake and output hourly and as ordered. Notify physician if below 10 mL/h or as specified for size of infant or child.
	These factors constitute the basic measures utilized in monitoring for decompensation of cardiac status. Closely related are respiratory function, hydration status, and hemodynamic status.

Continued

ACTIONS/INTERVENTIONS	RATIONALES

○ Excessive bleeding. If in postop status, notify physician if above 50 mL/h or as specified.
○ Tolerance of feedings.
○ Notify physician for:
  (1) Premature ventricular contractions (PVCs) or other arrhythmias
  (2) Limits of pulse, respiratory rate, output criteria as specified for individual patient
○ Use caution in the administration of medications as ordered, especially digoxin:
  (1) Have another RN check dose and medication order.
  (2) Validate and document the heart rate to be greater than specified lower limit parameter (e.g., 100 for infant) before administering.
○ Document if medication withheld because of heart rate.
○ Monitor for signs and symptoms of toxicity, e.g., vomiting.
○ Ensure potassium maintenance. Collaborate with physician regarding frequency of serum potassium measurement and immediately report results.
○ Maintain digitalizing protocol.
○ Make sure that parents understand patient's status and treatment.
○ Monitor patient's response to suctioning, x-ray, or other procedures.	

• Ensure availability of crash cart and emergency equipment as needed to include: ○ Cardiac or emergency drugs ○ Defibrillator ○ Ambu bag (pedi or infant size) ○ Appropriate suctioning equipment	Standard nursing care includes availability and appropriate use of equipment and meds in event of cardiac arrest. Anticipation for need of equipment with a child in high-risk status is required.
• Allow time for parents to voice concern on a regular basis. Set aside 10–15 min per shift for this purpose.	Verbalization of concerns helps reduce anxiety. Attempting to set aside time for this verbalization demonstrates the value it holds for the patient's care.
• Encourage parental input in care, such as with feeding, positioning, and monitoring of intake and output as appropriate.	Parental input assists in meeting parent's and child's emotional needs and augments the care of others. This action also allows for learning essential skills in a supportive environment.
• Encourage patient as applicable to participate in care. • Allow for sensitivity to time in understanding of diagnosis. The seemingly abstract nature of underlying cardiac physiology, especially in noncyanotic heart disease can be confusing.	Self-care enhances sense of autonomy and empowerment. Abstract aspects of an illness often prove more difficult to grasp. Congenital cardiac anomalies are often complex in nature, which requires health care personnel to use consistent terms and offer appropriate aids to depict key issues of anatomy.
• Support parents in usual appropriate coping mechanisms.	Emotional security may be afforded by encouragement of usual coping mechanisms for age and developmental status.
• Maintain appropriate technique in dressing change (asepsis and cautious handwashing). • Limit visitors in immediate postoperative status as applicable.	Standard care requires universal precautions, which minimize risk factors for infection. Visitation may prove overwhelming to all when unlimited in immediate postoperative period. Remember that numerous nursing-medical therapies must be attended to during this time also.
• Help reduce patient and parental anxiety by touching and allowing patient to be held and comforted.	Comforting allows parent and child to feel more secure and will decrease feeling of intimidation parents might perceive from numerous pieces of equipment and activity. Human caring helps offset high tech.

- Provide teaching with sensitivity to patient and parental needs regarding equipment, procedures, or routines, e.g, use a doll for demonstration with toddler.
- Encourage parents to meet parents of similarly involved cardiac patients.

- Address need for parents to continue with activities of daily living with confidence regarding knowledge of restrictions in child's status.

Individualized teaching with appropriate aids will most likely serve to reinforce desired learning and enlist the patient's cooperation.

Sharing with similarly involved clientele or families affords a sense of unity, hope, and affirmation of the future far beyond what nurses or others may offer.

Aim should be for normalcy within parameters dictated by the child's condition. Strive to restrain family from labeling child or encouraging child to become a "cardiac cripple."

Women's Health

ACTIONS/INTERVENTIONS	RATIONALES
• Assist patient with relaxation techniques.	Assists in stress reduction.
NOTE: Caution the patient to never begin a new vigorous exercise plan while pregnant. Teach the patient to exercise slowly, in moderation, and according to the individual's ability. A good rule of thumb is to use moderation and with the consent of the physician continue with the pre-pregnant established exercise plan. Most professionals discourage aerobics and hot tubs because of the heat. It is not known at this time if overheating by the mother is harmful to the fetus.	
• Assist in developing an exercise plan for cardiovascular fitness during pregnancy. Some good exercises are: ○ Swimming ○ Walking ○ Bicycling ○ Jogging (If patient has done this before and is used to it, jogging is probably not harmful, *but* remember that during pregnancy joints and muscles are more susceptible to strain. If patient feels pain, fatigue, or overheated, she should slow down or stop exercise.)	Assists in increasing cardiovascular fitness during pregnancy.
• Refer patient to support groups that understand the physiology of pregnancy and have developed exercise programs based on this physiology, such as swimming classes for pregnant women at the local YWCA, childbirth education classes, or exercise videotapes specifically directed and produced for use during pregnancy.	
• Teach patient and significant others how to avoid "supine hypotension" during pregnancy (particularly the later stages).	The expanded uterus causes pressure on the large blood vessels.
• Prior to the start of labor, encourage patient to attend childbirth education classes to learn how to work with her body during labor.	
• During the second stage of labor[34–36]: ○ Allow patient to assume whatever position aids her in the second stage of labor (i.e., upright, squatting, kneeling position, etc.). ○ Provide patient with proper physical support during the second stage of labor. This support might include allowing the partner or support person to sit or stand beside her and support her head or shoulders or to stand behind her supporting her with his or her body. The partner might also stand in front of her allowing her to lean on his or her shoulders with her arms about his or her neck. Patient may also use a birthing bed or chair, pillows, over-the-bed table, or bars.	

Continued

ACTIONS/INTERVENTIONS	RATIONALES

• **Do not** urge the woman to "push, push" or to hold breath during the second stage of labor. Allow the woman to bear down with her contractions at her own pace:
  ○ Encourage spontaneous bearing down only if fetal head has not descended low enough to stimulate Ferguson's reflex.
  ○ Encourage mother to push when she feels the urge and to rest between contractions.
  ○ Discourage prolonged maternal breath-holding (more than 6–8 s) during pushing.
  ○ Assist mother to accomplish 4 or more pushing efforts per contraction.
  ○ Support mother's efforts in pushing, and validate the normalcy of sensations and sounds mother is verbalizing. (These sounds may include grunting, groaning, and exhaling during the push or breath-holding less than 6 s.)
	Avoids straining and the Valsalva maneuver.
	
	Breath-holding involves the Valsalva maneuver. Increased intrathoracic pressure due to a closed glottis causes a decrease in cardiac output and blood pressure. The fall in pressure causes a decrease in placental perfusion causing fetal hypoxia.[28,37]

Psychiatric Health

ACTIONS/INTERVENTIONS	RATIONALES

• Monitor risk factors:
  ○ Medications
  ○ Past history of cardiac problems
  ○ Age
  ○ Current condition of the cardiovascular system
  ○ Weight
  ○ Exercise patterns
  ○ Nutritional patterns
  ○ Psychosocial stressors
	Early identification and intervention helps assure better outcome.

• Monitor every (number) hours (depends on level or risk, can be anywhere from 2–8 h) the client's cardiac functioning (list times to observe here):
  ○ Vital signs
  ○ Chest sounds
  ○ Apical-radical pulse deficit
  ○ Mental status
• Report alterations to medical practitioner immediately.
• If acute situation develops, notify medical practitioner and implement adult health nursing actions.
• If client's condition or other factors necessitate client's remaining in the mental health area beyond the acute stage, refer to adult health nursing actions for care on an ongoing basis. This is not recommended due to the lack of equipment and properly trained staff to care for this situation on most specialized care units.
	Basic database for further intervention.

• If client is placed on unit while in the rehabilitation stage of this diagnosis, implement the following nursing actions: (Discuss with client current rehabilitation schedule and record special consideration here.)	Promotes client's perceived control and supports self-care activities.
• Provide appropriate rest periods following activity. This varies according to the client's stage in rehabilitation. Most common times of needed rest are after meals and after any activity (note specific limits here).	Prevents excessive stress on the cardiovascular system and prevents fatigue.

- Assist client with implementation of exercise program. List types of activity, time spent in activity, and times of activity here. Also list special motivators the client may need, such as a companion to walk for 30 min 3 times a day at (times).

  Promotes cardiovascular strength and well-being.

- Provide diet restrictions, e.g., low sodium, low calorie, low fat, low cholesterol, or fluid restrictions.

  Decreases dietary contributions to increased risk factors.

- Monitor intake and output each shift.

  Medications can impact fluid balance, and excessive fluid can increase demands on the cardiovascular system. Increases client's perceived control and promotes early recognition and treatment of problem.

- Assess for and teach client to assess for:
  - Potassium loss (muscle cramps)
  - Chest pain
  - Sudden weight gain
  - Decreased urine output
  - Increased fatigue
- Assess increased risk factors, and assist client in developing a plan to reduce these, e.g., smoking, obesity, or stress—refer to appropriate nursing diagnosis for assistance in developing interventions.

  Increases client's perceived control and decreases risk for further damage to the cardiovascular system.

- Spend 30 min twice a day teaching client deep muscle relaxation and practicing this process (list times here).

  Relaxation decreases stress on the cardiovascular system.

- Discuss with patient's support system the lifestyle alterations that may be required.
- Develop stress reduction program with client and provide necessary environment for implementation. This could include massage therapy, meditation, aerobic exercise as tolerated, hobbies, or music (note specific plan here).

  Enhances possibility for continuation of behavior change.[30]

Gerontic Health

ACTIONS/INTERVENTIONS	RATIONALES
• Monitor for possible side effects of diuretic therapy.	Older adults may have excessive diuresis on normal diuretic dosage.
• Review the health history for liver or kidney disease in patients on diuretic therapy.	Diuretics may need to have adjusted dosages in those with preexisting kidney or hepatic disease to avoid complications.
• Whenever possible, give diuretics in the morning.	Decreases problems with nocturia and consequent disturbed sleep-rest pattern or high risk for injury from falls.
• Teach proper medication usage, e.g., dosage, side effects, dangers related to missed doses, and food/drug interactions.	Basic safety for medication administration.

• Teach patients who are on potassium-wasting diuretics:
  ○ The need for potassium replacement
  ○ Foods that are high in potassium, e.g., bananas
  ○ Signs and symptoms of potassium depletion	

• Assist patient and/or family to determine environmental conditions that may need to be adapted to promote energy.	Assists in conservation of energy and balancing oxygen demands with resources.[26]

Home Health

NOTE: If this diagnosis is suspected when caring for a client in the home, it is imperative that a physician referral be obtained immediately. If the client has been referred to home health care by a physician, the nurse will collaborate with the physician in the treatment of the client.

ACTIONS/INTERVENTIONS	RATIONALES

• Teach patient and significant others:
  ○ Risk factors, e.g., smoking, hypertension, or obesity
  ○ Medication regimen, e.g., toxicity or effects
  ○ Need to balance rest and activity
  ○ Monitoring of:
    (1) Weight, daily
    (2) Vital signs
    (3) Intake and output
  ○ When to contact health care personnel:
    (1) Chest pain
    (2) Dyspnea
    (3) Sudden weight gain
    (4) Decreased urine output
    (5) Increased fatigue
  ○ Dietary adaptations, as necessary:
    (1) Low sodium
    (2) Low cholesterol
    (3) Caloric restriction
    (4) Soft foods
	Provides for early recognition and intervention for problem.

• Assist patient and family in identifying lifestyle changes that may be required:
  ○ Eliminating smoking
  ○ Cardiac rehabilitation program
  ○ Stress management
  ○ Weight control
  ○ Dietary restrictions
  ○ Decreased alcohol
  ○ Relaxation techniques
  ○ Bowel regimen to avoid straining and constipation
  ○ Maintenance of fluid and electrolyte balance
  ○ Changes in role functions in family
  ○ Concerns regarding sexual activity
  ○ Monitoring activity and responses to activity
    (*Note*: Level of damage to left ventricle should be determined before exercise program is initiated.[38])
  ○ Providing diversional activities when physical activity is restricted (see Diversional Activity Deficit)
  ○ Pain control
	Provides basic information for client and family that promotes necesssary lifestyle changes.

• Teach family basic CPR. • Teach client and family purposes and side effects of medications and proper administration techniques. • Teach client and family to refrain from activities that increase the demands on the heart, e.g., snow-shoveling, lifting, or Valsalva maneuver.	Locus of control shifts from nurse to client and family, thus promoting self-care.
• Assist client and family to set criteria to help them to determine when a physician or other intervention is required. • Consult with or refer patient to appropriate assistive resources as indicated.	Provides additional support for client and family and uses already available resources in a cost-effective manner.

Cardiac Output, Decreased

FLOWCHART EVALUATION: EXPECTED OUTCOME 1

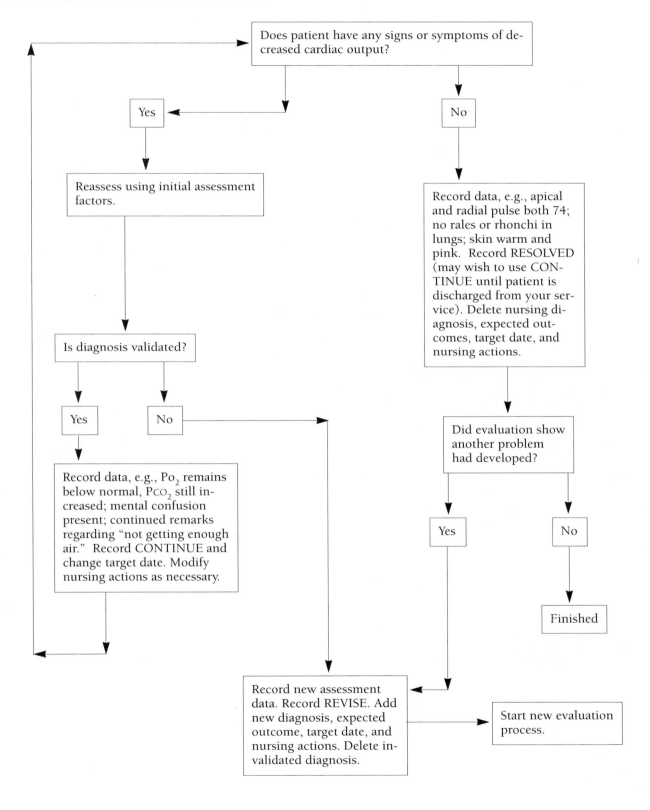

Cardiac Output, Decreased

FLOWCHART EVALUATION: EXPECTED OUTCOME 2

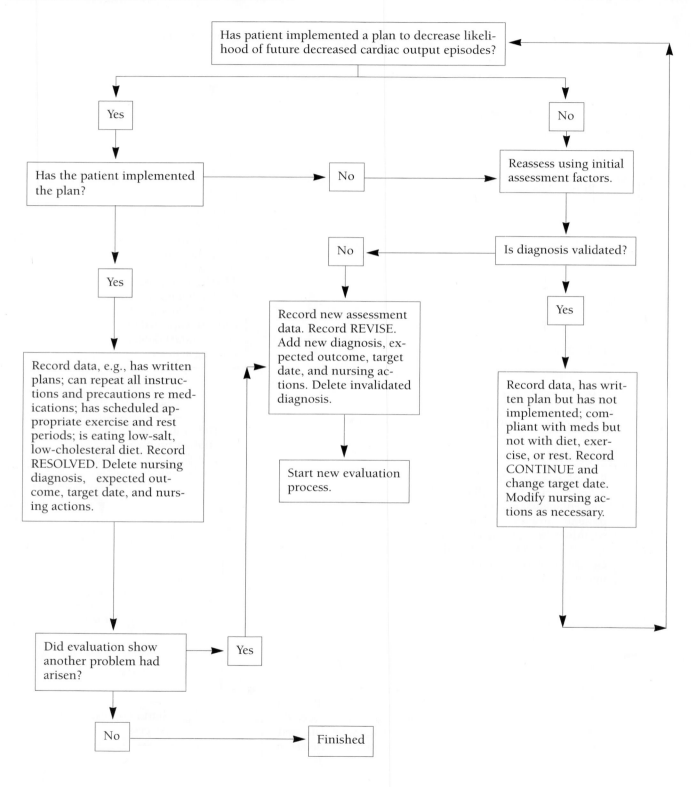

Disorganized Infant Behavior, Actual, Risk for, Potential for Enhanced Organized

DEFINITION[10]

DISORGANIZED INFANT BEHAVIOR Alteration in integration and modulation of the physiologic and behavioral systems of functioning, that is, autonomic, motor, state, organizational, self-regulatory, and attention-interaction systems.[10]

DISORGANIZED INFANT BEHAVIOR, RISK FOR Risk for alteration and modulation of the physiologic and behavioral systems of functioning, that is, autonomic, motor, state, organizational, self-regulatory, and attention-interaction systems.[10]

ORGANIZED INFANT BEHAVIOR, POTENTIAL FOR ENHANCED A pattern of modulation for the physiologic and behavioral systems of functioning of an infant, that is, autonomic, motor, state, organizational, self-regulatory, and attention-interaction systems, which is satisfactory but can be improved, resulting in higher levels of integration in response to environmental stimuli.[10]

NANDA TAXONOMY: MOVING 6.8.1, 6.8.2, AND 6.8.3

DEFINING CHARACTERISTICS[10]

1. Disorganized Infant Behavior
   a. Major defining characteristics
      (1) Change from baseline physiologic measures
      (2) Tremors, startles, or twitches
      (3) Hyperextension of arms and legs
      (4) Diffuse or unclear sleep
      (5) Deficient self-regulatory behaviors
      (6) Deficient response to visual or auditory stimuli
   b. Minor defining characteristics
      (1) Yawning
      (2) Apnea
2. Risk for Disorganized Infant Behavior
   a. Major risk factors
      (1) Pain
      (2) Oral or motor problems
      (3) Environmental overstimulation
      (4) Lack of containment or boundaries
      (5) Prematurity
      (6) Invasive or painful procedures
3. Potential for Enhanced Organized Infant Behavior
   a. Major defining characteristics
      (1) Stable physiologic measures
      (2) Definite sleep-wake states
      (3) Use of some self-regulatory behaviors
      (4) Response to visual-auditory stimuli
   b. Minor defining characteristics
      None given

RELATED FACTORS[10]

1. Disorganized Infant Behavior
   a. Pain
   b. Oral or motor problems
   c. Feeding intolerance
   d. Environmental overstimulation
   e. Lack of containment or boundaries
   f. Prematurity
   g. Invasive or painful procedures
2. Risk for Disorganized Infant Behavior
   The risk factors also serve as the related factors.
3. Potential for Enhanced Organized Infant Behavior
   a. Prematurity
   b. Pain

RELATED CLINICAL CONCERNS

1. Hospitalization
2. Any invasive procedure
3. Prematurity
4. Neurologic disorders
5. Respiratory disorders
6. Cardiovascular disorders

EXPECTED OUTCOMES

1. Will return to more organized behavioral response by (date) and/or
2. Parents can verbally describe measures that assist in modifying disorganized behavior by (date)

TARGET DATES

Disorganized infant behavior is very tiring, physically and emotionally, to both the infant and parents. Therefore, the initial target date should be within 24 hours of the diagnosis. As the infant's behavior becomes more organized, target dates can be increased in increments of 72 hours.

NURSING ACTIONS/INTERVENTIONS WITH RATIONALES

Adult Health

For this diagnosis, the Child Health nursing actions serve as the generic actions. This diagnosis would probably not arise on an adult health care unit.

Child Health

ACTIONS/INTERVENTIONS	RATIONALES
• Monitor for all possible contributing factors related to infant's status, including: ○ Prenatal course ○ Birth history and Apgars ○ Known medical diagnoses ○ All genetically relevant data ○ Actual description of problem/triggering cues ○ Treatment modalities (monitors, medications, special equipment, and/or special care related)	Inclusion of all contributing factors will result in an individualized plan of care.
• Determine mother's and father's (parental) perception of infant's status. • Identify specific parameters (according to etiologic or known cause of problem) for appropriate management of infant; i.e., lab ranges and respiratory rate (ABGs) or lab range as applicable. • Evaluate parental capacity to assume caregiving role of infant by: ○ Asking parent to verbalize special care infant requires ○ Observing parent in care behaviors while still in hospital setting for appropriateness; e.g., feeding, handling, or as necessary, giving meds, suctioning, etc. ○ Assessing problem-solving skills related to infant's care, i.e., when to call for assistance ○ Risk factor analysis of total 24-h care of infant ○ Ability to identify infant's cues ○ Ability to respond to infant's cues ○ Ability to handle, emotionally and otherwise, demands of infant's status ○ Verbalization of expected prognosis or developmental potential ○ Evidence of realistic planning for respite care backup after discharging from hospital	Ultimate responsibility will better be assumed by caregiver if planning is long term and considers parental input. Treatment of condition will be enhanced with a specific, individualized plan of care. Inclusion of early childhood developmental specialist, occupational therapist, physical therapist, dietitian, home health nurse, and others as required will offer essential specialized care. Anticipatory planning will enhance likelihood of adequate timing and gradual relinquishment of care to parents or, when necessary, other primary caregivers.
• Provide anticipatory care, including positioning, in planning for feedings, if necessary with safety-mindedness as dictated by infant's status, including possibility of cardiac or respiratory arrest. • Provide stimulation only as tolerated by infant, to include minimal gentle touching, decreased sound, decreased light, decreased strong chemical odors, gentle suctioning of oropharynx as necessary. • Support infant in basic physiologic needs as required, including: ○ Dietary needs (p.o., g-tube, hyperal, etc.) ○ Respiratory functioning or maintenance (O₂, trach, endotracheal + ventilation + pulmonary toileting) ○ Urinary/elimination (self-toileting, diapering, Foley)	Appropriate anticipation of possible cardiac or respiratory arrest and/or related dysfunction of vital functions will best identify degree of physiologic support required to sustain infant. Protection of infant from undue environmental stressors during acute phase will decrease the possibility of increased levels or length of time when disorganized behavior is present. Support of adaptive potentials may help restore patterns of organized behavior or at least maintain a more enhanced organized behavior pattern with individualized allowances as a basis for determining effective care.

- ○ Cardiac homeostasis (self-regulatory, medication, pacemaker, monitoring)
- ○ Neuromuscular requisites (positioning in alignment, protection from injury in event of seizure, use of splints, special equipment for adaptive needs, administration of seizure meds if needed)
- ○ Communication augmentation (close and continuous observation, interpretation of cues, adaptive aids ranging from musical toys to developmentally appropriate interactive toys)
- ○ Tolerance of stimulation (satisfactory O_2 sats, ability to rest at intervals, etc.)

POTENTIAL FOR ENHANCED

- Monitor for all factors contributing to disorganized behavior that can be controlled, e.g., sounds, sights, and other stimuli.
- Develop a plan for identifying adaptation behaviors for evaluating effectiveness of current treatment and redefinition.
- Once enhancement behaviors are able to be identified, redefine plan of care to best incorporate desired behaviors to degree possible.

Inclusion of all factors contributing will most likely offer potential to influence infant's behavior on an individualized basis.
Ongoing evaluation will serve the purpose of substantiation of progress and thereby define enhancement behaviors and patterns.

NOTE: Case management becomes an issue of paramount importance with a need to keep family updated as changes occur. Also, in the event of compromise and/or ultimate death, there should be consideration for:

Spiritual Distress, Risk for
Alteration in Grieving, Risk for
Parent, Infant, Child Attachment, Altered, Risk for

all of which are related to the status of the infant.

    Also, it could be that this infant requires long-term care with allowance for acute exacerbations made worse by underlying disorganized infant behavior.

Women's Health

NOTE: This diagnosis will relate to the delivery room and the immediate postpartum period (48 to 72 hours). For further clarification beyond this period, see Child Health.

ACTIONS/INTERVENTIONS	RATIONALES

• Monitor the infant's cardiovascular and respiratory system by use of Apgar score, at 1 and 5 min after birth.
• Prepare for neonatal resuscitation by having all equipment and supplies ready. Be prepared to support neonatal staff, if available, and/or pediatrician. Support and reassure parents by keeping them informed of infant's condition.
• Support the parents of the ill neonate by being available to listen and answer questions:
  ○ Act as a liaison between NICU and the parents, assisting both parties by clarifying and explaining.
  ○ Accompany and/or transport the patient to NICU the first time, to provide guidance and support, as well as introducing them to the NICU staff.
	Apgar score is an indicator of the infant's condition at birth and provides a baseline for determining the need for appropriate interventions and neonatal resuscitation.
	If there is a compromised infant, then it is appropriate for the nurse in the delivery room to support and assist the neonatal staff in stabilizing the infant. If no neonatal staff is available, the labor-delivery staff need to be well versed in neonatal stabilization and resuscitation.
	Parents often need to verbalize what they have been told by the neonatologist and the NICU staff. This helps them cope and can provide clarification of any information they have been given. The nurse who listens can correct inaccurate perceptions and keep NICU staff informed of the parents' understanding so that they can better understand and provide support where mother and family are physically and emotionally capable.

Continued

ACTIONS/INTERVENTIONS	RATIONALES
○ If the infant is transported to another hospital, keep the mother informed by establishing contact with the NICU staff.	
○ Obtain pictures of the infant and telephone numbers so the mother can call and talk with NICU staff.	
• Monitor and document the infant's physiologic parameters during periods of reactivity:	Confidence and infant caretaking activities are increased by utilizing every opportunity to teach new parents about their newborn.
○ Assist new parents in utilizing the normal periods of reactivity in the neonate to begin breast-feeding and the parent-infant attachment process.	
○ Perform a complete physical assessment of the newborn, documenting findings in an organized manner (usually head to toe).	
○ Note and inform parents of aspects of normal newborn appearance, especially noting such items as milia, normal newborn rash, or stork bites.	
○ Explain the importance of thermoregulation, voiding patterns, and neurologic adaptations during the immediate newborn period.	
○ Practice good handwashing techniques before touching the newborn, and explain the importance of this to parents in preventing infection.	
○ Monitor the infant for ability to feed (breast or bottle), intake, output, and weight loss or gain.	
○ Encourage parent participation in the care and observation of the infant.	
○ Be available to answer questions and demonstrate techniques of baby care to new parents.	
• Prevent heat loss by immediately drying the infant and laying it on a warmed surface (best place is skin to skin with mother).	Drying decreases the incidence of iatrogenic hypothermia in the newborn. (Infant's temperature can drop as much as 2.6°C in the delivery room.)[39]

IMMEDIATE POSTPARTUM PERIOD

• Perform a gestational age assessment, and compare the infant's gestational age and weight. Based upon this exam, determine if infant is[40]:	Gestational age and the size (AGA, SGA, LGA) of the infant can affect the transition to extrauterine life.
○ Average for gestational age (AGA)	
○ Small for gestational age (SGA)	
○ Large for gestational age (LGA)	
• Review the mother's prenatal history and labor-delivery history for factors that would interfere with the normal transitional physiologic process by the neonate such as metabolic disorders (diabetes, etc., and/or use of medications, both therapeutic and abusive).	The use of drugs during labor or prenatally and maternal diseases such as diabetes may inhibit the thermoregulatory system, cardiovascular responses, or respiratory effort.[40]
• Continue to monitor the infant's vital signs frequently.	

Psychiatric Health

Mental health interventions for this diagnosis would focus on family support. Refer to the following diagnoses for care plans:

Management of Therapeutic Regimen, Families, Ineffective

Caregiver Role Strain

Family Coping, Ineffective, Compromised or Disabling

Family Coping, Potential for Growth

Parenting, Altered or Risk for

The practitioner should review the definition and defining characteristics of these diagnoses to determine which one relates to those characteristics being demonstrated by the infant's family and/or support system.

Gerontic Health

This diagnosis would probably not be used in gerontic health.

Home Health

ACTIONS/INTERVENTIONS	RATIONALES

• Assist client and family in lifestyle changes that may be required. Provide for:
  ○ Supportive environment
  ○ Consistent care provider
  ○ Appropriate stimulation
  ○ Control of pain
  ○ Understanding of normal growth and development
	Home-based care requires involvement of the family. Disorganized infant behavior can disrupt family schedules. Adjustment in family activities may be required.

• Assist family to set criteria to help them determine when additional intervention is required, for example, change in baseline physiologic measures.	Provides family background knowledge to seek appropriate assistance as need arises.
• Refer patient to appropriate assistive resources as indicated.	Additional assistance may be required for the family to care for the infant. Use of readily available resources is cost-effective.

Disorganized Infant Behavior, Actual, Risk for, Potential for Enhanced Organized

FLOWCHART EVALUATION: EXPECTED OUTCOME 1

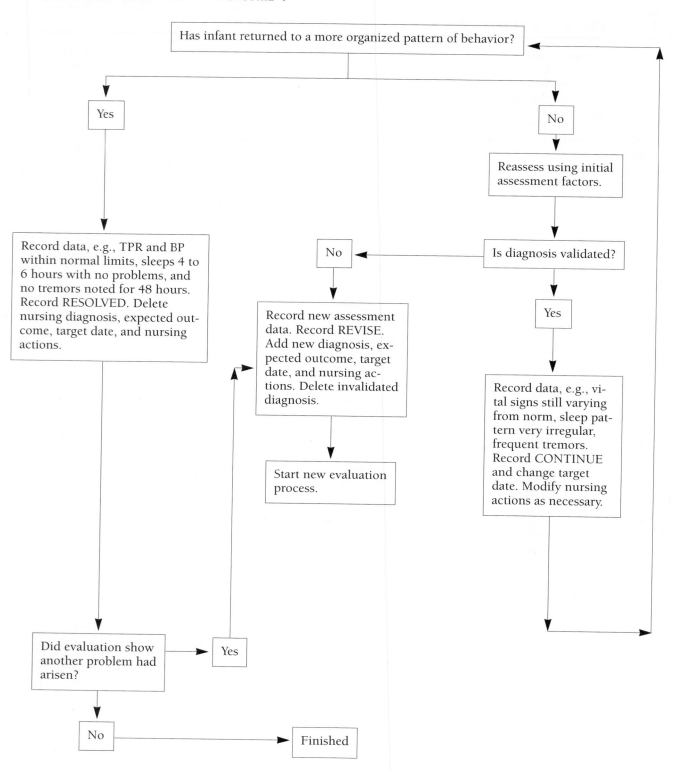

Disorganized Infant Behavior, Actual, Risk for, Potential for Enhanced Organized

FLOWCHART EVALUATION: EXPECTED OUTCOME 2

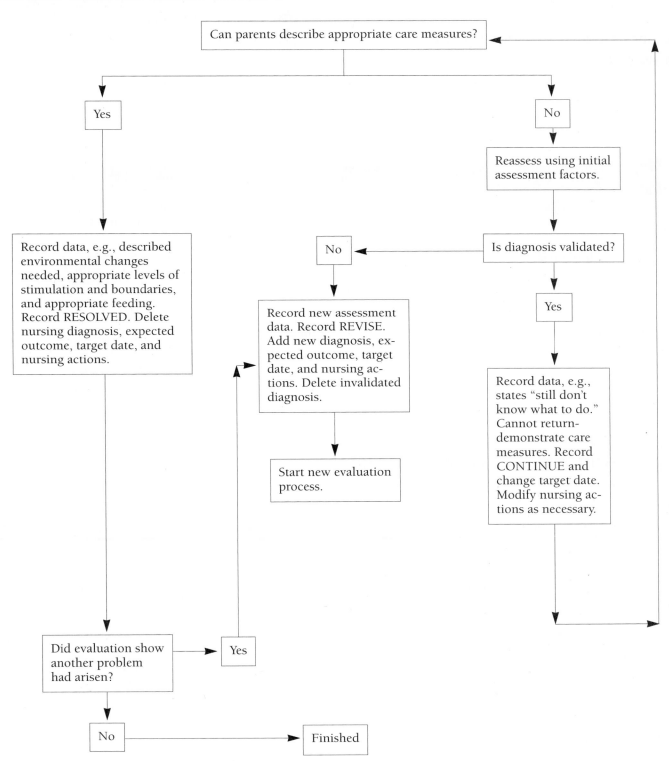

Can parents describe appropriate care measures?

Yes

No

Reassess using initial assessment factors.

Record data, e.g., described environmental changes needed, appropriate levels of stimulation and boundaries, and appropriate feeding. Record RESOLVED. Delete nursing diagnosis, expected outcome, target date, and nursing actions.

No

Is diagnosis validated?

Record new assessment data. Record REVISE. Add new diagnosis, expected outcome, target date, and nursing actions. Delete invalidated diagnosis.

Yes

Start new evaluation process.

Record data, e.g., states "still don't know what to do." Cannot return-demonstrate care measures. Record CONTINUE and change target date. Modify nursing actions as necessary.

Did evaluation show another problem had arisen?

Yes

No

Finished

Disuse Syndrome, Risk for

DEFINITION

A state in which an individual is at risk for deterioration of body systems as the result of prescribed or unavoidable musculoskeletal inactivity.[10]*

NANDA TAXONOMY: EXCHANGING 1.6.1.5

DEFINING CHARACTERISTICS[10]

1. Presence of risk factors
   a. Paralysis
   b. Mechanical immobilization
   c. Prescribed immobilization
   d. Severe pain
   e. Altered level of consciousness

RELATED FACTORS[10]

The risk factors also serve as the related factors.

RELATED CLINICAL CONCERNS

1. Cerebrovascular accident
2. Fractures
3. Closed head injury
4. Spinal cord injury or paralysis
5. Rheumatoid arthritis
6. Amputation
7. Cerebral palsy

HAVE YOU SELECTED THE CORRECT DIAGNOSIS?

Activity Intolerance   This diagnosis implies that the individual is freely able to move but cannot endure or adapt to the increased energy or oxygen demands made by the movement or activity.

Impaired Physical Mobility   With this diagnosis the individual could move independently if something was not limiting the motion. Impaired Physical Mobility could very well be a predisposing factor to Risk for Disuse Syndrome.

EXPECTED OUTCOMES

1. Will exhibit no signs or symptoms of disuse syndrome by (date) and/or
2. Will demonstrate (specify activities) to prevent development of disuse syndrome by (date)

TARGET DATES

Disuse syndrome can develop rapidly after the onset of immobilization. The initial target date, therefore, should be no more than 2 days.

NURSING ACTIONS/INTERVENTIONS WITH RATIONALES

Adult Health

ACTIONS/INTERVENTIONS	RATIONALES
• Monitor for contributing factors to pattern of disuse.	Can offset development of disuse syndrome or worsening of condition.
• According to patient's status, determine realistic potential and actual levels of functioning with regard to general physical condition: ○ Cognition ○ Mobility, head control, positioning ○ Communication, receptive and expressive, verbal or nonverbal ○ Augmentive aids for daily living	Improves planning and allows for setting of more realistic goals.
• Turn and anatomically position patient every 2 h on the (odd/even) hour.	

*Complications from immobility can include pressure ulcer, constipation, stasis of pulmonary secretions, thrombosis, urinary tract infection or retention, decreased strength or endurance, orthostatic hypotension, decreased range of joint motion, disorientation, body image disturbance, and powerlessness.

- Perform active and passive ROM exercises to all joints at least twice a shift while awake. State times here.
- Teach patient relaxation and pain reduction techniques every shift, and have patient return-demonstrate.
- Demonstrate and have patient return-demonstrate isotonic exercises.
- Encourage patient to perform isotonic exercises at least every 4 h at (state times here).
- Arrange daily activities with appropriate regard for rest as needed.
- Maintain adequate nutrition and fluid balance on daily basis.
- Orient patient to environment as necessary.
- Monitor patient and family for perceived and actual health teaching needs, including:
  - Patient's status
  - Patient's daily care
  - Equipment required for patient's care
  - Signs or symptoms to be reported to physician
  - Medication administration, instructions, and side effects
  - Plans for follow-up
- Refer to Impaired Physical Mobility for more detailed nursing actions.

Promotes circulation, prevents venous stasis, and helps to prevent thrombosis.
Relaxes muscles and promotes circulation.

Helps avoid syndrome; offsets complications of immobility.

Provides fluid and nutrients necessary for activity.

Maintains mental activity and reality.
Initiates appropriate home care planning.

Child Health

ACTIONS/INTERVENTIONS	RATIONALES
• Assist family in development of an individualized plan of care to best meet child's potential. • Assist family in identification of factors that will facilitate progress as well as those factors that may hinder progress in meeting child's potentials. List those factors here, and assist family in planning how to offset factors that hinder progress and encourage factors that facilitate progress. • Encourage patient and family to ventilate feelings that may relate to disuse problem by scheduling of 15–20 min each nursing shift for this activity. • Assist family in identification of support system for best possible follow-up care.	Family is the best source for individual preferences and needs as they can be related to the child's daily life. Identifies learning needs and reduces anxiety. Fosters a plan that can be adhered to if all involved participate in its development. Empowers family. Ventilation of feelings assists in reducing anxiety and promotes learning about condition. Promotes coordination of care and cost-effective use of already available resources.

Women's Health

This nursing diagnosis will pertain to women the same as to men. Refer to nursing actions for Risk for Activity Intolerance to meet the needs of women with the diagnosis of Risk for Disuse Syndrome.

Psychiatric Health

NOTE: The nursing actions in this section reflect the Risk for Disuse Syndrome related to mental health. This would include use of restraints and seclusion. If the inactivity is related to a physiologic or physical problem, refer to the Adult Health nursing actions.

ACTIONS/INTERVENTIONS	RATIONALES
• Attempt all other interventions before considering immobilizing the client. (See Risk for Violence, Chap. 9, for appropriate actions.)	Promotes client's perceived control and self-esteem.
• Carefully monitor client for appropriate level of restraint necessary. Immobilize the client as little as possible while still protecting the client and others.	Client safety is of primary importance while maintaining, as much as possible, client's perceived control and self-esteem.
• Obtain necessary medical orders to initiate methods that limit the client's physical mobility.	Provides protection of client's rights. This should be done in congruence with the state's legal requirements.
• Carefully explain to client in brief, concise language the reasons for initiating the intervention and what behavior must be present for the intervention to be terminated.	High levels of anxiety interfere with the client's ability to process complex information. Maintains relationship and promotes client's perceived control.
• Attempt to gain client's voluntary compliance with the intervention by explaining to client what is needed accompanied by a "show of force" (having the necessary number of staff available to force compliance if the client does not respond to the request).	Communicates to client that staff has the ability to maintain control over the situation and provides client with an opportunity to maintain perceived control and self-esteem.
• Initiate forced compliance only if there is an adequate number of staff to complete the action safely. (See Risk for Violence for a detailed description of intervention and forced compliance.)	Staff and client safety are of primary importance.
• Secure the environment the client will be in by removing harmful objects such as accessible light bulbs, sharp objects, glass objects, tight clothing, metal objects, or shower curtain rods.	Provides safe environment by removing those objects client could use to impulsively harm self.
• If client is placed in four-point restraints, maintain one-to-one supervision.	Promotes client safety and communicates maintenance of relationship while meeting security needs.
• If client is in seclusion or in bilateral restraints, observe client at least every 15 min, more frequently if agitated. (List observation schedule here.)	Assures client safety.
• Leave urinal in room with client or offer toileting every hour.	Meets client's physiologic needs and communicates respect for the individual.
• Offer client fluids every 15 min while awake.	
• Discuss with client his or her feelings about the initiation of immobility, and review at least twice a day the kinds of behavior necessary to have immobility discontinued (note behaviors here).	Promotes client's regaining control and clearly provides the client with alternative behaviors for coping.
• When checking client, let him or her know you are checking by calling him or her by name and orienting him or her to day and time. Inquire about client's feelings, and implement necessary reality orientation.	Promotes sense of security and provides information about client's mental status that will provide information for further interventions.
• Provide meals at regular intervals on paper containers, providing necessary assistance (amount and type of assistance required should be listed here).	Meets physiologic needs while maintaining client safety.
• If client is in restraints, remove restraints at least every 2 h one limb at a time. Have client move limb through a full ROM and inspect for signs of injury. Apply lubricants such as lotion to area under restraint to protect from injury.	Maintains adequate blood flow to the skin and prevents breakdown. Maintains joint mobility and prevents contractures and muscle atrophy.
• Pad the area of the restraint that is next to the skin with sheepskin or other nonirritating material.	Protects skin from mechanical irritation from the restraint.
• Check circulation in restrained limbs in the area below the restraint by observing skin color, warmth, and swelling. Restraint should not interfere with circulation.	Early assessment and intervention prevent long-term damage.
• Change client's position in bed every 2 h on the (odd/even) hour. Have client cough and deep breathe during this time.	Protects skin from ischemic and shearing pressure damage. Promotes normal clearing of airway secretions.
• Place body in proper alignment to prevent complications and injury. Use pillows for support if client's condition allows.	

- If client is in four-point restraints, place on stomach or side or elevate head of bed.

- Place client on intake and output monitoring to ensure that adequate fluid balance is maintained.

- Have client in seclusion move around the room at least every 2 h on the (odd/even) hour. During this time initiate active ROM and have client cough and take deep breaths.

- Administer medications as ordered for agitation.

- Monitor blood pressure before administering antipsychotic medications.

- Have client change position slowly, especially from lying to standing.

- Assist client with daily personal hygiene.

- Have environment cleaned on a daily basis.

- Remove client from seclusion as soon as the contracted behavior is observed for the required amount of time. (Both of these should be very specific and listed here. See Risk for Violence, Chap. 9, for detailed information on behavior change and contracting specifics.)

- Schedule time to discuss this intervention with client and his or her support systems. Inform support system of the need for the intervention and about special considerations related to visiting with the client. This information must be provided with consideration of the support system before and after each visit.

Prevents aspiration or choking.

Promotes normal hydration, which prevents thickening of airway secretions and thrombus formation.[41]
Assesses client's risk for the development of orthostatic hypotension.

The combination of immobility and antipsychotic medications can place the client at risk for the development of orthostatic hypotension. Slowing position change allows time for blood pressure to adjust and prevents dizziness and fainting.
Gives client a sense of control.
Communicates respect for the client.
Promotes client's perception of control and provides positive reinforcement for appropriate behavior.

Promotes family understanding and optimizes potential for positive client response.[30]

Gerontic Health

ACTIONS/INTERVENTIONS	RATIONALES
• Monitor for iatrogenesis, especially in the case of institutionalized elderly.	Although OBRA regulations require the least restrictive measures and ideally restraint-free care, older adults in long-term care may be placed at risk for disuse syndrome secondary to geri-chairs, use of wheelchairs, and lack of properly functioning or fitted adaptive equipment. Additionally, there may be reluctance to prescribe occupational therapy or physical therapy based on costs.
• Advocate for older adults to ensure inactivity is not based on ageist perspectives.	Health care providers may be reluctant to ensure early mobilization of older patients, especially of the old-old clientele.
• In the event of impaired cognitive function, remind patient of the need for and assist the patient (or caregiver) in mobilizing efforts.	Prompting may encourage increased activity and decrease the risk for disuse.

Home Health

ACTIONS/INTERVENTIONS	RATIONALES

• Teach client and family appropriate monitoring of causes, signs, and symptoms of Risk for Disuse Syndrome:
  ○ Prolonged bedrest
  ○ Circulatory or respiratory problems
  ○ New activity
  ○ Fatigue
  ○ Dyspnea
  ○ Pain
  ○ Vital signs (before and after activity)
  ○ Malnutrition
  ○ Previous inactivity
  ○ Weakness
  ○ Confusion
  ○ Fracture
  ○ Paralysis
	Provides for early recognition and intervention for problem.

• Assist client and family in identifying lifestyle changes that may be required:
  ○ Progressive exercise to increase endurance
  ○ ROM and flexibility exercise
  ○ Treatments for underlying conditions (cardiac, respiratory, musculoskeletal, circulatory, neurologic, etc.)
  ○ Motivation
  ○ Assistive devices as required (walkers, canes, crutches, wheelchairs, ramps, wheelchair access, etc.)
  ○ Adequate nutrition
  ○ Adequate fluids
  ○ Stress management
  ○ Pain relief
  ○ Prevention of hazards of immobility (e.g., antiembolism stockings, ROM exercises, position changes)
  ○ Changes in occupations, family, or social roles
  ○ Changes in living conditions
  ○ Economic concerns
  ○ Proper transfer techniques
  ○ Bowel and bladder regulation
	Provides basic information for client and family that promotes necessary lifestyle changes.

• Teach client and family purposes and side effects of medications and proper administration techniques (e.g., anticoagulants or analgesics). • Assist client and family to set criteria to help them to determine when physician or other intervention is required.	Locus of control shifts from nurse to client and family, thus promoting self-care.
• Consult with or refer patient to appropriate resources as indicated.	Provides additional support for client and family and uses already available resources in a cost-effective manner.

Disuse Syndrome, Risk for

FLOWCHART EVALUATION: EXPECTED OUTCOME 1

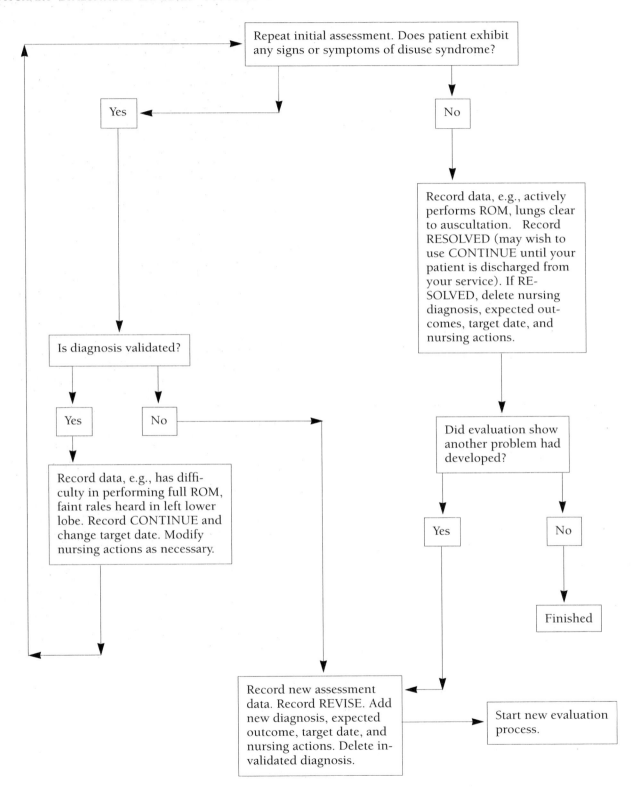

Disuse Syndrome, Risk for

FLOWCHART EVALUATION: EXPECTED OUTCOME 2

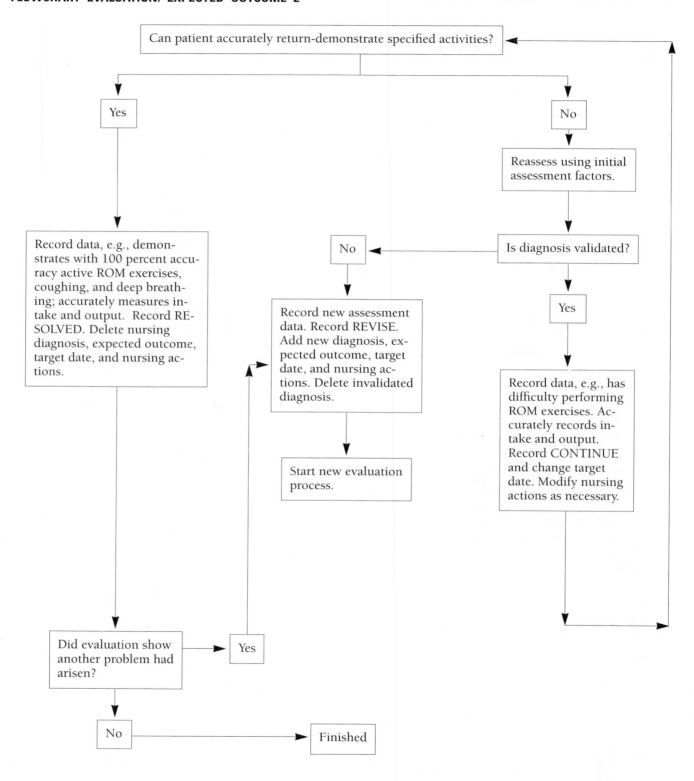

Diversional Activity Deficit

DEFINITION

The state in which an individual experiences a decreased stimulation from (or interest or engagement in) recreational or leisure activities.[10]

NANDA TAXONOMY: MOVING 6.3.1.1

DEFINING CHARACTERISTICS[10]

1. Major defining characteristics
   a. Patient's statements regarding boredom (wish there was something to do, to read, etc.)
   b. Usual hobbies not able to be undertaken in hospital
2. Minor defining characteristics
   None given

RELATED FACTORS[10]

1. Environmental lack of diversional activity, as in:
   a. Long-term hospitalization
   b. Frequent lengthy treatments

RELATED CLINICAL CONCERNS

Any medical diagnosis that could be connected to the related factors.

HAVE YOU SELECTED THE CORRECT DIAGNOSIS?

Activity Intolerance   If the nurse observes or validates reports of the patient's inability to complete required tasks because of insufficient energy, then Activity Intolerance is the appropriate diagnosis, not Diversional Activity Deficit.

Impaired Physical Mobility   When the patient has difficulty with coordination, range of motion, or muscle strength and control or has activity restrictions related to treatment, the most appropriate diagnosis is Impaired Physical Mobility. Diversional Activity Deficit is quite likely to be a companion diagnosis to Impaired Physical Mobility.

Social Isolation   This diagnosis should be considered if the patient demonstrates limited contact with community, peers, and significant others. When patient talks of loneliness rather than boredom, Social Isolation is the more appropriate diagnosis.

Sensory-Perceptual Alteration   This diagnosis would be best if the patient is unable to engage in his or her usual leisure-time activities due to loss or impairment of one of the senses.

EXPECTED OUTCOMES

1. Will have decreased number of complaints regarding boredom by (date) and/or
2. Will assist in designing and implementing a plan to overcome diversional activity deficit by (date)

TARGET DATES

Planning and accessing resources will require a moderate amount of time. A reasonable target date would be within 2 to 3 days.

NURSING ACTIONS/INTERVENTIONS WITH RATIONALES

Adult Health

ACTIONS/INTERVENTIONS	RATIONALES
• On admission, assist patient to review activity likes and dislikes.	Finds the activities the patient would most likely engage in.
• When this diagnosis is made, move patient to semiprivate room if possible and if patient is amenable to move.	Provides companionship, social interaction, and diversion.
• Encourage patient to discuss feelings regarding deficit and causes at least once per day at (time).	Helps patient identify feelings and begin to deal with them.
• Involve patient, to extent possible, in more daily self-care activities.	Increases self-worth and adequacy.

Continued

ACTIONS/INTERVENTIONS	RATIONALES
• Alter daily routine (e.g., bathe at different times or increase ambulation).	Creates change and provides some diversion.

• Rearrange environment as needed:
  ◦ Provide ample light.
  ◦ Place bed near window.
  ◦ Provide radio as well as television set.
  ◦ Place books, games, etc., within easy reach.
  ◦ Provide clear pathway for wheelchair, ambulations, etc.
  ◦ Move furniture.
	Facilitates activity.

• Provide change of environment at least twice a day at (times), e.g., out of room to sun deck or outside building. Add posters to room decor.	Creates change and broadens range of activities.

• Encourage significant others to assist in decreasing deficit:
  ◦ Bringing books, games, or hobby materials
  ◦ Visiting more frequently
  ◦ Encouraging other visitors
  ◦ Bringing a box of wrapped small items, one to be opened each day, e.g., paperback book, crossword puzzles, small jigsaw puzzle, or small handheld games
	Reinforces "normal" lifestyle, and encourages feelings of self-worth.

• Provide for appropriate adaptations in equipment or positioning to facilitate desired diversional activity.	
• Provide for scheduling of diversional activity at a time when patient is rested and without multiple interruptions.	
• Refer patient to individual health care practitioners who can best assist with problem.	

Child Health

ACTIONS/INTERVENTIONS	RATIONALES

• Monitor patient's potential for activity or diversion according to:
  ◦ Attention span
  ◦ Physical limitations and tolerance
  ◦ Cognitive, sensory, and perceptual deficits
  ◦ Preferences for gender, age, and interests
  ◦ Available resources
  ◦ Safety needs
  ◦ Pain
	Provides essential database for planning desired and achievable diversion.

• Encourage parental input in planning and implementing desired diversional activity plan. • Allow for peer interaction when appropriate through diversional activity.	Helps ensure that plan is attentive to child's interests, thus increasing the likelihood of the child's participation. Involvement of peers serves to foster self-esteem and meets developmental socialization needs.

Women's Health

NOTE: The following refers to those women placed on restrictive activities because of threatened abortions, premature labor, multiple pregnancy, or pregnancy-induced hypertension.

ACTIONS/INTERVENTIONS	RATIONALES
• Encourage family and significant others to participate in plan of care for patient.	Promotes socialization, empowers family, and provides opportunities for teaching.
• Encourage patient to list lifestyle adjustments that need to be made as well as ways to accomplish these adjustments.	Basic problem-solving technique that encourages patient to participate in care. Will increase understanding of current condition.
• Teach patient relaxation skills and coping mechanisms.	
• Maintain proper body alignment with use of positioning and pillows.	
• Provide diversional activities:	Provides a variety of options to offset deficit.
○ Hobbies, e.g., needlework, reading, painting, or television	
○ Job-related activities as tolerated (that can be done in bed), e.g., reading, writing, or telephone conferences	
○ Activities with children, e.g., reading to child, painting or coloring with child, allowing child to "help" mother (bringing water to mother or assisting in fixing meals for mother)	
○ Encourage help and visits from friends and relatives, e.g., visit in person, telephone visit, help with childcare, or help with housework	

Psychiatric Health

ACTIONS/INTERVENTIONS	RATIONALES
• Assess source of diversional activity deficit. Is the nursing unit appropriately stimulating for the level or type of clients, or is the problem the client's perceptions?	Recognizes the impact of physical space on the client's mood.
NURSING UNIT–RELATED PROBLEMS	
• Develop milieu therapy program:	
○ Include seasonal activities for clients such as parties, special meals, outings, or games.	Promotes here-and-now orientation and interpersonal interactions.
○ Alter unit environment by changing pictures, adding appropriate seasonal decorations, updating bulletin boards, or cleaning and updating furniture.	Enhances the aesthetics of the environment and has a positive effect on the client's mood.[22]
○ Alter mood of unit with bright colors, seasonal flowers, or appropriate music.	Colors and sounds impact the client's mood.[22]
○ Develop group activities for clients such as team sports, Ping-Pong, bingo games, activity planning groups, meal planning groups, meal preparation groups, current events discussion groups, book discussion groups, exercise groups, or craft groups.	Provides opportunities to build social skills and alternative methods of coping.
○ Decrease emphasis on television as primary unit activity.	Television does not provide opportunities for learning alternative coping skills and decreases physical activity.
○ Provide books, newspapers, records, tapes, and craft materials.	These resources assist the client in meeting belonging needs by facilitating interaction with others on the unit and the world around him or her.
○ Use community service organizations to provide programs for clients.	Provides varied sensory stimulation.
• Collaborate with occupational therapist for ideas regarding activities and supplies.	
• Collaborate with physical therapist regarding physical exercise program.	

Continued

ACTIONS/INTERVENTIONS	RATIONALES
CLIENT PERCEPTION–RELATED PROBLEMS	
• Discuss with client past activities, reviewing those that have been enjoyed and those that have been tried and not enjoyed.	Promotes client's sense of control.
• List those activities that the client has enjoyed in the past with information about what keeps client from doing them at this time.	
• Monitor client's energy level and develop activity that corresponds to client's energy level and physiologic needs. For example, manic client may be bored with playing cards and yet physiologic needs require less physical activity than the client may desire, so an appropriate activity would address both these needs. Note assessment decision here.	Promotes development of alternative coping behaviors by assisting client in choosing appropriate activities.
• Develop with client a plan for reinitiating a previously enjoyed activity. Note that plan here.	Promotes client's sense of control.
• Develop time in the daily schedule for that activity, and note that time here.	
• Relate activity to enjoyable time such as a time for interaction with the nurse alone or interaction with other clients in a group area.	Interaction can provide positive reinforcement for engaging in activity.
• Provide positive verbal feedback to client about his or her efforts at the activity.	Positive verbal reinforcement encourages appropriate coping behaviors.
• Assist client in obtaining necessary items to implement activity, and list necessary items here.	Facilitate appropriate coping behaviors.
• Develop plan with client to attempt one new activity—one that has been interesting for him or her but which he or she has not had time or direction to pursue. Note plan and rewards for accomplishing goals here.	Promotes client's perceived control and provides positive reinforcement for the behavior.
• Have client set realistic goals for activity involvement (e.g., one cannot paint like a professional in the beginning).	Promotes client's strengths and self-esteem.
• Discuss feelings of frustration, anger, and discomfort that may occur as client attempts a new activity.	Verbalization of feelings and thoughts provides opportunities for developing alternative coping strategies.
• Frame mistakes as positive tools of learning new behavior.	Promotes client's strengths.

Gerontic Health

ACTIONS/INTERVENTIONS	RATIONALES
• Ask patient if activities were decreased prior to hospitalization.	If decreased activities were noted prior to admission, there may be ongoing problems that are not related to the acute care setting.
• Provide at least 10–15 min per shift, while awake, to engage in reminiscing with patient.	Increases self-esteem and focuses on strengths the patient has developed over his or her lifetime.[42]

Home Health

ACTIONS/INTERVENTIONS	RATIONALES
• Monitor factors contributing to diversional activity deficit.	Provides database for prevention and/or early intervention.

• Involve client and family in planning, implementing, and promoting reduction in diversional activity deficit:
  ○ Family conference
  ○ Mutual goal setting
  ○ Communication
	Involvement improves motivation and improves the outcome.

• Assist client and family in lifestyle adjustments that may be required:
  ○ Time management
  ○ Work, family, social, and personal goals and priorities
  ○ Rehabilitation
  ○ Learning new skills or games
  ○ Development of support systems
  ○ Stress management techniques
  ○ Drug and alcohol use
	Provides basic information for client and family that promotes necessary lifestyle changes.

• Refer patient to appropriate assistive resources as indicated.	Provides additional support for client and family and uses already available resources in a cost-effective manner.

Diversional Activity Deficit

FLOWCHART EVALUATION: EXPECTED OUTCOME 1

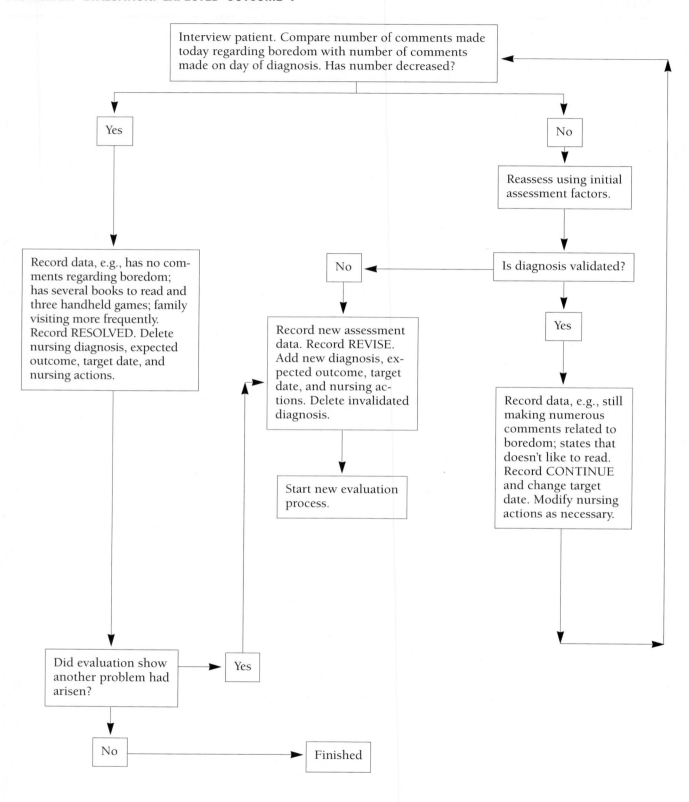

Diversional Activity Deficit

FLOWCHART EVALUATION: EXPECTED OUTCOME 2

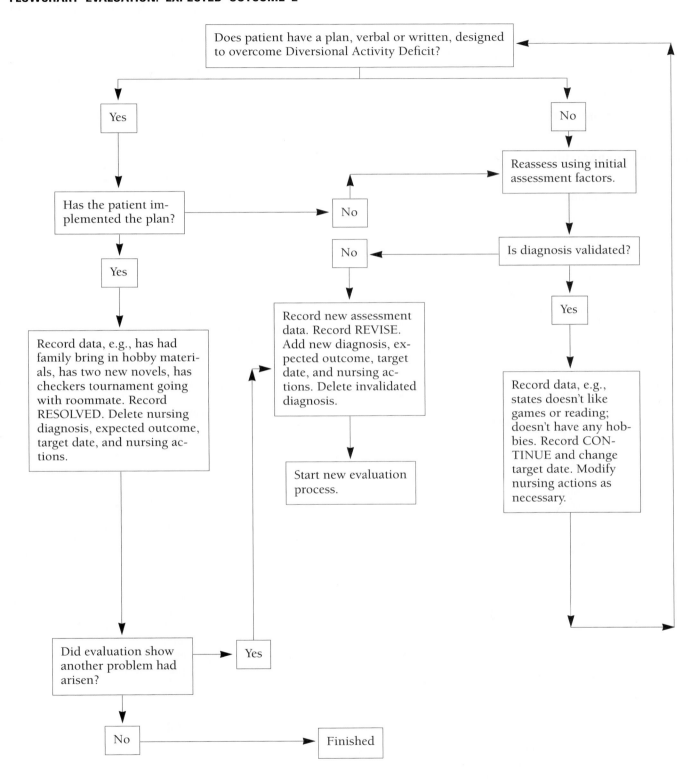

Dysfunctional Ventilatory Weaning Response (DVWR)

DEFINITION

A state in which a patient cannot adjust to lowered levels of mechanical ventilator support, which interrupts and prolongs the weaning response.[10]

NANDA TAXONOMY: EXCHANGING 1.5.1.3.2

DEFINING CHARACTERISTICS[10]

1. Mild DVWR
   a. Major defining characteristics
      (1) Responds to lowered levels of mechanical ventilator support with:
         (a) Restlessness
         (b) Slight increased respiratory rate from baseline
   b. Minor defining characteristics
      (1) Responds to lowered levels of mechanical ventilator support with:
         (a) Expressed feelings of increased need for oxygen
         (b) Breathing discomfort
         (c) Fatigue
         (d) Warmth
         (e) Queries about possible machine malfunction
         (f) Increased concentration on breathing
2. Moderate DVWR
   a. Major defining characteristics
      (1) Responds to lowered levels of mechanical ventilator support with:
         (a) Slight increase from baseline blood pressure <20 mm Hg
         (b) Slight increase from baseline heart rate <20 beats per minute
         (c) Baseline increase in respiratory rate <5 breaths per minute
   b. Minor defining characteristics
      (1) Hypervigilance to activities
      (2) Inability to respond to coaching
      (3) Inability to cooperate
      (4) Apprehension
      (5) Diaphoresis
      (6) Eye widening, "wide-eyed look"
      (7) Decreased air entry on auscultation
      (8) Color changes
      (9) Pale; slight cyanosis
      (10) Slight respiratory accessory muscle use
3. Severe DVWR
   a. Major defining characteristics
      (1) Responds to lowered levels of mechanical ventilator support with:
         (a) Agitation
         (b) Deterioration in arterial blood gases from current baseline
         (c) Increase from baseline blood pressure >20 mm Hg
         (d) Increase from baseline heart rate >20 beats per minute
         (e) Respiratory rate increased significantly from baseline
   b. Minor defining characteristics
      (1) Profuse diaphoresis
      (2) Full respiratory accessory muscle use
      (3) Shallow, gasping breaths
      (4) Paradoxical abdominal breathing
      (5) Discoordinated breathing with the ventilator
      (6) Decreased level of consciousness
      (7) Adventitious breath sounds
      (8) Audible airway secretion
      (9) Cyanosis

RELATED FACTORS[10]

1. Physical
   a. Ineffective airway clearance
   b. Sleep pattern disturbance
   c. Inadequate nutrition
   d. Uncontrolled pain or discomfort
2. Psychological
   a. Knowledge deficit of the weaning process and patient's role
   b. Patient-perceived inefficacy about the ability to wean
   c. Decreased motivation
   d. Decreased self-esteem
   e. Anxiety (moderate or severe)
   f. Fear
   g. Hopelessness
   h. Powerlessness
   i. Insufficient trust of the nurse
3. Situational
   a. Uncontrolled episodic energy demands or problems
   b. Inappropriate pacing of diminished ventilator support
   c. Inadequate social support
   d. Adverse environment (noisy, active environment, negative events in the room, low nurse-patient ratio, extended nurse absence from bedside, or unfamiliar nursing staff)
   e. History of ventilator dependence >1 week
   f. History of multiple unsuccessful weaning attempts

RELATED CLINICAL CONCERNS

1. Closed head injury
2. Coronary bypass
3. Respiratory arrest
4. Cardiac arrest
5. Cardiac transplant

Ineffective Breathing Pattern   In this diagnosis the patient's respiratory effort is insufficient to maintain the cellular oxygen supply. This diagnosis would contribute to the patient's being placed on ventilatory assistance; however, DVWR occurs after the patient has been placed on a ventilator and efforts are being made to reestablish a regular respiratory pattern. The key difference is whether or not a ventilator has been involved in the patient's therapy.

Impaired Gas Exchange   This diagnosis refers to the exchange of oxygen and carbon dioxide in the lungs or at the cellular level. This probably has been a problem for the patient and is one of the reasons the patient was placed on a ventilator. DVWR would develop after the patient had received treatment for the impaired gas exchange via the use of a ventilator.

EXPECTED OUTCOMES

1. Will be able to stay off the ventilator for at least (number) minutes by (date) and/or
2. Will be weaned from the ventilator by (date)

TARGET DATES

Initial target dates should be in terms of hours as the patient is going through the weaning process. As the patient improves, the target date could be expressed in increasing intervals from 1 to 3 days.

NURSING ACTIONS/INTERVENTIONS WITH RATIONALES

Adult Health

ACTIONS/INTERVENTIONS	RATIONALES
• Coach patient to take maximum inspiration and then to exhale all the air that he or she can. Check vital capacity measures (should be at least 10 mL/kg).	Encourages patient to initiate respiration.
• Measure inspiratory force with pressure manometer (the force needed to optimize successful weaning is -20 to -30).	Measures respiratory muscle strength.
• Assess PaO_2 (should be 60 or greater at 40% oxygen) and O_2 saturation (with pulse oximeter—should be equal to or more than 94).	Indicates amount of oxygen in alveoli.
• Determine positive end-expiratory pressure (PEEP). Physiologic PEEP is generally 5 cm of water.	PEEP should be sufficient to prevent collapse of alveoli.
• Assess tidal volume. Should be at least 3 mL/kg.	Essential for maintenance of adequate ventilation.
• Assess vital signs and respiratory pattern during weaning.	Essential monitoring of changes in respiratory effort and oxygenation.
• Use weaning technique ordered by physician (T-Piece or IMV technique).	
• Plan goals for weaning, and explain weaning procedure. Start weaning process at scheduled time off ventilator. Stay with patient during weaning process. Stop weaning process before patient becomes exhausted.	Ensures continuous monitoring of weaning success. Enables nurse to be able to place patient back on ventilator as soon as necessary.
• Reassure the patient that you are there in case of problems and that he or she can breathe on his or her own.	Instills trust, decreases anxiety, and increases motivation.
• If unable to wean while patient is still in the hospital, assess resources and support systems at home. Refer patient to home health or public health department at least 3 days prior to discharge.	Coordinates team efforts and allows sufficient planning time for home care.

Child Health

ACTIONS/INTERVENTIONS	RATIONALES

• Monitor for all contributing factors as applicable[43]:
  ◦ Pathophysiologic health concerns, e.g., infections, anemia, fever, or pain
  ◦ Previous respiratory history, especially risk indicators of reactive airway disease and bronchopulmonary dysplasia
  ◦ Previous cardiovascular history, especially risk indicators such as increased or decreased pulmonary blood flow associated with congenital deficits
  ◦ Previous neurologic status
  ◦ Recent surgical procedures
  ◦ Current medication regimen
  ◦ Psychological and emotional stability of parents as well as child
	Provides a database that will assist in generating the most individualized plan of care.

• Determine respirator parameters that suggest readiness to begin weaning process.[44] Collaborate with physician, respiratory therapist, and other health care team members:
  ◦ Spontaneous respirations for age, e.g., rate or depth
  ◦ Oxygen saturations in normal range for condition, e.g., spontaneous tidal volume of 5 mL/kg body weight, vital capacity per Wright Respirometer of 10 mL/kg body weight, effective oxygenation with PEEP of 4–6 cm of water. An exception to the normals would exist if an infant had transposition of the great vessels.
  ◦ Blood gases in normal range
  ◦ Stable vital signs
  ◦ Parental or patient anxiety regarding respirator
  ◦ Patient's facial expression and ability to rest
  ◦ Resolution of the precipitating cause for intubation and mechanical support
  ◦ Tolerance of suctioning and ambuing
  ◦ Central nervous system and cardiovascular stability
  ◦ Nutritional status, muscle strength, pain, drug-induced respiratory expression, or sleep deprivation
	Specific ventilator-related criteria will offer the best decision-making support for determining the best plan of ventilator weaning.

NOTE: Oxygen saturation, blood gases, and vital signs may be abnormal secondary to chronic lung damage with accompanying hypoxemia and hypercapnia, but the pH may be normal with metabolic compensation for chronic respiratory acidosis. In this instance acceptable ranges would be defined.

ACTIONS/INTERVENTIONS	RATIONALES
• Provide constant one-on-one attention to the patient, and focus primarily on cardiorespiratory needs. Have CPR backup equipment readily available.	Hierarchy of needs for oxygenation must be met for all vital functions to be effective in homeostasis. Anticipatory safety for a patient on a ventilator demands backup equipment in case of failure of the current equipment. Expression of feelings will assist in monitoring family concerns and help reduce anxiety.
• Monitor the anxiety levels of the patient and family at least once per shift.	Assists in further planning for weaning.

• Monitor patient's specific parameters during actual attempts at weaning:
  ◦ Arterial blood gases
  ◦ Vital signs
  ◦ Chest sounds
  ◦ Pulse oximetry
  ◦ Chest x-ray
  ◦ Hematocrit	

• Provide teaching as appropriate for patient and family with emphasis on the often slow pace of weaning.	Assessment and individualized learning needs allow appropriate focus on the patient. Explanation regarding the slow pace encourages a feeling of success rather than failure when each session does not meet the same time limits as the previous session.
• Provide attention to the rising of related emotional problems secondary to the association of ventilators with terminal life-support.	With the need to implement intubation and ventilation there can arise a myriad of concerns regarding the patient's prognosis.
• Refer patient for long-term follow-up as needed.	Fosters long-term support and coping with care at home.
• Administer medications as ordered with appropriate attention to preparation for weaning, e.g., careful use of paralytic agents or narcotics.	The best chance for successful weaning includes appropriate consciousness, no respiratory depression, and adequate neuromuscular strength. Special caution must be taken in positioning the patient receiving neuromuscular blocking agents so that dislocation of joints does not arise.[45]
• Maintain a neutral thermal environment.	Altered oxygenation and metabolic needs occur in instances of hyperthermia and hypothermia.
• Provide parents the option to participate in care as permitted.	Family input offers emotional input and security for the child in times of great stress, thereby allowing for growth in parent-child coping behaviors.
• Communicate with infant or child using age-appropriate methods, e.g., an infant will enjoy soft music, familiar voice while an older child may be able to use a small magic slate or point to key terms.	Effective communication serves to allow for expression of or reception of messages of cares or concerns, thereby acknowledging value of the patient.

Women's Health

The nursing actions for Women's Health with this diagnosis are the same as those for Adult Health.

Psychiatric Health

This diagnosis is not appropriate for the mental health care unit.

Gerontic Health

ACTIONS/INTERVENTIONS	RATIONALES

• Monitor patient for presence of factors that make weaning difficult such as[46]:
  ○ Poor nutritional status
  ○ Infection
  ○ Sleep disturbances
  ○ Pain
  ○ Poor positioning
  ○ Large amounts of secretions
  ○ Bowel problems
	These factors can significantly contribute to a delay in the weaning process.

• Ensure that communication efforts are enhanced by the proper use of sensory aids such as glasses, hearing aids, or adequate light, and decrease the noise level in room, speak in a low-pitched tone of voice, and face patient when speaking. If written instructions are used, make sure that they are brief, jargon free, printed or written in dark ink, and printed or written in large letters.	Effective communication is critical to success of weaning efforts. Lack of information or misinterpreted information may result in increased anxiety and decreased weaning success.
• Maintain same staff assignments whenever possible.[47]	Facilitates communication and decreases anxiety and fear caused by unfamiliarity with caregivers.
• Contract with patient for short-term and long-term weaning goals, providing reinforcements and rewards for progress. Use wall chart or diary to record progress.	

Home Health

Clients are discharged to the home health setting with ventilators; however, the nursing care required is the same as those actions covered in Adult Health and Gerontic Health.

Dysfunctional Ventilatory Weaning Response (DVWR)

FLOWCHART EVALUATION: EXPECTED OUTCOME 1

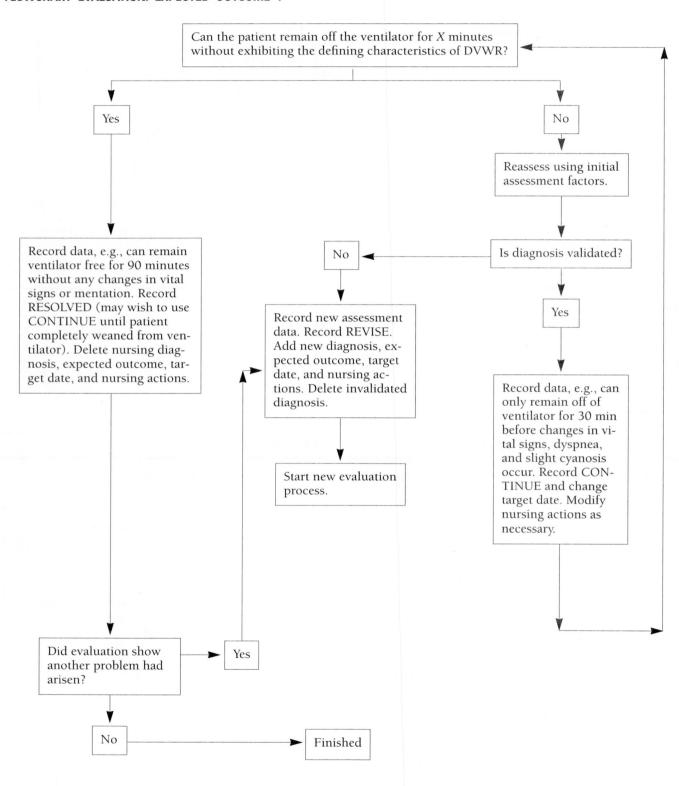

Dysfunctional Ventilatory Weaning Response (DVWR)

FLOWCHART EVALUATION: EXPECTED OUTCOME 2

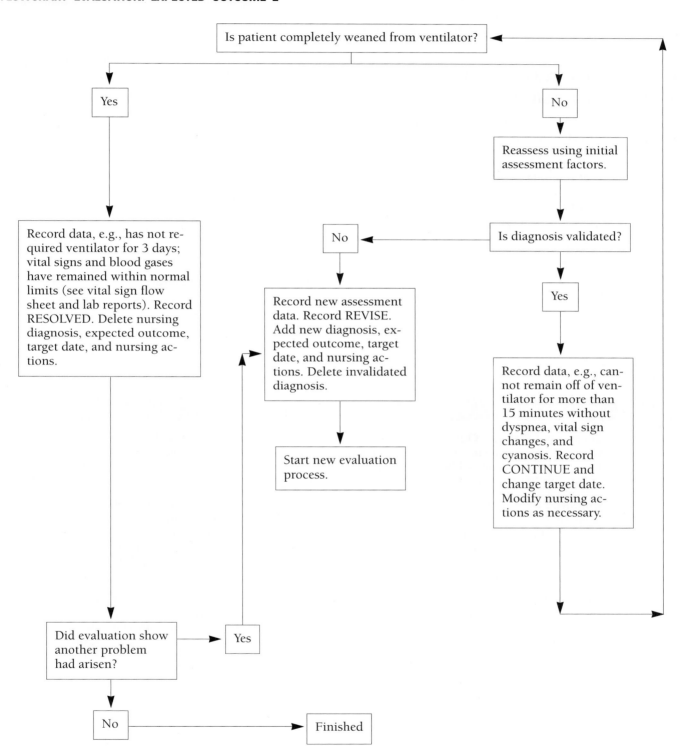

Dysreflexia

DEFINITION

The state in which an individual with a spinal cord injury at T7 or above experiences a life-threatening uninhibited sympathetic response of the nervous system to a noxious stimulus.[10]

NANDA TAXONOMY: EXCHANGING 1.2.3.1

DEFINING CHARACTERISTICS[10]

1. Major defining characteristics for individual with spinal cord injury (T7 or above) with:
   a. Paroxysmal hypertension (sudden periodic elevated blood pressure where systolic pressure is over 140 mm Hg and diastolic is above 90 mm Hg)
   b. Bradycardia or tachycardia (pulse rate of less than 60 or over 100 beats per minute)
   c. Diaphoresis (above the injury)
   d. Red splotches on skin (above the injury)
   e. Pallor (below the injury)
   f. Headache (a diffuse pain in different portions of the head and not confined to any nerve distribution area)

2. Minor defining characteristics:
   a. Chilling
   b. Conjunctival congestion
   c. Horner's syndrome (contraction of the pupil, partial ptosis of the eyelid, enophthalmus and sometimes loss of sweating over the affected side of the face)
   d. Paresthesia
   e. Pilomotor reflex (gooseflesh formation when skin is cooled)
   f. Blurred vision
   g. Chest pain
   h. Metallic taste in mouth
   i. Nasal congestion

RELATED FACTORS[10]

1. Bladder distention
2. Bowel distention
3. Skin irritation
4. Lack of patient and caregiver knowledge

RELATED CLINICAL CONCERNS

1. Spinal cord injury at T7 or above

HAVE YOU SELECTED THE CORRECT DIAGNOSIS?

Decreased Cardiac Output   Dysreflexia occurs only in spinal cord–injured patients and represents an emergency situation that requires immediate intervention. Decreased Cardiac Output may be suspected because of the changes in blood pressure or arrhythmias[48,49]; but if the patient has a spinal cord injury at T7 or above, Dysreflexia should be considered first.

Impaired Skin Integrity   Occasionally symptoms of Dysreflexia are precipitated by skin lesions such as pressure sores and ingrown or infected nails.[50] If the patient has a spinal cord injury at T7 or above in combination with impaired skin integrity, the nurse must be extremely alert to the possible development of Dysreflexia. In addition, one of the defining characteristics of Dysreflexia is red splotches which could lead to a misdiagnosis of Risk for Impaired Skin Integrity.

Urinary Retention   Dysreflexia should be suspected in patients with spinal cord injuries at T7 or above who experience bladder spasms, bladder distention, or untoward responses to urinary catheter insertion or irrigation.[50,51] Bowel distention or rectal stimulation may also lead to Dysreflexia.

EXPECTED OUTCOMES

1. Will have no signs or symptoms of Dysreflexia by (date) and/or
2. Will actively cooperate in care plan to prevent development of Dysreflexia by (date)

TARGET DATES

Dysreflexia is a life-threatening response. For this reason, the target date should be expressed in hours on a daily basis.

NURSING ACTIONS/INTERVENTIONS WITH RATIONALES

Adult Health

ACTIONS/INTERVENTIONS	RATIONALES
• Monitor vital signs, especially BP, every 3–5 min until stable; then every hour for 24 h; then every 2 h for 24 h; then every 4 h around the clock.	Extreme rises in BP are indicative of sympathetic nervous system stimulation and may lead to cerebrovascular accident and cardiac problems.
• Immediately locate source that may have triggered dysreflexia, e.g., bladder distention (76–90% of all instances), bowel distention (8% of all instances),[52–54] fractures, acute abdomen, narcotic withdrawal, pressure ulcers, childbirth, sunburn, invasive procedures below the level of the spinal cord injury, ingrown toenails, and poor patient positioning.	Finding precipitating causes prevents worsening of condition and allows further prevention of dysreflexia.
• Explain to patient reasons for procedures.	Reduces anxiety.
• Empty bladder slowly with straight catheter (**do not** use Crede's or tap bladder[52,53]), or manually remove impacted feces from rectum as soon as possible.	Alleviates precipitating causes.
• Elevate head of bed 90 degrees immediately if not contraindicated by spinal injury.	Creates orthostatic hypotension.
• Send urine specimen to lab for culture and sensitivity.	Assists in determining if infection is a possible cause of episode.
• Collaborate with physician regarding the administration of emergency antihypertensive therapy.	Facilitates lowering of BP; encourages teamwork.
• Keep patient warm; avoid chilling at all times.	Decreases sensory nervous stimulation.
• Monitor intake and output every hour for 48 h, then every 2 h for 48 h; then every 4 h. Note time schedule and dates here.	Monitors adequate functioning of bowel and bladder, which are common causative factors for dysreflexia.
• Collaborate with physician regarding daily monitoring of electrolyte balance.	Maintains fluid balance and prevents complications that could impact cardiovascular functioning.
• Turn, cough, and deep breathe patient every 2 h on the (odd/even) hour; keep in anatomic alignment.	Alleviates precipitating causes.
• Perform ROM (active or passive) exercises every 4 h while awake at (times). Pad bony prominences.	Alleviates precipitating causes; stimulates circulation and muscular activity; decreases incidence of pressure ulcers.
• Instruct patient on isotonic exercises. Encourage patient to perform isotonic exercises at least every 2 h on (odd/even) hour.	Increases circulation and prevents complications of immobility.
• Instruct patient on bladder and bowel conditioning. Monitor for bladder and bowel distention every 4 h at (times).	Eliminates the two primary precipitating causes.
• Catheterize as necessary; use rectal tube if not contraindicated to assist with flatus reduction.	Eliminates precipitating causes.
• Provide appropriate skin care each time patient is turned. Monitor skin integrity at least once per shift at (times).	Prevents and monitors for pressure ulcers.
• Maintain adequate food and fluid balance on a daily basis.	Assists in avoiding constipation.
• Involve family in care such as positioning, feeding, and exercising.	Assists in teaching and preparing of family for home care.
• Be consistent and supportive in approach.	Decreases anxiety and instills confidence in caregivers.
• Use abdominal binders and antiembolic stockings as needed.	Assists in preventing precipitating causes through providing cardiovascular support.
• Administer medications as required.	Medication therapy is generally instituted to help control BP, control heart rate, and block excessive autonomic nerve transmission.
• Encourage family to use community resources. Make referrals as soon as possible after admission.	Cost-effective use of available resources; provides long-range support for patient and family.

Child Health

ACTIONS/INTERVENTIONS	RATIONALES
• Administer medications as required to help control the blood pressure at appropriate levels for age and weight. • Monitor the pulse as needed and BP every 5 min until stable. Determine parameters for the patient according to the norms for age, site, and condition. • Monitor family's understanding and perception of the problem. Ensure that proper attention is paid to the family's needs for support during this emergency phase. • Teach patient, as capable, and family routine for care including the prevention of infection (particularly urinary and integumentary).	Assists in preventing seizures and provides appropriate intervention to maintain pressure within desired ranges. Basic monitoring for initial indications of problem development. Assists in preventing misunderstandings and will assist in identifying learning needs. Education enhances care and provides an opportunity for care to be practiced in a supportive environment.

Women's Health

> **NOTE:** This nursing diagnosis will pertain to women the same as to any other adult. The following precautions should be taken when the victim is pregnant.

ACTIONS/INTERVENTIONS	RATIONALES

• Position the patient to prevent supine hypotension by:
  ○ Placing the patient on her left side if possible
  ○ Using a pillow or folded towel under the right hip to tip to left
  ○ If neck injury is suspected, placing the patient on a back board and then tipping the board to the left
• Start an intravenous line for replacement of lost fluid volume.
 	
• Monitor fetal status continuously. Monitor for uterine contractions at least once per hour.
	Keeps the weight of the uterus off the inferior vena cava.
	
	The pregnant woman has 50% more blood volume, and her vital signs may not change until there is a 30% reduction in circulating blood volume.
	Basic data needed to ensure positive outcome.

Psychiatric Health

The expected outcomes and nursing actions for the mental health client are the same as those for the adult patient.

Gerontic Health

The nursing actions for the gerontic patient are the same as those for the adult patient.

Home Health

ACTIONS/INTERVENTIONS	RATIONALES
• Teach client and family measures to prevent Dysreflexia[54–56]: ○ Bowel and bladder routines ○ Prevention of skin breakdown (e.g., turning, transfer, or prevention of incontinence) ○ Use and care of indwelling urinary catheter ○ Prevention of infection	Basic care techniques that can assist in preventing the occurrence of dysreflexia.
• Assist client and family in identifying signs and symptoms of Dysreflexia[54]: ○ Teach family how to monitor vital signs and how to recognize tachycardia, bradycardia, and paroxysmal hypertension. ○ Assist client and family in identifying emergency referrals: (1) Physician (2) Emergency room (3) Emergency medical system	Provides for early recognition of and intervention for problem.
• Teach patient and family appropriate uses and side effects of medications as well as proper administration of the medications. • Obtain available wallet-sized card that briefly outlines effective treatments in an emergency situation.[57] Have client carry this card with him or her at all times. Family members must be familiar with content and location of card. **NOTE:** Labeled a Treatment Card, this card contains information related to pathophysiology, common signs and symptoms, stimuli that trigger AD, problems, and recommended treatment.	Locus of control shifts from nurse to client and family, thus promoting self-care.

Dysreflexia

FLOWCHART EVALUATION: EXPECTED OUTCOME 1

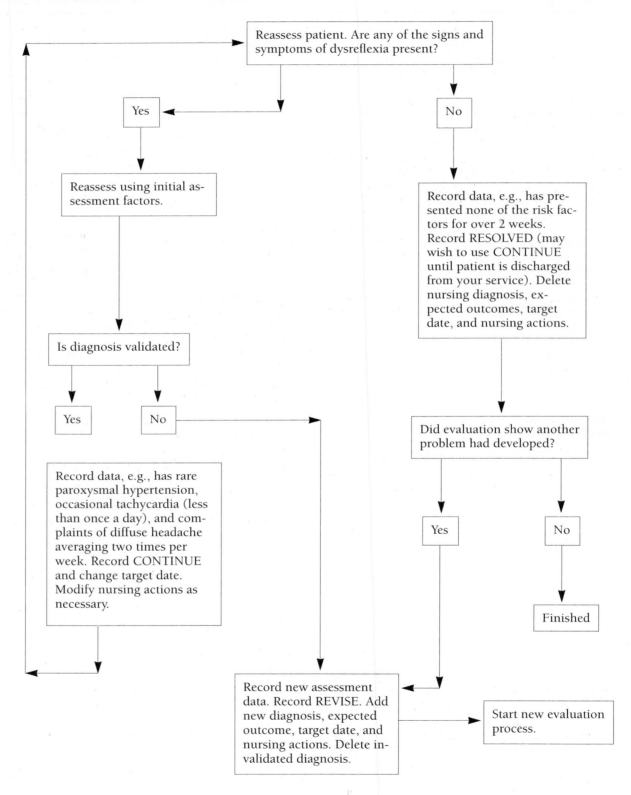

Reassess patient. Are any of the signs and symptoms of dysreflexia present?

Yes

No

Reassess using initial assessment factors.

Record data, e.g., has presented none of the risk factors for over 2 weeks. Record RESOLVED (may wish to use CONTINUE until patient is discharged from your service). Delete nursing diagnosis, expected outcomes, target date, and nursing actions.

Is diagnosis validated?

Yes

No

Record data, e.g., has rare paroxysmal hypertension, occasional tachycardia (less than once a day), and complaints of diffuse headache averaging two times per week. Record CONTINUE and change target date. Modify nursing actions as necessary.

Did evaluation show another problem had developed?

Yes

No

Finished

Record new assessment data. Record REVISE. Add new diagnosis, expected outcome, target date, and nursing actions. Delete invalidated diagnosis.

Start new evaluation process.

Dysreflexia

FLOWCHART EVALUATION: EXPECTED OUTCOME 2

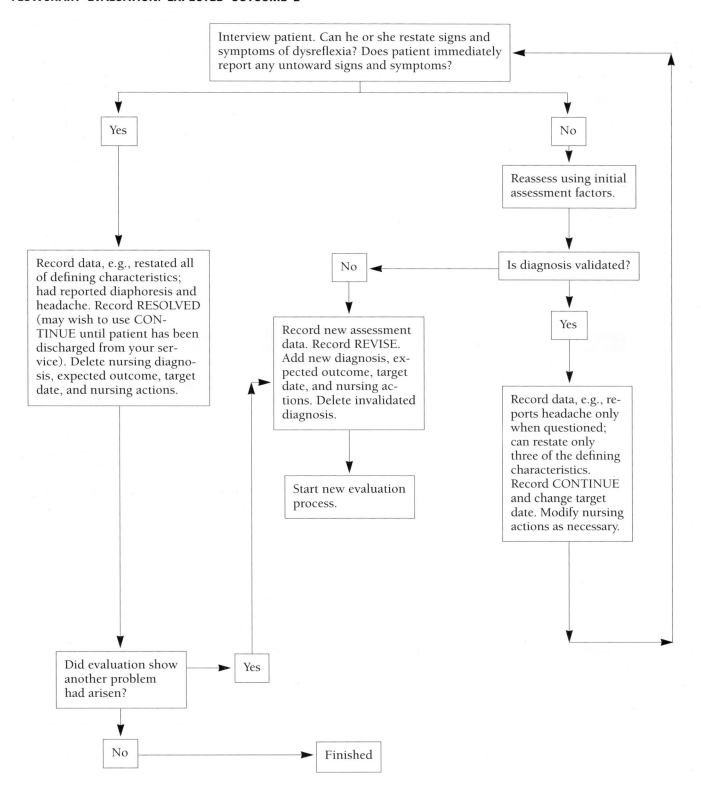

Fatigue

DEFINITION

An overwhelming sustained sense of exhaustion and decreased capacity for physical and mental work.[10]

NANDA TAXONOMY: MOVING 6.1.1.2.1

DEFINING CHARACTERISTICS[10]

1. Major defining characteristics
   a. Verbalization of an unremitting and overwhelming lack of energy
   b. Inability to maintain usual routines
2. Minor defining characteristics
   a. Perceived need for additional energy to accomplish routine tasks
   b. Increase in physical complaints
   c. Emotionally labile or irritable
   d. Impaired ability to concentrate
   e. Decreased performance
   f. Lethargic or listless
   g. Disinterest in surroundings; introspection
   h. Decreased libido
   i. Accident prone

RELATED FACTORS[10]

1. Decreased or increased metabolic energy production
2. Overwhelming psychologic or emotional demands
3. Increased energy requirements to perform activities of daily living
4. Excessive social and/or role demands
5. States of discomfort
6. Altered body chemistry (e.g., medications, drug withdrawal, or chemotherapy)

RELATED CLINICAL CONCERNS

1. Acquired immune deficiency syndrome
2. Hyper- or hypothyroidism
3. Cancer
4. Menopause
5. Depression
6. Anemia

HAVE YOU SELECTED THE CORRECT DIAGNOSIS?

Sleep Pattern Disturbance Fatigue is defined as a sense of exhaustion and decreased capacity for mental work regardless of adequate sleep. In this sense Fatigue may be considered an alteration in quality, not quantity, of sleep and is subjective.

Decreased Cardiac Output Decreased oxygenation to the muscles, brain, and so on, could result in a sense of fatigue.

Altered Nutrition, Less Than Body Requirements Decreased nutrition will ultimately lead to decreased muscle mass and decreased energy, which will result in Fatigue.

EXPECTED OUTCOMES

1. Will have decreased complaints of fatigue by (date) and/or
2. Will have implemented plan to offset fatigue by (date)

TARGET DATES

Fatigue can have far-reaching impact. For this reason the initial target date should be set at no more than 4 days.

NURSING ACTIONS/INTERVENTIONS WITH RATIONALES
Adult Health

ACTIONS/INTERVENTIONS	RATIONALES
• Collaborate with diet therapist for in-depth dietary assessment and planning. Monitor patient's food and fluid intake daily.	Adequate, balanced nutrition assists in reducing fatigue.
• Monitor for contributory factors on a daily basis at (time).	Assists in identifying causative factors, which then can be treated.

- Carefully plan activities of daily living and daily exercise schedules with detailed input from patient. Determine how to best foster future patterns that will maintain optimal sleep-rest patterns without fatigue through planning ADL with patient and family.
- Assign staff on a consistent basis.

- Provide frequent rest periods. Schedule at least 30 min for rest after any strenuous activity.
- Assist patient with self-care as needed. Plan gradual increase in activities over several days.
- Provide adequate input about usual sleep pattern versus current pattern associated with fatigue.
- Promote rest at night:
  ○ Warm bath at bedtime
  ○ Warm milk at bedtime
  ○ Back massage
- Avoid sensory overload or sensory deprivation. Provide diversional activities.

- Instruct patient is stress reduction techniques. Have patient return-demonstrate at least once a day through day of discharge.
- Assist patient to realistically appraise personal short- and long-term goals.
- Collaborate with physician regarding medical status and condition and its impact on promoting chronic fatigue.
- Assist patient to schedule at least 1 recreational night per week and 1 rest evening per week. Have patient sign contract with significant other to promote compliance with this schedule.
- Refer patient to local exercise center for assistance with regular exercise plan.

Realistic schedules based on patient's input promotes participation in activities and a sense of success.

Promotes adherence to planned schedule and facilitates patient's understanding of the need to be consistent in plan.
Allows patient to gradually increase strength and tolerance for activities.

Increases quantity and quality of rest and sleep.

Sensory aspects can deplete energy stores. Diversional activities help prevent overload or deprivation by focusing patient's concentration on an activity he or she personally enjoys.
Mental and physical stress greatly contribute to sense of fatigue.

Feeling overwhelmed by too many or unrealistic goals can increase fatigue.
Several medical diagnoses include fatigue as a symptom that can be offset by careful planning of care.

Provides distraction from overfocus on work or other such demands. Assists in reducing stress, which contributes to fatigue.

Regular exercise decreases fatigue.

Child Health

ACTIONS/INTERVENTIONS	RATIONALES
• Determine a plan to best address contributory factors as determined by verbalized perceptions of fatigue (may be related to parents' perceptions).	Parents are best able to describe objective behaviors that offer cues to fatigue factors, especially when the patient cannot speak or describe his or her feelings.
• Provide daily feedback regarding progress, and reassess child's and family's perception of fatigue.	Due to the ever-changing fatigue factors, close attention to progress will aid in a sense of mastery and objectify concerns.
• Ensure safety needs according to child's or infant's age and developmental capacity.	Standard accountability is to provide for safety needs with special attention to the child's age, developmental capacity, parental education, compliance, etc.

Women's Health

ACTIONS/INTERVENTIONS	RATIONALES
• During pregnancy, schedule rest periods during day.	Realistic planning to offer brief rest periods during the day.
• Find restful area, one time in the morning and one time in the afternoon, to get away from work area, and rest 5–10 min with feet propped above the abdomen.	
• During lunch, leave work area to rest 10–15 min with feet propped above the abdomen or lying on left side.	
• Have patient research the possibility of split time or job sharing at work during pregnancy.	
• Teach patient relaxation techniques.	Techniques induce a restful state and can be used for short periods of rest as well as more extended periods of rest.
• Teach patient to use music of preference during rest periods.	Assists with relaxation.
• Plan for at least 6–8 h of sleep during night. (See Sleep Pattern Disturbance, Chap. 6, for nursing actions to promote sleep.)	
• Involve significant others in discussion and problem-solving activities regarding lifestyle changes needed to reduce fatigue.	Family can assume more responsibilities to assist in increasing rest time for the patient.
• After delivery, identify a support system that can assist patient with infant care and household duties.	Assists in alleviating fatigue related to trying to manage household as always as well as trying to care for a new baby.
• Learn to rest and sleep when the infant sleeps.	Conserves energy and increases amount of time available for rest.
• Plan daily activities to alleviate unnecessary steps and to allow for frequent rest periods: ○ If bottle-feeding, prepare formula for 24 h at a time. ○ If breast-feeding, let spouse get up at night and bring baby to mother. ○ If breast-feeding, sleep with baby in bed. ○ Prepare extra when cooking meals for family and freeze extra for future meals (e.g., prepare big batch of stew or spaghetti on one day and freeze portions for future meals).	Baby begins to feed for longer periods and begins to sleep longer more quickly. Both mother and infant get more rest.
• Plan return to work on a gradual basis (e.g., work part-time for the first 2 wk, gradually increasing time at work until full-time by end of 4 wk).	Provides gradual return to activities and decreases likelihood of fatigue.

Psychiatric Health

NOTE: All goals established for the nursing actions should be achievable and adjusted as client's condition changes.

ACTIONS/INTERVENTIONS	RATIONALES
• Client must be out of bed and dressed by (note time here). Initially this goal may be limited to client getting out of bed without dressing.	Provides goal client can achieve and enhances self-esteem.
• Assist client with grooming activities (note here the degree of assistance needed as well as any special items needed).	Promotes client's sense of control and enhances self-esteem.
• While assisting client with grooming activities, teach performance of tasks in energy-efficient ways, e.g., placing all necessary items in one place before grooming is begun.	Promotes client's control by providing increased opportunity for self-care.

- Provide client with appropriate rewards for accomplishing established goals (note special goals here with the reward for achievement of goal). Establish rewards with client input.

- Establish time for client to rest during the day. Initially this will be more frequent and diminish as client's condition changes. Note times and duration of rest periods here.

- Walk with client on unit (number) of minutes (number) times a day.

- Have client identify pleasurable activities that cannot be performed because of fatigue.

- Identify one pleasurable activity, and develop a gradually escalating plan for client involvement in this activity. Provide rewards for accomplishment of each step in this plan.

- Provide client with foods that are high in nutritional value and easy to consume.

- Talk with client 30 min twice a day. Topics for this discussion should include:
  ○ Client's perception of the problem
  ○ Identification of thoughts that support the feeling of fatigue
  ○ Identification of thoughts that decrease feelings of fatigue
  ○ Identification of unrealistic goals
  ○ Client's evaluation of and attitudes toward self
  ○ Identification of circumstances in the client's environment that support continuing feelings of fatigue (e.g., family stressors or secondary gain from fatigue).
  ○ Identification of client's accomplishments

- After client has verbalized the effects negative thoughts have on feelings and behavior, teach client how to stop negative thoughts and replace them with positive thoughts.

- Reward client for positive self-statements.

- Assign client tasks on the unit, and provide positive reinforcement for task accomplishment. Note task assigned and reward established here.

- Involve client in group activity with other clients for (number) of minutes (number) times a day.

- Meet with client and client's family to evaluate interaction patterns and provide information that would assist them in assisting the client.

- Have client identify those factors that will maintain feeling of well-being after discharge and develop a specific behavioral plan for implementing them. Note plan here.

Positive reinforcement encourages appropriate behavior.

Meets physiologic need for rest. Also provides client with an opportunity for perceived control in determining when these rest periods should be provided.

Promotes cardiorespiratory fitness and promotes self-esteem by providing a goal the client can meet. Interaction with the nurse can provide positive reinforcement for this activity.
Promotes positive orientation by connecting client with images of past pleasures and provides material for developing positive imaging.
Promotes positive orientation by providing client with a goal to work toward. This will increase motivation. Positive reinforcement encourages behavior.

Meets physiologic needs for nutrition in a manner that conserves energy.
Promotes client's sense of control by providing time for his or her input into plan of care on a daily basis. Also provides positive reinforcement through social interaction with the nurse and verbal feedback about accomplishments.

Cognitive maps impact feelings and behavior. When cognitive maps are used inappropriately, they can promote maladaptive thinking, behaving, and feeling. Recognition of dysfunctional maps provides the client with the opportunity for developing positive orientation and adaptive cognitive maps.[22]
Positive reinforcement encourages appropriate behavior.

Interaction with peers provides opportunities to increase the patient's social network, learn problem-solving strategies, and test perceptions of self and experiences with peers.
Family support enhances probability of behavior changes being maintained after discharge.

Reinforces behavior change and new coping skills while providing positive feedback and enhancing self-esteem.[22]

Gerontic Health

ACTIONS/INTERVENTIONS	RATIONALES
• Review medications for side effects or possible drug interactions.	Many medications can contribute to the sensation of fatigue.
• Collaborate with physician regarding assessing patient for depression.	Depression is often underreported and undertreated in older adults.
• Monitor for activities that interrupt the patient's sleep pattern such as vital signs, body weight, or medical treatments.	Environmental noises and inattention to patient's usual sleep pattern may result in sleep fragmentation.
• Plan care activities around periods of least fatigue.	Gives attention to patient's circadian rhythm.

Home Health

ACTIONS/INTERVENTIONS	RATIONALES

• Assist patient and family in identifying risk factors pertinent to the situation:
  ○ Chronic disease (e.g., arthritis, cancer, or heart disease)
  ○ Medications
  ○ Pain
  ○ Role strain
• Teach client and family measures to promote capacity for physical and mental work:
  ○ Use assistive devices as appropriate (wheelchairs, crutches, canes, walkers, adaptive eating utensils, etc.).
  ○ Maintain sufficient pain control (analgesics, imagery, meditation, etc.).
  ○ Provide a safe environment to reduce barriers to activity and decrease potential for accidents (throw rugs, stairs, blocked pathways, etc.).
  ○ Provide balance of work and recreational activities.
  ○ Provide housekeeping assistance as appropriate (e.g., homemaker or meals-on-wheels).
• Provide diversional activity as appropriate (visiting friends or family, doing hobbies or schoolwork, etc.).
• Consult with or refer patient to appropriate resources as indicated.
	Provides additional support for client and family and uses already available resources in a cost-effective manner.

Fatigue

FLOWCHART EVALUATION: EXPECTED OUTCOME 1

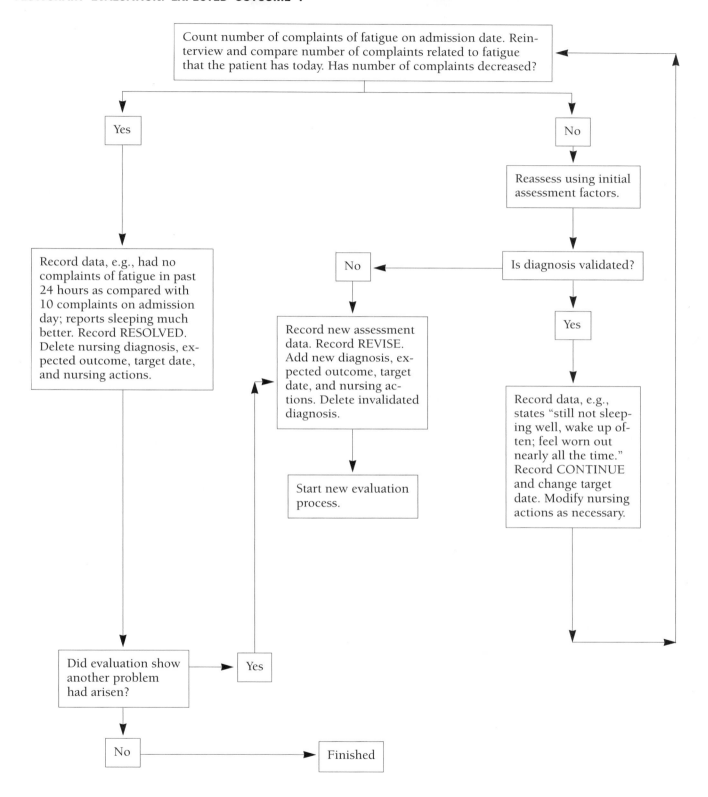

Fatigue

FLOWCHART EVALUATION: EXPECTED OUTCOME 2

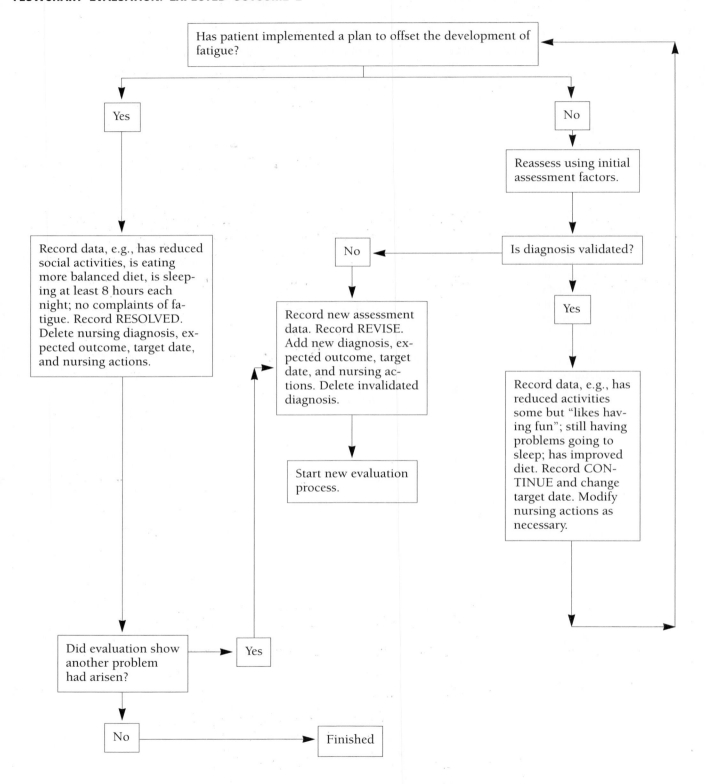

Gas Exchange, Impaired

DEFINITION

The state in which an individual experiences an excess or deficit in oxygenation and/or carbon dioxide elimination at the alveolar-capillary member (specify: hypercapnia or hypoxemia).[10]

NANDA TAXONOMY: EXCHANGING 1.5.1.1

DEFINING CHARACTERISTICS[10]

1. Major defining characteristics
   a. Dyspnea
   b. Confusion
   c. Abnormal ABGs
   d. Hypoxia
   e. Hypercapnia
      Headache upon awakening
      Vision disturbances
   f. Cyanosis (in neonates only)
   g. Somnolence
   h. Restlessness
   i. Irritability
2. Minor defining characteristics
   None given

RELATED FACTORS[10]

1. Ventilation perfusion imbalance

RELATED CLINICAL CONCERNS

1. Chronic obstructive pulmonary disease
2. Congestive heart failure
3. Asthma
4. Pneumonia
5. Pulmonary tuberculosis

HAVE YOU SELECTED THE CORRECT DIAGNOSIS?

Ineffective Airway Clearance This diagnosis means that something is blocking the air passage but that when and if air gets to the alveoli, there is adequate gas exchange. In Impaired Gas Exchange, the air (oxygen) that reaches the alveoli is not sufficiently diffused across the alveoli-circulatory membrane.

Ineffective Breathing Pattern This diagnosis suggests that the rate, rhythm, depth, and type of ventilatory effort is insufficient to bring in enough oxygen or get rid of sufficient amounts of carbon dioxide. These gases are sufficiently exchanged at the alveoli-circulatory membrane, but the pattern of ventilation makes breathing ineffective.

Decreased Cardiac Output In this diagnosis, the heart is not pumping a sufficient amount of blood through the lungs to take up enough oxygen or release enough carbon dioxide to meet the body requirements. There is no impairment in the gas exchange, but there is not enough circulating blood to combine with sufficient amounts of oxygen to supply the body's needs.

EXPECTED OUTCOMES

1. Will have no signs or symptoms of impaired gas exchange by (date) and/or
2. Will demonstrate improved blood gases and vital signs by (date). Note initial blood gas measurements and vital signs here.

TARGET DATES

Because of the extreme danger of Impaired Gas Exchange, progress should be evaluated at least every 8 hours until the client has stabilized. Thereafter, target dates at 3 to 5 days would be acceptable.

NURSING ACTIONS/INTERVENTIONS WITH RATIONALES

Adult Health

ACTIONS/INTERVENTIONS	RATIONALES

• Monitor and document:
  ○ Respiratory pattern, rate, and depth at least every 2 h on (odd/even) hour
  ○ Symptoms noted with respirations, such as pain, difficulty in breathing, retraction of sternum or flaring of nares, or allergies
  ○ Equipment used in ventilation, including ventilator settings for rate, oxygen (FiO_2), peak pressure (PP), and if continuous positive airway pressure (CPAP) is needed
  ○ Auscultation of breath sounds every 1 h or as needed, with follow-up chest x-ray as needed
  ○ Tolerance of chest physiotherapy
  ○ Suctioning tolerance, especially pulse rate
  ○ Nature of secretions obtained via suctioning
  ○ Observations of skin and mucous membranes for cyanosis
	Baseline factors that will allow assessment of patient's progress toward improvement or lack of progress.

• Maintain fluid and electrolyte balance:
  ○ Administer appropriate fluids and electrolytes as ordered.
  ○ Monitor hourly intake and output.
  ○ Administer potassium only after voiding is noted.
  ○ Monitor specific gravity 4 times a day at (times).	

• Administer or assist with intermittent positive-pressure breathing (IPPB) or continuous positive airway pressure (CPAP) as ordered. Stay with patient during treatment. In between treatments, administer oxygen as ordered.	Opens airways and alveoli and improves gas exchange. Oxygen reduces the work of breathing and thus enhances gas exchange.
• Perform nursing actions to maintain effective airway clearance. (See Ineffective Airway Clearance for nursing actions and enter those actions here.)	Clearing airways of secretions improves ventilation-perfusion relationship.

• Decrease patient's anxiety during periods of increased distress by:
  ○ Talking in a calm, slow voice
  ○ Reassuring patient that you can provide the necessary assistance
  ○ Having patient take slow, deep breaths and follow proper breathing techniques
  ○ Staying with client until episode resolves	

• Schedule at least 15 min with patient every 2 h on the (odd/even) hour for discussing concerns.	Assists in reducing fear and anxiety.
• Raise head of bed to 30 degrees or more if not contraindicated.	Facilitates chest expansion.
• Reduce chest pain by using noninvasive techniques and analgesics.	Relaxes muscle tension, decreases oxygen consumption, and decreases carbon dioxide production.
• Encourage drinking 2–3 L of fluid per day unless contraindicated by other medical problems, e.g., congestive heart failure.	Assists in liquefying secretions, which makes them easier to expel.
• Maintain adequate nutrition (high protein, low fat, and low carbohydrates) on a daily basis. Collaborate with diet therapist regarding several small meals per day rather than 3 large meals.	Decreases energy demand for digestion and prevents constriction of chest cavity due to a full stomach.
• Instruct in diaphragmatic deep breathing and pursed-lip breathing. Give patient information in clear, concise manner, providing written notes if necessary. This is especially true for the patient who has altered mental status as a result of hypoxia.	

- Have patient practice proper breathing once every hour while awake. These sessions should be supervised by the nurse until the patient masters the technique. Note schedule for practice sessions here.
- Provide teaching regarding respiratory exercises:
  ◦ Assume a sitting position with back straight and shoulders relaxed.
  ◦ Use conscious, controlled deep-breathing techniques that expand diaphragm downward (abdomen should rise).
  ◦ Breathe in deeply through the nose, hold for 2–3 s, then breathe out slowly through pursed lips. Abdomen will sink down with the exhalation.
- Instruct the patient (practice with and supervise until confident patient can perform exercises accurately) to perform exercises at least twice an hour while awake.
- Provide teaching regarding bronchial hygiene:
  ◦ Breathe deeply and slowly while sitting up.
  ◦ Use diaphragmatic breathing.
  ◦ Hold the breath for 3–5 s, and then slowly exhale through the mouth as much of the breath as possible.
  ◦ Take another deep breath, hold, and cough forcefully from deep in the chest. Repeat 2 times.
  ◦ Rest 15–20 min after coughing session.
- Assist with postural drainage and cupping and clapping exercises. Teach these exercises to significant other.
- Administer bronchodilators and mucolytic agents as ordered.
- Collaborate with physician regarding monitoring of blood gases. Report abnormal results immediately.
- Turn every 2 h on the (odd/even) hour. Encourage patient's mobility to the extent tolerated without dyspnea.
- Develop a schedule, on day of admission, for activity and rest that provides the patient with the greatest amount of activity with the least amount of fatigue, e.g., have chair in bathroom for being seated while doing daily hygiene. Note schedule here.
- Discuss with patient the effects smoking has on the respiratory system, and refer patient to a stop smoking group if patient is motivated to stop smoking; if not, instruct patient not to smoke 15 min before meals and physical activity.
- Review the patient's resources and home situation regarding long-term management of Impaired Gas Exchange prior to discharge. Refer to appropriate community resources.

Essential knowledge needed for patient to control situation. Will assist in expelling secretions.

PCO_2, PO_2, and O_2 saturation are indicators of the efficiency of gas exchange.
Position changes modify ventilation-perfusion relationships and enhance gas exchange.

Conserves energy needed for breathing and gas exchange.

Smoking, or passive smoke for the nonsmoker, greatly increases the risk for development of respiratory and cardiovascular diseases. Smoking immediately before eating or exercise causes vasoconstriction, leading to decreased gas exchange and compounding condition. Initiates appropriate home care planning and long-range support for patient and family.

Child Health

ACTIONS/INTERVENTIONS	RATIONALES

- Ensure availability of emergency equipment:
  ◦ Ambu bag
  ◦ Endotracheal tube appropriate for age and size of infant (3.5)
  ◦ Suctioning unit and catheters
  ◦ Infant, 5 or 8 Fr; child, 8 or 10 Fr
  ◦ Crash cart with appropriate drugs
  ◦ Defibrillation unit with guidelines
  ◦ O_2 tank (check amount of oxygen left)
	Basic emergency preparedness.

Continued

ACTIONS/INTERVENTIONS	RATIONALES
○ Tracheostomy sterile set ○ Sterile chest tube tray • Provide for parental input in planning and implementing care, e.g., comfort measures, assisting with feedings, and daily hygienic measures. • Allow at least 10–15 min per shift for family to verbalize concerns regarding child's status and changes. Encourage parents to ask questions as often as needed. • Collaborate with related health care team members as needed. • While the child is still in the hospital, provide opportunities for parents and child to master essential skills necessary for long-term care such as suctioning. • Ensure that parents and family receive CPR training well before dismissal from hospital. • Encourage parents to use support system to aid in coping with illness and hospitalization. • Allow for sibling visitation as applicable within institution or specific situation.	Parental involvement provides emotional security for child's parents and offers empowerment and allows practicing of care techniques in a supportive environment. Assists in reducing anxiety and provides teaching opportunity. Promotes coordination care without undue duplication and fragmentation of care. Learning of essential skills is enhanced when opportunities for practice are allowed in a safe, secure environment. Compliance is also fostered. Anticipatory need for CPR should better prepare parents and other family members in the event of pulmonary arrest. Having this basic knowledge will assist in reducing anxiety regarding home care. Reliance on others should afford parents some degree of relief from constant worry based on the likelihood of primary needs with a chronically ill child. Sibling visitation enhances the opportunity for family coping and growth. Provides moral support to both siblings.

Women's Health

NOTE: This nursing diagnosis will pertain to women the same as in any other adult. The following nursing actions will focus only on the fetal-placental unit during pregnancy. Placental function is totally dependent on maternal circulation; therefore, any process that interferes with maternal circulation will affect the oxygen consumption of the placenta and, in turn, the fetus.

ACTIONS/INTERVENTIONS	RATIONALES
• Assist patient in developing an exercise plan during pregnancy. • Teach patient and significant others how to avoid "supine hypotension" during pregnancy (particularly during the later stages): ○ Lying on right or left side to reduce pressure on vena cava ○ Taking frequent rest breaks during the day • Assist patient in identifying lifestyle adjustments that may be needed due to changes in physiologic function or needs during pregnancy: ○ Stop smoking. ○ Reduce exposure to secondhand smoke. ○ Avoid lying in supine position. ○ Take no drugs unless advised to do so by physician. • Identify underlying maternal diseases that will affect the fetal-placental unit during pregnancy. ○ Maternal origin: (1) Maternal hypertension (2) Drug addiction (3) Diabetes mellitus with vascular involvement (4) Sickle cell anemia (5) Maternal infections	Increases cardiovascular fitness and therefore increases oxygenation and nutrition to placenta and fetus. These disorders have a direct impact on the gas exchange in the fetal-placental unit.

(6) Maternal smoking
(7) Hemorrhage (abruptio placentae or placenta previa)
○ Fetal origin:
(1) Premature or prolonged rupture of membranes
(2) Intrauterine infection
(3) Rh disease
(4) Multiple pregnancy

Psychiatric Health

ACTIONS/INTERVENTIONS	RATIONALES
• If client is demonstrating alterations in mental status, assess for increased hypoxia.	The central nervous system is particularly sensitive to impaired gas exchange because of its reliance on simple sugar metabolism for energy production.[41]
• Observe client for signs of respiratory infection.	Infection will increase mucus production, which decreases airway clearance.[41]
• Protect client from respiratory infection by: ○ Maintaining proper humidity in environment ○ Placing him or her in private room or monitoring roommate closely for signs and symptoms of respiratory infection and, if present, moving client to another room ○ Assigning staff members to client who are free of infection ○ Keeping client away from crowds ○ Assisting client in obtaining appropriate immunizations against influenza ○ Having client inform staff of signs or symptoms of respiratory infection when the earliest symptoms appear ○ Keeping environment as free of respiratory irritants as possible, e.g., dust, allergens, or pollution	Prevents further injury to a system that is stressed and promotes airway patency.
• Discuss with client the effects of alcohol and other depressant drugs on the respiratory system. Refer to a drug-abuse recovery program as necessary.	The sedative effects of some drugs decrease airway clearance, increasing the risk for the development of infection. Diffusion is also decreased with chronic alcoholism.[58]
• Collaborate with physician regarding supplemental vitamins, especially thiamine, if the impaired gas exchange is secondary to alcohol abuse.	Thiamine is essential for the conversion of glucose to metabolically useful forms. Nerve cell function depends on this glucose. This compensates for the nutritional deficits that result when nutritional calories are replaced by alcohol.[57]
• Spend 30 min twice a day with client discussing feelings and reactions to current situation. As feelings are expressed, begin to explore lifestyle changes with client. Refer to Ineffective Individual Coping (Chap. 11) and Powerlessness (Chap. 8) for specific care plans related to coping styles.	Promotes client's sense of control by facilitating understanding of factors that contribute to maladaptive coping behaviors.
• Develop with client a plan for gradually increasing physical activity (see Activity Intolerance for specific behavioral interventions).	Improves cardiorespiratory functioning, thus improving gas exchange.

Gerontic Health

ACTIONS/INTERVENTIONS	RATIONALES
• Ensure that oxygen delivery system is properly functioning and fits well. Avoid face mask if patient is emaciated. Check proper positioning of nasal cannula (prongs turned inward).	Basic care standards.
• Monitor skin color, mental status, and vital signs every 2 h on the (odd/even) hour.	
• Check oxygen flow and amount every 4 h around the clock at (times).	The patient may increase the liter flow during acute episodes of impaired gas exchange and cause respiratory system depression with retention of carbon dioxide.
• Monitor for potential carbon dioxide narcosis, e.g., changes in level of consciousness, changes in oxygen and carbon dioxide blood gas levels, flushing, decreased respiratory rate, and headaches. This is especially important for patient on long-term oxygen therapy.[33]	
• Teach patient and family the signs and symptoms of carbon dioxide narcosis, especially those on long-term oxygen therapy.	Decreases potential for carbon dioxide narcosis.

Home Health

NOTE: If this diagnosis is suspected when caring for a client in the home, it is imperative that a physician referral be obtained immediately. If the client has been referred to home health care by a physician, the nurse will collaborate with the physician in the treatment of the client. Preliminary research[58] indicates that women with chronic bronchitis or chronic obstructive pulmonary disease (COPD) cannot walk as far as men. Activity should be planned according to tolerance, keeping in mind gender differences. There is no doubt that better control of dyspnea is a pressing need, with research[59] indicating that a client's subjective report of health status is a better predictor of level of functioning than is objective measure of the lung function.

ACTIONS/INTERVENTIONS	RATIONALES

• Teach client and family appropriate monitoring of signs and symptoms of Impaired Gas Exchange:
  ○ Pursed-lip breathing
  ○ Respiratory status: Cyanosis, rate, dyspnea, or orthopnea
  ○ Fatigue
  ○ Use of accessory muscles
  ○ Cough
  ○ Sputum production or change in sputum production
  ○ Edema
  ○ Decreased urinary output
  ○ Gasping
	Provides for early recognition and intervention for problem.

• Assist client and family in identifying lifestyle changes that may be required: ○ Prevention of Impaired Gas Exchange: Stopping smoking, prevention or early treatments of lung infections, avoidance of known irritants and allergens, obtaining influenza and pneumonia immunizations	Provides basic information for client and family that promotes necessary lifestyle changes.

- ○ Pulmonary hygiene: Clearing bronchial tree by controlled coughing, decreasing viscosity of secretions via humidity and fluid balance, and postural drainage
- ○ Daily activity as tolerated (remove barriers to activity)
- ○ Breathing techniques to decrease work of breathing (diaphragmatic, pursed lips, or sitting forward)
- ○ Adequate nutrition intake
- ○ Appropriate use of oxygen (dosage, route of administration, or safety factors)
- ○ Stress management
- ○ Limiting exposure to upper respiratory infections
- ○ Avoiding extreme hot or cold temperatures
- ○ Keeping area free of animal hair and dander or dust
- ○ Assistive devices required (oxygen, nasal cannula, suction, ventilator, etc.)
- ○ Adequate hydration (monitoring intake and output)
- Teach client and family purposes, side effects, and proper administration technique of medications.
- Assist client and family to set criteria to help them to determine when physician or other intervention is required, e.g., change in skin color, increased difficulty with breathing, increase or change in sputum production, or fever.
- Teach family basic CPR.
- Refer patient to community resources as needed.

Locus of control shifts from nurse to client and family, thus promoting self-care.

Provides additional support for client and family and uses already available resources in a cost-effective manner.

Gas Exchange, Impaired

FLOWCHART EVALUATION: EXPECTED OUTCOME 1

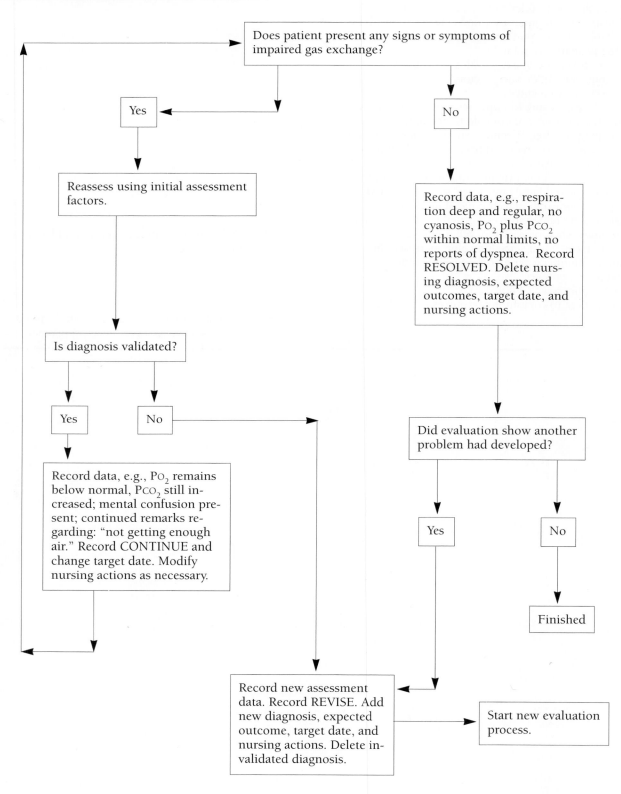

Does patient present any signs or symptoms of impaired gas exchange?

Yes

No

Reassess using initial assessment factors.

Record data, e.g., respiration deep and regular, no cyanosis, P_{O_2} plus P_{CO_2} within normal limits, no reports of dyspnea. Record RESOLVED. Delete nursing diagnosis, expected outcomes, target date, and nursing actions.

Is diagnosis validated?

Yes

No

Record data, e.g., P_{O_2} remains below normal, P_{CO_2} still increased; mental confusion present; continued remarks regarding: "not getting enough air." Record CONTINUE and change target date. Modify nursing actions as necessary.

Did evaluation show another problem had developed?

Yes

No

Finished

Record new assessment data. Record REVISE. Add new diagnosis, expected outcome, target date, and nursing actions. Delete invalidated diagnosis.

Start new evaluation process.

Gas Exchange, Impaired

FLOWCHART EVALUATION: EXPECTED OUTCOME 2

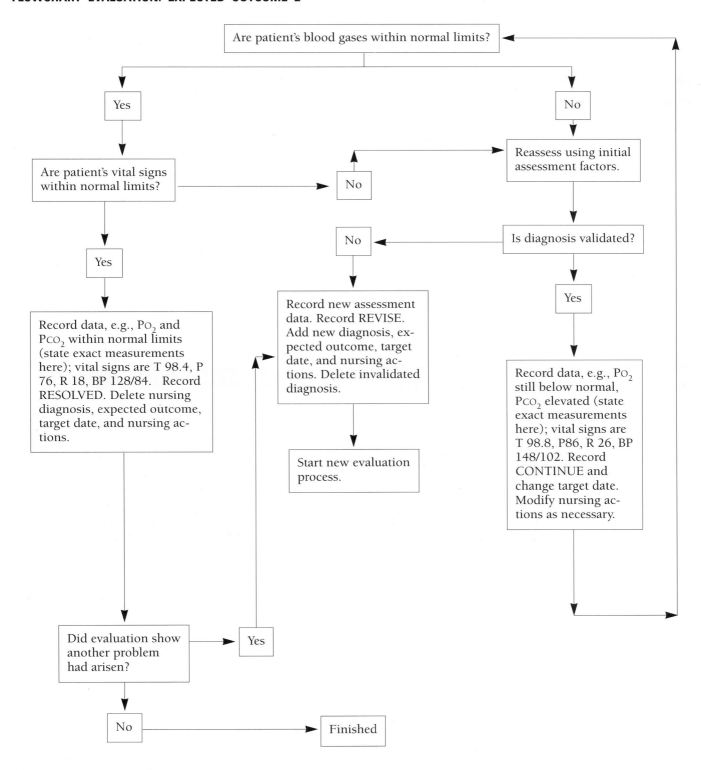

Are patient's blood gases within normal limits?

Yes

No

Are patient's vital signs within normal limits?

No

Reassess using initial assessment factors.

Yes

Is diagnosis validated?

No

Yes

Record data, e.g., P_{O_2} and P_{CO_2} within normal limits (state exact measurements here); vital signs are T 98.4, P 76, R 18, BP 128/84. Record RESOLVED. Delete nursing diagnosis, expected outcome, target date, and nursing actions.

Record new assessment data. Record REVISE. Add new diagnosis, expected outcome, target date, and nursing actions. Delete invalidated diagnosis.

Record data, e.g., P_{O_2} still below normal, P_{CO_2} elevated (state exact measurements here); vital signs are T 98.8, P86, R 26, BP 148/102. Record CONTINUE and change target date. Modify nursing actions as necessary.

Start new evaluation process.

Did evaluation show another problem had arisen?

Yes

No

Finished

Growth and Development, Altered

DEFINITION

The state in which an individual demonstrates deviations in norms from his or her age group.[10]

NANDA TAXONOMY: MOVING 6.6

DEFINING CHARACTERISTICS[10]

1. Major defining characteristics
   a. Delay or difficulty in performing skills (motor, social, or expressive) typical of age group
   b. Altered physical growth
   c. Inability to perform self-care or self-control activities appropriate to age
2. Minor defining characteristics
   a. Flat affect
   b. Listlessness
   c. Decreased responses

RELATED FACTORS[10]

1. Inadequate caretaking
2. Indifference
3. Inconsistent responsiveness
4. Multiple caretakers
5. Separation from significant others
6. Environmental and stimulation deficiencies
7. Effects of physical disability
8. Prescribed dependence

RELATED CLINICAL CONCERNS

1. Hypothyroidism
2. Failure to thrive syndrome
3. Leukemia
4. Deficient growth hormone
5. Personality disorders
6. Schizophrenic disorders
7. Substance abuse
8. Dementia
9. Delirium

HAVE YOU SELECTED THE CORRECT DIAGNOSIS?

Sensory-Perceptual Alterations This diagnosis should be considered when blindness, deafness, or neurologic impairment is present. Assisting the patient to adapt to these problems could resolve any developmental problems.

Impaired Physical Mobility When physical disabilities are present, they can definitely impact growth and development. In this example, Impaired Physical Mobility and Altered Growth and Development would be companion diagnoses.

Altered Nutrition, Less Than Body Requirements Lack of essential vitamins and minerals will also show a direct link to Altered Growth and Development. Assessment should be implemented for both diagnoses.

The nursing diagnoses grouped under self-perception and self-concept pattern, role-relationship pattern, and coping–stress tolerance pattern should also be considered when alterations in growth and development are present.

EXPECTED OUTCOMES

1. Will implement plan to offset, as much as possible, Altered Growth and Development factors by (date) and/or
2. Will return, as nearly as possible, to expected growth and development parameter for (specify exact parameter) by (date)

TARGET DATES

Assisting in modifying Altered Growth and Development factors will require a significant time; therefore, an initial target date of 7 to 10 days would be reasonable for evaluating progress.

NURSING ACTIONS/INTERVENTIONS WITH RATIONALES

Adult Health

NOTE: Nursing actions for this diagnosis are varied and complex and incorporate nursing actions associated with other nursing diagnoses. For example, the patient may have either a total self-care deficit or a subdeficit in hygiene, grooming, feeding, or toileting. For an adult, any of these would be an alteration in growth and development. Therefore, it would be appropriate to include the nursing actions associated with these nursing diagnoses in the nursing actions for Altered Growth and Development.

An adult is generally able to find or initiate diversional and social activities. However, if the adult does not participate in diversional or social activities, it could indicate Altered Growth and Development. Therefore, the nursing actions associated with Diversional Activity Deficit and Social Isolation would be appropriate to be included in the nursing actions for Altered Growth and Development.

ACTIONS/INTERVENTIONS	RATIONALES
• In general, the nurse should provide adequate opportunities for the patient to be successful in whatever task he or she is attempting.	Success increases motivation.
• Reward and reinforce success, however minor. Downplay relapses. Allow patient to be as independent as possible.	Increases self-esteem and active participation in care.
• Have consistent, nonjudgmental, caring people in the caregiving role.	Caring people can instill confidence in a patient and willingness to try new tasks.
• Work collaboratively with other health care professionals and with the patient and family in developing a plan of care.	Facilitates development of a plan that all will use consistently.

Child Health

ACTIONS/INTERVENTIONS	RATIONALES
• Monitor and teach parents to monitor child's growth and development status. Determine what alterations there are (i.e., delays or precocity).	As a rule, single assessments are not as revealing in growth and development parameters as are serial, longitudinal patterns. Parental involvement offers a more thorough monitoring, fosters their involvement with child, and empowers family.
• Determine what other primary health care needs exist, especially brain damage or residual of brain damage.	In instances of brain damage or retardation, it is often difficult to get an accurate assessment of cognitive capability. The general health of the patient will often influence, to a major degree, what alteration in cognitive functioning exists, e.g., sickle cell anemia with resultant infarcts to major organs such as the brain.
• Identify, with child or parents, realistic goals for growth and development.	A plan of care based on individual needs, with parental input, better reflects holistic care and increases probability of effective home management of problem.
• Collaborate with related health care team members as necessary.	Collaboration is required for meeting the special long-term needs for activities of daily living.
• Identify anticipatory safety for child related to Altered Growth and Development, e.g., ingestion of objects, falls, or use of wheelchair.	These children may be large physically due to chronological age, and there is a possibility of overlooking the developmental or mental age.
• In case of special diet due to a metabolic component, e.g., various enzymes lacking, provide appropriate health teaching for parents.	Appropriate diet can assist in preventing further deterioration or be essential to replace lacking vitamins, enzymes, or other nutrients.

Continued

ACTIONS/INTERVENTIONS	RATIONALES
• Refer child and parents to appropriate community resources to assist in fostering growth and development such as early childhood intervention services.	Offering early intervention assists in fostering development while preventing tertiary delays.
• Assist parents to provide for learning needs related to future development, including identification of schools for developmentally delayed children.	Appropriate match of services to needs enhances child's development to the level possible.
• Refer child and parents to state and national support groups such as National Cerebral Palsy Association.	Support groups assist in empowerment and advocacy at local, state, and national levels.
• Provide patient and family with long-term follow-up appointments before discharge.	Promotes implementation of management regimen and provides anticipatory resources and checkpoint for the patient and family.

Women's Health

NOTE: This nursing diagnosis will pertain to women the same as to any other adult. The following nursing actions pertain only to women with reproductive anatomic abnormalities.

ACTIONS/INTERVENTIONS	RATIONALES
• Obtain a thorough sexual and obstetric history, especially noting recurrent miscarriages in the first 3 mo of pregnancy.	Provides basic database for determining therapy needs.
• Collaborate with physician regarding assessment for infertility.	
• Refer to gynecologist for further testing if primary amenorrhea is present.	
• Encourage patient to verbalize her concerns and fears.	Decreases anxiety. Allows opportunity for teaching and allows correction of any misinformation.
• Encourage communication with significant others to identify concerns and explore options available.	Provides a base for teaching and long-range counseling.

Psychiatric Health

ACTIONS/INTERVENTIONS	RATIONALES
• Provide a quiet, nonstimulating environment or an environment that does not add additional stress to an already overwhelmed coping ability.	Too little or too much sensory input can result in a sense of disorganization and confusion and result in dysfunctional coping behaviors.[22]
• Sit with client (number) minutes (number) times per day at (list specific times) to discuss current concerns and feelings.	Attention from the nurse can enhance self-esteem. Expression of feelings can facilitate identification and resolutions of problematic coping behaviors.
• Provide client with familiar or needed objects. These should be noted here.	Promotes client's sense of control by providing an environment in which client feels safe and secure.
• Discuss with client perceptions of self, others, and the current situation. This should include client's perceptions of harm, loss, or threat. Assist client in altering perception of these situations so they can be seen as challenges or opportunities for growth rather than threats.	Provides positive orientation, which improves self-esteem and provides hope for the future.

- Provide client with an environment that will optimize sensory input. This could include hearing aids, eyeglasses, pencil and paper, decreased noise in conversation areas, appropriate lighting. (These interventions should indicate an awareness of sensory deficit as well as sensory overload, and the specific interventions for this client should be noted here, e.g., place hearing aid in when client awakens and remove before bedtime.)

Appropriate levels of sensory input promote contact with the reality of the environment, which facilitates appropriate coping.

- Provide client with achievable tasks, activities, goals (these should be listed here). These activities should be provided with increasing complexity to give client an increasing sense of accomplishment and mastery.

Provides positive reinforcement, which enhances self-esteem and provides motivation for working toward next goal.

- Communicate to client an understanding that all coping behavior to this point has been his or her best effort and asking for assistance at this time is not failure. Explain that a complex problem often requires some outside assistance in resolution. (This will assist client in maintaining self-esteem and diminish feelings of failure.)

Promotes positive orientation, which enhances self-esteem and promotes hope.

- Provide client with opportunities to make appropriate decisions related to care at his or her level of ability. This may begin as a choice between two options, which would then evolve into more complex decision making. It is important that this be at the client's level of functioning so that confidence can be built with successful decision-making experiences.

Promotes client's perception of control, which promotes self-esteem.

- Provide constructive confrontation for client about problematic coping behavior. (See Kneisl and Wilson[21] for guidelines on constructive confrontation.) The kinds of behavior identified by the treatment team as problematic should be listed here.

Provides opportunities for the client to question aspects of behavior that can promote desire to change.

- Provide client with opportunities to practice new kinds of behavior either by role playing or by applying them to graded real-life experiences.

Provides opportunities to practice new behavior in a safe environment where the nurse can provide positive feedback for gradual improvement of coping strategies. This increases probability for the success of the new behavior in real-life situation, which in turn serves as positive reinforcement for behavior change.
Positive reinforcement encourages appropriate behavior.

- Provide positive social reinforcement and other behavioral rewards for demonstration of adaptive behavior. (Those things that the client finds rewarding should be listed here with a schedule for use. The kinds of behaviors that are to be rewarded should also be listed.)

- Assist client in identifying support systems and in developing a plan for their use.

Support systems can provide positive reinforcement for behavior change, increasing the opportunities for client's success in enhancing self-esteem.

- Assist client with setting appropriate limits on aggressive behavior by (see Risk for Violence, Chap. 9, for detailed nursing actions if this is an appropriate diagnosis):
  - Decreasing environmental stimulation as appropriate (This might include a secluded environment.)

Excessive environmental stimuli can increase a sense of disorganization and confusion.

  - Providing client with appropriate alternative outlets for physical tension. (This should be stated specifically and could include walking, running, talking with a staff member, using a punching bag, listening to music, or doing a deep muscle relaxation sequence. These outlets should be selected with the client's input.)

Promotes a sense of control and teaches constructive ways to cope with stressors.

Continued

ACTIONS/INTERVENTIONS	RATIONALES
• Meet with client and support system to provide information on the client's situation and to develop a plan that will involve the support system in making changes that will facilitate the client's movement to age-appropriate behavior. Note this plan here. • Refer patient to appropriate assistive resources as indicated.	Enhances opportunities for success of the treatment plan.

Gerontic Health

The nursing actions for the gerontic patient with this diagnosis are the same as those for adult health and home health patients.

Home Health

ACTIONS/INTERVENTIONS	RATIONALES

• Monitor for factors contributing to the Alteration in Growth and Development.
• Involve client and family in planning, implementing, and promoting reduction or correction of the alteration in growth and development:
  ○ Family conference
  ○ Mutual goal setting
  ○ Communication
• Teach client and family measures to prevent or decrease alterations in growth and development:
  ○ Explain expected norms of growth and development with anticipatory guidance. If the caretakers realize, for example, that the newborn begins to roll over by 2–4 mo or that the 2-year-old can follow simple directions, then appropriate environmental and learning conditions can be provided to protect the child and to promote optimal development.
  ○ Alert parents to signs and symptoms of alterations in growth and development that may require professional evaluation, e.g., delay in language skills, delay in crawling or walking, or delay in growth below 50% on growth chart.
  ○ Discuss parenting skills, e.g., how to recognize developmental milestones and how to discipline effectively without violence.
  ○ Provide guidance on developmentally appropriate nutrition, e.g., how to introduce finger foods to toddlers, how to monitor calorie intake for expected developmental stage, and how to ensure a balanced diet.
• Assist client and family to identify lifestyle changes that may be required.
  ○ Care for handicaps (e.g., blindness, deafness, or musculoskeletal or cognitive deficit)
  ○ Proper use of assistive equipment
  ○ Adapting to need for assistance or assistive equipment
  ○ Determining criteria for monitoring client's ability to function unassisted
  ○ Time management
	Provides database for prevention and/or early intervention.
	Involvement improves motivation and improves the outcome.
	
	Locus of control shifts from nurse to client and family, thus promoting self-care.
	
	Provides basic information for client and family that promotes necessary lifestyle changes.

- ○ Stress management
- ○ Development of support systems
- ○ Learning new skills
- ○ Work, family, social, and personal goals and priorities
- ○ Coping with disability or dependency
- ○ Development of consistent routine
- ○ Mechanism for alerting family members to the need for assistance
- ○ Providing appropriate balance of dependence and independence
- Assist client and family to obtain assistive equipment as required (depending on alteration present and its severity):
  - ○ Adaptive equipment for eating utensils, combs, brushes, etc.
  - ○ Straw and straw holder
  - ○ Wheelchair, walker, motorized cart, or cane
  - ○ Bedside commode or incontinence undergarments
  - ○ Hearing aid
  - ○ Corrective lenses
  - ○ Dressing aids: Dressing stick, zipper pull, button hook, long-handled shoehorn, shoe fasteners, or Velcro closures
  - ○ Bars and attachments and benches for shower or tub
  - ○ Handheld shower device
  - ○ Medication organizers
  - ○ Magnifying glass
  - ○ Raised toilet seat
- Consult with appropriate assistive resources as indicated.

Assistive equipment improves function and increases the possibilities for self-care.

Provides additional support for client and family and uses already available resources in a cost-effective manner.

Growth and Development, Altered

FLOWCHART EVALUATION: EXPECTED OUTCOME 1

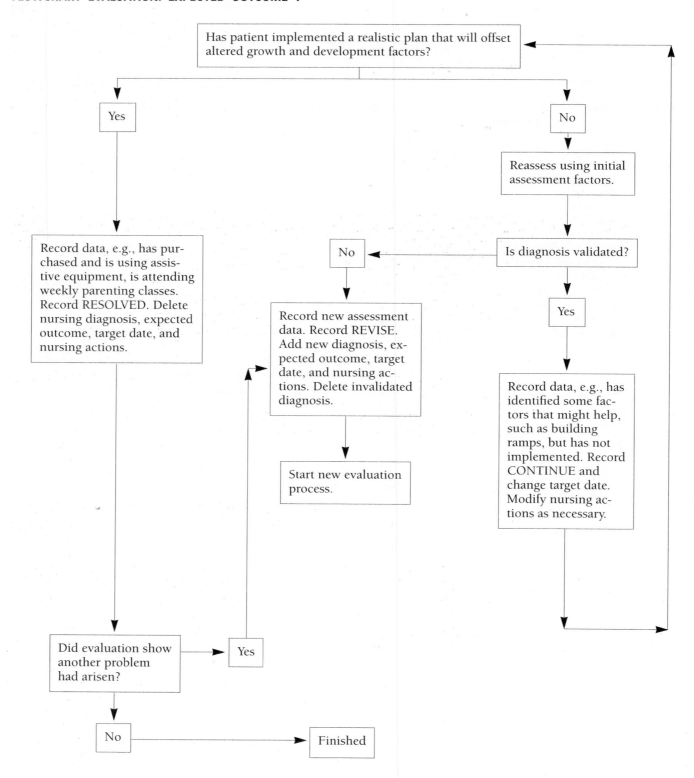

Growth and Development, Altered

FLOWCHART EVALUATION: EXPECTED OUTCOME 2

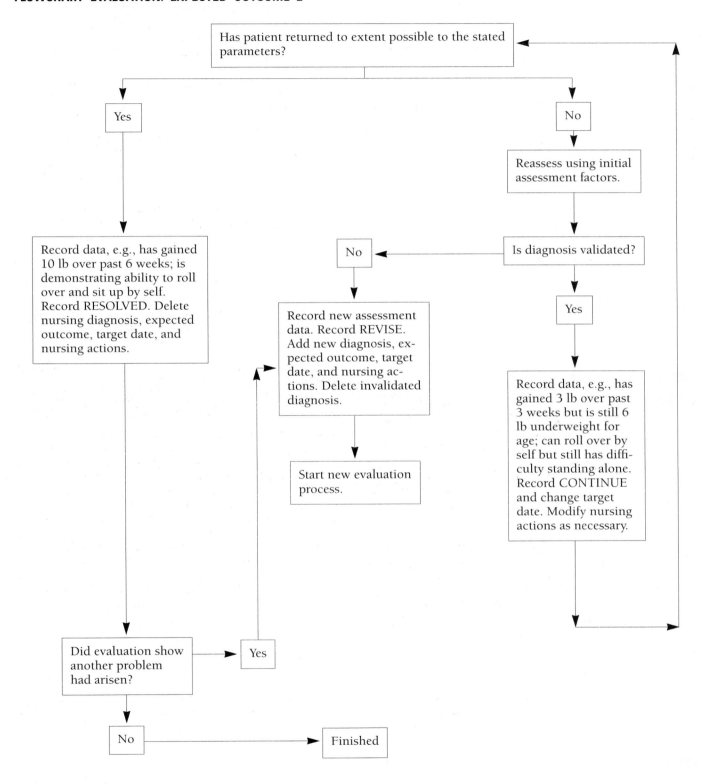

Home Maintenance Management, Impaired

DEFINITION

Inability to independently maintain a safe growth-promoting immediate environment.[10]

NANDA TAXONOMY: MOVING 6.4.1.1

DEFINING CHARACTERISTICS[10]

1. Subjective
   a. Household members express difficulty in maintaining their home in a comfortable fashion (critical).
   b. Household members request assistance with home maintenance (critical).
   c. Household members describe outstanding debts or financial crises (critical).
2. Objective
   a. Disorderly surroundings
   b. Unwashed or unavailable cooking equipment, clothes, or linen (critical)
   c. Accumulation of dirt, food wastes, or hygienic wastes (critical)
   d. Offensive odors

e. Inappropriate household temperature
f. Overtaxed family members, for example, exhausted or anxious (critical)
g. Lack of necessary equipment or aids
h. Presence of vermin or rodents
i. Repeated hygienic disorders, infestations, or infections (critical)

RELATED FACTORS[10]

1. Individual or family member disease or injury
2. Insufficient family organization or planning
3. Insufficient finances
4. Unfamiliarity with neighborhood resources
5. Impaired cognitive or emotional functioning
6. Lack of knowledge
7. Lack of role modeling
8. Inadequate support systems

RELATED CLINICAL CONCERNS

1. Dementia problems such as Alzheimer's disease
2. Rheumatoid arthritis
3. Depression
4. Cerebrovascular accident
5. Acquired immune deficiency syndrome

HAVE YOU SELECTED THE CORRECT DIAGNOSIS?

Activity Intolerance If the nurse observes or validates reports of the patient's inability to complete required tasks because of insufficient energy, then Activity Intolerance would be the more appropriate diagnosis.

Knowledge Deficit The problem with home maintenance may be due to the family's lack of education regarding the care needed and the environment that is essential to promote this care. If the patient or family verbalizes less-than-adequate understanding of home maintenance, then Knowledge Deficit is the more appropriate diagnosis.

Altered Thought Process If the patient is exhibiting impaired attention span, impaired ability to recall information, impaired perception, judgment, and decision making, or impaired conceptual and reasoning ability, the most proper diagnosis would be Altered Thought Process. Most likely, Impaired Home Management would be a companion diagnosis.

Ineffective Individual Coping or Ineffective Family Coping Suspect one of these diagnoses if there are major differences between reports by the patient and the family of health status, health perception, and health care behavior. Verbalizations by the patient or the family regarding inability to cope also require looking at these diagnoses.

Altered Family Processes Through observing family interactions and communication, the nurse may assess that Altered Family Processes should be considered. Poorly communicated messages, rigidity of family functions and roles, and failure to accomplish expected family developmental tasks are a few observations to alert the nurse to this possible diagnosis.

EXPECTED OUTCOMES

1. Will identify factors contributing to Impaired Home Maintenance Management by (date) and/or
2. Will demonstrate alterations necessary to reduce Impaired Home Maintenance Management by (date)

TARGET DATES

Target dates will depend on the severity of the Impaired Home Maintenance Management. Acceptable target dates for the first evaluation of progress toward meeting this outcome would be 5 to 7 days.

NURSING ACTIONS/INTERVENTIONS WITH RATIONALES

Adult Health

A nurse in an acute care facility might very well receive enough information, while the patient is hospitalized, to make this nursing diagnosis. However, nursing actions specific for this diagnosis will require implementation in the home environment; therefore, the reader is referred to the Home Health nursing actions for this diagnosis.

Child Health

ACTIONS/INTERVENTIONS	RATIONALES

• Monitor risk factors of or contributing factors to Altered Home Maintenance Management, to include:
  ○ Addition of a family member, e.g., birth
  ○ Increased burden of care due to child's illness or hospitalization
  ○ Lack of sufficient finances
  ○ Loss of family member, e.g., death
  ○ Hygienic practices
  ○ History of repeated infections or poor health management
  ○ Offensive odors
	Provides primary database for intervention.

• Identify ways to deal with home maintenance management alterations with assistance of applicable health team members.	Coordinated activities will be required to meet the entire range of needs related to improving problems with home maintenance management.
• Allow for individual patient and parental input in plan for addressing home maintenance management issues.	Parental input offers empowerment and attaches value to family preferences. This in turn increases the likelihood of compliance.
• Monitor educational needs related to illness and the demands of the situation, e.g., mom who must attend to a handicapped child and six other children with various school appointments, health care appointments, etc.	Monitoring of educational needs balanced with the home situation will best provide a base for intervention.
• Provide health teaching with sensitivity to patient and family situation, e.g, seeming inability to manage with overwhelming demands of child's need for care such as premature infant or child with cerebral palsy who has feeding difficulties.	Teaching to address identified needs will reduce anxiety and promote self-confidence in ability to manage.
• Provide 10–15 min each 8-h shift as a time for discussion of patient and family feelings and concerns related to health management.	Setting aside times for discussion shows respect and assigns value to the patient and family.
• Encourage patient and family to identify support groups in the community.	Support groups empower and facilitate family coping.
• If infant is at risk for sudden infant death by nature of prematurity or history of previous death in family, assist parents in learning about alarms and monitoring respiration, and institute CPR teaching. • Provide for appropriate follow-up after dismissal from hospital.	When risk factors for pulmonary arrest are present as, for example, for a SIDS infant, family members will be less anxious if they are taught CPR techniques and given opportunities to rehearse and master these techniques. Follow-up plans will provide a means of further evaluation for progress in coping with home maintenance management. Ideally, actual home visitation serves to allow the best opportunity for monitoring goal achievement.

Women's Health

ACTIONS/INTERVENTIONS	RATIONALES

• Assist the client to describe her perception or understanding of home maintenance as it relates to her lifestyle and lifestyle decisions. Include stress-related problems and effects of environment:
  ○ Allow patient time to describe work situation.
  ○ Allow patient time to describe home situation.
  ○ Encourage patient to describe how she manages her responsibilities as a mother and a working woman.
  ○ Encourage patient to describe her assets and deficits as she perceives them.
  ○ Encourage patient to list lifestyle adjustments that need to be made.
  ○ Monitor identified possible solutions, modifications, etc., designed to cope with each adjustment.
  ○ Teach client relaxation skills and coping mechanisms.
• Consider the patient's social network and significant others:
  ○ Identify significant others in patient's social network.
  ○ Involve significant others if so desired by patient in discussion and problem-solving activities regarding lifestyle adjustments.
	Provides database needed to plan changes that will increase ability in home maintenance management.

• Encourage patient to get adequate rest:
  ○ Take care of self and baby only.
  ○ Let significant other take care of the housework and other children.
  ○ Learn to sleep when the baby sleeps.
  ○ Have specific, set times for friends or relatives to visit.
  ○ If breast-feeding, significant other can change infant and bring infant to mother at night so that mother does not always have to get up for infant. Or mother can sleep with infant.
	Fatigue can be a major contributor to impaired home maintenance management.
	
	Both parents and infant get more rest. Baby begins to nurse longer and sleep for longer periods of time.

○ Cook several meals at one time and freeze them for later use.
  ○ Prepare baby formula for a 24-h period and refrigerate for later use.
  ○ Freeze breast milk, emptying breast after baby eats; significant other can then feed infant one time at night so that mother can get adequate, uninterrupted sleep.
  ○ Put breast milk into bottle and directly into freezer:
    (1) Milk can be added each time breasts are pumped until the needed amount is obtained.
    (2) Milk can be frozen for 6 wk if needed.
    (3) To use, milk should be removed from freezer and allowed to thaw to room temperature.
    (4) Once thawed, milk must be used within a 12- to 24-h period. **Do not refreeze**.	

Psychiatric Health

ACTIONS/INTERVENTIONS	RATIONALES
• Discuss with client his or her concerns about returning home. • Develop with client and significant others a list of potential home maintenance problems.	Promotes client's sense of control, which enhances self-esteem. Promotes client's and support system's sense of control, which increases the willingness of the client to work toward goals.

- Teach client and family those tasks that are necessary for home care. Note tasks and teaching plan here.
- Provide time to practice home maintenance skills, at least 30 min once a day. Medication administration could be evaluated with each dose by allowing client to administer own medications. The times and types of skills to be practiced should be listed here.
- If financial difficulties prevent home maintenance, refer to social services or a financial counselor.
- If client has not learned skills necessary to cook or clean home, arrange time with occupational therapist to assess for ability and to teach these skills. Support this learning on unit by (check all that apply):
  - Having client maintain own living area
  - Having client assist with the maintenance of the unit (state specifically those chores client is responsible for)
  - Having client assist with the planning and preparation of unit meals when this is a milieu activity
  - Having client clean and iron own clothing
- If special aids are necessary for client to maintain self successfully, refer to social services for assistance in obtaining these items.
- If client needs periodic assistance in organizing self to maintain home, refer patient to homemaker service or other community agency.
- If meal preparation is a problem, refer patient to community agency for meals-on-wheels, or assist family with preparing several meals ahead of time or exploring nutritious, easy ways to prepare meals.
- Determine with client a list of rewards for meeting the established goals for achievement of home maintenance, and then develop a schedule for the rewards. Note the reward schedule here.
- Assess environment for impairments to home maintenance, and develop with client and family a plan for resolving these difficulties (e.g., recipes that are simplified and written in large print to make them easier to follow).
- Provide appropriate positive verbal reinforcers for accomplishment of goals or steps toward the goals.
- Utilize group therapy once a day to provide:
  - Positive role models
  - Peer support
  - Reality assessment of goals
  - Exposure to a variety of problem solutions
  - Socialization and learning of social skills

Provides opportunities for positive reinforcement of approximation of goal achievement.

Provides opportunities to practice new skills in a safe environment and to receive positive reinforcement for approximation of goal achievement.

Positive reinforcement encourages the maintenance of new behavior.

Positive reinforcement encourages maintenance of new behaviors.

Gerontic Health

ACTIONS/INTERVENTIONS	RATIONALES
• Refer to local Alzheimer's and related diseases support group if dementia is present.	Alzheimer's support group can provide information on resources and techniques to continue home care.

Home Health

ACTIONS/INTERVENTIONS	RATIONALES
• Monitor factors contributing to impaired home maintenance management (items listed under related factors section).	Provides database for prevention and/or early intervention.
• Involve patient and family in planning, implementing, and promoting reduction in the impaired home maintenance management: ○ Family conference ○ Mutual goal setting ○ Communication ○ Family members given specified tasks as appropriate to reduce the impaired home maintenance management (shopping, washing clothes, disposing of garbage and trash, yard work, washing dishes, meal preparation, etc.)	Involvement improves motivation and the outcome.
• Assist patient and family in lifestyle adjustments that may be required: ○ Hygiene practices ○ Drug and alcohol use ○ Stress management techniques ○ Family and community support systems ○ Removal of hazardous environmental conditions such as improper storage of hazardous substances, open heaters and flames, breeding areas for mosquitos or mice, or congested walkways ○ Proper food preparation and storage	Provides basic information for client and family that promotes necessary lifestyle changes.
• Refer patient and family to appropriate assistive resources as indicated.	Provides additional support for client and family and uses already available resources in a cost-effective manner.

Home Maintenance Management, Impaired

FLOWCHART EVALUATION: EXPECTED OUTCOME 1

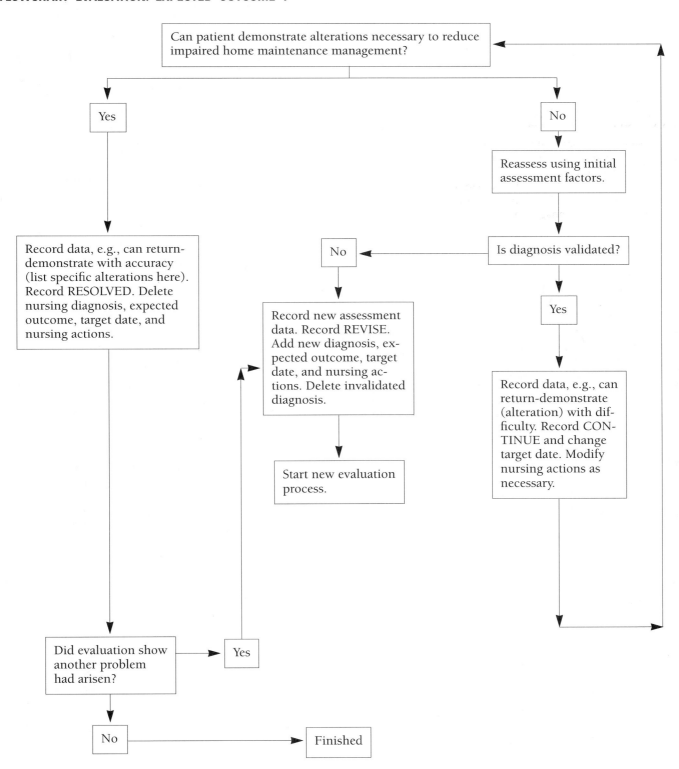

Home Maintenance Management, Impaired

FLOWCHART EVALUATION: EXPECTED OUTCOME 2

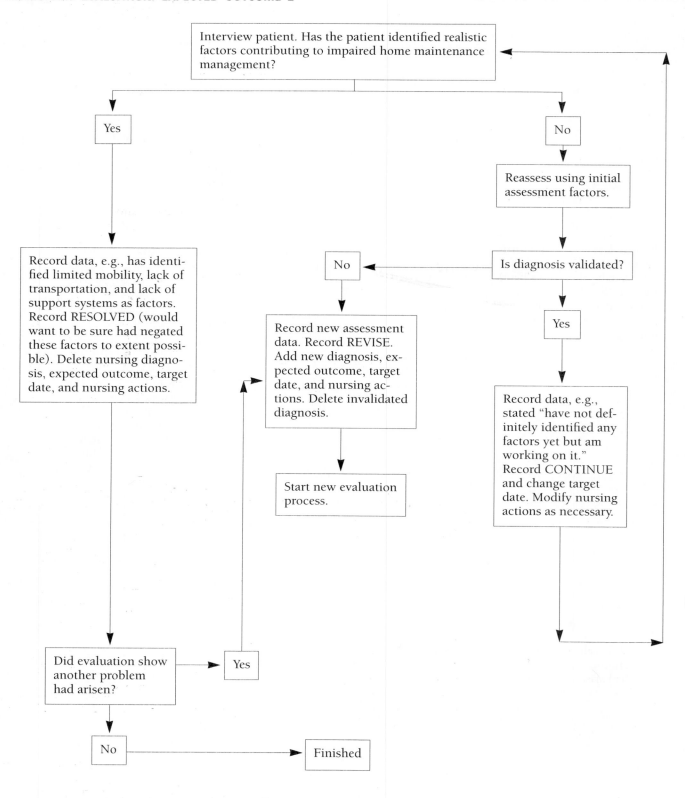

Interview patient. Has the patient identified realistic factors contributing to impaired home maintenance management?

Yes

No

Reassess using initial assessment factors.

Record data, e.g., has identified limited mobility, lack of transportation, and lack of support systems as factors. Record RESOLVED (would want to be sure had negated these factors to extent possible). Delete nursing diagnosis, expected outcome, target date, and nursing actions.

No

Is diagnosis validated?

Yes

Record new assessment data. Record REVISE. Add new diagnosis, expected outcome, target date, and nursing actions. Delete invalidated diagnosis.

Record data, e.g., stated "have not definitely identified any factors yet but am working on it." Record CONTINUE and change target date. Modify nursing actions as necessary.

Start new evaluation process.

Did evaluation show another problem had arisen?

Yes

No

Finished

Inability to Sustain Spontaneous Ventilation

DEFINITION

A state in which the response pattern of decreased energy reserves results in an individual's inability to maintain breathing adequate to support life.[10]

NANDY TAXONOMY: EXCHANGING 1.5.1.3.1

DEFINING CHARACTERISTICS[10]

1. Major defining characteristics
   a. Dyspnea
   b. Increased metabolic rate
2. Minor defining characteristics
   a. Increased restlessness
   b. Apprehension
   c. Increased use of accessory muscles
   d. Decreased tidal volume
   e. Increased heart rate
   f. Decreased pO_2
   g. Increased pCO_2
   h. Decreased cooperation
   i. Decreased SaO_2

RELATED FACTORS[10]

1. Metabolic factors
2. Respiratory muscle fatigue

RELATED CLINICAL CONCERNS

1. Chronic obstructive pulmonary disease
2. Asthma
3. Closed head injury
4. Respiratory arrest
5. Cardiac surgery
6. Adult respiratory distress syndrome

HAVE YOU SELECTED THE CORRECT DIAGNOSIS?

Ineffective Breathing Pattern   In this diagnosis the patient's respiratory effort is insufficient to maintain the cellular oxygen supply. Both diagnoses would contribute to the patient's being placed on ventilatory assistance; however, Inability to Sustain Spontaneous Ventilation would be a more life-threatening, critical diagnosis than an Ineffective Breathing Pattern. The major difference would be the criticalness of the patient's condition.

Impaired Gas Exchange   This diagnosis refers to the exchange of oxygen and carbon dioxide in the lungs or at the cellular level. Both this diagnosis and Inability to Sustain Spontaneous Ventilation demonstrate this characteristic, but an Inability to Sustain Spontaneous Ventilation is more critical than an impairment.

EXPECTED OUTCOMES

1. Blood gases will return to normal range by (date) and/or
2. Will not require ventilator support by (date)

TARGET DATES

Due to the life-threatening potential of this diagnosis, initial target dates will need to be stated in terms of hours. After the patient's condition has improved and stabilized, the target date can be increased in increments of 1 to 3 days.

NURSING ACTIONS/INTERVENTIONS WITH RATIONALES

Adult Health

ACTIONS/INTERVENTIONS	RATIONALES
• Monitor negative pressure (pneumobelt or pneumowrap) or positive pressure (intermittent or continuous) ventilators at least hourly.	Ensures correct functioning of equipment.
• Continuously monitor patient's response to ventilator.	Fear of ventilator malfunction can alter respiratory efforts.
• Provide sedation if needed.	Prevents patient from working against ("bucking") the ventilator.
• Verify ventilator settings every hour.	Ensures adequate functioning of equipment.

Continued

ACTIONS/INTERVENTIONS	RATIONALES
• Schedule at least 15 min every hour to talk with the patient. • Reassure patient's family while patient is on ventilator.	Decreases anxiety and helps prevent patient from working against the ventilator. Essential monitoring of respiratory and ventilator effectiveness.
• Monitor vital signs, especially respiratory status, at least every hour and every time nurse is with patient. • Collaborate with physician regarding frequency of ABG measurements. • Use pulse oximeter to determine oxygen saturation, and monitor every 15–30 min. • Elevate head of bed 30 degrees if not contraindicated. • Suction as needed. • Observe closely for oxygen toxicity. • Turn every 2 h on (odd/even) hour.	Monitors effectiveness of therapy. Facilitates diaphragmatic excursion. Removes secretions that may block airways. Inappropriate functioning of ventilator can cause greater oxygen consumption than the body can tolerate. Facilitates lung expansion, helps to mobilize secretions, improves circulation to extremities, and prevents pressure ulcers.
• Explain all procedures and manipulations of ventilator to patient prior to implementing. Keep call light within reach. • Provide alternative methods of communication, e.g., magic slate, pad and pencil, or flash cards of usual requests (bedpan, urinal, pain, etc.) • Provide adequate hydration. Monitor and document intake and output at least every shift and total every 24 h. Weigh patient daily at same time and in same-weight clothing. • Monitor for respiratory function, e.g., temperature, culture, and sensitivity of respiratory secretions. • Provide chest physiotherapy and postural drainage if not contraindicated. • Plan activity-rest schedule on a daily basis. Allow at least 2 h of uninterrupted rest during the day. • Review patient's resources and support systems for management of ventilator at home. • Collaborate with respiratory therapists as needed.	Assists in reducing anxiety. Avoids fluid-volume deficit, assists in liquefying secretions, and prevents development of pulmonary edema. Infection increases the respiratory demand and increases secretions. It will also decrease gas exchange. Loosens and mobilizes secretions. Conserves energy and promotes REM sleep. Initiates timely home care planning. Ensures coordination of care.

Child Health

ACTIONS/INTERVENTIONS	RATIONALES

• Determine parameters for respiratory status:
  ◦ Range of acceptable rate, rhythm, and quality of respiration
  ◦ Limits for apnea monitor setting.[60] The settings should be set for a range of safety according to age-related norms:
    (1) Neonates: 30–60
    (2) Infants: 25–60
    (3) Toddlers: 24–40
    (4) Preschoolers: 22–34
    (5) Adolescents: 12–16
  ◦ Arterial blood gases
  ◦ Oxygen saturation levels
  ◦ Respiratory testing, e.g., pneumogram
	A specific respiratory assessment will help to individualize the plan of care.

- Other indicators of respiratory functions, e.g., cyanosis, mottling, diminished pulses, listless behavior, poor feeding, or vital signs
- Provide one-on-one care for infants and children at high risk for apnea or pulmonary arrest.

In high-risk respiratory patients, the possibility of arrest should be planned for. Identification of the actual arrest is a major factor in successful resuscitation.

- Keep emergency medications and equipment (ambu bag, airway, suctioning equipment, crash cart, ventilator, and oxygen) in close proximity.

Success in appropriate treatment of pulmonary arrest requires anticipatory planning with standard treatment modalities according to the American Heart Association guidelines and Pediatric Advanced Life Support guidelines.

- Administer medication as ordered, being careful in administration of medications that might affect respirations, e.g., narcotics, bronchodilators, or vasoconstrictors. Monitor blood levels for therapeutic parameters of aminophylline-theophylline. Report levels above or below the desired range.

Anticipatory planning for the possibility of respiratory depression or arrest will lessen the likelihood of actuality in many instances and serve to allow for more success in treatment of these problems. If neuromuscular blocking agents are utilized, exercise caution in positioning due to the possibility of dislocation.[45]

- Encourage family to ventilate concerns about patient's respiratory status.

Verbalization of concerns helps reduce anxiety and provides subjective data for assessment and an opportunity for teaching.

- Allow parental input as an option when it is realistic.

Parental involvement will provide emotional security for the child and will reinforce parental coping.

- Carry out teaching according to inquiries by patient or family.

Individualized learning is facilitated when it is directed toward stated needs.

- Check level of consciousness (responsiveness) at least every 30 min.

Decreased responsiveness is indicative of onset of respiratory failure.

- Monitor and document episodes of crying that result in apnea or loss of usual color for prolonged periods (15 s or above).

Breath-holding or crying may seem to cause hypoxia, but often there are underlying causes. Attention to underlying cause can be carried out, but vigilance for possible arrest is necessary.

- Exercise caution in feeding or offering fluids.

Possible aspiration is likely if the infant is apneic, unable to suck well, or has problems swallowing.

- Monitor for factors contributing to problem:
  - Central nervous system status
  - Airway
  - Chest wall
  - Respiratory muscles
  - Lung tissue

Alteration in any aspect of respiratory anatomy will effect adequate ventilation.

ADDITIONAL INFORMATION

In the event of a decision to withhold or cease use of the ventilator for the purpose of determining brain death, be aware of the major nursing implications involved in legal acts related to brain death determination in children.

Women's Health

The nursing actions for Women's Health are the same as those for Adult Health.

Psychiatric Health

If the client develops this diagnosis while being cared for in a mental health unit, he or she should immediately be transferred to an intensive care unit or adult health unit. A mental health unit is not equipped to handle this type of emergency.

Gerontic Health

ACTIONS/INTERVENTIONS	RATIONALES
• Monitor for iatrogenic reactions to medications.	Medication reactions may decrease respiratory drive and effort.
• Observe for signs and symptoms of sleep-pattern disturbance.	Decreased rest secondary to sleep pattern disturbances further diminishes physiologic reserves in older patients.[61]

Home Health

Should the home health client develop this diagnosis, the nurse should immediately have the client transferred to an acute care setting for the proper care.

Inability to Sustain Spontaneous Ventilation

FLOWCHART EVALUATION: EXPECTED OUTCOME 1

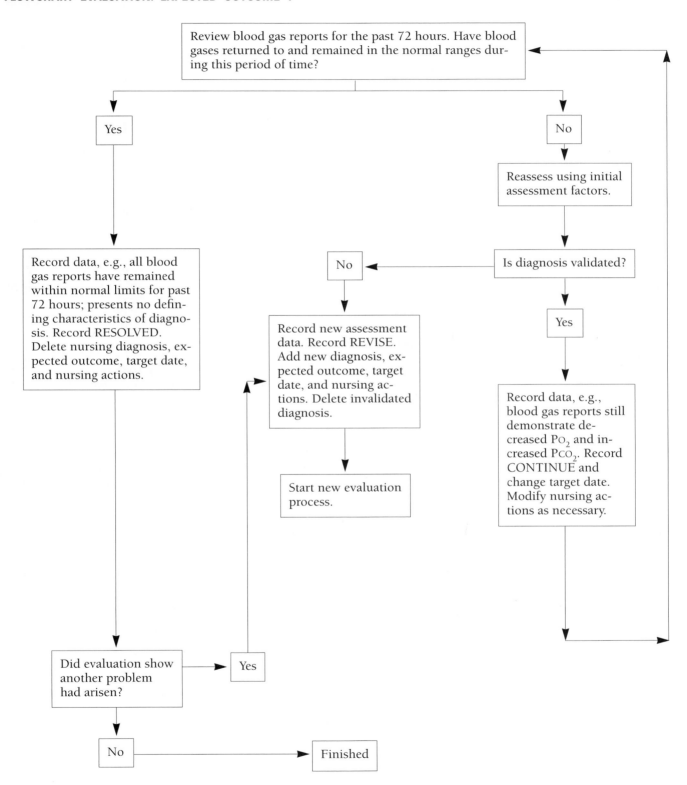

Inability to Sustain
Spontaneous Ventilation

FLOWCHART EVALUATION: EXPECTED OUTCOME 2

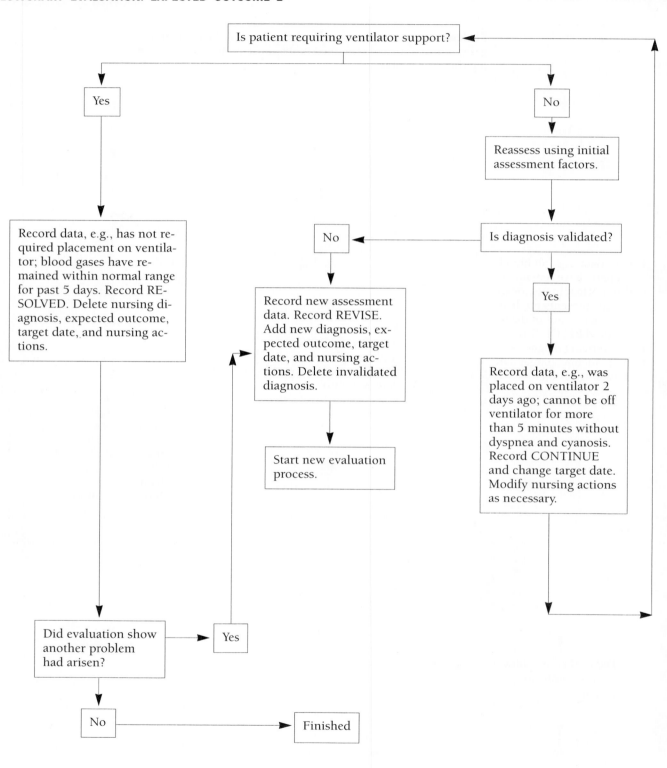

Peripheral Neurovascular Dysfunction, Risk for

DEFINITION

A state in which an individual is at risk of experiencing a disruption in circulation, sensation, or motion of an extremity.[10]

NANDA TAXONOMY: MOVING 6.1.1.1.1

DEFINING CHARACTERISTICS[10]

1. Risk factors
   a. Fractures
   b. Mechanical compression, for example, tourniquet, cast, brace, dressing, or restraint
   c. Orthopedic surgery
   d. Trauma
   e. Immobilization
   f. Burns
   g. Vascular obstruction

RELATED FACTORS[10]

The risk factors also serve as the related factors for this diagnosis.

RELATED CLINICAL CONCERNS

1. Fractures
2. Buerger's disease
3. Thrombophlebitis
4. Burns
5. Cerebrovascular accident

 HAVE YOU SELECTED THE CORRECT DIAGNOSIS?

Altered Tissue Perfusion Altered Tissue Perfusion is an actual diagnosis and indicates that a definite problem has developed. Risk for Peripheral Neurovascular Dysfunction indicates that the patient is in danger of developing a problem if appropriate nursing measures are not instituted.

EXPECTED OUTCOMES

1. Will develop no problems with peripheral neurovascular function by (date) and/or
2. Will be performing at least (number) of activities to offset development of peripheral neurovascular dysfunction by (date)

TARGET DATES

Initial target dates should be stated in hours. After the patient is able to be more involved in self-care and prevention, the target date can be expressed in increments of 3 to 5 days.

NURSING ACTIONS/INTERVENTIONS WITH RATIONALES

Adult Health

ACTIONS/INTERVENTIONS	RATIONALES
• Assist patient to do ROM exercise every 2 h on the (odd/even) hour.	Increases circulation and maintains muscle tone and movement.
• Instruct patient regarding isometric and isotonic exercises. Have patient exercise every 4 h while awake at (times).	Increases circulation and maintains muscle tone.
• Collaborate with dietitian regarding a low-fat, low-cholesterol diet. Maintain fluid and electrolyte balance.	Maintains hydration and assists in preventing development of atherosclerosis.
• Complete traction checks and peripheral assessments every 2 h on the (odd/even) hour.	Helps monitor deviations from baseline before problem reaches a serious state.
• Keep extremities warm.	Promotes circulation.
• Turn every 2 h on the (odd/even) hour.	Prevents sustained pressure on any pressure point.
• Monitor skin integrity every 2 h on the (odd/even) hour.	Allows intervention before skin breakdown occurs.
• Plan activity-rest schedule on a daily basis.	Increases circulation and maintains muscle tone without fatiguing patient.
• Monitor patient's understanding of the effect of smoking or, if nonsmoker, the effects of passive smoke on peripheral circulation.	Smoking constricts peripheral circulation, leading to increased problems with peripheral neurologic and vascular functioning.

Child Health

ACTIONS/INTERVENTIONS	RATIONALES
• Determine exact parameters to be used in monitoring risk concerns, e.g., if the patient is without sensation in specific levels of anatomy, document what the known deficits are: High level of myelomeningocele, lumbar 4, with apparent sensation in peroneal site.	Specific parameters for assessment of neurodeficits can guide caregivers in choosing the best precautionary treatment.
• Carry out treatments with attention to the neurodeficits, e.g., using warm pads for a child unable to perceive heat would require constant attention for signs or symptoms of burns.	Common safety measure.
• Provide teaching according to the patient and family needs, especially with regard to safety.	Appropriate assessment will best foster learning and help prevent injury.
• Include family in care and use of equipment, e.g., braces.	Family involvement assuages the child's emotional needs and empowers the parents.
• Provide dismissal follow-up.	Long-term follow-up validates the need for rechecking and offers a time to reassess progress in goal attainment or altered patterns.

Women's Health

NOTE: Women are at risk for thrombosis in lower extremities during pregnancy and the early postpartum period. Because of decreased venous return from the legs, compression of the large vessels supplying the legs during pregnancy and during pushing in the second stage of labor, patients need to be continuously assessed for this problem.[62]

ACTIONS/INTERVENTIONS	RATIONALES
• Closely monitor patient at each visit, and teach patient to self-monitor size, shape, symmetry, color, edema, and varicosities in the legs.	Knowledge of the problem and its causative factors can assist in planning and carrying out good health habits during pregnancy. This knowledge can assist in preventing thrombotic complications during pregnancy.
• Encourage the patient to walk daily during the pregnancy and to wear supportive hosiery.	
• Assist the patient to plan a day's schedule during pregnancy that will allow her time to rest. The schedule should also include several times during the day for her to elevate her legs.	
• Encourage the patient to use a small stool when sitting, e.g., at a desk to keep feet elevated and lessen compression on upper thighs and knees.	
• In the event that thrombophlebitis develops:	Basic assessment for early detection of complications.
○ Monitor legs for stiffness, pain, paleness, and swelling in the calf or thigh every 4 h around the clock.	
○ Place patient on strict bedrest with affected leg elevated.	Basic safety measure to avoid dislodging of clots.
• Provide analgesics as ordered for pain relief, and assess for effectiveness within 30 min of administration.	
• Place a bed cradle on the bed.	Keeps pressure of bed linens off the affected leg.
• Administer and monitor the effects of anticoagulant therapy as ordered. Collaborate with physician regarding the frequency of laboratory exams to monitor clotting factors. *Note:* Breast-feeding mothers on heparin can continue to breast-feed. Breast-feeding mothers on dicumarol should **stop** breast-feeding since it is passed to the infant in the breast milk.	

- **Do not** rub, massage, or bump affected leg. Handle leg with care when changing linens or giving bath.
- Assist family to plan for care of infant; include mother in planning process.

- Encourage verbalizations of fears and discouragement of mother and family.

Basic safety measures to avoid dislodging clots.

Assists patient and family in coping with illness. Promotes effective implementation of home care. Provides support and teaching opportunity.

Psychiatric Health

The mental health client with this diagnosis would require the same type of nursing care as the adult client. A review of the nursing actions for Activity Intolerance, Impaired Physical Mobility, and Inadequate Tissue Perfusion would also be of assistance.

Gerontic Health

ACTIONS/INTERVENTIONS	RATIONALES
• Avoid the use of restraints if at all possible.	Restraint use in older adults can lead to physical and mental deterioration, injury, and death.[63]
• Monitor restraints, if used, at least every 2 h on the (odd/even) hour. Release restraints, and perform ROM exercises before reapplying.	Frequent monitoring decreases the risk of injury.

Home Health

Nursing actions for the home health client with this diagnosis would be the same as those for the adult health client.

Peripheral Neurovascular Dysfunction, Risk for

FLOWCHART EVALUATION: EXPECTED OUTCOME 1

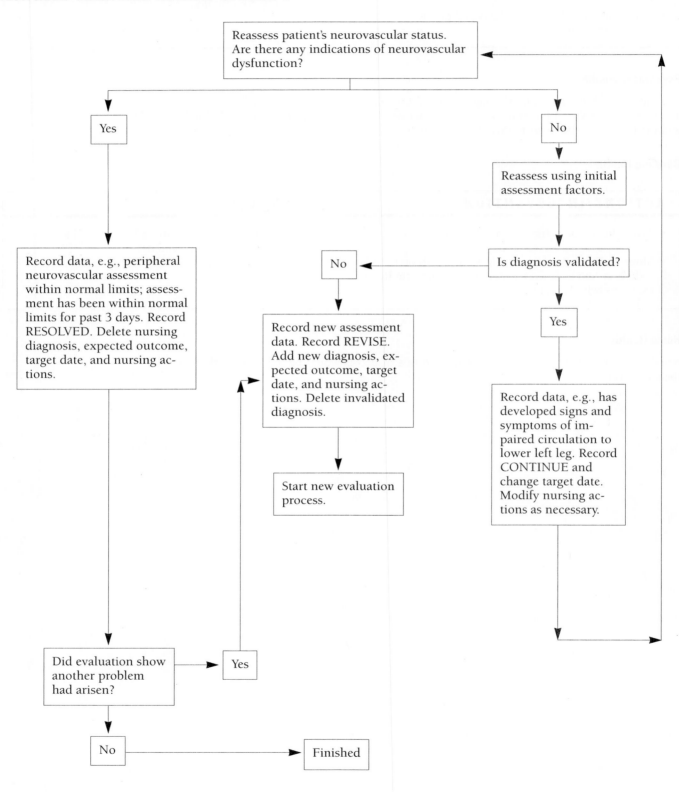

Reassess patient's neurovascular status. Are there any indications of neurovascular dysfunction?

Yes

No

Reassess using initial assessment factors.

Record data, e.g., peripheral neurovascular assessment within normal limits; assessment has been within normal limits for past 3 days. Record RESOLVED. Delete nursing diagnosis, expected outcome, target date, and nursing actions.

No

Is diagnosis validated?

Record new assessment data. Record REVISE. Add new diagnosis, expected outcome, target date, and nursing actions. Delete invalidated diagnosis.

Yes

Start new evaluation process.

Record data, e.g., has developed signs and symptoms of impaired circulation to lower left leg. Record CONTINUE and change target date. Modify nursing actions as necessary.

Did evaluation show another problem had arisen?

Yes

No

Finished

Peripheral Neurovascular Dysfunction, Risk for

FLOWCHART EVALUATION: EXPECTED OUTCOME 2

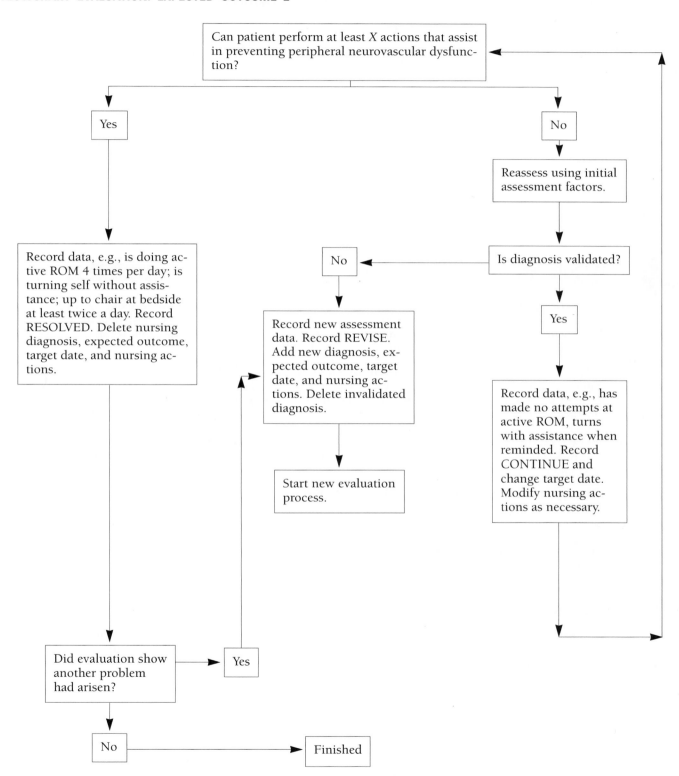

Physical Mobility, Impaired

DEFINITION

A state in which the individual experiences a limitation of ability for independent physical movement.†[10]

NANDA TAXONOMY: MOVING 6.1.1.1.

DEFINING CHARACTERISTICS[10]

1. Major defining characteristics
   a. Inability to purposefully move within the physical environment, including bed mobility, transfer, and ambulation
   b. Reluctance to attempt movement
   c. Limited range of motion
   d. Decreased muscle strength, control, and/or mass
   e. Imposed restrictions of movement, including mechanical or medical protocol
   f. Impaired coordination

2. Minor defining characteristics
   None given

RELATED FACTORS[10]

1. Intolerance to activity or decreased strength and endurance
2. Pain or discomfort
3. Perceptual or cognitive impairment
4. Neuromuscular impairment
5. Musculoskeletal impairment
6. Depression or severe anxiety

RELATED CLINICAL CONCERNS

1. Fractures that require casting or traction
2. Rheumatoid arthritis
3. Cerebrovascular accident
4. Depression
5. Any neuromuscular disorder

HAVE YOU SELECTED THE CORRECT DIAGNOSIS?

Activity Intolerance   This diagnosis implies that the individual is freely able to move but cannot endure or adapt to the increased energy or oxygen demands made by the movement or activity. Impaired Physical Mobility indicates that an individual would be able to move independently if something were not limiting the motion.

Impaired Physical Mobility   This diagnosis also needs to be differentiated from the respiratory (Impaired Gas Exchange and Ineffective Breathing Pattern) and cardiovascular (Decreased Cardiac Output and Altered Tissue Perfusion) nursing diagnoses. Mobility depends on effective breathing patterns and effective gas exchange between the lungs and the arterial blood supply. Muscles have to receive oxygen and get rid of carbon dioxide for contraction and relaxation. Since oxygen is transported and dispersed to the muscle tissue via the cardiovascular system, it is only logical that the respiratory and cardiovascular diagnoses could impact mobility.

Altered Nutrition, More or Less Than Body Requirements   Nutritional deficit would indicate that the body is not receiving enough nutrients for its metabolic needs. Without adequate nutrition, the muscles cannot function appropriately. With More Than Body Requirements, mobility may be impaired simply because of the excess weight. In someone who is grossly obese, range of motion is limited, gait is altered, and coordination and tone are greatly reduced.

EXPECTED OUTCOMES

1. Will demonstrate measures (identify specifics) to increase mobility by (date) and/or
2. Will demonstrate increased strength and endurance by (date)

TARGET DATES

These dates may be short term or long term based on the etiology of the diagnosis. An acceptable first target date would be 5 days.

---

†Suggested Functional Level Classification
0 = Completely independent.
1 = Requires use of equipment or device.
2 = Requires help from another person, for assistance, supervision, or teaching.
3 = Requires help from another person and equipment device.
4 = Dependent, does not participate in activity.
Code adapted by NANDA from E Jones, et al, Patient Classification for Long-Term Care: Users' Manual, HEW, Publication No HRA-74-3107, November 1974.

NURSING ACTIONS/INTERVENTIONS WITH RATIONALES
Adult Health

ACTIONS/INTERVENTIONS	RATIONALES
• Maintain proper body alignment at all times; support extremities with pillows, blankets, towel rolls, or sandbags. Use footboards, firm mattress, and bed boards as necessary to support positioning.	Prevents flexion contractures.
• Implement measures to prevent falls such as keeping bed in low position, raising siderails, and having items within easy reach.	Basic safety measures.
• Teach patient how to move body in bed.	Prevents shearing forces. Participation promotes self-esteem.
• Perform ROM exercises (passive, active, and functional) every 2 h on the (odd/even) hour.	Increases circulation, maintains muscle tone, and prevents joint contractures.
• Turn, cough, and deep breathe every 2 h on a schedule opposite from the ROM exercises, e.g., if ROM is on even hour, then turn, cough, and deep breathe on odd hour. Massage pressure points after turning.	Increases circulation, promotes maintenance of lung functioning, keeps airways clear, and assists in preventing hypostatic pneumonia. Improves tissue oxygenation.
• Monitor skin over pressure areas every 4 h while awake at (times).	Basic monitoring of skin integrity.
• Implement nursing actions specific to traction, casts, braces, prostheses, slings, and bandages.	Each of these therapies also has complicating side effects.
• Provide progressive mobilization as tolerated. Schedule increased mobilization on a daily basis, e.g., increase ambulation length by 25 ft each day.	Maintains muscle tone and prevents complications of immobility.
• Medicate for pain as needed, especially before activity. Document effectiveness of medication within 30 min after administering medication.	Pain interferes with ability to ambulate by inhibiting muscle movement.
• Apply heat or cold as ordered.	Aids in muscle healing and promotes relaxation.
• Maintain adequate nutrition on a daily basis.	Provides nutrients for energy and prevents protein loss due to immobility.
• Collaborate with physical therapist regarding exercise program.	Coordinates team approach to care.
• Observe for complications of immobility, e.g., negative nitrogen balance or constipation.	Allows early detection and prevention of complications.
• Provide health teaching: ◦ Transfer methods ◦ Use of assistive devices ◦ Safety precautions ◦ Positioning and body mechanics ◦ Prescribed exercise ◦ Self-care activities	Facilitates understanding of care. Encourages participation in care. Promotes effective management of therapeutic regimen.
• Include patient and family or significant other in carrying out plan of care.	Allows time for practice under supervision. Increases likelihood of effective management of therapeutic regimen.

Child Health

ACTIONS/INTERVENTIONS	RATIONALES
• Monitor alteration in mobility each 8-h shift according to: ◦ Actual movement noted and tolerance for the movement ◦ Factors related to movement, e.g., braces used or progress in use	Provides the primary database for an individualized plan of care.

Continued

ACTIONS/INTERVENTIONS	RATIONALES
○ Situational factors, e.g., previous status, current health needs, or movement permitted ○ Pain ○ Circulation check to affected limb ○ Change in appearance of affected limb or joint • Include related health team members in care of patient as needed. • Consider patient and family preferences in planning to meet desired mobility goals. • Encourage family members, especially parents, to participate in care of patient according to needs and situation (feeding and comfort measures). • Provide diversional activities appropriate for age and developmental level. • Maintain appropriate safety guidelines according to age and developmental guidelines. • Devote appropriate attention to traction or related equipment in use, e.g., weights hanging free or rope knots tight. • Monitor patient and family needs for education regarding patient's situation and any future implications. • Attend to intake and output to ensure adequate fluid balance for each 24-h period. • Address related health issues appropriate for patient and family.	The nurse is in the prime position to coordinate health team members to best match needs and resources. Consideration of preferences increases likelihood of plan success. Involving family in care serves to enhance their skills in care required at home. Diversional activity, when appropriately planned, serves to refresh and relax the patient. Basic requirements for maintaining standards of care. Ensures therapeutic effectiveness of equipment and provides for safety issues related to these interventions. Allows timely planning for home care and allows practice of care in a supportive environment. Strict intake and output will assist in monitoring hydration status, which is crucial for healing and circulatory adequacy. Appropriate attention to related health issues fosters holistic care; e.g., child may need braces but may also have need for healing, or speech follow-up secondary to meningitis, and developmental delays.

Women's Health

NOTE: The following nursing actions apply to those women placed on restrictive activities because of threatened abortions, premature labor, multiple pregnancy, or pregnancy-induced hypertension.

ACTIONS/INTERVENTIONS	RATIONALES
• Encourage family and significant others to participate in plan of care for patient. • When resting in bed, have patient rest in left lateral position as much as possible. • Encourage patient to list lifestyle adjustments that will need to be made. • Teach patient relaxation skills and coping mechanisms. • Encourage adequate protein intake. • Maintain proper body alignment with use of positioning and pillow. • Provide diversionary activities, e.g., hobbies, job-related activities that can be done in bed, or activities with children. • Encourage help and visits from friends and relatives: ○ Visit in person ○ Telephone visit ○ Help with childcare ○ Help with housecare	Will prevent supine hypotension and will allow adequate renal and uterine perfusion. Decreases anxiety and muscle tension. Replaces protein lost due to decreasing muscle contraction during immobility. Decreases anxiety and reduces muscle tension. Provides appropriate amounts of activity without danger to pregnancy.

Psychiatric Health

ACTIONS/INTERVENTIONS	RATIONALES
NOTE: The following actions and interventions are related to impose restrictions.	
• Attempt all other interventions before considering immobilizing client as an intervention (see Risk for Violence, Chap. 9, for appropriate nursing actions).	Promotes client's sense of control and supports self-esteem.
• Carefully monitor client for appropriate level of restraint necessary. Immobilize the client as little as possible while still protecting the client and others.	
• Obtain necessary medical orders to initiate methods that limit the client's physical mobility.	
• Carefully explain to client in brief, concise language reasons for initiating this intervention and what behavior must be present for the intervention to be terminated.	Excessive stimuli can increase confusion. Explanation provides client with sense of control.
• Attempt to gain client's voluntary compliance with the intervention by explaining to client what is needed and with a "show of force" (have the necessary number of staff available to force compliance).	Promotes client's sense of control and safety, which promotes self-esteem.
• Initiate forced compliance only if there is an adequate number of staff to complete the action safely. (See Risk for Violence, Chap. 9, for a detailed description of intervention with forced compliance.)	Client and staff safety is of primary concern.
• Secure the environment the client will be in by removing harmful objects such as accessible light bulbs, sharp objects, glass objects, tight clothing, and metal objects such as clothes hangers or shower curtain rods.	Prevents injury by protecting client from impulsive actions of self-harm.
• If client is placed in four-point restraints, maintain one-to-one supervision.	Client safety is of primary concern.
• If client is in seclusion or in bilateral restraints, observe client at least every 15 min, more frequently if agitated (list observation schedule here).	
• Leave urinal in room with client or offer toileting every hour.	
• Offer client fluids every 15 min.	Maintains adequate hydration.
• Discuss with client his or her feelings about the initiation of immobility and review with him or her again, at least twice a day, the behavior necessary to have immobility discontinued.	Exploration of feelings in an accepting environment helps client to identify and explore maladaptive coping behaviors. Promotes client's sense of perceived control.
• When checking client, let him or her know you are checking by calling him or her by name and orienting him or her to day and time. Inquire about client's feelings and implement necessary reality orientation.	Promotes perceived control and promotes an environment of trust.
• Provide meals at regular intervals on paper containers providing necessary assistance (amount and type of assistance required should be listed here).	Meets biophysical need while providing consistency in a respectful manner, which promotes self-esteem and trust.
• If client is in restraints, remove restraints at least every 2 h, one limb at a time. Have client move limb through a full ROM and inspect for signs of injury. Apply lubricants such as lotion to area under restraint to protect from injury.	Promotes normal circulation and motion, which prevent injury to the limb.
• Pad the area of the restraint that is next to the skin with sheepskin or other nonirritating material.	Protects skin from mechanical irritation.
• Check circulation in restrained limbs in the area below the restraint by observing skin color, warmth, and swelling. Restraint should not interfere with circulation.	Early assessment and intervention prevents serious injury.
• Change client's position in the bed every 2 h on the (odd/even) hour.	Prevents disuse syndrome.

Continued

ACTIONS/INTERVENTIONS	RATIONALES
• Place body in proper alignment. Use pillows for support if client's condition allows.	Prevents complications and injury.
• If client is in four-point restraints, place him or her on stomach or side.	Prevents aspiration or choking.
• Place client on intake and output monitoring.	Assures that adequate fluid balance is maintained.
• Have client in seclusion move around the room at least every 2 h on the (odd/even) hour, and during this time initiate active ROM.	Prevents complications of immobility.
• Administer medications as ordered for agitation.	Medications reduce anxiety and facilitate interaction with others.
• Monitor blood pressure before administering antipsychotic medications.	Psychotropic medications can cause orthostatic hypotension.
• Assist client with daily personal hygiene (record time for this here).	Communicates positive regard for the client by the nurse, which facilitates the development of positive self-esteem.
• Have environment cleaned on a daily basis.	Promotes sanitary conditions and provides an orderly environment, which can decrease the client's disorganization and confusion.
• Review with client the purpose for restraint or seclusion as required, and discuss alternative kinds of behavior that will express feelings without threatening self or others.	Promotes client's sense of control by providing him or her with behavioral alternatives and establishing clear limits.
• Remove client from seclusion as soon as the contracted behavior is observed for the required amount of time (both of these should be very specific and listed here). See Risk for Violence, Chap. 9, for detailed information on behavior change and contracting specifics.	Provides positive reinforcement for appropriate coping behavior and promotes client's sense of control.
○ Schedule time to discuss this intervention with client and his or her support system. Inform support system of the need for the intervention and about special considerations related to visiting with the client. This information must be provided with consideration of client confidentiality. Plan to spend at least 5 min with the members of the support system before and after each visit.	Support system understanding and support of treatment goals have a positive effect on client outcome.
○ Arrange consultations with appropriate resources after client is released from mobility limitations to assist client with developing alternative coping behavior. This could include a physical therapist, an occupational therapist, or a social worker.	Facilitates the development of trust as well as respect for the client, which can have a positive effect on the client's self-esteem.
NOTE: The following interventions are related to restrictions due to psychogenic causes	
○ If restrictions are due to anxiety, refer to Chap. 8 and the diagnosis of anxiety.	
○ If restrictions are due to depressed mood, implement the following interventions:	
(1) Sit with client for (number) minutes (number) times per shift. Initially these times will be brief but frequent, e.g., 5 min per hour.	
(2) Establish clear expectations for these interactions; e.g., client is not expected to talk and it is ok for these times to be spent in silence.	Communicates respect for the client and facilitates the client's perception of control.
• Explain to client in simple concrete terms the positive effects of physical activity on mood. Note person responsible for this teaching here.	Physical activity can stimulate endorphin production, which has a positive effect on mood.
• Talk with client about activities he or she has enjoyed in the past.	Promotes a positive expectational set based on past positive experiences.

• Develop with client a program for increasing physical activity. Note that contact here. Also note rewards for accomplishing goals, e.g., will walk from bed to door once per hour. If accomplished, client can remain in bed during visiting hours. Activities can increase as client masters each step.

Promotes client's sense of control. Positive reinforcement encourages behavior and enhances self-esteem.

• Provide positive verbal reinforcement for accomplishing tasks.

• Recognize client's perceptions about the difficulty of physical activity in the initial stages of recovery.

• Pair physical activity with situations the client finds rewarding. Note these situations here, e.g., walking with client to get a cup of coffee. This pairs walking with two things the client finds rewarding: (1) time with nurse and (2) coffee.

Positive recognition from significant others enhances self-esteem.

Communicates acceptance of client and facilitates the development of a trusting relationship.

Promotes positive expectational set by pairing physical exercise with a positive stimuli.

• Have client identify perceived barriers to increased physical activity. Note those here and develop with client plan for reducing these. Note plan here.

• Teach support system the importance of client's increasing physical activity, and have them identify ways they could assist with this. Note here the person responsible for this, and record the plan when it is developed.

Promotes client's sense of control and increases the client's commitment to the plan since he or she has contributed to the plan.

Support system involvement increases the probability for positive outcome.

Gerontic Health

ACTIONS/INTERVENTIONS	RATIONALES
• Monitor for complications of immobility such as: ○ Orthostatic hypotension ○ Thrombosis ○ Urinary tract infections ○ Constipation	Normal aging changes in combination with immobility can leave the older adult at increased risk for complications.[64]
• Observe patient when he or she is changing position, pushing a wheelchair, or toileting for Valsalva maneuver (increased intrathoracic pressure induced by forceful exhalation against a closed glottis).	Valsalva maneuver can produce increased pulse rate and increased BP. This adversely affects patients with cardiovascular disorders, which may lead to their choosing not to engage in physical activity.[64]
• Monitor for behavioral changes that may result from decreased sensory stimulation or decreased socialization, e.g., depression, hostility, confusion, or anxiety.	Psychologic changes not addressed may increase problems of physical mobility and lead to prolonged periods of immobility.
• Observe when increasing mobility, transferring, or during early ambulation stage for the high risk for falls.	Older adults may be at risk for falls secondary to orthostatic BP changes or problems with balance especially after prolonged periods of immobility.
• Teach client to perform isometric muscle contraction, namely, tightening of muscle group as hard as possible and then relaxing the muscles.	Isometric contraction helps maintain muscle strength, which can decrease with immobility as much as 5% per day.[64]

Home Health

ACTIONS/INTERVENTIONS	RATIONALES
• Assist patient and family in identifying risk factors pertinent to the situation: ○ Immobility ○ Malnourishment ○ Confusion or lethargy ○ Physical barriers ○ Neuromuscular deficit ○ Musculoskeletal deficit ○ Trauma ○ Pain ○ Medications that affect coordination and level of arousal ○ Debilitating disease (cancer, stroke, diabetes, muscular dystrophy, multiple sclerosis, arthritis, etc.) ○ Depression ○ Lack of or improper use of assistive devices ○ Casts, slings, traction, IVs, etc. ○ Weather hazards	Locus of control shifts from nurse to client and family, thus promoting self-care.
• Teach client and family measures to promote physical activity: ○ Use of assistive devices (wheelchairs, crutches, canes, walkers, prostheses, adaptive eating utensils, devices to assist with activities of daily living, etc.) ○ Providing safe environment (reducing barriers to activity such as throw rugs, furniture in pathway, electric cords on floor, doors, or steps) ○ Maintaining skin integrity ○ Use of safety devices (ramps, lift bars, tub rails, tub or shower seat) ○ Proper transfer techniques	
• Assist patient and family in identifying lifestyle changes that may be required. ○ Alteration in living space (ramps, assistive devices, etc.) ○ Changes in role functions ○ Range of motion exercises ○ Positioning and transferring techniques ○ Pain control ○ Progressive activity ○ Use of assistive devices ○ Prevention of injury ○ Maintenance of skin integrity ○ Assistance with activities of daily living ○ Special transportation needs ○ Financial concerns	Provides basic information for client and family that promotes necessary lifestyle changes.
• Consult with or refer patient to appropriate assistive resources as indicated.	Provides additional support for client and family and uses already available resources in a cost-effective manner.

Physical Mobility, Impaired

FLOWCHART EVALUATION: EXPECTED OUTCOME 1

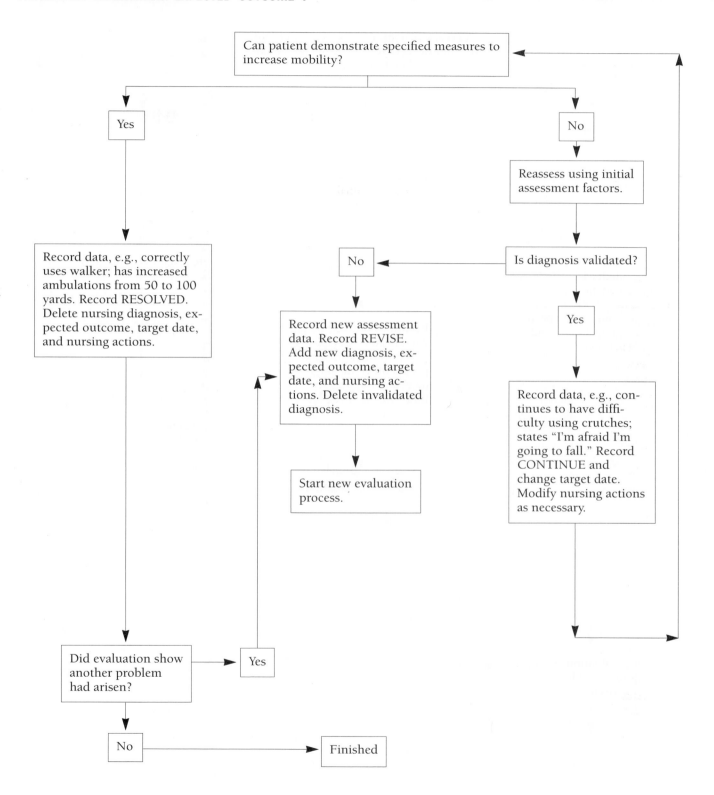

Physical Mobility, Impaired

FLOWCHART EVALUATION: EXPECTED OUTCOME 2

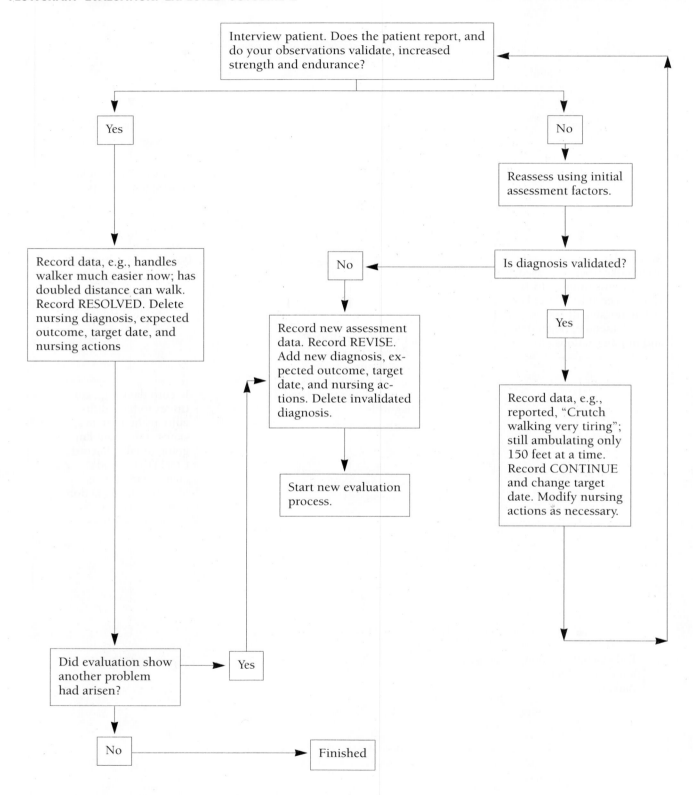

Self-Care Deficit
(Feeding, Bathing-Hygiene, Dressing-Grooming, Toileting)

DEFINITION

A state in which an individual experiences an impaired ability to perform complete feeding, bathing-hygiene, dressing-grooming, or toileting activities for himself or herself.[10]

NANDA TAXONOMY: MOVING 6.5.1, 6.5.2, 6.5.3, AND 6.5.4

DEFINING CHARACTERISTICS[10]

1. Feeding Self-Care Deficit‡
   a. Major defining characteristics
      (1) Inability to bring food from a receptacle to the mouth
   b. Minor defining characteristics
      None given
2. Bathing-Hygiene Self-Care Deficit‡
   a. Major defining characteristics
      (1) Inability to wash body or body parts (critical defining characteristic)
      (2) Inability to obtain or get to water source
      (3) Inability to regulate temperature or flow
   b. Minor defining characteristics
      None given
3. Dressing-Grooming Self-Care Deficit‡
   a. Major defining characteristics
      (1) Impaired ability to put on or take off necessary items of clothing (critical defining characteristic)
      (2) Impaired ability to obtain or replace articles of clothing
      (3) Impaired ability to fasten clothing
      (4) Inability to maintain appearance at a satisfactory level
   b. Minor defining characteristics
      None given
4. Toileting Self-Care Deficit‡

   a. Major defining characteristics
      (1) Unable to get to toilet or commode (critical defining characteristic)
      (2) Unable to sit on or rise from toilet or commode (critical defining characteristic)
      (3) Unable to manipulate clothing for toileting (critical defining characteristic)
      (4) Unable to carry out proper toilet hygiene (critical defining characteristic)
      (5) Unable to flush toilet or commode
   b. Minor defining characteristics
      None given

RELATED FACTORS[10]

1. Feeding, Bathing-Hygiene, or Dressing-Grooming Self-Care Deficit
   a. Intolerance to activity; decreased strength and endurance
   b. Pain or discomfort
   c. Perceptual or cognitive impairment
   d. Neuromuscular impairment
   e. Musculoskeletal impairment
   f. Depression or severe anxiety
2. Toileting Self-Care Deficit
   a. Impaired transfer ability
   b. Impaired mobility status
   c. Intolerance to activity
   d. Decreased strength and endurance
   e. Pain or discomfort
   f. Perceptual or cognitive impairment
   g. Neuromuscular impairment
   h. Musculoskeletal impairment
   i. Depression of severe anxiety

RELATED CLINICAL CONCERNS

1. Cerebrovascular accident
2. Spinal cord injury
3. Dementia
4. Depression
5. Rheumatoid arthriti

HAVE YOU SELECTED THE CORRECT DIAGNOSIS?

Activity Intolerance This diagnosis implies that the individual is freely able to move but cannot endure or adapt to the increased energy or oxygen demands made by the movement or activity. Activity Intolerance can be a contributing factor to the development of self-care deficits.

Impaired Physical Mobility This diagnosis is quite often a contributing factor to the development of Self-Care Deficit. It is probable that any time a patient has Impaired Physical Mobility, he or she will also have some degree of Self-Care Deficit.

Altered Thought Process If the patient is exhibiting impaired attention span, impaired ability to recall information, impaired perception, judgment, and decision making, or impaired conceptual and reasoning ability, the most proper diagnosis would be Altered Thought Process. Most likely, Self-Care Deficit would be a companion diagnosis.

---

‡Level 0 to 4: Use same code as in Impaired Physical Mobility.

> **Ineffective Individual Coping or Ineffective Family Coping** Suspect one of these diagnoses if there are major differences between reports by the patient and the family of health status, health perception, and health care behavior. Verbalizations by the patient or the family regarding inability to cope also require looking at these diagnoses.
>
> **Altered Family Processes** Through observing family interactions and communication, the nurse may assess that Altered Family Processes should be considered. Poorly communicated messages, rigidity of family functions and roles, and failure to accomplish expected family developmental tasks are a few observations to alert the nurse to this possible diagnosis.

EXPECTED OUTCOMES

1. Will implement a self-care plan by (date) and/or
2. Will return-demonstrate, with 100 percent accuracy, (specify) self-care by (date)

TARGET DATES

Overcoming a self-care deficit will take a significant investment of time; however, 7 days from the date of diagnosis would be appropriate to check for progress.

NURSING ACTIONS/INTERVENTIONS WITH RATIONALES

Adult Health

NOTE: Self-care deficits range from a total self-care deficit to very specific areas of self-care deficits such as bathing-hygiene or feeding. The nursing actions presented are general in nature and would need to be adapted to fit the exact self-care deficit of the individual. Collaboration with a rehabilitation nurse clinician and/or review of rehabilitation literature would be excellent sources for current and specific nursing actions related to a patient's particular self-care deficit. Review of the nursing actions for Altered Urinary Elimination Patterns, Activity Intolerance, Impaired Physical Activity, Impaired Skin Integrity, and Altered Nutrition will also be helpful.

ACTIONS/INTERVENTIONS	RATIONALES

• Provide extra time for giving daily care and include:
  ○ Emotional support
  ○ Teaching
  ○ Return-demonstration of self-care activities
	Instills trust, avoids overwhelming patient, facilitates self-motivation, and allows immediate feedback on self-care.

• Provide privacy and safety for patient to practice self-care.	Avoids embarrassment for patient, provides basic safety, and allows practice under closely supervised situation.
• Remind patient to wear corrective appliances, e.g., braces, dentures, glasses, or hearing aid.	Promotes self-care by offsetting present limitations.
• Provide positive reinforcement for each self-care accomplishment.	Increases self-esteem and motivation.
• Perform ROM exercises, or assist patient with them every 4 h while awake at (times).	Increases circulation and maintains muscle tone and joint mobility.

• Assist patient and significant others in planning measures to overcome or adapt to self-care deficits:
  ○ Gradual increments in self-care responsibility, e.g., getting up in chair independently before ambulating to bathroom by self
  ○ Self-care assistive devices, e.g., helping hand
	Promotes timely home care planning and encourages participation in care.

• Assist significant others to provide assistive devices, e.g., raised toilet seat, buttonhook, or angled extension comb and brush.	

• Place visual aid in room to help document progress:
  ○ Chart that allows placement of stars for each day patient accomplishes goal in self-care
  ○ Calendar to document progress
	Visually documents succeess.

• Monitor:
  ○ Vital signs every 4 h while awake at (times)
  ○ Ambulation: Increase, to extent possible, on a daily basis
	Baseline data needed to validate progress and assist in determining physiologic impact of progress.

• Collaborate with physician regarding pain management	Pain inhibits muscle movement and activity.
• Measure intake and output. Total every 8 h and every 24 h	Basic monitoring of fluid and electrolyte status that impacts mobility and self-care.
• Monitor bowel elimination at least once daily at (time).	Baseline data that assist in determining bowel functioning pattern.
• Establish bowel- and bladder-retraining programs as necessary. See Altered Bowel and Urinary Elimination, Chap. 4.	Provides basic education, practice, and reinforcement that facilitates patient's control of these functions.
• Collaborate with dietitian regarding diet, e.g., foods to facilitate self-feeding.	Promotes self-care and provides motivation to continue striving for improvement.
• Refer patient to community support services.	Provides for long-time support.

• Have visiting nurse service assist significant others to adapt home environment, at least 3 days prior to discharge:
  ○ Nonskid rugs
  ○ Ramps
  ○ Handrails
  ○ Safety strips in tub and shower
	Provides time to adapt home for basic safety measures.

Child Health

ACTIONS/INTERVENTIONS	RATIONALES
• Monitor patient's and parent's potential for self-care measures appropriate to age and developmental factors.	Provides a database for an individualized plan of care.
• Allow patient and parents to participate in planning for care when possible to help ensure best compliance.	Enhances satisfaction and increases likelihood that care will be continued after discharge from hospital.
• Teach the appropriate skills necessary for self-care in the child's terms with sensitivity to developmental needs for practice, repetition, or reluctance.	Individualized teaching is the best way to reinforce learning. Sensitivity to special needs attaches value to the patient and family's needs.
• Provide opportunities that will enhance the child's confidence in performing self-care.	Confidence in self-care will enhance self-esteem.

Women's Health

ACTIONS/INTERVENTIONS	RATIONALES
• Encourage patient to list lifestyle adjustments that need to be made	Promotes gradual assumption of self-care while avoiding overwhelming patient with activities that must be accomplished.

• Encourage progressive activity and increased self-care as tolerated:
  ○ Ambulation
  ○ Bathing
  ○ Body image and early postpartum exercises
  ○ Bowel care
  ○ Breast care
  ○ Perineal care	

• Encourage patient to get adequate rest:
  ○ Take care of self and baby only.
  ○ Let significant other take care of the housework and other children.
  ○ Learn to sleep when the baby sleeps.
  ○ Have specific, set times for friends or relatives to visit.	

Continued

ACTIONS/INTERVENTIONS	RATIONALES
∘ If breast-feeding, significant other can bring infant to mother at night (mother doesn't have to get up every time for infant).	
• Provide quiet, supportive atmosphere for interaction with infant.	Promotes attachment.
• Instruct patient in infant care, and have her return-demonstrate:	Basic teaching measures for care of newborn.
∘ Bathing	
(1) **Never** leave infant or small child alone in bath.	
(2) Bathe infant in small area (kitchen sink is good) for first weeks.	
(3) Use warm area in house.	
(4) Use area convenient for mother.	
(5) Be sure area is not drafty.	
(6) Never run water directly from faucet onto infant, and always test it with forearm before placing infant in it (water should be warm, but not too hot).	
∘ Cord care	
(1) Clean cord with alcohol and cotton swabs when changing diaper.	
(2) Clean around base of cord.	
(3) Leave cord alone until it drops off by itself.	
(4) Alert mother that there will be a small amount of spotting (bleeding) at cord site when it drops off.	
∘ Clothing	
(1) To determine if infant is warm enough, feel infant's chest or back with hand; never judge infant's body temperature by feeling infant's hands or feet.	
(2) Use mild detergent when laundering infant's clothing.	
∘ Diapering	
(1) Cloth diapers	
(2) Disposable diapers	
(3) Cleaning of infant when changing diapers	
∘ Circumcision care—Yellen clamp (metal clamp)	
(1) Gently wash penis with water to remove urine and feces.	
(2) Reapply fresh, sterile petrolatum gauze around glans.	
(3) It is best to use cloth diapers until completely healed (approximately 7–10 days).	
∘ Circumcision care—Plastic bell	
(1) Gently wash penis with water to remove urine and feces.	
(2) **Do not** apply petrolatum gauze.	
(3) Leave plastic circle on penis alone until tissue heals and circle falls off.	
∘ Taking baby's temperature and reading a thermometer:	
(1) Axillary	
(2) Rectal	
• Explain infant alert and rest states and how caretaker can best interact with infant during these states.	Promotes attachment.

Psychiatric Health

ACTIONS/INTERVENTIONS	RATIONALES
• Determine client's optimum level of functioning and note here.	This information assists in establishing realistic goals.
• Develop behavioral short-term goals by:	Goal accomplishment provides positive reinforcement and enhances self-esteem.
○ Listing those activities client can assume	
○ Breaking these activities into their component parts	
○ Determining how much of each activity client could successfully complete and listing achievable activities here with goal achievement dates	
○ Discussing expectations with client	
• Keep instructions simple.	Inappropriate levels of sensory stimuli can contribute to the client's sense of disorganization and confusion. Interaction with the nurse can be a source of positive reinforcement.
• Provide support to client during tasks by:	
○ Spending time with client while he or she is completing the task	
○ Having all items necessary to achieve task readily available	Increases possibility for client's successfully completing the task.
○ Assisting client in focusing on the task at hand	
○ Providing positive verbal feedback as each step of the task is achieved	Positive feedback encourages behavior.
• Keep environment uncluttered, presenting only those items necessary to complete the task in the order needed.	Inappropriate levels of sensory stimuli can contribute to the client's sense of disorganization and confusion.
• Develop a reward schedule for achievement of goals. Discuss with client possible rewards, and list those things client finds rewarding here with the goal to be achieved to gain the reward.	Promotes client's sense of control, and positive feedback encourages behavior.
• Schedule adequate time for client to accomplish task (depressed client may need 2 h to bathe and dress).	Communicates acceptance of the client, which facilitates the development of trust and self-esteem.
• Decrease environmental stimuli to the degree necessary to assist client in focusing on task.	Promotes client's sense of control.
• Present activities of daily living on a regular schedule, and note that schedule here. This schedule should be developed in consultation with the client.	
• Spend (number) minutes with client twice a day discussing feelings and reactions to current progress and expectations. Times for this and person responsible for this activity should be listed here.	Expression of feelings in a safe environment can facilitate problem identification and the development of coping strategies.
• Allow client to perform activities even though it might be easier at times for staff to complete the task for the client.	Communicates trust and promotes client's sense of control.
• Communicate expectations and goals to all staff members.	Promotes consistency in the treatment and communicates respect for the client.
• Discuss with family and other support systems and the client the plan and goals. Spend at least 5 min with family after each visit to answer questions and explain treatment plan.	Increases potential for success of treatment plan.
• Have support systems identify how they can assist client in achieving established goals.	
• Spend time with client discussing alternative ways of coping with the frustration that may occur while attempting to reach established goals.	Promotes client's sense of control when he or she encounters these difficulties. Successful coping will promote positive self-esteem.
• Collaborate with occupational therapist or physical therapist regarding special adaptations needed to assist client with task accomplishment, e.g., exercises to increase muscle strength when the muscles have not been used for a period of time.	

Continued

ACTIONS/INTERVENTIONS	RATIONALES
• Monitor effects medications might have on goal achievement, and collaborate with physician regarding problematic areas. • Develop goals and schedules with client, communicating that he or she does have responsibility and control in issues related to care. • Discuss with client and significant others those things that will facilitate continuance of self-care at home, and develop a plan that will assist client in obtaining necessary items. • Refer patient to community resources as necessary for continued support.	Facilitates the development of positive coping strategies and increases potential for success when the client returns home. Successful accomplishment of this transition promotes positive self-esteem.

Gerontic Health

ACTIONS/INTERVENTIONS	RATIONALES
• Teach self-monitoring skills such as maintaining a journal or diary to record what factors may increase the self-care deficit.	Encourage patient to identify areas that may need improvement or changes in lifestyle.[65]
• Contract with the patient for achievement of specific incremental goals, and provide rewards or reinforcements when goals are met.	Enhances motivation to increase self-care.

Home Health

ACTIONS/INTERVENTIONS	RATIONALES
• Monitor factors contributing to self-care deficit of (specify). This includes items in the related factors section.	Provides database for prevention and/or early intervention.

• Involve client and family in planning, implementing, and promoting reduction in the specific self-care deficit:
  ○ Family conference
  ○ Mutual goal setting
  ○ Communication
	Involvement improves motivation and improves the outcome.

• Assist client and family to obtain assistive equipment as required:
  ○ Raised toilet seat
  ○ Adaptive equipment for eating utensils, combs, brushes, etc.
  ○ Rocker knife
  ○ Suction device under plate or bowl
  ○ Wrist or hand splints
  ○ Blender, crockpot, or microwave
  ○ Long-handled reacher (helping hand)
  ○ Box on seat of chair
  ○ Raised ledge on utility board
  ○ Straw and straw holder
  ○ Washcloth with soap
  ○ Wheelchair, walker, motorized cart, or cane
  ○ Bedside commode, incontinence undergarments
  ○ Bars and attachments and benches for shower or tub
  ○ Handheld shower device
  ○ Long-handled sponge
	Assistive equipment improves function and increases the possibilities for self-care.

- ○ Shaver holder
- ○ Medication organizers or magnifying glass
- ○ Diet supplements
- ○ Hearing aid
- ○ Corrective lenses
- ○ Dressing aids: Dressing stick, zipper pull, buttonhook, long-handled shoehorn, shoe fasteners, or Velcro closures.
- Teach client and family signs and symptoms of overexertion:
  - ○ Pain
  - ○ Fatigue
  - ○ Confusion
  - ○ Decrease or excessive increase in vital signs
  - ○ Injury
- Assist client and family in lifestyle adjustments that may be required:
  - ○ Proper use of assistive equipment
  - ○ Adapting to need for assistance or assistive equipment
  - ○ Determining criteria for monitoring client's ability to function unassisted
  - ○ Time management
  - ○ Stress management
  - ○ Development of support systems
  - ○ Learning new skills
  - ○ Work, family, social, and personal goals and priorities
  - ○ Coping with disability or dependency
  - ○ Providing environment conducive to self-care privacy, pain relief, social contact, and familiar and favorite surroundings and foods
  - ○ Prevention of injury (falls, aspiration, burns, etc.)
  - ○ Monitoring of skin integrity
  - ○ Development of consistent routine
  - ○ Mechanism for alerting family member to need for assistance
- Refer patient to appropriate assistive resources as indicated.

Planning activities around physical capabilities prevents further reduction in self-care capacity.

Provides basic information for client and family that promotes necessary lifestyle changes.

Provides additional support for client and family and uses already available resources in a cost-effective manner.

Self-Care Deficit
(Feeding, Bathing-Hygiene, Dressing-Grooming, Toileting)

FLOWCHART EVALUATION: EXPECTED OUTCOME 1

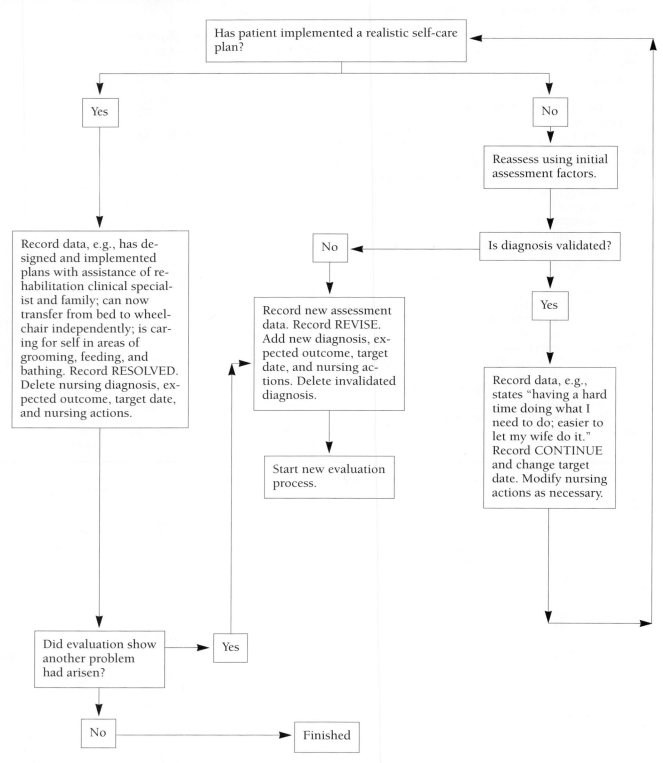

Self-Care Deficit
(Feeding, Bathing-Hygiene,
Dressing-Grooming, Toileting)

FLOWCHART EVALUATION: EXPECTED OUTCOME 2

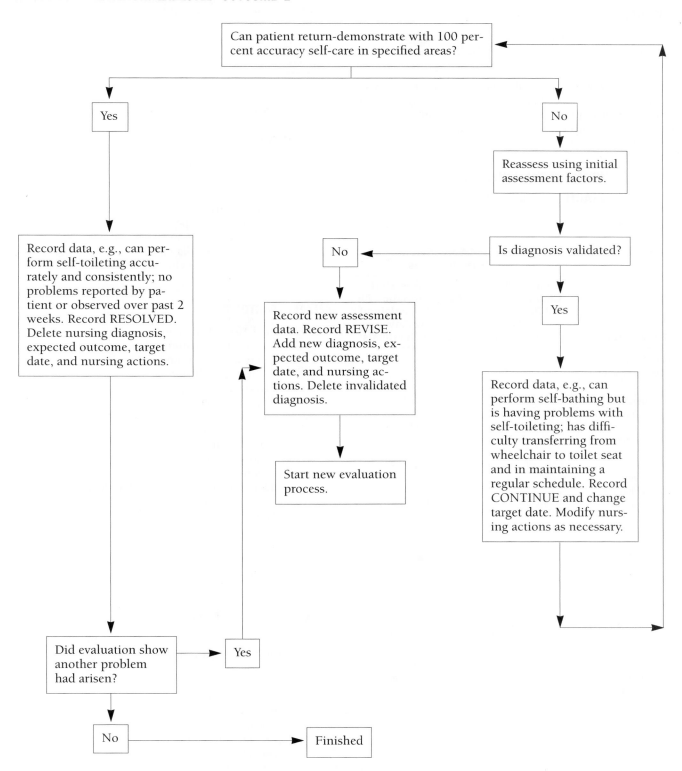

Tissue Perfusion (Specify Type), Altered (Renal, Cerebral, Cardiopulmonary, Gastrointestinal, Peripheral)

DEFINITION

The state in which an individual experiences a decrease in nutrition and oxygenation at the cellular level due to a deficit in capillary blood supply.[§,10]

Decreased Coronary Tissue Perfusion: A decrease in nutrition and oxygenation at the cellular level of the myocardium due to a deficit in the coronary arterial blood supply, an imbalance between myocardium demand and coronary arterial blood flow.

NANDA TAXONOMY: EXCHANGING 1.4.1.1

DEFINING CHARACTERISTICS[10]

1. Altered Tissue Perfusion

Estimated Sensitivities and Specifications

Characteristic	Chances That Characteristic Will Be Present in Given Diagnosis	Chances That Characteristic Will Not Be Explained by Any Other Diagnosis
Skin temperature, cold extremities	High	Low
Skin color		
Dependent blue or purple	Moderate	Low
Pale on elevation, color does not return on lowering of leg (critical)	High	High
Diminished arterial pulsations (critical)	High	High
Skin quality: Shining	High	Low
Lack of lanugo	High	Moderate
Round scars covered with atrophied skin	High	Moderate
Gangrene	Low	High
Slow-growing, dry brittle nails	High	Moderate
Claudication	Moderate	High
Blood pressure changes in extremities	Moderate	Moderate

Estimated Sensitivities and Specifications

Characteristic	Chances That Characteristic Will Be Present in Given Diagnosis	Chances That Characteristic Will Not Be Explained by Any Other Diagnosis
Bruits	Moderate	Moderate
Slow healing of lesions	High	Low

2. Decreased Coronary Tissue Perfusion
   a. Chest pain, with/without radiation
   b. Chest heaviness/pressure/tightness
   c. Shortness of breath, with feeling of suffocation
   d. EKG changes: inverted T wave, elevated ST segment
   e. Dysrhythmias
   f. Palpitations
   g. Dizziness/syncope
   h. Apprehension/sense of "impending doom"
   i. Acute onset of diaphoresis and vomiting, especially in the elderly

RELATED FACTORS[10]

1. Altered Tissue Perfusion
   a. Interruption of arterial flow
   b. Interruption of venous flow
   c. Exchange problems
   d. Hypovolemia
   e. Hypervolemia
2. Decreased Coronary Tissue Perfusion
   a. Artherosclerosis
   b. Coronary artery spasm
   c. Diabetes mellitus
   d. Dysrhythmias
   e. Tachycardia; e.g., paroxysm atrial tachycardia
   f. Left ventricular hypertrophy
   g. Hyperthyroidism
   h. Systemic hypertension
   i. Familial hyperlipidemia
   j. Anemia
   k. Hypoxia

RELATED CLINICAL CONCERNS

1. Thrombophlebitis
2. Amputation reattachment
3. Varicosities
4. Diabetes mellitus
5. Cardiac infections
6. Anemia
7. Myocardial infarction
8. Coronary artery disease
9. Kawasaki's disease
10. Congestive heart failure
11. Congenital cardiac anomalies
12. Coronary artery aneurysm

§Further work and development are required for the subcomponents, specifically cerebral, renal, and gastrointestinal.

HAVE YOU SELECTED THE CORRECT DIAGNOSIS?

Decreased Cardiac Output   Altered Tissue Perfusion relates to deficits in the peripheral circulation with cellular impact. Altered Cardiac Output relates specifically to a heart malfunction. Tissue perfusion problems may develop secondary to decreased cardiac output but can also exist without cardiac output problems.[32]

EXPECTED OUTCOMES

1. Will have no signs or symptoms of altered tissue perfusion (or decreased coronary tissue perfusion) by (date) and/or
2. Will implement a plan to decrease the likelihood of future alterations in tissue perfusion (or decreased coronary tissue perfusion) by (date)

TARGET DATES

A maximum target date would be 2 days from the date of admission because of the dangers involved. A patient who develops this diagnosis should be referred to a medical practitioner immediately.

ADDITIONAL INFORMATION

Perfusion is the movement of blood to and from a body part. Adequate perfusion determines cell survival and depends on an adequate pump and vascular volume as well as adequate functioning of the precapillary sphincters. The adequacy of these structures is affected by, among others, vasomotor, metabolic, and neural factors.[33,66]

The basic function of the cardiovascular system is to transport water, oxygen, nutrients, and hormones to the cells and to remove carbon dioxide, waste products, and heat from the cells. The size of the blood vessels decreases along the length of the arterial system, which increases resistance to fluid flow. To perfuse the cells adequately, the mean arterial blood pressure is maintained within a relatively narrow range by such regulatory systems as the baroreceptors, sympathetic nerves, and the cardiac branch of the vagus nerve.[33,66]

NURSING ACTIONS/INTERVENTIONS WITH RATIONALES

Adult Health

ACTIONS/INTERVENTIONS	RATIONALES
Altered Tissue Perfusion • Monitor, initially every 2 h on the (odd/even) hour, then increasing to every 4 h at (times): ○ Peripheral pulses ○ Capillary refill ○ Skin temperature ○ Edema: Measure circumference (abdomen and ankles) with tape measure. ○ Motor and sensory status ○ Vital signs ○ For signs and symptoms of pulmonary edema	Determines changes in physiologic baselines. Permits early detection and treatment of complications.
• Weigh daily at 7 a.m. • Measure intake and output. Total every 8 and 24 h. • Monitor bowel elimination at least daily. • Position patient carefully, and change position at least every hour while awake: ○ Arterial interference: Head and chest elevated, and extremities in dependent position ○ Venous interference: Extremities elevated ○ Combined arterial-venous interference: Supine ○ Apply sheepskin, alternating air mattress, or egg crate mattress applied to bed ○ Provide heel and elbow protectors ○ Provide bed cradle to avoid linen pressure on extremities ○ **Not** to be used: Knee gatch or pillows under knees	Allows monitoring of fluid balance. Permits assessment of nutritional status and bowel functioning. Promotes circulation. Prevents pressure ulcers and venous stasis.

Continued

ACTIONS/INTERVENTIONS	RATIONALES

• Provide skin and foot care at least once per shift at (times):
   ○ Cleanse and dry well.
   ○ Apply lotion.
   ○ Do not massage if possibility of emboli exists.
 • Collaborate with enterostomal therapist regarding care of open lesions:
   ○ Cleansing
   ○ Medicated ointments, etc.
   ○ Dressings
	Prevents skin integrity problems.

• Exercise extremities at least every 4 h while awake at (times):
   ○ Range of motion
   ○ Buerger-Allen exercises
 • Collaborate with physical therapist regarding gradually increasing total exercise program.
	Facilitates circulation and assists in preventing complications of immobility.

• Apply supportive or antiembolic hose. Remove for at least 30 min each shift at (times), and cleanse skin underneath.	Promotes venous return. Avoids skin integrity problems.

• Collaborate with physician regarding frequency of each of the following laboratory examinations, and monitor results:
   ○ Electrolytes
   ○ Arterial blood gases
   ○ Blood urea nitrogen
   ○ Cardiac enzymes
   ○ Coagulation time
	Allows determination of any changes in physiologic indicators of tissue perfusion.

• Administer, as ordered, and monitor results of medications:
   ○ Analgesics
   ○ Anticoagulants
   ○ Vasodilators
   ○ Antilipemics
	Basic monitoring of the various drugs used in the variety of situations related to altered tissue perfusion.

• Apply, and monitor closely, warm packs for phlebitis.
 	
 • Collaborate with dietitian regarding dietary adaptations:
   ○ Calorie restrictions
   ○ Lowered cholesterol
   ○ Decreased saturated fats
   ○ Decreased caffeine and alcohol intake
	Promotes venous return and awareness of possibility of burn injury.
	 Nutritional changes that may assist in avoiding future episodes of tissue perfusion.

• Teach patient and assist in implementation at least once per shift while awake at (times):
   ○ Stress management techniques
   ○ Relaxation techniques
	Decreases anxiety and modifies sympathetic nervous system response.

• Teach patient and significant others:
   ○ Exercise program
   ○ Dietary adaptations
   ○ Smoking cessation
   ○ Avoidance of extremes in temperature
   ○ Avoidance of prolonged standing, sitting, or crossing of legs
   ○ Avoiding use of over-the-counter medications
   ○ Continued use of stress management and relaxation techniques
   ○ Skin and foot care
   ○ Prescribed medication regimen: Effects and toxicity
	Basic home care planning. Promotes participation in care and implementation of prescribed regimen.

• Refer patient to visiting nurse service.	Provides long-term support.

Decreased Coronary Tissue Perfusion[67-79]

- Monitor every 5 minutes × 4, then every 15 minutes × 4, then every 30 minutes × 4, then hourly. Advance only if patient is pain free. Communicate any changes to physician.

  Determines changes in physiological baselines; permits early detection and treatment of complications.

  ○ Signs and symptoms of M.I.

  Pre-infarction, intra-infarction, post-infarction, life threatening.

  ○ Level of consciousness

  Determines level and extent of body systems compromise. Decreased cerebral perfusion.

  ○ Vital signs:

  Determines changes in physiologic baseline.
    (1) temperature
    (2) pulse
    (3) respirations
    (4) blood pressure—orthostatic blood pressures (lying, sitting, standing)
  ○ Cardiac rhythm, regularity and effectiveness:

  As indicators of cardiac function, irritability and/or failure.
    (1) atrial, sinus, ventricular

  Determines function of the conduction system.
    (2) normal, abnormal

  Determines rhythms' effects on the patient.
    (3) bradycardia, tachycardia
    (4) blocks: first, second, third degree
    (5) patient tolerating/not tolerating
    (6) life-threatening
  ○ ST segment monitoring:

  Determines the presence of ischemia and/or silent M.I.
    (1) elevation
    (2) inversion
    (3) symptomatic
    (4) nonsymptomatic
  ○ Level of comfort, agitation, and restlessness

  Determines if cardiac damage is still on-going; as a rough indicator of the severity of the evolving M.I. versus angina.

  ○ Apical pulse compared to peripheral pulse

  Determines decrease in peripheral perfusion.
  ○ Capillary refill

  As an indicator of hypoxia.
  ○ Hourly urinary intake and output; totals every 8 and 24 hours.

  As an indicator of fluid retention and overload.
  ○ Daily weight at the same time each day.

  Rough indicator of fluid retention (increased weight).
- Administer, as ordered, and monitor results of medications:

  Basic monitoring of the various drugs used in the variety of situations related to altered tissue perfusion, coronary.
  ○ analgesics
  ○ thrombolytics.
  ○ vasodilators
  ○ anticoagulants
  ○ antiarrhythmics
  ○ sedatives
  ○ antilipidemics
  ○ antiplatelet aggregants
  ○ antihypertensives
- Monitor bowel sounds every 4 hours; monitor bowel elimination at least daily.

  Determine decreased blood flow to the small and large bowel.
- Collaborate with physicians regarding frequency of each of the following lab tests and monitor the results.

  Allows determination of any change in physiologic indicators of tissue perfusion to various organs.
  ○ chemistry profile
  ○ cardiac enzymes
  ○ cardiac isoenzymes
  ○ pro time
  ○ partial thromboplastin time
  ○ arterial blood gases
- Collaborate with physicians regarding frequency of each of the following:

  Allows for further evaluation of the cardiac and respiratory function.
  ○ chest x-ray
  ○ electrocardiogram
  ○ echocardiogram

Continued

ACTIONS/INTERVENTIONS	RATIONALES

• Position patient carefully and change position at least hourly. Exercise extremities at least every 4 hours, including range of motion.
  ○ Arterial interface: head and chest elevated, and extremities in dependent position.
  ○ Venous interface: extremities elevated.
  ○ Combined arterial-venous interface: supine.
  ○ Apply sheepskin, alternating pressure mattress to bed.
  ○ Provide heel and elbow protectors.
  ○ Provide bed caradle to avoid linen pressure to extremities.
  ○ Do not use knee gatch or pillows under knees.
  ○ Trendelenberg position if blood pressure is low.
• Provide skin and foot care at least once per shift.
 	
• Monitor data provided by and effects of invasive lines.
  ○ Swan-Ganz catheter
  ○ arterial lines
  ○ femoral sheaths
  ○ intra-aortic balloon pump
  ○ subclavian catheter
• Apply supportive or antiembolic hose. Remove for at least 30 minutes each shift and cleanse skin underneath.
• Collaborate with cardiac rehabilitation nurse on patient activity, education, and support. Include family at all times.
  ○ Gradually increase activity.
  ○ Stop activity if not pain free.
  ○ Need for regular exercise program.
  ○ Changes in life style, less stress.
  ○ Smoking cessation.
  ○ Weight reduction.
  ○ Relaxation methods, time out stress management techniques.
  ○ Purpose/use of medications, side effects of, complications of, interactions of (with other drugs and food)
  ○ Warning signs of impending cardiac problems.
  ○ Have rapid response system in place.
  ○ What support patient has, from whom, from where, inside and outside the family; e.g., groups—professional and layman.
• Collaborate with physical therapist regarding gradually increasing total exercise program.
• Collaborate with dietitian regarding dietary modifications:
  ○ calorie restrictions
  ○ low cholesterol
  ○ decreased saturated fats
  ○ decreased caffeine and alcohol intake.
• Teach patient and significant other:
  ○ exercise program
  ○ dietary modifications
  ○ avoidance of extreme temperatures
  ○ avoidance of over-the-counter medications
  ○ continued use of stress management and relaxation techniques
  ○ skin and foot care
• Refer to visiting nurse service.
	Promotes circulation; prevents pressure ulcers and prevents arterial and venous stasis.
	
	Maintains skin integrity; allows for determination of compromised circulation to lower extremities. Determines complications caused by or adverse effects of various lines; determines changes in patient's baseline condition.
	
	Promotes venous return; avoids skin integrity problems.
	
	Allows for determination of patient/family's level of understanding of disease state, what areas need further education, and what familial support systems are available to the patient; increases level of health and wellness; increases control of life.
	
	Promotes return to function life style.
	
	Decrease risk of future problems.
	
	Basic home care planning; promotes participation in care and implementation of prescribed regimen.
	
	Provides long-term support.

Child Health

ACTIONS/INTERVENTIONS	RATIONALES
• Perform appropriate monitoring and documentation for contributory factors to include: ○ Circulatory monitoring of anatomic site or general signs and symptoms related to peripheral pulses ○ Apical pulse, blood pressure, temperature, and respiration (Monitor at least every hour or as ordered, and check cardiac monitor if applicable.) ○ Intake and output every hour ○ Nausea or vomiting ○ Constipation or diarrhea ○ Tolerance of feeding ○ Pain or discomfort ○ Skin color and temperature; any integrity problems ○ Circulatory pattern: Notify physician for any change in the pattern that suggests lack of oxygenation, e.g., cyanosis, arterial blood gas results, or decreased pulses. ○ Appropriate functioning of equipment such as ventilator, arterial line, or intravenous pump ○ Maintenance of intravenous line for administration of fluids ○ Positional demands ○ Pain or discomfort ○ Sensory input appropriate for age and developmental status ○ Fluid and electrolytes	Provides basic database to ascertain progress and to individualize plan of care.
• Collaborate with other health care providers as needed.	Coordination and implementation of plan of care may involve numerous professionals according to the cause of alteration and the treatment modalities available. Basic emergency preparedness.
• Provide for appropriate availability of resuscitative equipment including: ○ Ambu bag ○ Crash cart for pediatrics with drugs and defibrillator ○ Appropriate respiratory intubation equipment	
• Provide for parental and child health teaching needs by allowing 10–15 min per 8-h shift for verbalization of concerns.	Verbalization of health-related concerns may serve as cue for teaching needs and also reduce anxiety.
• Allow for parental participation in care of child at appropriate level, e.g., giving comfort or assisting with feeding.	Parental involvement in care puts child at ease and provides self-esteem and empowerment for parents.
• Encourage rest by scheduling procedures together with devotion to ample time between activities.	Appropriate attention to rest needs helps prevent further metabolic demands on already less than ideal homeostasis scenario.
• Allow for patient and parental preferences in plan of care.	Individualization shows value attached to parents' input.
• Deal with appropriate related factors associated with altered tissue perfusion, e.g, minimizing crying by anticipating needs.	All efforts to lessen workload on heart and respiratory system will assist in preventing further decompensation.
• Provide appropriate safety precautions for age, e.g., keeping siderails up or positioning as ordered.	Safety is a standard part of care and ought to be planned for according to health status, age, and development.
• Maintain proper use of equipment such as Clinitron bed or special K-pads.	Assists circulation.
• Provide for appropriate follow-up via scheduled appointments after hospitalization.	Encourages consistency in long-range care. Demonstrates how to schedule appointments and provides support for parents.

Continued

ACTIONS/INTERVENTIONS	RATIONALES
• Provide patient with teaching appropriate to needs of illness and family, e.g., if activities and daily care are to be modified, consider use of pulse oximeter to monitor perfusion and explain how to check circulation after cast application.	Assists in reducing anxiety and facilitates home management of care.
• Ensure that parents have been certified in CPR before child is dismissed from hospital.	Basic need for home care when perfusion problem is present.
NOTE: A major effort will be that of follow up with appropriate specialized care to include pediatric cardiology and as needed, other expertise to anticipate long course. Every aim is directed at early diagnosis, especially in instances of any congenital cardiac anomaly; i.e., simple coronary artery malformation versus that associated with other related physiologic malformation of the heart and vasculature. A specific concern is Kawasaki's disease with a residual concern of coronary artery aneurysm. Periodic echocardiography is mandated for these individuals.	

Women's Health

ACTIONS/INTERVENTIONS	RATIONALES

• Assist patient in identifying lifestyle adjustments that may be needed due to changes in physiologic function or needs during experiential phases of life (e.g., pregnancy, birth, and postpartum and those realted to gynecology):
  ○ Avoid prolonged sitting and sitting with crossed legs or standing.
  ○ Develop exercise plan for cardiovascular fitness during pregnancy.
  ○ Avoid wearing constrictive clothing.
  ○ Maintain a balanced diet with adequate hydration.
  ○ Avoid constipation and bearing down to prevent hemorrhoids.
	Decreases factors that could lead to decreased perfusion of oxygen to uterus, placenta, and fetus.

• Monitor patient for signs of pregnancy-induced hypertension (PIH)
  ○ Prenatal weight
  ○ Blood pressure
  ○ Presence of edema
  ○ Proteinuria
  ○ Preeclampsia
  ○ Headaches
  ○ Visual changes such as blurred vision
  ○ Increased edema of face and pitting edema of extremities
  ○ Oliguria
  ○ Hyperreflexia
  ○ Nausea or vomiting
  ○ Epigastric pain
  ○ Eclampsia
  ○ Convulsions
  ○ Coma
	Allows early intervention to avoid perfusion problems and development of complications.

• Monitor for edema:
  ○ Swelling of hands, face, legs, or feet.
  ○ **Caution:** Patient may have to remove rings.
  ○ May need to wear loose shoes or a bigger shoe size.
	Provides early warning of perfusion problems and promotes early intervention.

- ○ Schedule rest breaks during day when patient can elevate legs.
- ○ When lying down, lie on left side to promote placental perfusion and prevent compression of vena cava.
- In collaboration with physician (as appropriate), monitor:
  - ○ Check intake and output (urinary output should not be less than 30 mL/h or 120 mL/4 h).
  - ○ Use magnesium sulfate ($MgSO_4$) and hydralazine hydrochloride (Apresoline) therapy according to physician's orders. Have antidote for $MgSO_4$ (calcium gluconate) available at all times during $MgSO_4$ therapy.
  - ○ Assess deep tendon reflexes (DTR).
  - ○ Check respiratory rate, pulse, and BP at least every 2 h on the (odd/even) hour.
  - ○ Evaluate for possibility of seizures.
  - ○ Limit the amount of noise in the patient's environment.
  - ○ Fetal heart rate and well-being.
- Provide quiet, nonstimulating environment for patient.

Reduces anxiety and promotes rest. Both measures will assist in maintaining peripheral circulation by avoiding vasoconstriction.

- Provide patient and family with factual information and support as needed.

Reduces anxiety and provides teaching opportunity.

- Monitor and teach patient to monitor and report any signs of PIH immediately:
  - ○ Rapid rise in BP
  - ○ Rapid weight gain
  - ○ Marked hyperreflexia, especially transient or sustained ankle clonus
  - ○ Severe headache
  - ○ Visual disturbances
  - ○ Epigastric pain
  - ○ Increase in proteinuria
  - ○ Oliguria, with urine output of less than 30 mL/h
  - ○ Drowsiness

Allows early detection of problem and more rapid intervention.

- In collaboration with dietitian:
  - ○ Obtain nutritional history.
  - ○ Provide high-protein diet (80–100 g of protein).
  - ○ Provide low-sodium diet (not above 6 g daily or below 2.5 g daily).

Dietary measures that assist in controlling BP.

ORAL CONTRACEPTIVE THERAPY

- Monitor for factors that contraindicate use of oral birth control pills:
  - ○ Family history of stroke, diabetes, or reproductive cancer
  - ○ History of thromboembolic disease or vascular problems, hypertension, hepatic disease, and smoking
  - ○ Presence of any breast disease, nodule, or fibrocystic disease

These factors will promote side effects and untoward effects from birth control pills.

PREMENSTRUAL SYNDROME

- Assist patient to identify symptoms that occur premenstrually that interfere with normal activities of daily living:
  - ○ Constipation

Provides database necessary to plan appropriate intervention.

Continued

ACTIONS/INTERVENTIONS	RATIONALES

◦ Bloating (abdominal)
   ◦ Edema in hands and feet
   ◦ Headaches or vertigo
   ◦ Oliguria
   ◦ Irritability
   ◦ Depression
• Provide patient with literature on premenstrual syndrome.
• In collaboration with dietitian:
   ◦ Obtain nutritional history.
   ◦ Provide diet high in complex carbohydrates and protein.
   ◦ Provide low-sodium diet (not above 6 g daily or below 2.5 g daily).
• Teach and encourage patient to:
   ◦ Utilize an exercise program.
   ◦ Utilize biofeedback for severe symptoms.
   ◦ Stop smoking.
   ◦ Utilize relaxation techniques to reduce stress.
 	
NOTE: In instances of decreased coronary tissue perfusion, the women's health client should immediately be transferred to a coronary care unit.
	Dietary measures that assist in reducing the effects of premenstrual syndrome.

Psychiatric Health

NOTE: The nursing actions in this section reflect alteration in tissue perfusion related to the cerebral and peripheral vascular systems since these are the systems most commonly affected in the mental health setting. If the client develops decreased coronary tissue perfusion, he or she should immediately be transferred to a coronary care unit.

ACTIONS/INTERVENTIONS	RATIONALES

• Check on orthostatic hypotension by taking blood pressure while client is lying down, then taking blood pressure just after client stands or sits up (provide support for client to prevent injury from a fall).
• Monitor client's mental status. If compromised, provide information in a clear, concise manner.
• Discuss with client causes of decreased cerebral blood flow.
• Have client get out of bed slowly by:
   ◦ Sitting up
   ◦ Swinging legs over edge of bed
   ◦ Resting in this position for at least 2 min
   ◦ Standing up slowly
   ◦ Walking slowly
• Teach client to avoid situations in which he or she changes position quickly, e.g., bending over to pick something up off the floor or standing quickly from a sitting position.
• Have client supported while changing positions that cause vertigo until problem is resolved.
• Assist client in getting in and out of the bathtub.
• Collaborate with physician regarding alterations in medications.
	Psychotropic medications can predispose client to orthostatic hypotension.
	
	Assists in explaining reasons for therapies to client.
	
	Allows time for cardiovascular system to adapt, thus preventing fainting or dizziness to orthostatic hypotension.
	
	Promotes changing to a medication that would not interfere with perfusion.

- If situation persists, have client:
  ○ Sleep sitting up or with head elevated.
  ○ Use elastic stockings that are waist high.
  ○ Apply stockings while client is still in bed.
  ○ Have client raise legs for several minutes.
  ○ Apply stockings slowly and evenly.
  ○ Remove stockings after client is lying down at least every 8 h.

Provides external support for venous system.

- Develop with client a plan for daily exercise that is very modest, e.g., walking the length of the hall for 15 min twice a day for 3 days, then increasing distance and time gradually until client is walking for 30 min twice a day. Note client's exercise regimen here.

Improves cardiovascular strength. Assists in maintaining muscle tone that assists in supporting the venous circulation.

- Develop with the client a reward schedule for implementing exercise plan. List rewards and the reward schedule here.
- Provide the client with positive verbal support for goal accomplishment.
- Do not allow client to participate in unit activities that could produce injury until the condition is resolved, e.g., cooking or using sharp objects while standing.

Basic safety measures.

- Discuss with client the effects of alcohol and smoking on blood flow, and assist him or her to develop alternative coping behavior if necessary. Note plan for this here.
- Provide decaffeinated beverages for the client. Consult with dietary department about this adaptation.
- Increase client's fluid intake during times of increased loss such as exercise or periods of anxiety. Instruct client in the need for this.
- Observe client carefully after injecting medications that have a high potential for producing hypotension. This is especially true for those clients who are very agitated and physically active.

Basic measure to offset the possibility of falling secondary to orthostatic hypotension.

- Inform client of need to change position slowly after injecting medication.
- Teach client and support system about over-the-counter medications that alter blood flow, e.g., cold medications, antihistamines, or diet pills.
- Monitor peripheral pulses on affected limbs every 8 h at (times).
- Avoid and teach client to avoid pressure in points on affected limbs to include:
  ○ Changing position frequently when sitting or lying down
  ○ Avoiding pressure in the area behind the knee
  ○ Not crossing legs while sitting
  ○ Making sure shoes fit properly and do not rub feet
  ○ Elevating feet when sitting to reduce pressure on backs of legs

Avoids compromising circulation by pressure or constriction.

- Keep feet clean and dry, and teach client to do the same by assessing foot condition once a day at (time). This assessment should include:
  ○ Washing feet
  ○ Checking for sores, reddened areas, and blisters
  ○ Keeping toenails trimmed and caring for ingrown nails
  ○ Applying lotion to feet
  ○ Rubbing reddened areas if client does not have a history of emboli
  ○ Applying clean, dry socks

Avoids lower extremity skin integrity problems and possible infection with the resultant impact on circulation.

Continued

ACTIONS/INTERVENTIONS	RATIONALES
◦ Teaching significant others to assist with foot care of elderly client ◦ Keeping limbs warm (but do not use external heating sources such as heating pads or hot-water bottles) • Develop with the client an exercise program and note that program here. Begin slowly, and gradually increase time and distance, e.g., walk for 15 min 2 times per day for 1 wk. This should be increased until client is walking 1 mi in 30–45 min 3 times a week.	Promotes normal venous return.

• Instruct client to discontinue exercise if:
   ◦ Pulse does not return to resting rate within 3 min after exercise.
   ◦ Shortness of breath continues for more than 10 min after stopping exercise.
   ◦ Fatigue is excessive.
   ◦ Muscles are painful.
   ◦ Client experiences dizziness, pain in the chest, light-headedness, loss of muscle control, or nausea.
	Client safety is of primary importance.

• Encourage client's exercise by:
   ◦ Walking with him or her
   ◦ Determining things that the client would find rewarding and supplying these as goals are achieved
   ◦ Providing positive verbal support as goals are achieved. Note client's specific reward system here.
• Monitor client's nutritional status, and refer to nutritionist for teaching if necessary.	

• Discuss with client the effects of smoking on peripheral blood flow, and assist him or her in decreasing or eliminating this by:
   ◦ Referring client to a stop-smoking group
   ◦ Encouraging him or her not to smoke before meals or exercise
   ◦ Decreasing amount smoked per day
	Nicotine causes vasospasm and vasoconstriction.

• Discuss special needs with client and support system before discharge. • Refer client to community agencies to provide ongoing care as needed.	Increases probability of client's behavior change being maintained after discharge.

Gerontic Health

The nursing actions for the gerontic patient with this diagnosis are the same as those for adult health and home health patients.

Decreased Coronary Tissue Perfusion: Nursing interventions found in the Adult Health section are appropriate to this age group, in addition to the following interventions.

ACTIONS/INTERVENTIONS	RATIONALES
• Monitor for signs of dyspnea, chronic fatigue, behavioral changes, evidence of acute cerebral insufficiency.	Older clients with decreased cardiac perfusion often present with these symptoms.
• Plan physical activities, such as hygiene, meals, ambulation, with rest periods.	Decreases cardiac workload.
• Instruct in use of oxygen, if prescribed.	Supplemental oxygen may be prescribed to help decrease cardiac workload.
• Teach client relaxation methods to help decrease anxiety.	Decreasing anxiety helps to decrease the release of catecholamines. An increase in catecholamines results in increased cardiac workload.

Home Health

NOTE: If this diagnosis is suspected when caring for a client in the home, it is imperative that a physician referral be obtained immediately. If the client demonstrates symptoms of decreased coronary perfusion, the client should be transferred immediately to a coronary care unit. If the client has been referred to home health care by a physician, the nurse will collaborate with the physician in the treatment of the client.

ACTIONS/INTERVENTIONS	RATIONALES
• Teach client and family appropriate monitoring of signs and symptoms of alteration in tissue perfusion. ○ Pulse (lying, sitting, and standing) ○ Skin temperature and turgor ○ Edema ○ Motor status ○ Sensory status ○ Blood pressure (lying, sitting, standing, and pulse pressure) ○ Respiratory status (dyspnea, cyanosis, and rate) ○ Weight fluctuations ○ Urinary output ○ Leg pain with walking	Provide database for prevention and/or early intervention.
• Assist client and family in identifying lifestyle changes that may be required: ○ Eliminating smoking ○ Decreasing caffeine ○ Decreasing alcohol ○ Avoiding over-the-counter medications ○ Protecting skin and extremities from injury due to decreased sensation (burns, frostbite, etc.) ○ Protecting skin from pressure injury (making frequent position changes and using sheepskin for pressure areas and foot cradle) ○ Improving arterial blood flow (keeping extremities warm, elevating head and chest, avoiding crossing legs or sitting for long periods of time, wiggling fingers and toes every hour, and performing ROM exercises) ○ Performing exercise program as tolerated ○ Improving venous blood flow (elevating extremity, using antiembolus stockings, and avoiding pressure behind the knees) ○ Performing skin and foot care ○ Decreasing cholesterol and saturated fat intake ○ Performing diversional activities as needed ○ Practicing stress management	Provide basic information for client and family that promotes necessary lifestyle changes.
• Teach family basic CPR. • Teach client and family purposes, side effects, and proper administration techniques of medications. • Assist client and family to set criteria to help them to determine when a physician or other intervention is required.	Locus of control shifts from nurse to client and family, thus promoting self-care.
• Consult with or refer patient to appropriate assistive resources as indicated.	Provides additional support for client and family and uses already available resources in a cost-effective manner.

Tissue Perfusion, Altered (Specify Type), Altered (Renal, Cerebral, Cardiopulmonary, Gastrointestinal, Peripheral)

FLOWCHART EVALUATION: EXPECTED OUTCOME 1

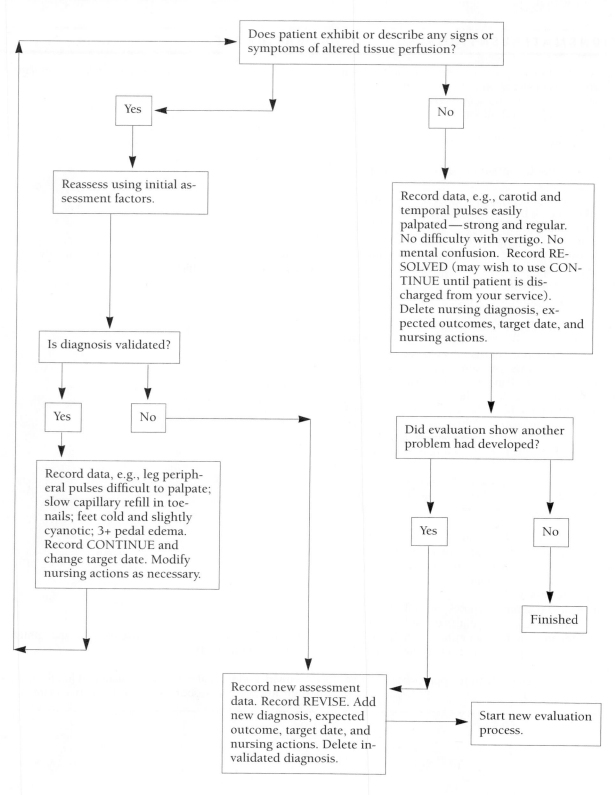

Tissue Perfusion, Altered (Specify Type), Altered (Renal, Cerebral, Cardiopulmonary, Gastrointestinal, Peripheral)

FLOWCHART EVALUATION: EXPECTED OUTCOME 2

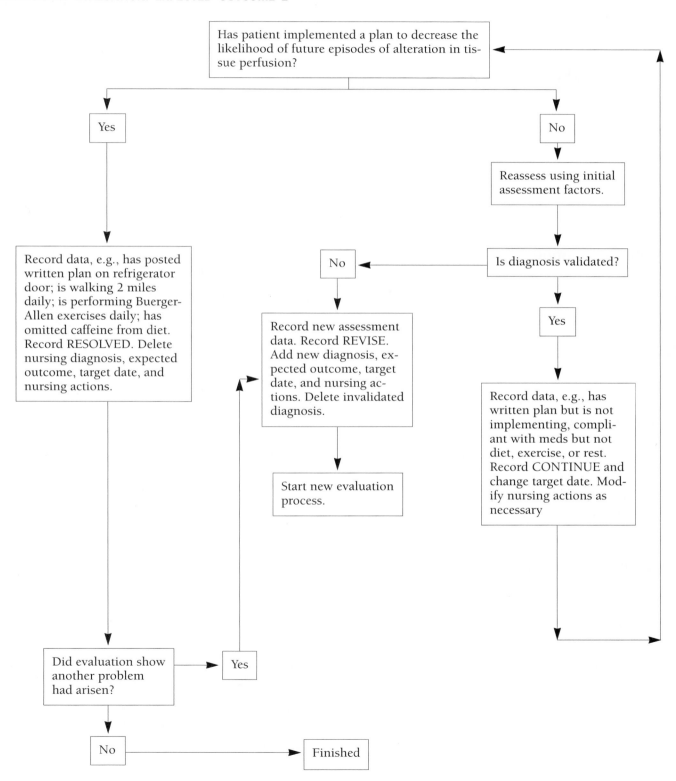

CHAPTER

6

Sleep-Rest Pattern

Pattern Description

The sleep-rest pattern includes relaxation in addition to sleep and rest. The pattern is based on a 24-hour day and looks specifically at how an individual rates or judges the adequacy of his or her sleep, rest, and relaxation in terms of both quantity and quality. The pattern also looks at the patient's energy level in relation to the amount of sleep, rest, and relaxation described by the patient as well as any aids to sleep the patient uses.

Pattern Assessment

1. Does the patient report a problem falling asleep?
   a. Yes (Sleep Pattern Disturbance)
   b. No
2. Does the patient report interrupted sleep?
   a. Yes (Sleep Pattern Disturbance)
   b. No

Conceptual Information

A person at rest feels mentally relaxed, free from anxiety, and physically calm. *Rest* need not imply inactivity, and inactivity does not necessarily afford rest. Rest is a reduction in bodily work that results in the person's feeling refreshed, with a sense of readiness to perform activities of daily living.

Sleep is a state of rest that occurs for sustained periods. The reduced consciousness during sleep provides time for essential repair and recovery of body systems. A person who sleeps has temporarily reduced interaction with the environment. Sleep restores a person's energy and sense of well-being.

Recent studies confirm that sleep is a cyclical phenomenon. The most common sleep cycle is the 24-hour, diurnal day-night cycle. This 24-hour cycle is also referred to as the *circadian rhythm*. In general, the 24-hour circadian rhythm is governed by light and darkness. Additional factors that influence the sleep-wake cycle of the individual are biological, such as hormonal and thermoregulation cycles. Most individuals attempt to synchronize activity with the demands of modern society. The two specialized areas of the brain stem that control the cyclical nature of sleep are the *reticular activating system* in the brain stem, spinal cord, and cerebral cortex, and the *bulbar synchronizing portion* in the medulla. These two systems function intermittently by activating and suppressing the higher centers of the brain.

After falling asleep, a person passes through a series of stages that afford rest and recuperation physically, mentally, and emotionally. In Stage 1, the individual is in a relaxed, dreamy state, aware of his or her surroundings. In Stages 2 and 3, there is progression to deeper levels of sleep in which the individual becomes unaware of his or her surroundings but wakens easily. In Stage 4, there is profound sleep characterized by little body movement and difficult arousal. Stage 4 restores and allows the body to rest. These stages are known as *non–rapid eye movement (NREM)*. Stage 5 is called *rapid eye movement (REM)*. It is in this stage that the individual dreams. Other characteristics of this stage of sleep are irregular pulse, variable blood pressure, muscular twitching, profound muscular relaxation, and an increase in gastric secretion.[1] After REM, the individual progresses back through Stages, 1, 2, and 3 again.

A person's age, general health status, culture, and emotional well-being will dictate the amount of sleep he or she requires. On the whole, older persons require less sleep while young infants require the most sleep. As the nurse assesses the patient's needs for sleep and rest, he or she makes every effort to individualize the care according to this sleep-rest cycle. A major emphasis is to provide patient education regarding the influence of the disease process on sleep-rest patterns.

Reports of the occurrence of excessive and pathologic sleep most commonly relate to narcolepsy and hypersomnia. *Narcolepsy* is characterized by an attack of irresistible sleep of brief duration with "auxiliary" symptoms. In sleep paralysis, the narcoleptic patient is unable to speak or move and breathes in a shallow manner. Auditory or visual hypnagogic hallucinations may occur. *Cataplexy*, a brief form of narcolepsy, is an abrupt and reversible decrease or loss of muscle tone and is most often elicited by emotion. The attacks may last several seconds and almost go undetected, or they may last as long as 30 minutes with muscular weakness being evident. In the initial stage of the attack, consciousness remains intact.[2]

Hypersomnia, on the other hand, is characterized by daytime sleepiness and sleep states that are less imperative and of longer duration than those in narcolepsy. Often a deepening and lengthening of night sleep is also noted. Sleep apnea and the Kleine-Levin syndrome are two examples of the hypersomnia disorders.[2]

Sleep apnea may occur in patients with a damaged respiratory center in the brain, brain stem infarction, drug intoxication (barbiturates, tranquilizers, etc.), bilateral cordotomy, and Ondine's curse syndrome. Patients with the typical pickwickian syndrome show marked obesity and associated alveolar hypoventilation, sleep apnea, and hypersomnia. There are several forms of this condition that may exist without obesity. One such syndrome is Ondine's curse syndrome, which involves the loss of the automaticity of breathing and manifests during sleep as a recurrent apnea. Another is the Kleine-Levin syndrome, which is associated with periods of hypersomnia accompanied by bulimia or polyphagia and mental disturbances. There is also a cyclic hypersomnia reported that is related to the premenstrual periods. The typical syndrome, pickwickian, is rare while the atypical variants seem more common.[2]

Various factors influence a person's capability to gain adequate rest and sleep. For the home setting, it is appropriate for the nurse to assist the patient in developing behavior conducive to rest and relaxation. In a health care setting, the nurse must be able to provide ways of promoting rest and relaxation in a stressful environment. Loss of privacy, unfamiliar noises, frequent examinations, tiring procedures, and a general upset in daily routines culminate in a threat to the client's achievement of essential rest and sleep.

Developmental Considerations

In general, as age increases, the amount of sleep per night decreases. The length of each sleep cycle—active (REM) and quiet (NREM)—changes with age. For adults, there is no particular change in the actual number of hours slept, but there is a change in the amount of deep sleep and light sleep. As age increases, the amount of deep sleep decreases and the amount of light sleep increases. This helps explain why the older patient wakens more easily and spends time in sleep throughout the day and night. REM sleep decreases in amount from the time of infancy (50 percent) to late adulthood (15 percent). The changes in sleep pattern with age development are[3]:

Infant: Awake 7 hours; NREM sleep 8.5 hours; REM sleep, 8.5 hours

Age 1: Awake 13 hours; NREM sleep, 7 hours; REM sleep, 4 hours

Age 10: Awake 15 hours; NREM sleep, 6 hours; REM sleep, 3 hours

Age 20: Awake 17 hours; NREM sleep, 5 hours; REM sleep, 2 hours

Age 75: Awake 17 hours; NREM sleep, 6 hours; REM sleep 1 hour

INFANT

The development of sleep and wakefulness can be traced to intrauterine life. A gestational age of 36 weeks seems to be a landmark, for it is at this time that the behavioral states in the fetus and preterm infant begin to take on a more mature character. The joining of physiologic variables results in identification of recurrent behavioral states with various parameters. Term birth leads to a number of profound changes, especially in respiratory regulation, but more evidence suggests continuity of development, rather than discontinuity, prevails.[4]

The newborn begins life with a regular schedule of sleep and activity that is evident during periods of reactivity. For the first hour infants born of unmedicated mothers spend 60 percent of the time in the quiet, alert state and only 10 percent of the time in the irritable, crying state. Five distinct sleep-activity states for the infant have been noted[5]: (1) regular sleep, (2) irregular sleep, (3) drowsiness, (4) alert inactivity, and (5) waking and crying.

After 1 month of age, sleep and wakefulness change dramatically as do a large number of physiologic variables. This period of CNS reorganization (with a likely increased vulnerability) is immediately following by a short transient interval at 3 months of age, in which play and wakefulness and, within it, the basic rest-activity cycle, show excessive regularity. This regularity may carry its own risk.

The study of mobility has proven worthwhile in detecting the origin of the basic rest-activity cycle in the fetus. Neonatologists, who deal with the immature infant, often use mobility in prognosis.

Apneas during sleep are common in normal infants and occur most often during the newborn period with a marked decrease in the first 6 months of life. Long apneas, above 15 seconds, are not usually observed during sleep in laboratory conditions. Obstructive apneas of 6 to 10 seconds are also rarely observed. However, in laboratory studies, paradoxical breathing is observed in neonates, and periodic breathing is associated with REM sleep in normal infants.[4]

Infants found not breathing, by parents, are usually rushed to the hospital. Causes for life-threatening apnea to be investigated include: congenital conditions especially cardiac disease or arrhythmias; cranial, facial, or other conditions affecting the anatomy of the airway; infections such as sepsis, meningitis, pneumonia, botulism, and pertussis; viral infections such as respiratory syncytial virus; metabolic abnormalities; administration of sedatives; seizures; and chronic hypoxia. If these causes are ruled out, the infant is diagnosed as having "apnea of infancy." Sleep studies, with polygraphic recordings, are required. The term *Near Miss Sudden Infant Death Syndrome* (Near Miss SIDS) implies that the child is found limp, cyanotic, and not breathing, and would have died had caretakers not intervened. Because the relation of the Near Miss SIDS event to SIDS is speculative, *apnea of infancy* is the preferred term.[4]

Obstructive and central apnea identification, hypopnea, prolonged expiration, apnea and reflux, and apnea and cardiac arrhythmia are the current issues being studied in trying to solve this problem. For any infant-related apnea, hospitalization, with special observation for all possible contributing factors, and close monitoring of cardiac and respiratory function are recommended. Attention must be given to parents for the extreme anxiety this problem creates.

The newborn and young infant spend more time in REM sleep than adults. As the infant's nervous system develops, the infant will have longer periods of sleep and wakefulness that become more regular. At approximately 8 months of age, the infant goes through the stage of separation anxiety with potentially altered sleep patterns. Teething, ear infections, or other disorders affect sleep patterns. Respirations are quiet with minimal activity noted during deep sleep. The infant sleeps an average of 12 to 16 hours per day.

TODDLER AND PRESCHOOLER

The toddler needs approximately 10 to 12 hours of sleep at night with an approximate 2-hour nap in the afternoon. The proportion of REM sleep is 25 percent. Rituals for preparation for sleep are important, with bedtime associated as separation from family and fun. Quiet time to gradually unwind, a favorite object for security, and a relatively consistent bedtime are suggested. Nightmares may begin to occur due to magical thinking.

The preschooler sleeps approximately 10 to 12 hours per day. Dreams and nightmares may occur at this time, and resistance to bedtime rituals is also common. Unwinding or slowing down from the many activities of the day is recommended to lessen sleep disturbances. Actual attempts to foster relaxation by mental imaging at this age have proved successful. The proportion of REM sleep is 20 percent.

Special needs may be prompted for the toddler during hospitalization. When at all possible, a parent's presence should be encouraged throughout nighttime to lessen fears. Limit setting with safety in mind is also necessary for the toddler due to his or her surplus of energy and desire for constant activity. The preschooler may be at risk for fatigue. Sleep may not be necessary at nap time, but rest without disturbance is recommended to supplement night sleep and to prevent fatigue.

SCHOOL-AGE CHILD

The school-age child seems to do well without a nap and requires approximately 10 hours of sleep per day, with REM sleep being approximately 18.5 percent. Individualized rest needs are developed by this age with a reliable source being the child who can express his or her feelings about rest or sleep. Health status would also determine to a great extent how much sleep the child at this age requires. Permission to stay up late must be weighed against the potential upset to routine and demands of the next day. When bedtime is assigned a status, peer pressure and power issues may ensue.

When the school-ager alters the usual routines of sleep and rest, fatigue may be a result. Attempts should be made to maintain usual routines even when school is not in session to best maintain the usual sleep-rest pattern.

ADOLESCENT

Irregular sleep patterns seem to be the norm for the adolescent due to high activity levels and usual peer-related activities. There may be a tendency to overexertion, which is made more pronounced by the numerous physiologic changes that create increased demands on the body. Fatigue may occur during this time. On the average, the adolescent sleeps approximately 8 to 10 hours per day with REM sleep being 20 percent.

Rest may be necessary to supplement sleep. Supplementing sleep with rest serves to assist in preventing illness or the risk of illness. Extracurricular activities may also need to be prioritized.

ADULT

The adult sleeps approximately 8 hours per day with REM sleep being 22 percent. Sleep patterns may be subject to young infants or children in the household or after-hours professional and social demands.

The adult may be at high risk for fatigue due to increasing role expectations, especially in the instance of a new baby being cared for. Sleep deprivation is not a positive means of coping with the many expectations the adult may feel.

Research has shown that women of all ages have higher rates of sleep disturbance than men. Some speculation has occurred that relates this to the reproductive lives of women and hormonal changes. It is well documented that the psychosocial and hormonal changes that accompany pregnancy lead to sleep disturbances.[6] That sleep deprivation occurs during postpartum periods is a well-known fact. A new baby does not allow for uninterrupted sleep for approximately 4 to 6 weeks after birth.[7,8]

The major cause of sleep disturbance in menopause is frequent nocturnal hot flashes coupled with early morning awakenings.[6]

OLDER ADULT

The older adult requires less sleep on the average, approximately 5 to 7 hours of sleep per day. The proportion of REM sleep may vary from 20 to 25 percent; however, deep sleep, Stage 4 NREM sleep, is decreased.[9] Older adults report problems in falling asleep and increased periods of waking during the night. Periodic leg movement is also a phenomenon that is reported in sleep disturbances of older adults. The etiology is unknown, and the prevalence is estimated at anywhere from 25 to 37 percent. Those suffering from periodic leg movement have symptoms of leg kicks, insomnia, motor restlessness, and increased daytime sleepiness.[10] Institutionalized older adults may report problems with sleep if their usual sleep pattern does not coincide with the facility schedule. A number of older adults may report taking more naps in the daytime. Safety needs during sleep and rest periods should be kept in mind.

The actual decreased need for sleep may result in fatigue when the older adult is not allowed to divide the sleep time between day and night as he or she might if he or she were residing in his or her own home. Individualized attention to sleep and potential fatigue is critical to best prevent further loss of activity and self-worth for this client.

Since fatigue plays a major role in determining the quality and amount of musculoskeletal activity undertaken, consideration of the factors that influence fatigue are essential parts of the assessment for the sleep-rest pattern.

APPLICABLE NURSING DIAGNOSIS

Sleep Pattern Disturbance

DEFINITION

Disruption of sleep time causes discomfort or interferes with desired lifestyle.[11]

NANDA TAXONOMY: MOVING 6.2.1

DEFINING CHARACTERISTICS[11]

1. Major defining characteristics
   a. Verbal complaints of difficulty falling asleep (*critical*)
   b. Awakening earlier or later than desired (*critical*)
   c. Interrupted sleep (*critical*)
   d. Verbal complaints of not feeling well rested (*critical*)

e. Changes in behavior and performance (increasing irritability, restlessness, disorientation, lethargy, or listlessness)
f. Physical signs (mild fleeting nystagmus, slight hand tremor, ptosis of eyelid, expressionless face, dark circles under eyes, frequent yawning, or changes in posture)
g. Thick speech with mispronunciation and incorrect words
2. Minor defining characteristics
   None given

RELATED FACTORS[11]

1. *Sensory alterations:* Internal (illness or psychologic stress)
2. *Sensory alterations:* External (environmental changes or social cues)

RELATED CLINICAL CONCERNS

1. Colic
2. Hyperthyroidism
3. Anxiety
4. Depression
5. Chronic obstructive pulmonary disease
6. Any postoperative state
7. Pregnancy; postpartum

HAVE YOU SELECTED THE CORRECT DIAGNOSIS?

Sleep Pattern Disturbance rarely requires differentiation from any other diagnosis and is quite often a companion diagnosis for any hospitalization.

Ineffective Individual Coping   In some instances, patients will use sleep as an avoidance mechanism and might report a sleep pattern disturbance when in reality there is no disturbance. Review of the number of hours of sleep would indicate the patient has a normal sleep pattern but desires to increase the amount of sleep to avoid having to deal with stress, anxiety, fear, and so on. These patients will invariably be requesting "a sleeping pill."

Fatigue   With this diagnosis the patient will talk about lack of energy and difficulty in maintaining his or her usual ADL. However, when questioned, this fatigue will exist in spite of the amount of sleep.

Activity Intolerance   Again, a lack of energy will be reported, but there will be no report of inadequate sleep. Indeed, the hours of sleep may have increased.

EXPECTED OUTCOMES

1. Will demonstrate at least 6 to 8 hours of uninterrupted sleep each night by (date) (**NOTE:** Actual hours of uninterrupted sleep will depend on patient's age and developmental level) and/or
2. Will verbalize decreased number of complaints regarding loss of sleep by (date)

TARGET DATES

The suggested target date is no less than 2 days after the date of diagnosis and no more than 5 days. This length of time will allow for initial modification of the sleep pattern.

NURSING ACTIONS/INTERVENTIONS WITH RATIONALES

Adult Health

ACTIONS/INTERVENTIONS	RATIONALES
• Teach relaxation exercises as needed.	Decreases sympathetic response and decreases stress.
• Suggest sleep preparatory activities such as quiet music, warm fluids, decreased active exercise at least 1 h prior to scheduled sleep time. Provide a high-carbohydrate snack.	These winding-down activities promote sleep. Carbohydrates stimulate secretion of insulin. Insulin decreases all amino acids but tryptophan. Tryptophan in larger quantities, in the brain, increases production of serotonin, a neurotransmitter that induces sleep.[12]
• Provide warm, noncaffeinated fluids after 6 p.m.; limit fluids after 8 p.m.	Warm drinks are relaxing. Limiting fluid reduces the chance of midsleep interruption to go to the bathroom.
• Assist to bathroom or bedside commode, or offer bedpan at 9 p.m.	The urge to void may interrupt the sleep cycle during the night. Voiding immediately before going to bed lessens the probability of this occurring.
• Schedule all patient therapeutics prior to 9 p.m.	Promotes uninterrupted sleep.
• Maintain room temperature at 68 to 72°F.	Environment temperature that is the most conducive to sleep.
• Notify operator to hold telephone calls starting at 9 p.m.	Promotes uninterrupted sleep.
• Ensure adherence, as closely as possible, to patient's usual bedtime routine.	Follows patient's established pattern, promotes comfort, and allows patient to wind down.
• Close door to room; limit traffic into room beginning at least 1 h prior to scheduled sleep time.	Reduces environmental stimuli.
• Administer required medication, e.g., analgesics, sedative, after all daily activities and therapeutics are completed. Monitor effectiveness of medication 30 min after time of administration.	Promotes action and effect of medication. Allows evaluation of medication effectiveness and provides data for suggesting changes in medication if needed.
• Give back massage immediately after administering medication. If no medications are needed, give back massage after toileting.	Relaxes muscles and promotes sleep.
• Place patient in preferred sleeping position; support position with pillows.	Promote patient's comfort and follows patient's usual routine.
• Ascertain if patient would like a night light.	Promotes sense of orientation in an unfamiliar environment.
• Once patient is sleeping, place do-not-disturb sign on door.	Promotes uninterrupted sleep.
• Increase exercise and activity during the day as appropriate for patient's condition.	Promotes regular diurnal rhythm.
• When appropriate, discuss reasons for sleep pattern disturbance; teach appropriate coping mechanisms.	Promotes adaptation that can increase sleep.

Child Health

ACTIONS/INTERVENTIONS	RATIONALES
• Give warm bath 30 min to 1 h before scheduled sleep time.	Promotes relaxation and provides quiet time as a part of the sleep routine.
• Feed 15–30 min before scheduled sleep time—formula, snack of protein and simple carbohydrate, no fats.	In young infants and small children, a sense of fullness and satiety, without difficulty in digestion, promotes sleep without the likelihood of upset or disturbances.
• Implement usual bedtime routine: Rocking, patting, child's cuddling of favorite stuffed animal, or using special blanket.	A structured approach to setting limits while honoring individual preference. Provides security and promotes sleep.
• Read a calm, quiet story to child immediately after putting to bed.	Reading allows a passive, meaningful enjoyment that occupies the attention of the young child while creating a bond between caretaker and child. Serendipitous relaxation often follows.

• Provide environment conducive to sleep: Room temperature of 74–78°F, soft, relaxing music, or night light.	Lack of unpleasant stimuli will provide sensory rest, as well as a change to tune out need for cognitive-perceptual activity.
• Restrict loud physical activity at least 2–3 h before scheduled sleep time.	Overstimulating physical activity may signal the central nervous system to activate bodily functions.
• Schedule therapeutics around sleep needs. Complete all therapeutics at least 1 h before scheduled sleep time.	The nurse's valuing of the sleep schedule will convey respect for the importance of sleep to the patient and family.
• Assist parents with defining and standardizing general waking and sleeping schedule.	Parents will be able to cope better with developmental issues given the knowledge and opportunity to inquire about sleep-related issues. It is reported that limit setting with confidence, by parents, is the most effective way to develop healthy patterns of sleep when no related health problems exist.
• Teach parents and child appropriate age-related relaxation techniques, e.g., imagination of the "most-quiet-place game" and other imaging techniques.	Improves parents' coping skills in dealing with common developmental issues that affect sleep.

• Discuss with parents difference between inability to sleep and fears related to developmental crises:
  ○ Infant and toddler: Separation anxiety
  ○ Preschooler: Fantasy versus reality
  ○ School age: Ability to perform at expected levels
  ○ Adolescent: Role identity versus role diffusion	

• Ensure child's safety according to developmental and psychomotor abilities, e.g., infant placed on side or back; no plastic, loose-fitting sheets; and bedrails to prevent falling out of bed.	Basic safety standards for infants and children.

Women's Health

ACTIONS/INTERVENTIONS	**RATIONALES**
• Assist patient to schedule rest breaks throughout day.	Knowledge and proper planning can help patient reduce fatigue during pregnancy and the immediate postpartum period.
• Review daily schedule with patient, and assist patient to adjust sleep schedule to coincide with infant's sleep pattern.	Knowledge of life changes can help in planning and implementing mechanisms to reduce fatigue and sleep disturbance.
• Identify a support system that can assist patient in alleviating fatigue.	

• Assist patient in identifying lifestyle adjustments that may be needed due to changes in physiologic function or needs during experiential phases of life, e.g., pregnancy, postpartum, or menopause:
  ○ Possible lowering of room temperature
  ○ Layering of blankets or covers that can be discarded or added as necessary
  ○ Practicing relaxation immediately before scheduled sleep time
  ○ Establishing a bedtime routine, e.g., bath, food, fluids, or activity	

• Involve significant others in discussion and problem-solving activities regarding life-cycle changes that are affecting work habits and interpersonal relationships, e.g., hot flashes, pregnancy, or postpartum fatigue.	
• Teach patient to experiment with restful activities when she cannot sleep at night rather than lying in bed and thinking about not sleeping.	

Psychiatric Health

ACTIONS/INTERVENTIONS	RATIONALES
• Provide only decaffeinated drinks during all 24 h.	Caffeine stimulates the central nervous system.
• Spend (amount) minutes with client in activity of client's choice at least twice a day.	Increases mental alertness and activity during daytime hours.
• Provide appropriate positive reinforcement for achievement of steps toward reaching a normal sleep pattern.	Positive reinforcement encourages behavior.
• Talk client through deep muscle relaxation exercise for 30 min at 9 p.m.	Facilitates relaxation and disengagement from the activities and thoughts of the day to prepare the client both physically and mentally for sleep.
• Sit with client for (amount) minutes 3 times a day in a quiet environment, and provide positive reinforcement for client's accomplishments. (*Note:* This is for clients with increased activity.)	Positive reinforcement encourages calm behavior and enhances self-esteem.
• Go to client's room and walk with him or her to the group area 3 times a day.	Stimulates wakefulness during daytime hours and facilitates the development of a trusting relationship.
• Spend time out of the room with the client until he or she demonstrates ability to tolerate 30 min of interaction with others. (*Note:* This is for clients with depressed mood.)	Stimulates wakefulness during daytime hours.
• Spend 30 min with client discussing concerns 2 h prior to bedtime.	Facilitates problem solving during daytime hours at a time when normal sleep patterns will not be disturbed.
• If client does not fall asleep within 45 min after retiring, have him or her get up and move around the unit, sit at nurses' station and read, or engage in some other activity that does not focus on working or going to sleep and that is not exciting for the client.	Sleep is a spontaneous behavior and cannot be achieved by "working on it." Refocuses client's behavior from "trying to go to sleep."[13]

Gerontic Health

ACTIONS/INTERVENTIONS	RATIONALES
• Collaborate with the physician and the pharmacist if a sleeping medication is prescribed to ensure that the drug is one that minimally interferes with the normal sleep cycle.	This assures that the older adult has as natural a sleep pattern as possible.
• Monitor for the presence of pain prior to bedtime and if the patient is found awake frequently during the night.	Untreated pain may prevent the onset of sleep and interrupt the individual's usual sleep pattern.
• Monitor for symptoms of depression,[14] especially if the older adult reports waking very early in the morning with an inability to fall back to sleep and experiencing feelings of anxiety upon awakening.	Depression is frequently underreported and undertreated in older adults.

Home Health

ACTIONS/INTERVENTIONS	RATIONALES

• Involve client and family in planning, implementing, and promoting restful environment and sleep routine:
  ○ Close door to room.
  ○ Turn room lights off, and provide small night light.
  ○ Pull blinds to block out streetlights (at night) or sunlight (daytime).
	Household involvement is important to ensure that the environment is conducive for sleep and rest.

- ○ Limit activity in room beginning at least 30 min before scheduled sleep time.
- ○ Unplug telephone in room, or adjust volume control on bell.
- ○ Coordinate family activities and client's sleep needs to maximize both schedules.
- ○ Request that visits and calls be made at specified times so that sleep time is not interrupted.
- ○ Provide favorite music, pillows, bedclothes, teddy bears, etc.
- ○ Provide optimal room temperature and ventilation.
- ○ Support usual bedtime routine as much as possible in relation to medical diagnosis and client's condition.
- ○ Assist client with bedtime routine as necessary.
- • Maintain pain control via appropriate medications, body positioning, and relaxation.

Pain disturbs or prevents sleep and rest.

- • Encourage self-care, exercise, and activity as appropriate and based on medical diagnosis and client's condition.

Sleep-rest patterns are stabilized by a balance of activity and exercise.

Sleep Pattern Disturbance

FLOWCHART EVALUATION: EXPECTED OUTCOME 1

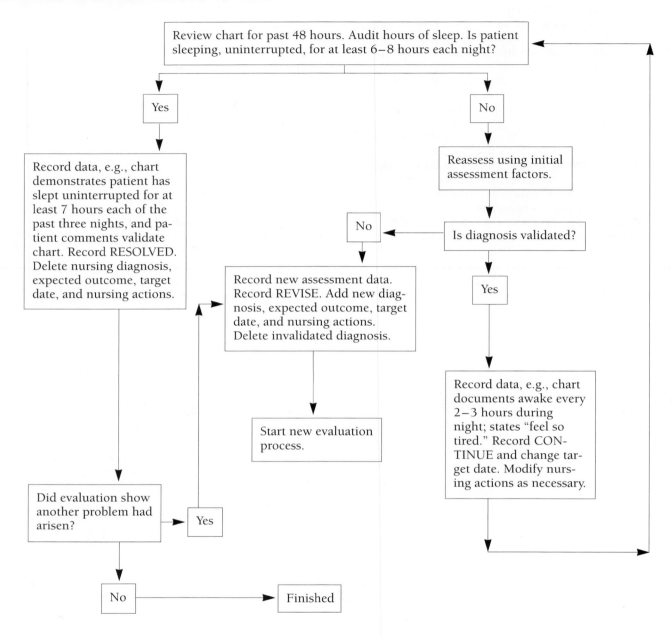

Sleep Pattern Disturbance

FLOWCHART EVALUATION: EXPECTED OUTCOME 2

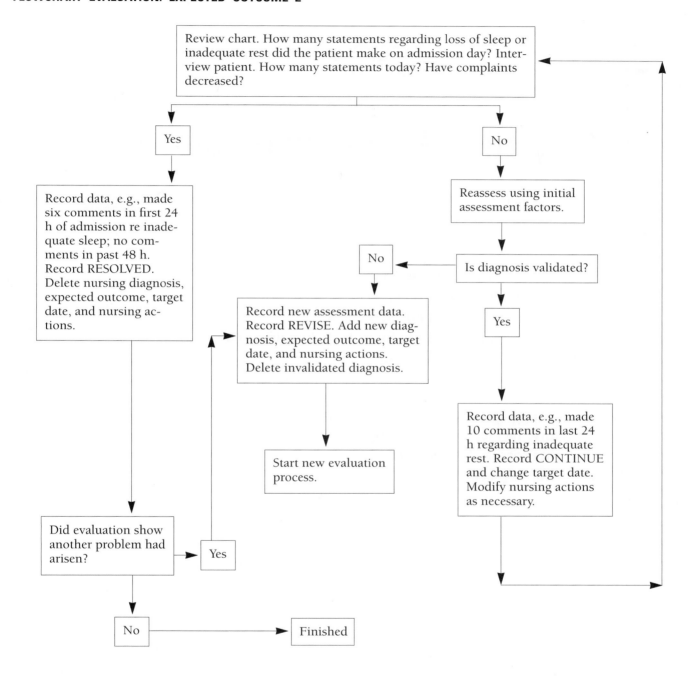

7

Cognitive-Perceptual Pattern

Pattern Description

Rationality, the ability to think, has often been described as the defining attribute of human beings. Thus, the cognitive-perceptual pattern becomes the essential premise for all other patterns used in the practice of nursing. Since this pattern deals with the adequacy of the sensory modes and adaptations necessary to negate inadequacies in the cognitive functional abilities, any failure in recognizing alterations in this pattern will hamper assessment and intervention in all of the other patterns. The nurse must be aware of the cognitive-perceptual pattern as an integral and important part of holistic nursing.

The cognitive-perceptual pattern deals with thought, thought processes, and knowledge as well as the way the patient acquires and applies knowledge. A major component of the process is perceiving. *Perceiving* incorporates the interpretation of sensory stimuli. Understanding how a patient thinks, perceives, and incorporates these processes to best adapt and function is paramount in assisting the patient to return to or maintain the best health state possible. Alterations in the process of cognition and perception are an initial step in any assessment.

Additionally, the nurse-patient relationship identifies human response as a major premise for the nursing process. Ultimately, then, it is this very notion of thought and learning potential that facilitates the self-actualization of human beings.

Pattern Assessment

1. Does ICP fluctuate following a single activity?
   a. Yes (Decreased Adaptive Capacity, Intracranial)
   b. No
2. Does the patient have a problem with appropriate response to stimuli?
   a. Yes (Confusion)
   b. No
3. Does the patient have a problem with fluctuating levels of consciousness (in presence of inappropriate response to stimuli)?
   a. Yes (Acute Confusion)
   b. No (Chronic Confusion)
4. Does the patient indicate difficulty in making choices between options for care?
   a. Yes (Decisional Conflict [Specify])
   b. No
5. Is the patient delaying decision making regarding care options?
   a. Yes (Decisional Conflict [Specify])
   b. No
6. Has the patient been disoriented to person, place, and time for over 3 months?
   a. Yes (Impaired Environmental Interpretation Syndrome)
   b. No
7. Can the patient respond to simple directions or instructions?
   a. Yes
   b. No (Impaired Environmental Interpretation Syndrome)

8. Does the patient indicate lack of information regarding his or her problem?
   a. Yes (Knowledge Deficit [Specify])
   b. No
9. Can the patient restate regimen he or she needs to follow for improved health?
   a. Yes
   b. No (Knowledge Deficit [Specify])
10. Can the patient remember events occurring within past 4 hours?
    a. Yes
    b. No (Impaired Memory)
11. Review the mental status examination. Is the patient fully alert?
    a. Yes
    b. No (Altered Thought Processes or Sensory-Perceptual Alteration)
12. Does the patient or his or her family indicate that the patient has any memory problems?
    a. Yes (Altered Thought Process)
    b. No
13. Review sensory examination. Does the patient display any sensory problems?
    a. Yes (Sensory-Perceptual Alteration [Specify])
    b. No
14. Does the patient use both sides of body?
    a. Yes
    b. No (Unilateral Neglect)
15. Does the patient look at and seem aware of affected body side?
    a. Yes
    b. No (Unilateral Neglect)
16. Does the patient verbalize that he or she is experiencing pain?
    a. Yes (Pain or Chronic Pain)
    b. No
17. Has the pain been experienced for more than 6 months?
    a. Yes (Chronic Pain)
    b. No (Pain)
18. Does the patient display any distraction behavior (moaning, crying, pacing, or restlessness)?
    a. Yes (Pain)
    b. No

Conceptual Information

A person who is able to carry out the activities of a normal cognitive-perceptual pattern experiences conscious thought, is oriented to reality, solves problems, is able to perceive via sensory input, and responds appropriately in carrying out the usual activities of daily living in the fullest level of functioning. All of these functions rely on a healthy nervous system that contains receptors to detect input accurately, a brain that can interpret the information correctly, and transmitters that can transport decoded information. Bodily response is also a basic requisite to respond to the sensory and perceptual demands of the individual.

Cognition is the process of obtaining and using knowledge about one's world through the use of perceptual abilities, symbols, and reasoning. For this reason it includes the use of human sensory capabilities to receive input about the environment. This process usually leads to *perception*, which is the process of extracting information in such a way that the individual transforms sensory input into meaning. Cognition incorporates knowledge and the process used in its acquisition; therefore, ideas (concepts of mind symbols) and language (verbal symbols) are two tools of cognition. Learning may be considered the dynamic process in which perceptual processing of sensory input leads to concept formation and change in behavior. Cognitive development is highly dependent on adequate, predictable sensory input.

There are two general approaches to contemporary cognitive theory. The information-processing approach attempts to understand human thought and reasoning processes by comparing the mind to a sophisticated computer system that is designed to acquire, process, store, and use information according to various programs or designs.

The second approach is based on the work of the Swiss psychologist Jean Piaget, who considered cognitive adaptation in terms of two basic processes: assimilation and accommodation. *Assimilation* is the process by which the person integrates new perceptual data or stimulus events into existing schemata or existing patterns of behavior. In other words, in assimilation, a person interprets reality in terms of his or her own model of the world based on previous experience. *Accommodation* is the process of changing that model the individual has of the world by developing the mechanisms to adjust to reality. Piaget believed that representational thought does not originate in a social language but in unique symbols that provide a foundation later for language acquisition.[1]

The American psychologist Jerome Bruner broadened Piaget's concept by suggesting that the cognitive process is affected by three modes: The *enactive mode* involves representation through action, the *iconic mode* uses visual and mental images, and the *symbolic mode* uses language.[1]

Cognitive dissonance is the mental conflict that takes place when beliefs or assumptions are challenged or contradicted by new information. The unease or tension the individual may experience as a result of cognitive dissonance usually results in the person's resorting to defense mechanisms in an attempt to maintain stability in his or her conception of the world and self.

In a broad sense, thinking activities may be considered internally adaptive responses to intrinsic and extrinsic stimuli. The thought processes serve to express inner impulses, but they also serve to generate appropriate goal-seeking behavior by the individual. This behavior is enhanced by perceptual processes as well.

Perception is the process of extracting information in such a way that the individual transforms sensory input into meaning. The senses that serve as the origin of perceptual stimuli are as follows:

1. Exteroreceptors (distance sensors)
   a. Visual
   b. Auditory
2. Proprioceptors (near sensors)
   a. Cutaneous (skin senses that detect and communicate or transduce changes in touch, e.g., pressure, temperature, and pain)
   b. Chemical sense of taste
   c. Chemical sense of smell

3. Interoceptors (deep sensors)
   a. Kinesthetic sense that senses changes in the position of the body and motions of the muscles, tendons, and joints
   b. Static or vestibular sense that senses changes related to maintaining position in space and the regulation of organic functions such as metabolism, fluid balance, and sensual stimulation

It is important to note that since perceptual skill processing is an internal event, its presence and development are inferred by changes in overt behavior. For full appreciation of the cognitive-perceptual pattern, it is also necessary to understand the normal physiology of the nervous system.

Developmental Considerations

INFANT

The full-term newborn has several sensory capacities. The neonate should have a pupillary reflex in response to light and a corneal reflex in response to touch. The sensory myelinization is best developed at birth for hearing, taste, and smell.

VISION   The eye is not structurally completely differentiated from the macula. The newborn has the capacity to momentarily fixate on a bright or moving object held within 8 inches and in the midline of the visual field. By approximately 4 months of age, the infant is capable of 20/200 visual acuity. Binocular fixation and convergence to near objects is possible by approximately 4 months of age. In a supine position, the infant follows a dangling toy from the side to past midline.

HEARING   The neonate is capable of detecting a loud sound of approximately 90 decibels and reacts with a startle. At birth all of the structural components of the ear are fully developed. However, the lack of cortical integration and full myelination of the neural pathways prevents specific response to sound. The infant will usually search to locate sounds. By approximately 15 months of age the infant is beginning to acquire eye-hand coordination and is capable of accommodation to near objects. Of concern at this age would be any abnormalities noted in any of these tasks plus rubbing of eyes, self-rocking, or other self-stimulating behavior. By approximately 2 months the infant will turn to the appropriate side when a sound is made at ear level. By approximately 20 months the infant will localize sounds made below the ear. A cause for concern might be failure to be awakened by loud noises or any of the above findings being abnormal. Speech or the uttering of sounds by the age of 6 to 8 months would also be a component.

SMELL   Smell seems to be a factor in breast-fed infant's response to the mother's engorgement and leaking. Newborns will turn away from strong odors such as vinegar and alcohol. By approximately 6 to 9 months, the infants associate smell with different foods and familiar people of their circle of activity. Avoidance of strong, unpleasant odors occurs also.

TASTE   The newborn responds to various solutions with the following gustofacial reflexes:

1. A tasteless solution elicits no facial expression.

2. A sweet solution elicits an eager suck and look of satisfaction.

3. A bitter liquid produces an angry, upset expression.

By 1 year of age the infant shows marked preferences, with similar responses to different flavors, as did the young neonate.

TOUCH   At birth the neonate is capable of perception of touch, and the mouth, hands, and soles of the feet are the most sensitive. There is increasing support for the notion that touch and motion are essential to normal growth and development.

By 1 year of age the infant has a preference for soft textures over rough, grainy textures. The infant relies on the sense of touch for comforting. Overresponse or underresponse to stimuli, for example, pain, is a cause for concern.

PROPRIOCEPTION   The infant, at birth, is limited in perceiving itself in space, as this requires deep myelination and total integration of cortical activity. There is momentary head control. In general, referral to more exacting neurologic reflexes of the neonate will provide in-depth supplementary data. In essence, primitive reflexes, which are protective in nature, serve to assist the neonate in adjustment to extrauterine life and identification of congenital anomalies. A critical appreciation of organic and operational synergy for the CNS is necessary as sensory deficits are considered.

By approximately 3 months of age the infant will, when suspended in a horizontal prone position with the head flexed against the trunk, reflexively draw up the legs—this is known as the *Landau reflex*. It remains present until approximately 12 to 24 months of age. Another related reflex is the *parachute reflex* in which the infant, on being suspended in a horizontal prone position and suddenly thrust downward, will place hands and fingers forward in an attempt to protect himself or herself from falling. This reflex appears at approximately 7 months and persists indefinitely.

The neonate responds with total body reaction to a painful stimulus. The primitive reflexes demonstrate this, especially the *Moro or startle response* to sudden loss of support or loud noises. The neonate is dependent on others for protection from pain. The mother of a newborn is most often the person who assumes this task, along with the father and other primary caregivers. For this reason, management of pain must also include the parents. Distraction, for example, a pacifier, is useful in dealing with painful stimuli.

The infant gradually offers localized reaction in response to pain at approximately 6 to 9 months of age. Still, the cognitive abilities of the infant remain limited with respect to pain. Often a physical tugging of the painful body part proves to be the clue of pain for the infant, as with an earache. The infant is incapable of offering cooperation in procedures and must be physically restrained as he or she is largely incapable of resisting painful stimuli. Crying and irritability may also be manifestations of pain, particularly when the nurse is sure that the infant's other basic needs have been attended to.

If chronic pain comes to be a way of life for the infant soon after birth or before much development has occurred, there may be alterations in any of the subsequent development. In some instances, infants adapt and develop high tolerances for pain.

The neonate is dependent on others for appropriate care and health maintenance. Values for health care are being formed through this provision of care by others. The infant will gradually continue to learn values of health care. Safety becomes an ongoing concern as has been previously acknowledged. Parents or primary caregivers assume this responsibility. The infant is capable of object permanence but cannot be expected to remember abstract notions.

The neonate subjected to hypoxia in the perinatal period is at risk for possible future developmental delays. Apgar scores are typically used as criteria, in addition to neurologic reflexes. Seizures during the neonatal period must also be followed. In a general sense, the premature infant of less than 38 weeks' gestation should also be considered at risk for developmental delays. It is paramount that close examination be performed for basic primitive reflexes and general neonatal status as well as identification of any genetic syndromes or congenital anomalies.

The infant gradually incorporates symbols and interacts with the world through primary caregivers. Any major delays in development should be cause for further close follow-up. Sensory-perceptual deficiencies may indeed bring about impaired thought processes.

TODDLER AND PRESCHOOLER

Binocular vision is well established by now. The toddler can distinguish geometric shapes and can demonstrate beginning depth perception. Marked strabismus should be treated at this time to prevent amblyopia. The toddler can begin to name colors.

Smell, taste, and touch all become more related as the toddler initially sees an object and handles it while enjoying, via all the senses, what it is to "know." Regression to previous tactile behavior for comfort is common in this group, as exemplified by a preference for being patted and rocked to sleep during times of stress such as illness. Concerns by this time would be for secondary deficits in development that may arise. There is also a great concern for the toddler who shows greater response to movement than to sound or who avoids social interaction with other children. By this time speech should be sufficiently developed to validate a basic sense of the toddler's ability to use symbols. Proprioception is not perfected, but "toddling" represents a major milestone. Falls at this age are common.

There is an even greater incorporation of sensory activity in sequencing for the preschooler, in whom major myelination for the most part is fully developed. There is refinement of eye-hand coordination, and reading readiness is apparent. Visual acuity begins to approach 20/20, and the preschooler will know colors. Prior to the age of 5 the child should be screened for amblyopia; after age 5 there is minimal potential for development of amblyopia. Language becomes more sophisticated and serves to provide social interaction. By this age the child will remember and exercise caution regarding potential dangers, such as hot objects.

The toddler may regress to previous behavior levels with physical resistance in response to painful stimuli. This will be especially true with invasive procedures. On occasion a toddler may demonstrate tolerance for painful procedures on the basis of understanding benefits offered, for example, young children with a medical diagnosis of leukemia. This is not the usual case, however. Temper tantrums, outbursts, and avoidance of painful stimuli describe the usual behavior of the toddler. When the toddler must deal with chronic pain, he or she may regress to previous behavior as a means of coping.

The preschooler views any invasive procedure as mutilation and attempts to withdraw in response to pain. The preschooler cries out in pain and will express feelings in his or her own terms as descriptors of pain. The interpretation of pain is influenced greatly by the parental and familial value systems. In severe pain the potential for regression to previous behavior is high. The nurse should be aware that fears of abandonment, death, or the unknown will be brought out by pain for this age group. Also, the effect the pain has on others may serve to further frighten the child.

Play is an ideal noninvasive means of assessment. Difficulties in gait, balance, or the use of upper limbs in symmetry with lower limbs should be noted, as well as related holistic developmental components including speech, motor, cognitive, perceptual, and social components. Allowance should be made for regression to prior patterns as needed in times of stress such as illness and hospitalization. If a deficit exists, parents should be encouraged to continue appropriate follow-up and intervention.

The preschooler may be aware of how he or she is different from peers, although egocentrism continues. Of importance is the mastery of separation from parents for increasing periods of time. The likelihood of sibling integration should be considered also. At this time a known neglect of one side of the body may be problematic, as the child may rebel and fail to comply with desired therapy.

The toddler gradually learns to care for himself or herself and is strongly influenced by the family's value system. There is capacity for expression of beginning thoughts.

The preschooler has capacity for magical thinking and enjoys role-play of the parent of the same sex. At this age, beginning resistance to parental authority is common and the child is still egocentric in thought. This makes it difficult to apply universal understanding of the use of language and symbols for children of this age; for example, death may be perceived as "sleep."

By this age there should be a general notion of the cognitive capacity for the child. The child explores the world in a meaningful fashion and still relies closely on primary caregivers. If there are marked delays, they should be monitored with a focus on maintaining optimum functioning with developmental sequencing.

The preschooler will enjoy activity and is beginning to enjoy learning colors, using words in sentences, and gradually forming relationships with persons outside the immediate family. If there are delays, they should continue to be monitored. By now major deficits in cognition become more obvious.

SCHOOL-AGE CHILD

The school-ager has a significant ability to perform logical operations. More complete myelination and maturation enhance the basic physiologic functioning of the central nervous system. Generally, the school-age child can establish and follow simple rules. There is self-motivation with a gradual grasp of time in a more abstract nature. The concept of death is recognized as permanent.

The school-age child begins to interpret the experience of pain with a cognitive component—the cause or source of pain, as well as implications for possible recurrence. The child of this developmental category will attempt to hold still as needed, with an appearance of bravery. Expression of the experience of pain is to be expected by a school-ager. If the school-ager is particularly shy, special attempts should be made to establish a trusting relationship to best manage pain. A major fear is loss of control. The nurse must consider the need to completely evaluate chronic pain. In some instances, it may signal other altered patterns, especially a distressed family or inability to cope as well. Lower performance in school can be an indicator of chronic pain. Also, the nurse should be aware of the increased complexity required for daily activities of living. The child of this age may feel negative about himself or herself if he or she is unable to perform as peers do. The importance of group activities cannot be overstressed.

The school-age child will blossom with a sense of accomplishment. When school does not bring success, frustration follows. It is mandatory that caution be exercised in assessing for deficits versus behavioral manifestations of not liking school.

ADOLESCENT

VISION Acuity of 20/20 is reached by now. Squinting should be investigated, as should any symptoms of prolonged eyestrain.

HEARING Further investigation should be done on any adolescent who speaks loudly or who fails to respond to loud noises.

TOUCH Overreaction or underreaction to painful stimuli is cause for further investigation.

TASTE The adolescent may prefer food fads for a length of time, but concern would be appropriate if the adolescent overuses spices, especially salt or sugar, or complaints of foods not "tasting as they used to."

SMELL The adolescent should distinguish a full range of odors. The nurse should be concerned if the adolescent is unresponsive to noxious stimuli.

PROPRIOCEPTION There may be temporary clumsiness associated with growth spurts. The nurse should be concerned if he or she observes patterns of deteriorating gross and fine motor coordination and ataxia.

By now the adolescent is capable of formal operational thought and is able to move beyond the world of concrete reality to abstract possibilities and ideas. Problem solving is evident with inductive and deductive capacity. There is an interest in values with a tendency toward idealism. Attention must be given to the adolescent's sensitivity to others and potential for rejection if body image is altered. Of particular importance at this time are sports and peer-related activities. As feelings are explored more cautiously, there is a tendency to draw into oneself at this stage. There may be major conflicts over independence when self-care is not possible.

The adolescent fears mutilation and attempts to deal with pain as an adult might. Self-control is strived for with allowance for capitalization on gains from pain. Sexuality factors of role performance enter into this group as pain occurs. As with the adult, an attempt to discover the cause and implication of the pain is made. The adolescent experiencing chronic pain will be at risk for abnormal peer interaction and may potentially endure altered self-perception.

The adolescent will most often remain steady in cognitive functioning if there are no major emotional or sensory problems. Of concern at this age would be substance abuse that could impair thought processes.

ADULT AND OLDER ADULT

VISION   The adult is capable of 20/20 vision with a gradual decline in acuity and accommodation after approximately 40 years of age. There is a tendency toward farsightedness. Color discrimination decreases in later ages, with green and blue being the major hues affected. Depending on the cause, there is a great potential for the use of corrective aids. In examples of degenerative processes, though, such is not the case, as with macula degeneration. Eventually depth perception and peripheral vision are also affected. There may also be a sensitivity to light as with cataract formation. The nurse should be alert for all etiologic components, especially the retinopathy associated with diabetic alterations.

HEARING   The adult has a sensitivity to accurately discriminate 1600 different frequencies. There should be equal sensation of sounds for the left and right ear. The Rinne test may be done to validate air and bone conduction via a tuning fork. The Weber test may be used to assess lateralization. Equilibrium assessment will provide data regarding the vestibular branch.

With time, the acuity of what is heard gradually diminishes, with detection of high-pitched frequencies especially affected. The nurse should be concerned with a lack of response to loud noises and increased volume of speech and should be alert to cues of decreased hearing such as cupping of the hand on the "better" ear or leaning sideways to catch the conversation on the "better" side.

SMELL   There may be a gradual deterioration in sensitivity for smell after approximately age 60, although for the most part the sense of smell remains functional in the absence of organic disease. There may be altered gastrointestinal enzyme production, which ultimately interferes with usual perception of smells.

TASTE   The ability to taste is well differentiated in adulthood. Sweet and sour can be detected bilaterally. Concern may be raised if the client states the sense of taste has diminished or changed. There is a gradual loss of acuity in taste as aging occurs in later life. This is due in part to decreased enzymatic production and utilization in digestive processes. Oversalting or spicing of foods may serve as a clue to this loss of taste sensation. The use of dentures may also affect the sensation of taste and enjoyment of food.

TOUCH   The adult is able to discriminate on a wide range of tactile stimuli, including pressure, temperature, texture, and pain or noxious components. With aging, there is a decrease in subcutaneous fat, loss of skin turgor, increase in capillary fragility, and a decrease in conduction of impulses. All of these changes influence the sense of touch with a loss of acuity in aging.

PROPRIOCEPTION   The adult is well coordinated and has a keen sense of perception of his or her body in space. There are multiple protective mechanisms that aid in maintaining balance. Typically, even with eyes closed, the individual is able to stand and maintain balance.

By now the tolerance and threshold one has for pain is well established. The individual has learned various ways to cope with pain and thus may be equipped with a more stable base from which to respond. Paradoxically the adult may also experience unresolved conflicts of previous development levels as well. For this reason the required change may be subject to associated changes as the multiple demands of daily living are affected by pain and its response by the adult.

The adult is equipped to solve problems and apply principles to everyday living. There is emphasis on seeking a mate for life who is able to satisfy basic companionship needs. There may be difficulties in accepting life's challenges as parents or as adults juggling the many roles necessary. There is, in later life, a gradual decline in problem-solving capacity, which may be exaggerated by illness.

Allowing for potential decrease in bodily perception and functioning with age must be considered. As assessment is carried out, focus should be on risk factors such as chronic illness, financial deficits, resolution of ego integrity versus despair, and obvious etiologic components. The nurse should assist the patient to maintain self-care as the patient desires.

With aging there is a gradual loss of balance, perhaps most related to the concurrent vascular changes. For this reason proprioceptive data may provide an immediate basis for safety needs of the geriatric client.

In the absence of adversity, the adult enjoys the daily challenges of living. If coping is altered for whatever reason, a risk for impaired thought process exists. With the process of aging, there are potential risks for impaired thought process. In addition, there may be potential risks for some regarding degenerative brain and CNS disorders, which also include impaired thought processes. Two concerns for older adults related to altered thought process are dementia and delirium or acute confusional states.

APPLICABLE NURSING DIAGNOSES

Adaptive Capacity, Decreased, Intracranial

DEFINITION

A clinical state in which intracranial fluid dynamic mechanisms that normally compensate for increases in intracranial volumes are compromised, resulting in repeated disproportionate increases in intracranial pressure (ICP) in response to a variety of noxious and nonnoxious stimuli.[2]

NANDA TAXONOMY: EXCHANGING 1.7.1
DEFINING CHARACTERISTICS[2]

1. Major defining characteristics
   a. Repeated increases in ICP of greater than 10 mm

Hg for more than 5 minutes following any of a variety of external stimuli.
2. Minor defining characteristics
   a. Disproportionate increase in ICP following single environmental or nursing maneuver stimulus
   b. Elevated P2 ICP waveform
   c. Volume pressure response test variation (volume-pressure ratio > 2, pressure = volume index < 10)
   d. Baseline ICP equal to or greater than 10 mm Hg
   e. Wide amplitude ICP waveform

RELATED FACTORS[2]

1. Brain injuries
2. Sustained increase in ICP $\geq$ 10 to 15 mm Hg

3. Decreased cerebral perfusion pressure $\leq$ 50 to 60 mm Hg
4. Systemic hypotension with intracranial hypertension

RELATED CLINICAL CONCERNS

1. Head injury
2. Cerebral ischemia
3. Cranial tumors
4. Hydrocephalus
5. Cranial hematomas
6. AV formation
7. Vasogenic or cytotoxic cerebral edema
8. Hyperemia
9. Obstruction of venous outflow

HAVE YOU SELECTED THE CORRECT DIAGNOSIS?

Altered Protection   This diagnosis is typically associated with immune disorders or clotting disorders. However, maladaptive stress response and general neurosensory alterations are also associated with altered protection. Decreased Adaptive Capacity, Intracranial, is a specific diagnosis related to intracranial fluid dynamic mechanisms.

Fluid-Volume Excess   This diagnosis refers to the overall fluid in the body. Body fluid may be normal in Decreased Adaptive Capacity, Intracranial. However, the intracranial fluid volume and pressure are abnormal.

Altered Tissue Perfusion   This diagnosis defines a decrease in nutrition and oxygenation at the cellular level due to a deficit in capillary blood supply and may be a companion diagnosis to Decreased Adaptive Capacity, Intracranial, depending on the cerebral perfusion pressure and the secondary physiologic cellular damage brought on by the brain injury.

EXPECTED OUTCOMES

1. Will have an ICP within normal range by (date) and/or
2. Will have improved neurologic signs by (date)

TARGET DATES

Decreased Adaptive Capacity, Intracranial, is a life-threatening condition and should have target dates set in terms of hours. After stabilization, the time frame may be moved to 48-hour increments.

NURSING ACTIONS/INTERVENTIONS WITH RATIONALES

Adult Health

ACTIONS/INTERVENTIONS	RATIONALES
• Hyperventilate as necessary.	Decreased $PaCO_2$ leads to vasoconstriction and thus reduces cerebral blood flow.[3]
• Monitor ABGs. Maintain PaO_2 > 80 mm Hg; $PaCO_2$ at 25–33 mm Hg. Avoid hypoxia.	Hyperventilation produces systemic alkalosis, which passes through the blood-brain barrier to buffer the cerebral acidosis created by lactic acid buildup.[4] Hyperventilation can produce a paradoxical vasodilatation in areas of the brain.[3,4]
• Monitor cerebral blood flow and cerebral ischemia with xenon-enhanced CT as needed.	
• Give IV THAM as ordered.	THAM is a weak base that may produce a prolonged alkalization of the cerebrospinal fluid (CSF).[4,5]
• Monitor CSF for lactate and creatinine-kinase BB bands.	Reflects amount of brain tissue acidosis.[6]

- Monitor neurologic status: Glasgow Coma Scale for level of consciousness, motor power, and general sensory exam as needed or at least every 8 h; pupillary size and response every hour; and cardiovascular and respiratory status every hour.
- Monitor ECG. Watch for T-wave changes, shortened P-R interval, prolonged Q-T interval, PVCs, ventricular ectopy, sinus bradycardia, and ventricular or supra-ventricular tachycardia.
- Elevate head of bed 0–30 degrees. Keep head and neck in a neutral position, or slightly extend head and neck. Do not hyperextend head and neck. Do not turn head to right or left or place head and neck in a flexed position.[10] Avoid hip flexion of more than 90 degrees.
- Turn every 2 h. Have sufficient personnel to move patient. Keep body and head in alignment. Turn slowly. May use specialty beds and alternating pressure mattress.
- Give medications for sedation (e.g., midazolam IV drip) and chemical paralysis (e.g., atracurium IV drip) as ordered. Lubricate eyes or tape shut. Provide comfort measures. Gently touch hand or face. Talk quietly with patient.
- Prevent initiation of Valsalva's maneuver.

- Monitor fluid status. Patient should be normovolemic. Sometimes fluids are restricted, and other times they are not. Monitor I&O and electrolytes. Monitory CVP (should be at least 6–8 mm Hg) or pulmonary wedge pressure. Fluid volume should provide sufficient mean arterial pressure (MAP) to support a cerebral perfusion pressure (CPP) of 60–70 mm Hg (CPP = MAP − ICP).
- Give diuretics as ordered, e.g., mannitol or furosemide. Monitor serum osmolarity levels (should not exceed 320 mOsm).
- Monitor, PT, PTT, and platelet count.
- Monitor ICP (goal < 20 mm Hg) and CPP (CPP = MAP − ICP; normal = 80–100 mm Hg; range = 50–150 mm Hg; goal > 60 mm Hg). CPP (cerebral perfusion pressure) is an indirect index of cerebral blood flow.[12] Use ventricular catheter, subarachnoid screw, epidural monitor, continuous jugular venous bulb oxygen saturation ($SjbO_2$), arterial saturation of O_2, pulse oximetry, transcranial doppler studies, xenon-enhanced computerized tomography; cerebral oxygen extraction ratio (c $O_2ER = Sa\ O_2 − Sjb\ O_2/Sa\ O_2 \times 100$).
- Monitor patency and sterility of monitoring device. Used closed system. Change as per institution's protocol. Never allow fluid to backflow into cranial cavity. Do not use monitor (unless absolutely necessary) to obtain CSF. Assess insertion site when changing dressings. Keep site clean and dry. Monitor temperature, WBC, and differential as per protocol.
- Balance and recalibrate monitoring device as per institution protocol.

Reflects amount of brain tissue acidosis.[6]
Routine neuroassessment can cause slight increases in ICP.

Intracranial pathology is frequently associated with myocardial dysfunction.[7]

Promotes venous drainage from the head.[8] Some research indicates good outcomes with head of bed flat.[9]

Turning can cause increases in ICP by obstructing venous return from the brain.[11]

Relaxes and calms the patient. Keeps the patient from fighting or "bucking" the ventilator.[12] Drugs need to have a short half-life so that neuroassessments, when done, are not affected.[13] Stop drug approximately 1/2 hour before neuroassessment. Cover period with morphine.
Any activity—conversation about the patient's condition, either with the patient or at the bedside regarding the patient, coughing, sneezing, vomiting, bathing, giving medications, fever, pain, dressing change, agitation, spontaneous movement, etc.—can increase ICP.[11,14–16]
Light touch may decrease ICP.[17]
Decreases cerebral intravascular fluid.[18] Recent research discusses the use of hypertonic crystalloid solutions (NaCl 7.5% or 9%) with or without the addition of a colloid (dextran 70).[19]

Removes water from cerebral tissues.

Reduces the risk of intracranial hemorrhage.
Methods to measure ICP and CPP. Accurate monitoring of abnormal ICP enables health care providers to aggressively treat patients and results in improved patient outcomes.[20] Transcranial doppler studies assess cerebral blood flow regionally and detect focal areas of low flow or spasm.[21] Along with arterial saturation, can assess the relationship between the supply and use of O_2 by the brain, providing early detection of cerebral ischemia.[21] Cerebral oxygen extraction ratio is more indicative of oxygen supply and use by the brain.[22,23] Refer to reference 23 for protocol used with c O_2ER.
Invasive techniques of monitoring hold inherent risk of cranial infection.[20]

Continued

ACTIONS/INTERVENTIONS	RATIONALES
• Give anticonvulsants as ordered.	Prophylactic to prevent seizure activity as seizures cause elevation in ICP and increase metabolic demand for oxygen and glucose.[12]
• Assist with barbiturate coma as ordered. Monitor patient for decreased respirations and pneumonia.	Decreases metabolic activity of the brain. Also depresses cardiac function, thereby decreasing cardiac output and blood pressure.[12,18]
• Give neuroprotective agents as ordered: ∘ Oxygen-free radicals scavengers (antioxidants, e.g., PEG-SOD) ∘ Excitatory amino acid receptor (glutamate) antagonists (MK801 and D-CPP-ene) ∘ NMDA antagonists or calcium channel blockers specific to neural tissue, e.g., nimodipine ∘ High-dose synthetic steroids, e.g., methylprednisolone	Research in animals has shown that these drugs are effective in reducing ischemic damage and preserving cell function.[24-27] Further research is needed to evaluate effects of drugs and drug therapy in humans.
• Drain CSF from ventriculostomy based on ICP and c O_2ER.	Decreases ICP.
• Suction cautiously as needed. Prophylactic use of lidocaine HCl IV or endotracheally 5 min before suctioning has been recommended. Preoxygenate. Suction a maximum of 2 passes of 10 s, using less than 120 mm Hg of negative pressure. Use appropriate-size suction catheter. Oxygenate after suctioning with 100% oxygen. Caution in use of hyperventilation. Wait at least 5 min to allow ICP and CPP to return to normal before suctioning again.	Suctioning can cause increase in ICP.[12,14,28]
• Assist in hypothermia treatment as ordered. Best done within 6 h of trauma for 48 h. Mild to moderate (32-34°C).	Decreases cerebral metabolic rate and ICP.
• Minimize environmental stimuli (light, sounds, and odors).	Minimizes fluctuations in ICP and CPP.[15]
• Note ICP and CPP before and after activities.	
• Monitor response to nursing interventions.	
• Coordinate and schedule interventions of all members of the health care team.	Uncoordinated activities may dangerously increase ICP.
• Avoid chilling when bathing. Do passive ROM exercises when bathing.	Some research indicates bathing may be calming.[16]

Child Health

ACTIONS/INTERVENTIONS	RATIONALES
• Monitor for factors contributing to altered intracranial pressure, especially positioning, treatments, medications, suctioning, ventilation, etc.	Thorough evaluation for contributing factors allows for early detection of complications.
• Carry out thorough neurologic assessment according to degree of stimulation and movement permitted per infant's or child's status.	Deviations from norms will assist in differential workup and expedite treatment plan.
• Maintain head of bed > 30 degrees, with head in line with body—ideally not positioned from side to side unless specified. (Avoid use of pillows under head.) Recheck every 1–2 h.	Neutral body alignment will assist in stabilizing the intracranial adaptation.
• Offer a calm, supportive environment with attention to safety according to infant's or child's needs.	Few stimuli will enhance the infant's or child's likelihood of rest during acute phase, while safeguarding will minimize further injury.

- Develop a daily plan of care that best matches the developmental capacity of the infant or child, yet allows for possible regression.
- Incorporate parental input in daily plan of care as may be appropriate.

- Offer time (30 min each shift and as needed) for parents to ventilate feelings regarding infant's or child's status.
- Provide adequate teaching regarding equipment, procedures, surgery, etc.
- Offer gentle massage and monitor carefully skin integrity and tissue perfusion, especially when condition lasts more than 2 days.
- Check for potential untoward effects of meds, and exercise caution in appropriate dilution for IV administration.
- Maintain ongoing communication with family to offer updates on infant's or child's condition.
- Encourage parents to bring infant's or child's favorite blanket, small toy, or security object if possible.
- Arrange for appropriate follow-up, including home health, physical therapy, or neuro, especially when there may be a V-P shunt, for example.

Previous skills may be unable to be remastered or altered temporarily due to illness in the pediatric client.

Family will feel valued while their input will assist in providing some familiarity to infant or child and lessen effects of multiple caregivers.
Ventilation will assist in reducing anxiety and offer cues regarding parental concerns.
Knowledge allows for acceptance and understanding of infant's or child's status and power of masking unknown.
Likelihood of skin breakdown increases when repositioning is limited.

Likelihood of interaction increases with 3 or more medications, and inappropriate administration may likewise cause side effects.
Trust in caregivers will be enhanced if family can be kept abreast of activities on ongoing basis.
Familiar favored objects offer a sense of security in otherwise foreign setting, thereby reducing stress.
Appropriate referral will foster long-term continued regimen and offer goals over time.

Women's Health

ACTIONS/INTERVENTIONS	RATIONALES

For Women's Health, see Adult Health, except for the following:

ECLAMPSIA

- Place on continuous intensive monitoring (cardiac and fetal).
- Place in a darkened, quiet environment, to decrease external stimuli.

Reduction of external stimuli can reduce or prevent convulsions in these patients. They need the reduction of light to lessen eye pain and headache.

- Place padded tongue blade at head of bed.
- Carefully monitor $MgSO_4$ levels, if appropriate, for therapeutic dose and/or toxicity.

ONCE CONVULSION HAS BEEN CONTROLLED

- Monitor FHT
- Assist patient in orientation to time and place.

- Do not allow patient to ambulate alone. Provide assistance. Provide bedside commode.

Often lethargy and confusion are the result of $MgSO_4$ therapy for eclampsia.
These patients feel out of control, lethargic, confused, and cannot remember what has just been said to them as a result of both the convulsion and the medication. They need specific direction and a lot of support and understanding.

NEWBORN

- Carefully assess the newborn for cranial injury.
- Carefully examine the infant's skull. Note the anterior and posterior fontanels. Be especially alert for a bulging anterior fontanel indicative of:
  - Increased intracranial pressure
  - Major hemorrhage
  - Hydrocephalus

Psychiatric Health

The nursing actions for Psychiatric Health for this diagnosis are the same as the actions enumerated in the Adult Health section.

Gerontic Health

ACTIONS/INTERVENTIONS	RATIONALES
• Maintain head in neutral position, even while patient is side lying.	Prevents increases in pressure from flexion or extension of the head.

Nursing interventions found in the Adult Health section are appropriate to this age group. Caution must be used due to the potential for problems regarding hydration, hypothermia, pupillar reaction, deficits related to eye surgery, and risk for sensory deprivation with decreased activity.

Home Health

See Adult Health care plan. If patient with this diagnosis is in the home, professional home care will be required.

Adaptive Capacity, Decreased, Intracranial

FLOWCHART EVALUATION: EXPECTED OUTCOME 1

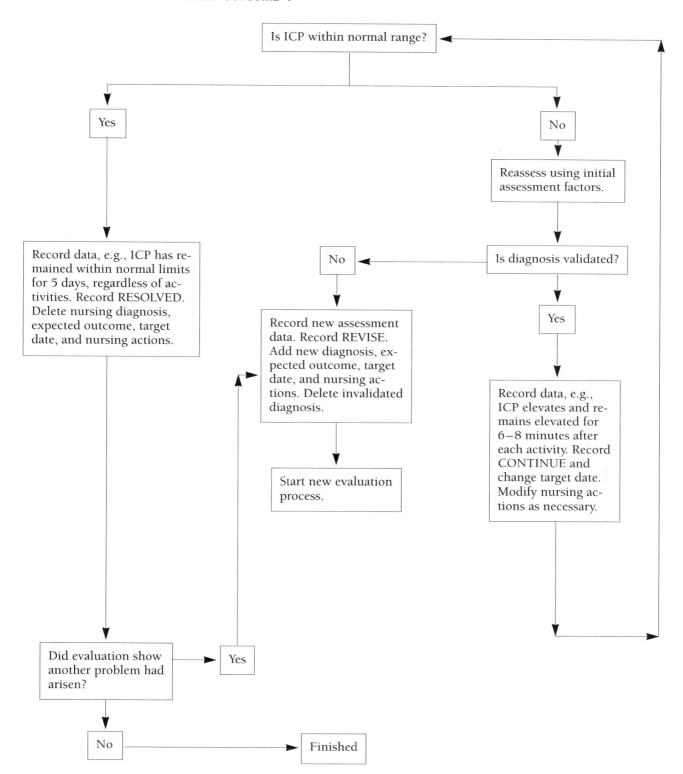

Adaptive Capacity, Decreased, Intracranial

FLOWCHART EVALUATION: EXPECTED OUTCOME 2

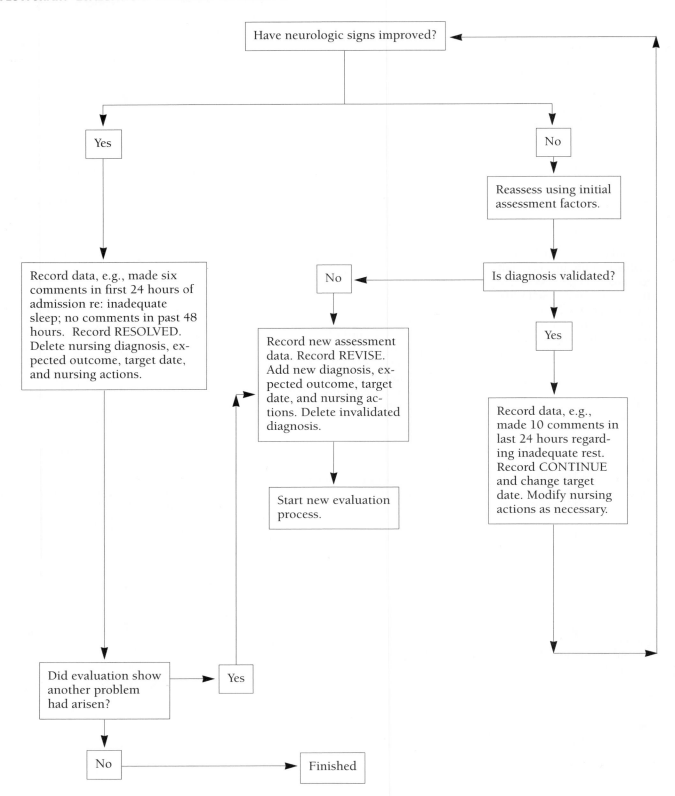

Confusion, Acute and Chronic

DEFINITION

ACUTE   The abrupt onset of a cluster of global, transient changes and disturbances in attention, cognition, psychomotor activity, level of consciousness, and/or sleep-wake cycle.[2]

CHRONIC   An irreversible, long-standing, and/or progressive deterioration of intellect and personality characterized by decreased ability to interpret environmental stimuli and decreased capacity for intellectual thought processes and manifested by disturbances of memory.

NANDA TAXONOMY: KNOWING 8.2.2 AND 8.2.3

DEFINING CHARACTERISTICS[2]

1. Acute
   a. Major defining characteristics
      (1) Fluctuation in cognition
      (2) Fluctuation in sleep-wake cycle
      (3) Fluctuation in level of consciousness
      (4) Fluctuation in psychomotor activity
      (5) Increased agitation or restlessness
      (6) Misperception
      (7) Lack of motivation to initiate and/or follow through with goal-directed or purposeful behavior
   b. Minor defining characteristics
      (1) Hallucination
2. Chronic
   a. Major defining characteristics
      (1) Clinical evidence of organic impairment
      (2) Altered interpretation or response to stimuli
      (3) Progressive and/or long-standing cognitive impairment
   b. Minor defining characteristics
      (1) No change in level of consciousness
      (2) Impaired socialization
      (3) Impaired memory (short term, long term)
      (4) Altered personality

RELATED FACTORS[2]

1. Acute
   a. Over 60 years of age
   b. Dementia
   c. Alcohol abuse
   d. Drug abuse
   e. Delirium
2. Chronic
   a. Alzheimer's disease
   b. Korsakoff's psychosis
   c. Multi-infarct dementia
   d. Cerebral vascular accident
   e. Head injury

RELATED CLINICAL CONCERNS

1. Head injury
2. CVA
3. Alzheimer's disease
4. Chemical abuse
5. Dementia

HAVE YOU SELECTED THE CORRECT DIAGNOSIS?

Sensory-Perceptual Alteration   An alteration in one of the senses could create a short-term confusion that is correctable. If a sensory deficit is found, the most correct diagnosis is Sensory-Perceptual Alteration.

Impaired Thought Process   The individual has a problem with cognitive operation and engages in nonreality thinking. Other functioning is normal. Confusion causes problems in both mental and physical functioning.

Impaired Memory   This diagnosis is related to memory only. Other cognitive functioning may be OK.

EXPECTED OUTCOMES

1. If acute, will return to nonconfused state by (date), and/or
2. If chronic, family will restate measures to work with confused state by (date)

TARGET DATES

For acute confusion, an appropriate target date would be 72 hours after admission. Chronic confusion may be permanent, but the family should be able to learn appropriate intervention techniques within 72 hours.

NURSING ACTIONS/INTERVENTIONS WITH RATIONALES

Adult Health

ACTIONS/INTERVENTIONS	RATIONALES
• Identify self and patient by name at the beginning of each interaction.	Memory loss necessitates frequent orientation to person, time, and environment.
• Speak slowly and in short, clear, concrete, simple sentences and words.	Allows time for information processing and avoids use of complex statements and abstract ideas.
• Periodically orient and/or reorient patient to the environment.	Helps alleviate anxiety brought on by changing levels of orientation and helps meet safety needs of patient.
• When patient is delusional, focus on underlying feelings and reinforce reality (have clocks, calendars, etc., on the wall). Do not argue with patient.	Recognizing and/or acknowledging feelings may decrease patient's anxiety and give him or her a sense of being understood. Arguing may increase patient's anxiety and reinforce intensity delusions.[29]
• When hallucinations and/or illusions are present, reinforce reality and attempt to identify underlying feelings or environmental stimuli.	False and/or distorted sensory experiences are common in confused states. To help decrease anxiety, focus on feelings underlying these experiences while calmly reinforcing reality.[29]
• If patient becomes aggressive, focus on underlying feelings and attempt to refocus interaction on topics more acceptable and/or less threatening to patient.	Focusing on feelings increases patient's feelings of being understood, and discussing nonthreatening topics increases patient's sense of competency and self-esteem.
• Keep patient's room well lighted. Maintain a calm environment.	Decreases possibility of environmental sensory misrepresentations and helps meet patient safety needs. Patients with confusion are experiencing increased levels of anxiety and can become physically and mentally exhausted. Promoting rest often means controlling environmental stimuli that contribute to the confusion.
• Encourage patient to wear and use personal devices (glasses or hearing aids).	These items increase accuracy of visual and auditory perceptions.
• During abusive episodes, ignore insults and focus on underlying feelings. Set limits on behavior if physically abusive.	Projection of fear and anger onto persons in the environment is common in confused states. Arguing or becoming defensive escalates the situation and adds to the patient's fear and anger.
• Teach family about patient's condition and how to interact more effectively with patient; i.e., provide ongoing orientation to surroundings and happenings within the family.	Assists family in understanding changes in patient's orientation, cognition, and behavior. Increases family's sense of competency in relating to patient.
• Recognize family responses to patient's condition and teach about reasons for condition and how to respond during acute episodes.	Family members often feel anxious and helpless about patient's behavior. Teaching them reasons for patient's condition and how to respond decreases their anxiety and may help decrease patient's confusion.
• Refer patient to psychiatric-mental health clinical nurse specialist. Make other referrals to community agencies as needed; i.e., Alzheimer's support group, adult day care, meals-on-wheels, etc.	The psychiatric-mental health CNS has the expertise to collaborate with the adult health nurse to plan nursing interventions for the patient that will help the patient and nursing staff deal with chronic confusion in the acute care setting.

Child Health

Although usually found in populations over 60 years of age, confusion may occur in younger people as well, due to similar causes. Uncertainty may be greater regarding potential for recovery due to age, exact cause of problem, and so on.

ACTIONS/INTERVENTIONS	RATIONALES

ACUTE

- Monitor for potential contributory factors, especially as applicable:
  - Prenatal influences, i.e., drugs or sepsis
  - Previous health status
  - Known conditions requiring treatment or not
  - Triggering event, trauma, surgery, emotional event
  - Daily routine or alterations
- Determine with parents previous patterns of development, and develop daily plan of care within capacity offered by infant's or child's status.
- Identify current plan of care to best suit infant's or child's capacities with input from all members of health care team, especially parents.
- Offer treatment within developmentally appropriate framework of infant or child.

- Provide a safe or calm environment with stimuli best suited to infant's or child's needs.

- Offer parents realistic plans for infant or child with frequent updates.

- Provide 30 min each shift for parents to ventilate feelings about infant or child.
- Identify discharge and follow-up needs with attention to all members of the health team.

Rationales:

A thorough assessment will offer the best basis for identification and treatment of confusion.

Parents are best able to provide previous development capacity cues within level of comfort for infant or child, thus enhancing likelihood of a sense of security for all. Best holistic plan of care reflects expertise of all who best know and interact with infant or child.

In all situations there is greater likelihood of success in care when the infant or child is approached from a developmentally appropriate stance to afford a sense of security.
Environment that is safe and developmentally appropriate will provide freedom from injury while allowing the infant or child to recover.
Parents will better be able to trust and accept infant's or child's status and caregivers when trusting relationships are based on communication that is honest and forthright.
Ventilation will help reduce anxiety and offers cues to parental concerns.
Support for parents upon the family's return to home will help them maintain plan for care and thereby attain treatment goals.

CHRONIC

- Offer resources for support groups and advocacy interest opportunities.
- Explore specific patterns of daily care needs and how best to offer care within the domain of resources available.

Rationales:

Specific support groups will assist parents in dealing with situation represented by infant's or child's status.
Realistic demands will best direct care according to existing time and constraints.

Note risk for Caregiver Role Strain due to demands over time.

Women's Health

See nursing actions for Adult Health. See magnesium sulfate therapy specific for pregnancy-induced hypertension (PIH) in Women's Health section for Adaptive Capacity, Intracranial, Decreased.

Psychiatric Health

ACTIONS/INTERVENTIONS	RATIONALES

ACUTE

Mental health clients at risk for this diagnosis include:
   Patients taking the following medications: Lithium, antianxiety agents, anticholinergics, phenothiazine, barbiturates, methyldopa, disulfiram, alcohol, cocaine, amphetamines, opiates, and hallucinogenics
   Patients experiencing: Drug withdrawal, ECT treatments, dementia, dissociative disorders, mood disorders, and thought disorders, and elderly clients with acute infections such as UTIs

Continued

ACTIONS/INTERVENTIONS	RATIONALES
• Place client in an environment with appropriate stimuli. Note level of stimulation and alterations in environmental stimuli here. For example, specific objects in the environment that stimulate illusions should be removed, and appropriate lighting, clocks and calendars, and holiday decorations should be used. Refer to day, date, and other orienting information during each interaction with client.	Increases patient safety and promotes orientation.[30,31]
• Assign client room that provides opportunities for careful observation while not providing a chaotic environment.	Promotes client safety and decreases environmental stimuli. High levels of stimuli can increase confusion and hyperactivity.[32–34]
• Place identifying information on patient and patient's room. Utilize patient's preferred name in each interaction. Note that name here.	Promotes safety and orientation.
• Remove harmful objects from the environment. This could include objects in walkways, cords, belts, and raised bedrails or other restraining devices. During periods of increased agitation, one-to-one observation should be instituted.	Protects client from falls and accidental injury. Clients attempting to free themselves can fall or be injured on the restraints.[30] Promotes client safety.
• Assign primary care nurse each shift. Note those persons here.	Promotes client orientation by providing familiar environment.[31,32]
• Observe every (number) of minutes. Inform client of this schedule, and provide client with written information as necessary. Note information necessary for client here.	Promotes client safety. Provides opportunities to reorient client to here and now and to assure client comfort.[34] Promotes client's sense of control.
• Replace the use of physical restraints with one-to-one observation, comfort measures, recliners, appropriate physical activity, visual barriers, secure unit, lower bed, or bed on floor. Note here those interventions specific to this client.[30]	Promotes safety and client's self-esteem by maintaining personal control and dignity. Frequent use of restraints can encourage clients to assume a passive approach to avoid further restraint or as an adaptation to daily use of restraints. At times physical restraints may increase agitation.[30,34,36]
• If physical restraints are used, check circulation every (number) minutes (should be at least 15), remove restraint one limb at a time every (number) hours (should be at least every 2), and provide ROM, opportunities to void, nourishment, brief clear explanations about the purpose of the restraint, and information about when they will be removed during each interaction.	Promotes client safety, sense of personal control, and self-esteem.[31,35] Promotes physical comfort, which decreases agitation.
• Utilize touch as appropriate to client. Note client's preferences here.	Client's touch preferences are very personal. Some clients may find it comforting while others may perceive it as an intrusion and respond with increased agitation.[34]
• Administer antipsychotic only if neurologic status indicates that this will not increase confusion.	Antipsychotic medications can increase confusion. These medications can also produce orthostatic hypotension, increasing client's fall risk.[30,33]
• Provide daily routine that closely resembles client's normal schedule. Note that schedule here.	Promotes orientation, increases client's sense of personal control, and orientation.
• Provide whatever aids the client needs to adequately perceive the environment (hearing or vision). Note necessary aids here and location for storing when not in use by the client.	Promotes orientation to the environment and sense of personal control.
• Assess mental status through normal interactions with client. Do not use formal mental status exams unless absolutely necessary. Note method and schedule for assessment here.	Repeated questioning can increase client's confusion, and inability to answer questions may have negative impact on self-esteem.[31,35]

- Limit client's choices, and provide information or direction in brief, simple sentences. Note level of client's ability to process information here; e.g., client can choose between two items. Support optimal cognitive functioning by (note here those interventions to be used with this client):
  - Responding to client's confused verbalizations (delusions, hallucinations, confabulations, illusions, etc.) in a calm manner
  - Utilizing refocusing and/or responding to the feelings underlying the content to respond to confused verbalizations
  - Utilizing I messages rather than arguments to reorient when necessary.
  - Providing clothing that is appropriate to time of day and situation, e.g., night clothes at night and street clothes during the day
  - Scheduling participation in groups that provide opportunities to remember, review current events, discuss seasonal activities, and socialize (note here the schedule and appropriate groups for this client)
  - Provide measures that promote rest and sleep. Note here those measures that are specific for this client with schedule for implementation.
- Provide clear feedback on appropriate behavior. Refer to Risk for Violence if client is at risk for violent behavior toward self or others. Assess expectations for being realistic with client's abilities. Note limits to be set here with specific consequences for unwanted behaviors and specific reinforcers for desired behaviors.
- Provide support system with information about client and how to best approach client. Note here the information to be provided and responsible person.

Increases orientation while preserving client's self-esteem. Large amounts of information provided at one time can increase confusion and agitation.[31,34]

Increased anxiety can increase confusion and agitation.[31,34]

Maintains self-esteem, relieves anxiety, and orients to present reality.[37]

Meets client's esteem needs by communicating respect while providing orientation.[31,35,37] Promotes here-and-now orientation.[31]

Promotes here-and-now orientation. Provides opportunities to maintain current cognitive skills.[31,37]

Inadequate sleep can increase confusion and disorientation.[31]

Positive reinforcement encourages behavior. Realistic goals increase opportunities for success, providing positive reinforcement and enhancing self-esteem.

Provides support system with positive coping strategies that enhance client's functioning.

CHRONIC

Mental health clients at risk for this diagnosis include those with Alzheimer's disease, Korsakoff's psychosis, and AIDS dementia. In addition to those interventions for acute confusion, the following interventions are included. It is important to remember that the primary difference between those two diagnoses is the irreversibility of the cognitive deficits in this diagnosis. It is also important to assess the client for depression because depression can appear as those illnesses that are related to this diagnosis, especially elderly clients.

- Maintain familiar environment by:
  - Providing objects from the client's home environment to include pictures, personal bedding, personal clothing, music, and other special objects with personal meaning. Note those objects important to the client here with those nursing actions necessary to maintain the objects.
  - Label room with name in large letters and a familiar picture or item.
  - Provide same room for entire hospital stay. Assign primary care personnel. Note those persons here.

  - Provide structured daily routines, and note client's routine here. This should parallel prehospital routine as much as possible.

Promotes orientation while promoting sense of safety and security.[35]

Maintains orientation while promoting a sense of personal control by maintaining independence.[31,35]
Maintains orientation by providing continuity of surroundings and staff familiar with client's needs, perspective, and treatment plan. Excessive stimulation can exacerbate cognitive or behavioral problems.
Promotes orientation by providing familiarity.[30,38]

Continued

ACTIONS/INTERVENTIONS	RATIONALES
• Provide opportunities for client to be involved in reminiscence, remotivation, current events, socialization, and other groups as appropriate by providing client with assistance needed to get to the groups. Note the client's group schedule here with the assistance needed from nursing staff.	Provide opportunities for clients to interact using current cognitive skills, which helps to decrease anxiety, maintain dignity, and prevent further deterioration and withdrawal.[37]
• Spend (number) minutes (number) times a day discussing client's past experiences. This activity can be facilitated with music, family photos, and other items that elicit memories. Note client's response to this activity, and if it appears to increase stress, discontinue. The process of this interaction is to provide positive cognitive reframes of past experiences.	Promotes positive reorientation, maintains client's dignity, and promotes positive self-esteem. It is important to note that some clients may have a great deal of difficulty coping with past experiences. If this process increases anxiety, the activity should be discontinued since high levels of anxiety can increase confusion.
• Identify and control underlying causes or triggers of increased cognitive and behavioral problems. This could include limiting visitors or certain topics of conversation, increasing rest or providing rest periods during the day, and assuring adequate hydration. Note the special adaptations here.	Preserves client's dignity and sense of control.[38] Each of these factors can decrease the client's ability to cope.
• Utilize nonconfrontational approaches for dealing with behavior extremes. This could include changing the client's context, responding to the feelings being expressed, or meeting comfort needs. Note here those responses that are most effective for the client.	Maintains client's dignity and recognizes the limitations of cognitive abilities.[38]
• Spend (number) minutes (number) times a day with client doing (this should be some activity client enjoys and provide an opportunity for success):	Positive environmental cues from staff have been shown to decrease problematic behaviors in these clients.[39]
• Spend (number) minutes (number) times a day involved in (type) exercise with client (choose exercise client enjoys and involves large motor activity if at all possible):	Increased physical activity decreases wandering behavior and improves client's rest.[36,39]
• Retrieve and divert client when wandering behavior presents risk or takes her or him into unobserved areas.	Decreases client's wandering behaviors.[39]

Gerontic Health

ACTIONS/INTERVENTIONS	RATIONALES
• Review pertinent lab work for possible imbalances.	Acute confusion may be related to changes in electrolytes, glucose, or drug levels.
• Obtain medication list from client or family of all prescribed and OTC medications used by client.	Medications are a frequent precipitant for acute confusion, especially in the very young or old.
• Decrease extraneous audible-visual input. Provide low-stimuli environment.	Decreases sensory overload and need to cope with a complex and noisy environment.
• Provide orienting cues to the physical layout of the care site (such as universal symbols for the bathroom, eating area, and client's room).	Promotes independence.
• Provide personalized surroundings (familiar pictures, clothing, or mementos).	Promotes identification with self.
• Use client photograph to identify personal space.	Increases connectedness with self. Provides sense of belonging.
• Address client by preferred name at each contact.	Reinforces sense of self.
• Introduce self by name at each contact.	Provides sense of the familiar.
• Arrange for family or significant others to be available during periods of increased anxiety or agitation.	Provides for familiar person in the care setting.
• Use name and orienting cues in conversations.	Enhances sense of self and connectedness.

• Provide physical contact and/or comfort along with verbal interactions.	Decreases anxiety generated when trying to cope with threatening environment. Assists client in sorting out environment and setting.
• Explore and explain briefly equipment used in care.	Decreases fearfulness.
• Disguise invasive equipment being used in care.	Prevents removal of needed equipment.
• Use familiar objects for activities such as glasses or cups for fluids rather than styrofoam cups or paper or plastic cartons.	Decreases complexity of coping with the unfamiliar.
• Assign consistent caregivers.	Provides sense of security.
• Limit choices to two in situations where client must make decisions such as dressing or eating.	Decreases stress of too many choices.
• Provide positive feedback for independent function.	Promotes self-esteem.
• Ensure quiet time or rest periods during the day.	Decreases stress.
• Approach and work with client in an unhurried manner.	Sense of urgency associated with speed perceived as threatening.
• Provide information in simple sentences and allow time for client to process information.	Decreases complexity.
• If repetition is needed, repeat information in the exact manner as originally stated.	Allows for processing of information.
• Encourage participation in failure-free activities such as singing, exercise, or uncomplicated crafts.	Enhances self-esteem.
• Monitor mental status for changes at least daily and every shift in acute care setting.	
• Monitor for increased confusion related to new medication usage.	

Home Health

NOTE: Onset of acute confusion may be an emergency requiring immediate referral for care.

ACTIONS/INTERVENTIONS	RATIONALES
• Assist client and family in identifying lifestyle changes that may be required: ○ Treatment or prevention of underlying problem (substance abuse, infection, pain, or nutritional deficits) ○ Providing for rest periods ○ Providing safe environment ○ Providing environmental cues to orient patient, e.g., clocks or calendars ○ Providing assistive resources as required; ○ Family response to changing behavior and mental status of affected person	Home-based care requires involvement of the family. Acute confusion disrupts family schedules and role relationships. Adjustments in family activities and roles may be required. Decreased vision or hearing acuity may contribute to confusion.
• Assist family to set criteria to help them determine when additional intervention is required, for example, change in baseline behavior.	Provides family background knowledge to seek appropriate assistance as need arises.
• Refer patient to appropriate assistive resources as indicated.	Additional assistance may be required for the family to care for the acutely confused person. Use of readily available resources is cost-effective.

Confusion, Acute and Chronic

FLOWCHART EVALUATION: EXPECTED OUTCOME 1

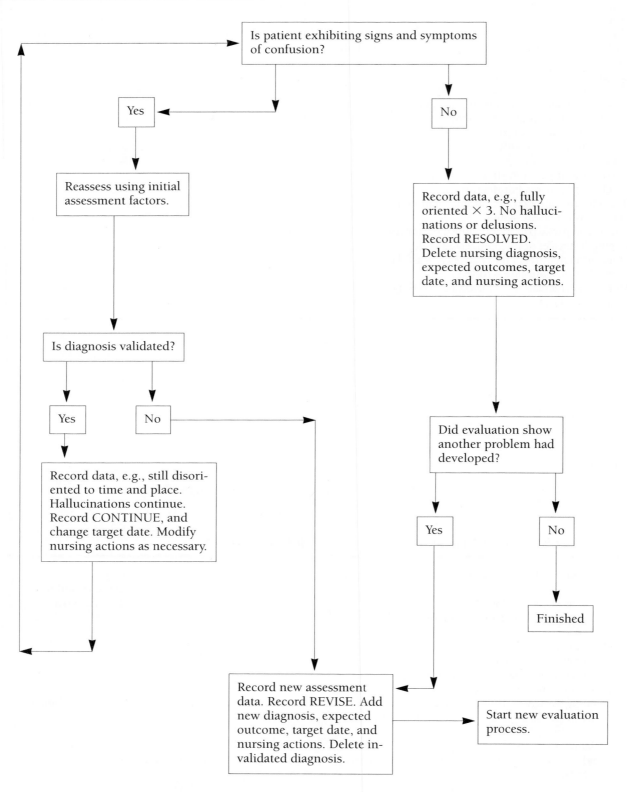

Confusion, Acute and Chronic

FLOWCHART EVALUATION: EXPECTED OUTCOME 2

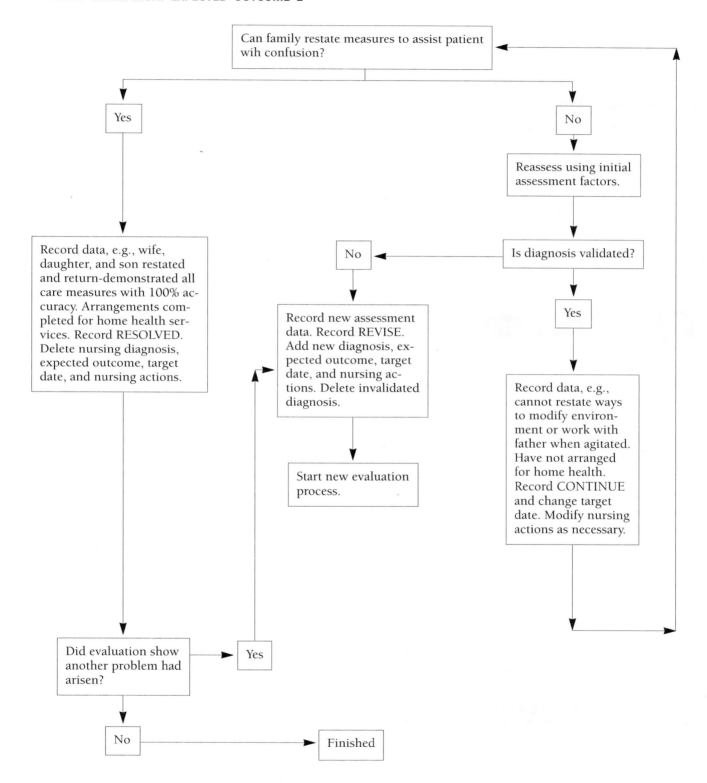

Decisional Conflict (Specify)

DEFINITION

The state of uncertainty about course of action to be taken when the choice among competing actions involves risk, loss, or challenge to personal life values.[2]

NANDA TAXONOMY: CHOOSING 5.3.1.1

DEFINING CHARACTERISTICS[2]

1. Major defining characteristics
   a. Verbalized uncertainty about choices
   b. Verbalization of undesired consequences of alternative actions being considered
   c. Vacillation between alternative choices
   d. Delayed decision making
2. Minor defining characteristics
   a. Verbalized feeling of distress while attempting a decision
   b. Self-focusing
   c. Physical signs of distress or tension (increased heart rate, increased muscle tension, restlessness, etc.)
   d. Questioning personal values and beliefs while attempting a decision

RELATED FACTORS[2]

1. Unclear personal values or beliefs
2. Perceived threat to value system
3. Lack of experience or presence of interference with decision making
4. Lack of relevant information
5. Support system deficit
6. Multiple or divergent sources of information

RELATED CLINICAL CONCERNS

1. Any surgery causing body image change
2. Any illness carrying a potential terminal prognosis
3. Any chronic disease
4. Dementia

HAVE YOU SELECTED THE CORRECT DIAGNOSIS?

Anxiety Anxiety is considered to be a feeling of threat that may not be known by the person as a specific causative factor. In Decisional Conflict, the patient knows the options but cannot decide between specifics.

Knowledge Deficit In Knowledge Deficit, the client does not have the information to make a decision. In Decisional Conflict, the information is known.

Ineffective Individual Coping This diagnosis is closely related in that adaptive behavior and problem-solving abilities are not able to meet the demands of the client's needs. Ineffective Individual Coping and Decisional Conflict may very well be companion diagnoses.

EXPECTED OUTCOMES

1. Will verbalize at least one concrete personal decision by (date) and/or
2. Will return-demonstrate at least (number) conflict resolution techniques by (date)

TARGET DATES

Value clarification, belief examination, and learning decision-making processes will require a considerable length of time and will require much support. Therefore, target dates in increments of weeks would be most appropriate.

NURSING ACTIONS/INTERVENTIONS WITH RATIONALES
Adult Health

ACTIONS/INTERVENTIONS	RATIONALES
• Instruct patient in stress-reduction techniques as needed. Have patient return-demonstrate specific techniques at least daily.	Reduces anxiety, enabling patient to better process problems.
• Assist patient to focus on problem-solving processes. Help patient to verbalize alternatives and advantages and disadvantages of solutions. Help patient to realistically appraise situations and set realistic short-term objectives daily.	Assists patient to learn to use the problem-solving process.

- Support patient's values as necessary. Do not be judgmental when interacting with patient. Help patient to clarify values and beliefs as needed.
- Assist patient to seek, find, and interpret relevant information about problem; refer patient to community resources for support.
- Refer to psychiatric nurse clinician as needed.

Helps patient focus on what is important to self in decision making rather than being concerned about pleasing others.
Assists patient to explore alternatives; coordinates care of patient.

A nurse specialist may be better able to help the patient focus on the underlying process.

Child Health

ACTIONS/INTERVENTIONS	RATIONALES
• Determine who will intervene on behalf of the infant or child: parents or appointed legal guardian.	For legal and ethical reasons, it is essential to clarify when the parent(s) are unable to assume the parental role and obligations and that this fact is known to all involved in the child's care. It is likewise essential for all caregivers to know who the legal guardian or spokesperson is.
• In instances of conflicting decision makers, ensure that the child's rights are protected according to legal statutes.	Irrespective of conflicts in decision making, the infant or child is entitled to appropriate care. In extreme cases of conflict a state or local judge may appoint guardians or foster parents to assume decision making regarding health matters. In other instances, e.g., withholding suggested treatment due to religious beliefs, individual states, and precedents must be sought by the parties involved.
• Ensure that appropriate documentation is carried out according to situational needs.	Legal documentation according to health care decisions and related matters is to be carried out as standard care with attention to the mandates of the institution regarding appropriate paper forms to complete.
• Although the child may be ill-equipped or unable to participate fully in decision making, encourage developmentally appropriate components for care to assist child in learning decision making.	Early involvement in decision making fosters safe support for the child, thereby increasing the likelihood of learning effective coping behaviors. Will also empower the child and foster a positive self-image.
• Be certain that choices or options indeed exist when the child is allowed to exercise decision making.	Preferences and individualization will be realistically valued when there are choices or options in the care plan. It is unethical to indicate that there are choices when none exists; e.g., medication cannot be given by any other route but intramuscular.
• Provide behavioral reinforcement that best fosters learning with appropriate follow-up when the child is involved in decisional conflict.	Appropriate reinforcement will serve to enhance learning and assist the patient in growth in decision making.
• Consider potential long-term residual or subsequent effects related to specific decisional conflict for the child or family.	Decision making often has far-reaching effects; e.g., in early childhood values of a lifetime are formulated. Appropriate regard to this fact should guide all involved in this aspect of child rearing and supportive aspects of health care.

Women's Health

Unwanted Pregnancy

ACTIONS/INTERVENTIONS	RATIONALES
• Provide an atmosphere that encourages patient to view her options in the event of an unwanted pregnancy. Assure the patient of confidentiality.	Provides information that allows the patient to make an informed choice.
• Give clear, concise, complete information to the patient, describing the choices available to her: ○ Carrying the pregnancy and keeping infant	

Continued

ACTIONS/INTERVENTIONS	RATIONALES
○ Adoption of infant ○ Abortion • Discuss with the patient the advantages and disadvantages of each option. • Encourage patient to discuss beliefs and practices in a nonthreatening atmosphere and include significant others in conversation and decision as the patient desires. • Refer patient to proper agency for guidance and treatment. • Discuss and review with patient the different methods of birth control. • Assess the patient's ability to correctly use the different methods of birth control. • Provide factual information, listing the advantages and disadvantages of each method. • Provide patient information on obtaining her method of choice. • Explore with patient and significant other their views on children and family.	Provides information and support to assist patient in planning future pregnancies.

Women's Health

Less-Than-Perfect Infant

NOTE: Families faced with the birth of a child with congenital anomalies or developmental defects experience decisional conflict and great confusion about choices that need to be made. Often there is a sense of urgency, as decisions need to be made quickly to save the life of the infant. Many times the infant was delivered by cesarean section, and it is the mother's partner who, alone, must often make crucial decisions that could affect the family and the life of the infant. Parents not only experience confusion but fear, guilt, helplessness, and inadequacy as parents.

ACTIONS/INTERVENTIONS	RATIONALES
• Provide accurate information to parents as soon as possible.	Provides information and supportive environment that helps parents to make decisions.[40,41]
STILLBORN OR FETAL DEMISE • Let parents see and hold infant if at all possible.	Promotes bonding and provides comfort for both parents and infant.
• Support parents in their grieving process for the loss of the perfect infant and perhaps the death of the infant.[42,43] • Keep the parents informed, continuously, and encourage the health care team to talk to them often. • Contact significant persons, of parent's choice, who can come and be of support to them.[44] • Give parents a private place to be with their support persons. • Encourage parents to visit infant in NICU as often as possible. • Collaborate with NICU staff to plan time for mother and infant activities together as much as possible. • Refer to support groups and agencies as needed for follow-up care when leaving hospital.	Support is essential in resolving decisional conflict.

Psychiatric Health

NOTE: The client who is experiencing a decisional conflict is faced with confusion about alternative solutions. When assisting these clients, the nurse should be careful not to connote the client's confusion negatively. Various authors[45-47] have supported the positive role confusion plays in the change process. Erickson[45] frequently encouraged confusion as a way to distract the conscious mind and allow the unconscious to develop solutions. It is from this theoretical base that the following interventions are developed.

ACTIONS/INTERVENTIONS	RATIONALES
• Assure the client that the difficulty he or she is experiencing in decision making is positive in that it has placed him or her in a position to look for new creative solutions. If he or she were not experiencing this difficulty, he or she might be tempted to remain in the same old problem solution set.	Promotes positive orientation, self-worth, and hope.
• Assist client in reducing the pressure of time on making a decision.	
• Have client explain the time he or she has given himself or herself to make a decision. Asking the client the following question may assist in this process: "What is the worst that will happen if a decision is not made right now?"	Provides time to develop alternative problem solution and decreases stress on the client.
• Assist client in verbalizing all the information that he or she currently has on the choices.	Aids in understanding client's perception of the situation.
• Have client explore feelings related to the choices and the information related to the choices. This process may extend over several days. The client may be reluctant to verbalize negative feelings related to certain choices if a trusting relationship has not yet been developed with the nurse.	The client's cognitive style and feelings about the situation impact their appraisal of both the situation and possible solutions.[48]
• Have the client discuss how significant others think and feel about the various choices. Have client evaluate the impact of the feelings of significant others on his or her decision-making process.	Support system involvement increases the probability of positive outcomes.
• Have client fantasize an ideal choice.	Accesses creative problem solutions that bypass the client's self-imposed limits.
• Have client construct a list of solutions (at least 20) that would produce the ideal choice. (These solutions are not to be evaluated at this time.) Encourage client to develop some unrealistic solutions. This may be promoted by asking the client what he or she might tell a friend to do in this situation or by having client generate three magic-wish solutions, e.g., "If you had a magic wand, what would you do to resolve this situation?"	
• Sort through developed list with client generating solutions from the ones listed. At this time the client can begin to combine and eliminate ideas after evaluation. Carefully evaluate each solution before it is eliminated. What appears to be a bizarre solution can become useful when altered or combined with another idea.	
• As each idea is evaluated, provide all information necessary to evaluate the idea.	Aids in assessing client's commitment to each possible solution.
• Explore client's thoughts and feelings about each idea.	
• Remind client that there are no perfect answers and each of us makes the best choice that can be made at the time.	Promotes positive orientation, self-worth, and hope for the future.

Continued

ACTIONS/INTERVENTIONS	RATIONALES
• Remind client that if a choice that is made does not resolve the problem, alternative solutions can then be tried.	Promotes positive orientation.
• Remind client that a solution that does not work provides more information about the problem that can be used in developing future solutions.	
• Meet with client and support system to allow the support system to be a part of the decision-making process if this is appropriate.	Support system involvement increases the probability of positive outcome.
• Discuss with client and support system any secondary gains from not making a decision.	Assess for positive reinforcement for not resolving problem.
• Once a decision is made, have client develop a behavioral plan for implementation.	Having a plan to cope with the anticipated situations promotes a perception of greater control over future situations and increases the probability of client's enacting new coping behaviors.

Gerontic Health

ACTIONS/INTERVENTIONS	RATIONALES
• Discuss with patient prior examples of decisional conflict and their outcomes.	Emphasizes ability to problem solve and reinforces successes.

Home Health

ACTIONS/INTERVENTIONS	RATIONALES
• Teach client and family measures to decrease decisional conflict: ○ Providing appropriate health information ○ Joining a support group ○ Clarifying values ○ Performing stress reduction activities ○ Seeking spiritual or legal assistance as needed ○ Identifying useful sources of information	Appropriate knowledge and values clarification between the client and family will reduce conflict.
• Assist client and family in identifying risk factors pertinent to the situation: ○ Lack of knowledge ○ Developmental or situational crisis ○ Role confusion ○ Excess stress ○ Excess stimuli	Early identification of risk factors provides opportunity for early intervention.
• Consult with or refer patient to appropriate assistive resources as indicated.	Use of the network of existing community services provides for effective utilization of resources.

Decisional Conflict (Specify)

FLOWCHART EVALUATION: EXPECTED OUTCOME 1

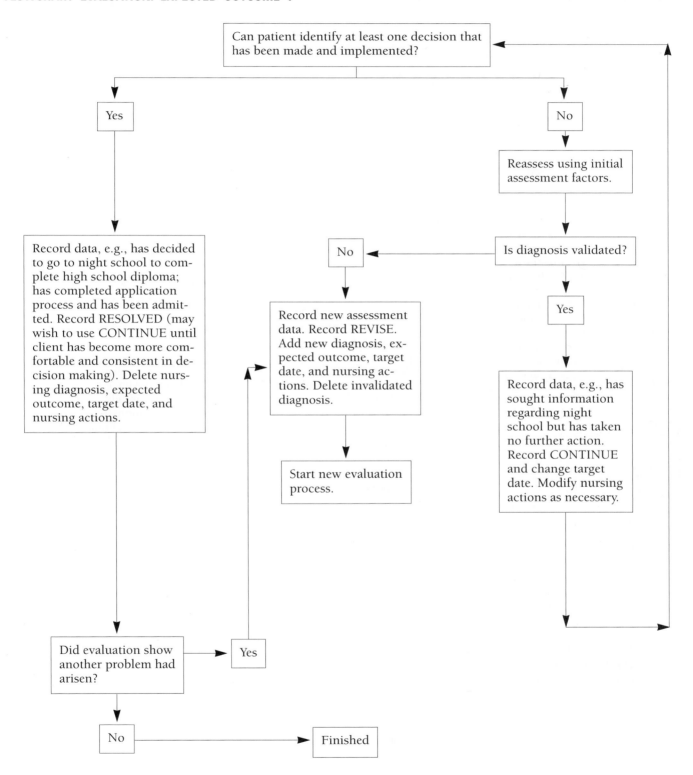

Decisional Conflict (Specify)

FLOWCHART EVALUATION: EXPECTED OUTCOME 2

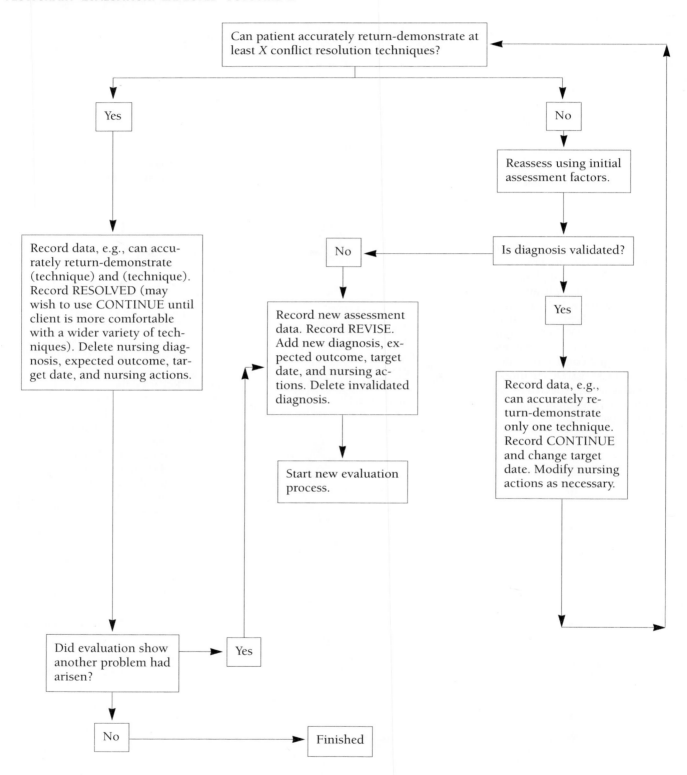

Environmental Interpretation Syndrome, Impaired

DEFINITION

Consistent lack of orientation to person, place, time, or circumstances over more than 3 to 6 months necessitating a protective environment.

NANDA TAXONOMY: KNOWING 8.2.1

DEFINING CHARACTERISTICS[2]

1. Major defining characteristics
   a. Consistent disorientation in known and unknown environments
   b. Chronic confusional states
2. Minor defining characteristics
   a. Loss of occupation or social functioning from memory decline
   b. Inability to follow simple directions or instructions
   c. Inability to reason
   d. Inability to concentrate
   e. Slow in responding to questions

RELATED FACTORS[2]

1. Dementia (Alzheimer's disease, multi-infarct dementia, Pick's disease, AIDS, dementia)
2. Parkinson's disease
3. Huntington's disease
4. Depression
5. Alcoholism

RELATED CLINICAL CONCERNS

See Related Factors.

HAVE YOU SELECTED THE CORRECT DIAGNOSIS?

There are several diagnoses that interface with this diagnosis, for example, Impaired Memory, Impaired Thought Process, or Confusion. This diagnosis refers to a long-term problem (3 to 6 months) that results in the patient having to be admitted to a protective environment. This diagnosis predominantly relates to an end result of the other diagnoses.

EXPECTED OUTCOMES

1. Will have decreased episodes of environmental confusion by (date) and/or
2. Will have no injuries related to environmental functioning by (date)

TARGET DATES

This is a long-term diagnosis, so an appropriate target date would be expressed in terms of weeks or months.

NURSING ACTIONS/INTERVENTIONS WITH RATIONALES

Adult Health

NOTE: These actions/interventions and rationales are essentially the same as those for Chronic Confusion.

ACTIONS/INTERVENTIONS	RATIONALES
• Identify self and patient by name at each interaction.	Short-term memory loss necessitates frequent orientation to person, time, and environment.
• Speak slowly and clearly in short, simple words and sentences.	Allows time for information processing and avoids use of complex statements and abstract ideas.
• When patient is delusional, focus on underlying feelings and reinforce reality (have clocks, calendars, etc., on the wall); do not argue with patient.	Recognizing and acknowledging feelings may decrease client's anxiety and give a sense of being understood. Arguing may increase patient's anxiety and reinforce intensity delusions.[49]
• If patient becomes aggressive, focus on underlying feelings and attempt to refocus interaction on topics more acceptable and/or less threatening to patient.	Focusing on feelings increases patient's feelings of being understood, and discussing nonthreatening topics increases patient's sense of competency and self-esteem.
• Keep patient's room well lighted. Maintain a calm environment.	Decreases possibility of environmental sensory misrepresentations and helps meet patient safety needs.

ACTIONS/INTERVENTIONS	RATIONALES
• Teach family about patient's condition and how to interact more effectively with patient; i.e., provide ongoing orientation to surroundings and happenings within the family.	Assists family in understanding changes in patient's orientation, cognition, and behavior. Increases family's sense of competency in relating to patient.
• Refer to psychiatric-mental health clinical nurse specialist. Make other referrals to community agencies as needed, i.e., Alheizmer's support group, adult daycare, meals-on-wheels, etc.	The psychiatric-mental health CNS has the expertise to collaborate with the adult health nurse to plan nursing interventions for the patient that will help the patient and nursing staff deal with chronic confusion in the acute care setting.

Child Health

This diagnosis may be present in children also; if so, the same basic plan of care as that of adults should be implemented, with attention to safe, developmentally appropriate interventions.

ACTIONS/INTERVENTIONS	RATIONALES
• Monitor for parental-infant reciprocity to determine nature of parent-infant or -child relationship.	Reciprocity will offer cues as to what match does or does not exist in the relationship.
• When there may be a genetic concern, offer appropriate counseling.	When a genetic component exists, there is an obligation for present and futuristic planning by all involved.
• Offer 30 min each shift for parents to ventilate specific concerns regarding infant or child.	Ventilation offers reduction in anxiety, plus an opportunity to note parental concerns.

Women's Health

See Adult Health nursing actions.

Psychiatric Health

Mental health clients who demonstrate this syndrome would include those with depression, alcoholism, and chronic thought disorders.

ACTIONS/INTERVENTIONS	RATIONALES
• Monitor client's level of anxiety and refer to Anxiety, Chap. 8, for detailed interventions related to this diagnosis.	Increased anxiety can negatively impact memory and orientation and contribute to further deficits.
• Place client in an environment with appropriate stimuli. Note level of stimulation and alterations in environmental stimuli here; i.e., specific objects in the environment that stimulate illusions should be removed, and appropriate lighting, clocks and calendars, and holiday decorations should be provided. Refer to day, date, and other orienting information during each interaction with the client.	Increases patient safety and promotes orientation.
• Place identifying information on patient and patient's room. Utilize client's preferred name in each interaction. Note that name here.	Provides safety and promotes orientation.
• Remove harmful objects from the environment. This could include objects in walkways, cords, belts, and raised bedrails or other restraining devices. Note here special precautions for this client.	Protects client from falls and accidental injury.

- Assign primary care nurse each shift. Note those persons here.
- Observe every (*number*) minutes. Inform client of this schedule, and provide client with written information as necessary. Note information necessary for client here. If client is depressed, this observation may be increased due to increased risk for self-harm. Refer to High Risk for Violence, Chap. 9, for specific interventions.
- Provide daily routine that closely resembles client's normal schedule. Note that schedule here.
- Assess mental status through normal interactions with client. Do not use formal mental status exams unless absolutely necessary. Note here the method and schedule for assessment.
- Limit client's choices, and provide information or direction in brief, simple sentences. Note here the level of client's ability to process information; i.e., client can choose between two items.
- Keep initial interactions short but frequent. Speak to client in brief, clear sentences. Note frequency and length of interactions here.
- Utilize I messages, rather than argument, to reorient when necessary.

- Respond to confused verbalizations by responding to the feelings being expressed.
- When client's ability to tolerate more complex situations increases, schedule his or her participation in groups that provide opportunities to remember, review current events, discuss seasonal activities, and socialize. Note here the schedule and appropriate groups for this client.
- Provide clear feedback on appropriate behavior. Set behavior goals that client can achieve. Note here those behaviors that are to be rewarded and the rewards that are to be given.
- Spend (*number*) minutes (*number*) times a day involved in exercise with client. (Choose exercise client enjoys and that involves large motor activity if at all possible.) Note the specific activity here.
- Spend (*number*) minutes (*number*) times per week providing information to client's support system. Note here the specific information to be provided and person responsible for this activity.

Promotes client orientation by providing familiar environment.
Promotes client safety. Provides opportunities to reorient client to here and now and to assure client comfort.
Promotes client's sense of control.

Promotes orientation, and increases client's sense of personal control and orientation.
Repeated questioning can increase client's confusion, and inability to answer questions may have negative impact on self-esteem.

High levels of stimulation can increase confusion, and inability to make choices may have negative impact on client's self-esteem.

Too much information can increase the client's confusion and disorganization.

Meets client's esteem needs by communicating respect while providing orientation. Promotes here-and-now orientation.
Maintains self-esteem, relieves anxiety, and orients to present reality.
Promotes here-and-now orientation. Provides opportunities to maintain current cognitive skills.

Positive reinforcement encourages behavior. Realistic goals increase opportunities for success, providing positive reinforcement and enhancing self-esteem.

Improves rest and increases release of natural endorphins.

Family and client involvement enhances effectiveness of intervention and promotes community support.

Gerontic Health

ACTIONS/INTERVENTIONS	RATIONALES
• Review mental status exam to identify areas of strengths and needs.	Depending on exam used, may indicate client's ability to read, interpret symbols, or process simple versus complex instructions.
• Survey current environment for potential unsafe areas.	Correcting unsafe areas decreases potential for client injury.
• Adapt environment to decrease risk for injury, e.g., access to exits, thermal injury potential, or ingestion of harmful substances.	
• Instruct caregiver in environmental adaptations to provide protective environment.	

Continued

ACTIONS/INTERVENTIONS	RATIONALES
• Use labeling or pictorial symbols to indicate specific areas or conveniences (such as universal symbols for food or restrooms or pictures to indicate client's room).	Assists client to interpret environment.
• Ensure identification of client (ID bracelet or necklace).	Provides means of identification in the event that client leaves the care setting.
• Provide conversational cues to person, place, and time.	Presents information in a nonquizzing, nonthreatening manner.

Home Health

ACTIONS/INTERVENTIONS	RATIONALES
• Assist client and family in identifying lifestyle changes that may be required: 　○ Provide consistent care provider. 　○ Provide for consistent daily schedule with structured activities. 　○ Have client wear identity bracelet; put name in client's clothing. 　○ Provide safe environment. 　○ Provide environmental cues to orient patient, e.g., clocks or calendars. 　○ Provide assistive resources as required. 　○ Monitor family response to changing behavior and mental status of affected person.	Home-based care requires involvement of the family. Impaired interpretation of the environment disrupts family schedules and role relationships. Adjustments in family activities and roles may be required.
	Decreased vision or hearing acuity may contribute to confusion.
• Assist family to set criteria to help them determine when additional intervention is required, for example, help them recognize signals indicating change in their ability to maintain a safe environment.	Provides family background knowledge to seek appropriate assistance as need arises.
• Refer client to appropriate assistive resources as indicated.	Additional assistance may be required for the family to care for the family member with impaired environmental interpretive syndrome.

Environmental Interpretation Syndrome, Impaired

FLOWCHART EVALUATION: EXPECTED OUTCOME 1

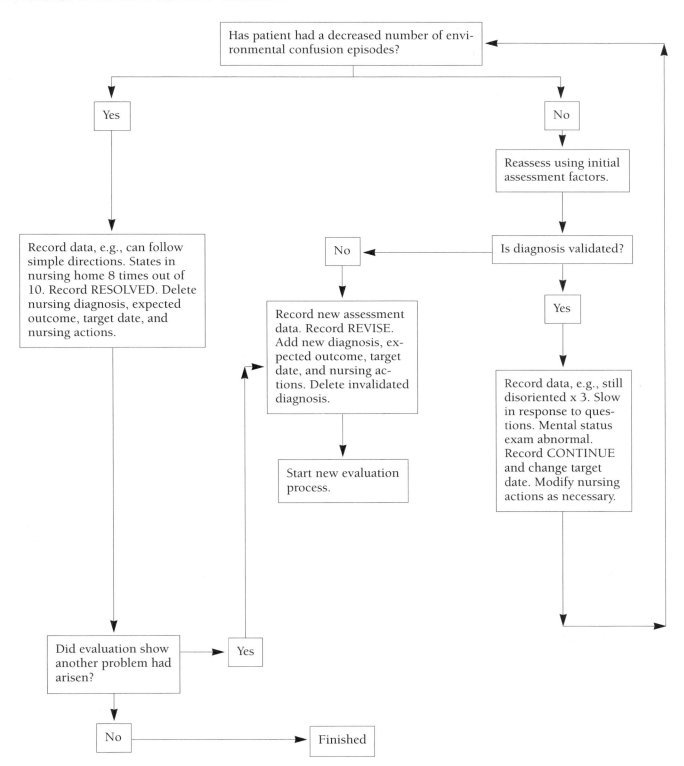

Environmental Interpretation
Syndrome, Impaired

FLOWCHART EVALUATION: EXPECTED OUTCOME 2

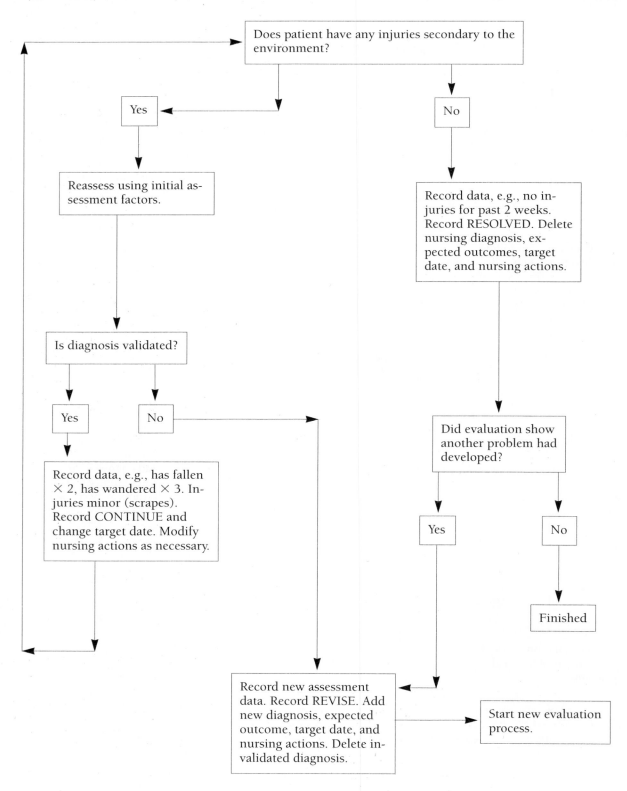

Knowledge Deficit (Specify)

DEFINITION

Absence or deficiency of cognitive information related to specific topic.[2]

> **NOTE:** The 1994 Preconference Workgroup for this diagnosis recommended the use of knowledge deficit as an etiology rather than as a nursing diagnosis.

NANDA TAXONOMY: KNOWING 8.1.1
DEFINING CHARACTERISTICS[2]

1. Major defining characteristics
   a. Verbalization of the problem
   b. Inaccurate follow-through of instruction
   c. Inaccurate performance of test
   d. Inappropriate or exaggerated behaviors, for example, hysterical, hostile, agitated, or apathetic

2. Minor defining characteristics
   None given

RELATED FACTORS[2]

1. Lack of exposure
2. Lack of recall
3. Information misinterpretation
4. Cognitive limitation
5. Lack of interest in learning
6. Unfamiliarity with information resources

RELATED CLINICAL CONCERNS

1. Any diagnosis that is entirely new to the patient
2. Mental retardation
3. Post head injury
4. Depression
5. Dementia

HAVE YOU SELECTED THE CORRECT DIAGNOSIS?

Noncompliance   In Noncompliance the patient can return-demonstrate skills accurately or verbalize the regimen needed but does not follow through on the care.

Altered Thought Process   This diagnosis would be evident by lack of immediate recall on return-demonstration rather than inaccurate or limited demonstration and recall.

Powerlessness   This diagnosis would be reflected by statements such as "How will this help?" "I have no control over this," or "I have to rely on others" rather than statements such as "I don't really understand," "I'm not really sure how," or "Is this right?"

Altered Health Maintenance   Altered Health Maintenance may include Knowledge Deficit, but it is broader in scope and includes such aspects as limited resources and mobility factors.

EXPECTED OUTCOMES

1. Will return-demonstrate (specific knowledge deficit activity) by (date) and/or
2. Will restate (specific knowledge deficit material) by (date)

TARGET DATES

Individual learning curves vary significantly. A target date ranging from 3 to 7 days could be appropriate based on the individual's previous experience with this material, education level, potential for learning, and energy level.

NURSING ACTIONS/INTERVENTIONS WITH RATIONALES

Adult Health

ACTIONS/INTERVENTIONS	RATIONALES
• Contract with patient regarding what the patient wants and needs to learn. Be sure to include a time frame in the contract. Have patient sign contract to ensure patient consent for teaching. Review the patient's and family's current level of knowledge regarding this illness, hospitalization, and cultural and value beliefs.	Incorporates patient into learning process and provides additional motivation for resolving deficit. Allows assessment of patient's readiness to learn. Improves learning since it is based on exactly where the patient or family is in their knowledge and avoids needless repetition.

Continued

ACTIONS/INTERVENTIONS	RATIONALES
• Design teaching plan specific to patient's deficit area, e.g., self-administration of medication, and specific to patient's level of education, e.g., eighth-grade reading level. Include significant others in teaching sessions. Be sure plan includes content, objectives, methods, and evaluation.	Provides new knowledge based on patient's perceived needs. Individuals learn in their own way and in their own time frame. Motivates learning and provides support and reinforcement for learning.
• Explain each procedure as it is being done, and give the rationale for procedure and the patient's role.	Incorporates another teaching method and reduces anxiety, thus promoting learning.
• Teach only absolutely relevant information first.	Patient will remember initial information more than subsequent information. Avoids overwhelming patient with information.
• Provide positive reinforcement as often as possible for patient's progress.	Reinforces learning achieved and promotes positive orientation.
• Design teaching to stimulate as many of the patient's senses as possible, e.g., visual, audio, touch, or smell. Have patient return-demonstrate any psychomotor activities.	Enhances learning and provides mechanism to evaluate learning, teaching effectiveness, and allows clarification of any misunderstandings.
• Have patient restate, in his or her own words, cognitive materials during teaching session. Have the patient repeat on each subsequent day until discharge.	Repeated practice of a behavior internalizes and personalizes the behavior.[49]
• Provide quiet, well-lighted, temperature-controlled teaching environment during teaching session.	Limits distractions.

• Ensure that basic needs are taken care of before and immediately after teaching sessions:
  ○ Food and fluids
  ○ Toileting
  ○ Pain relief
	Prevents distractions during teaching session due to basic needs not being met.

• Pace teaching according to patient's rate of learning and preference during teaching session.	Considers patient's learning style and ability to process new information.
• Encourage patient's verbalization of anxiety, concern, etc., about self-care. Listen carefully. Redesign plan to incorporate patient's concerns as needed.	Considers patient's input into plan of teaching. Increases likelihood of patient's retaining and using information. Expressing fear and anxiety helps reduce their levels and provides a means by which possible resources can be explored for dealing with the patient's health care issues.

• Incorporate into teaching plans, in addition to specifics (provide written information to reinforce verbal teaching):
  ○ Normal body functioning
  ○ Signs and symptoms of altered functioning
  ○ Diet (food and fluid)
  ○ Exercise and activity
  ○ Growth and development
  ○ Self-examination
  ○ Impact on environment, stress, and change in lifestyle on health
	Provides foundational knowledge on which to build more specific information.

• After first teaching session, start each teaching session with revalidation of the previous session. End each session with a summary.	Reinforces what is known. Builds new information on previous knowledge and organizes new knowledge for patient.
• Collaborate with and refer patient to appropriate assistive resources.	Coordinates team approach to health and provides means to follow up and reinforce learning.

Child Health

ACTIONS/INTERVENTIONS	RATIONALES
• Determine if there are ambiguities in the minds of parents or child.	Clarification and verification will ensure a greater likelihood of understanding and valuing aspects critical to patient teaching.
• Identify the learning capacity for the patient and family.	Realistic capacity for learning should be a primary factor in patient teaching since it serves as one major parameter in expectations of learning.
• Determine the scope and appropriate presentation for patient and family based on all of the above, plus developmental crises for each and all—do not overwhelm the patient	Developmental needs of all involved will best serve as an essential framework for teaching the patient and family. Potentials and capacity for use of all the sensory-perceptual aspects of cognition should be explored and used to ensure the best opportunity for effective teaching.

• Evaluate appropriately the effectiveness of the teaching-learning experience by:
  ○ Brief verbal discourse to provide concrete data
  ○ Written examination in brief to show progress
  ○ Observation of skills critical for care, e.g., change of dressing according to sterile technique
  ○ Allowing child to perform skills in general fashion with use of dolls
	Evaluation is an indicator of both teaching effectiveness and learning. It serves as another essential aspect of patient teaching with the appropriate focus on individualization by pointing out areas needing reteaching.

Women's Health

ACTIONS/INTERVENTIONS	RATIONALES

• Teach normal physiologic changes new mother can expect postpartum:
  ○ Lochia flow
    (1) Normal: Rubra 1–3 days; serosa 3–10 days; alba 10–14 days
    (2) Abnormal: Bright red blood and clots with firm uterus; foul odor; pain, fever; or persistent lochia serosa or pink to red discharge after 2 wk
  ○ Breast changes
    (1) Breast-feeding: Engorgement; comfort measures; clothing; positions for mother and infant comfort; and hygiene (also see actions for the Nutrition diagnoses in Chap. 3)
    (2) Non-breast-feeding: Suppression of lactation (medications, clothing such as tight-fitting bra, and comfort measures); importance of holding baby while bottle-feeding (do not prop bottle and burp baby often); formulas (different kinds and preparation)
  ○ Perineum and rectum: Episiotomy, hemorrhoids, hygiene, medications, and comfort measures
	Provides information to assist new mothers in postpartum adaptation.

• Demonstrate infant care to new parents:
  ○ Bathing
  ○ Feeding
  ○ Cord care
  ○ Holding, carrying, etc.
  ○ Safety
  ○ Sleep-wake states of infant
	Assists new parents in adapting to parenting role. Allows parents to practice new skills in a nonthreatening environment and to seek clarification from an informed source.

Continued

ACTIONS/INTERVENTIONS	RATIONALES

• Provide quiet, supportive atmosphere for interaction with infant to allow parent to:
  ○ Become acquainted with infant
  ○ Practice caretaking activities such as breast or formula feeding
  ○ Begin integration of infant into family
• Discuss infant care, taking into consideration age and cultural differences of parents:
  ○ Teenagers: Involve significant others. Have mother return-demonstrate infant care. Refer to support systems such as Young Parent Services and church groups.
  ○ First-time older mothers: Allow verbalization of fears. Involve significant others. Provide encouragement.
• Adjust teaching to take into consideration different cultural caretaking activities such as preventing the evil eye in the Hispanic culture or the mother's not holding the baby for several days immediately after birth in some Far Eastern Indian cultures.
• Demonstrate newborn skills to parents. Utilize different assessment skills to teach parents about their newborn's capabilities—gestational age assessment, physical examination of newborn, or Brazelton Neonatal Assessment Scale.
• Encourage parents to hold and talk to newborn.
 	
• Discuss different methods of birth control and the advantages and disadvantages of each method.
  ○ Chemical: Spermicides and pills
  ○ Mechanical: Condom, diaphragm, or intrauterine device (IUD)
  ○ Behavioral: Abstinence, temperature-ovulation-cervical mucus (Billing's method), or coitus interruptus
  ○ Sterilization: Vasectomy, tubal ligation, or hysterectomy.
	Promotes positive learning experience for mother, father, and baby.
	
	Helps parents gain confidence when caring for newborn. Provides opportunity for nurse to teach and reinforce teaching.
	Informs new mother (parents) of choices in birth control methods and gives them the opportunity to ask questions.

Psychiatric Health

ACTIONS/INTERVENTIONS	RATIONALES
• Ask client about previous learning experiences in general and about those related to the current area of concern; e.g., has client learned that he or she is a poor learner, that he or she does not have the intellectual ability to learn the type of information that is currently required, or that the smallest mistake in the activity to be learned could be fatal. • Monitor client's current level of anxiety. If level of anxiety will inhibit learning, assist client with anxiety reduction. Refer to Anxiety, Chap. 8, for detailed interventions. • Determine what client thinks is most important in the current situation.	Helps to determine aspects of the client's cognitive appraisal that could impact learning. Severe anxiety and impaired cognitive functioning can decrease the client's ability to attend to the environment in a manner that facilitates learning. Client's cognitive appraisal can impact the client's willingness to attend to the information. This is especially true of adult learners.

- Assist client in meeting those needs that represent lower-level needs on Maslow's hierarchy so that attention can be focused on the area of learning to be addressed; e.g., if the client is concerned that children are not being cared for while he or she is hospitalized, he or she may not be able to focus on learning. List the needs to be met here.

Promotes attention to learning. Reduces anxiety.

- Include client in group learning experiences, e.g., medication groups.

Provides client with opportunity to learn from others and to discuss new coping behaviors in a safe environment.

Gerontic Health

ACTIONS/INTERVENTIONS	RATIONALES
• Determine current knowledge base by interviewing patient and have patient state current knowledge regarding condition.	Provides a stepping-stone to pieces of information that may be incorrect or lacking.
• Ensure that adaptive equipment, if needed, is functioning and used.	Enhances communication process.
• Encourage patient to set the pace of the teaching sessions.[50]	Assists in keeping sessions focused on patient's ability to acquire new information.
• Monitor for fatigue.	Fatigue interferes with concentration, which decreases learning.
• Present small pieces of information in each session.	Avoids overwhelming the patient. Promotes learning.
• Use examples that can be related to the individual's life and lifestyle.	Adds realism to information and makes transferring of information easier.
• Determine if there is increased anxiety during teaching sessions, e.g., watch body language. If so, use relaxation techniques prior to session.	Anxiety decreases concentration and ability to learn.
• Use audiovisual aids that are appropriate for the individual in regard to print size, colors, volume, and tone pitch.	Promotes visual and sensory input according to individual's needs.
• Use repetition with positive feedback for correct responses.	Reinforces learning and allows evaluation of learning.

Home Health

NOTE: Many of the interactions between clients, families, and the nurse during the course of home health care are related to health education. Proper assessment by the nurse of the potential for or actual knowledge deficit is imperative. The nurse should use techniques based on learning theory to design teaching interventions that will be appropriate to the situation at hand. These techniques include, but are not limited to, using teaching materials that match the readiness of the participant, repeating the material using several senses, reinforcing the learner's progress, using a positive and enthusiastic approach, and decreasing barriers to learning, for example, language, pain, or physical illness.

ACTIONS/INTERVENTIONS	RATIONALES
• Teach the client and family measures to reduce knowledge deficit by seeking the following information and learning conditions: ○ Information regarding disease process ○ Rationale for treatment interventions ○ Techniques for improving the learning situation (motivation, teaching materials that match cognitive level of participants, reduction of discomfort, e.g., control of pain and use of familiar surroundings)	Conditions that support learning will decrease deficit. Provides client and family with necessary information.

Continued

ACTIONS/INTERVENTIONS	RATIONALES
○ Enhancement of self-care capabilities ○ Written materials to supplement oral teaching, i.e., written materials that are appropriate to cognitive level and to self-care management ○ Addressing client and family questions	
• Coordinate the teaching activities of other health care professionals who may be involved. Reinforce the teaching of ROM by the physical therapist, for example.	Coordination reduces duplication and enhances planning. Provides an opportunity for health care professionals to clarify any conflicting information before sharing it with the client.
• Involve client and family in planning, implementing, and promoting reduction in knowledge deficit: ○ Family conference ○ Mutual goal setting ○ Communication ○ Family members responsible for specific tasks or information	Involvement improves motivation and the outcome.
• Consult with or refer patient to assistive resources as indicated.	Use of the network of existing community services provides for effective utilization of resources.

Knowledge Deficit (Specify)

FLOWCHART EVALUATION: EXPECTED OUTCOME 1

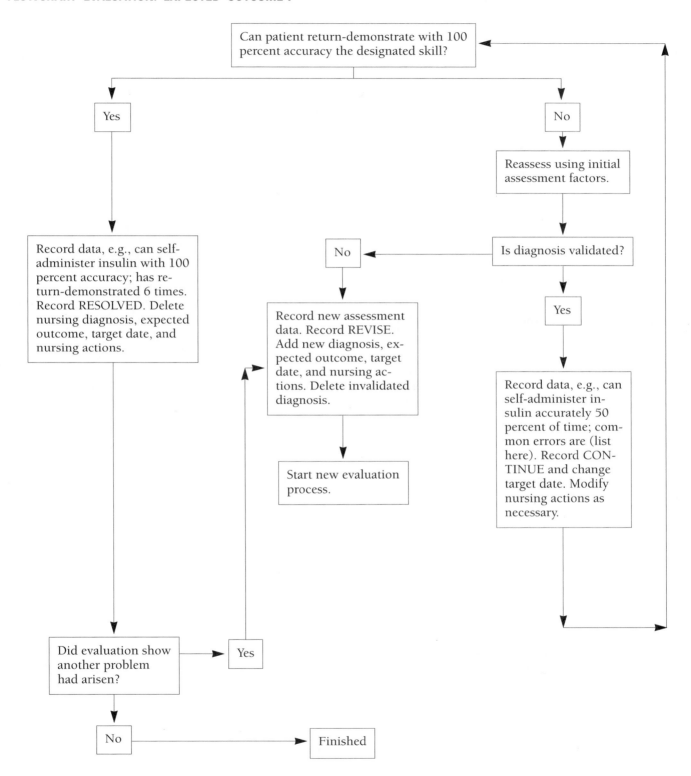

Knowledge Deficit (Specify)

FLOWCHART EVALUATION: EXPECTED OUTCOME 2

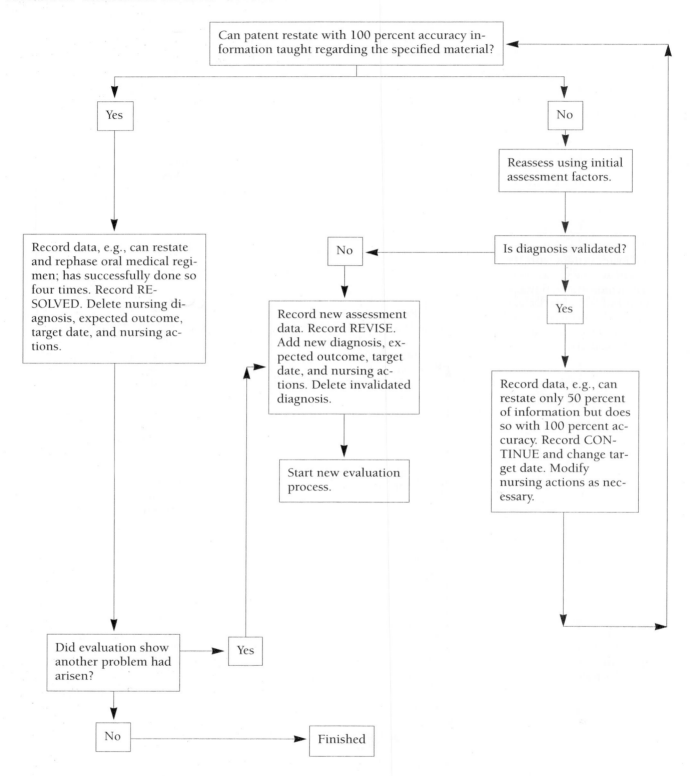

Memory, Impaired

DEFINITION

The state in which an individual experiences the inability to remember or recall bits of information or behavioral skills. Impaired memory may be attributed to pathophysiologic or situational causes that are either temporary or permanent.[2]

NANDA TAXONOMY: KNOWING 8.3.1

DEFINING CHARACTERISTICS[2]

1. Major defining characteristics
   a. Observed or reported experiences of forgetting
   b. Inability to determine if a behavior was performed
   c. Inability to learn or retain new skills or information
   d. Inability to perform a previously learned skill
   e. Inability to recall factual information
   f. Inability to recall recent or past events

2. Minor defining characteristics
   a. Forgets to perform a behavior at a scheduled time

RELATED FACTORS[2]

1. Acute or chronic hypoxia
2. Anemia
3. Decreased cardiac output
4. Fluid and electrolyte imbalance
5. Neurologic disturbances
6. Excessive environmental disturbances

RELATED CLINICAL CONCERNS

1. Hypoxia
2. Anemia
3. Congestive heart failure
4. Alzheimer's disease
5. Cerebral vascular accident
6. Dementia

HAVE YOU SELECTED THE CORRECT DIAGNOSIS?

This diagnosis is very similar to other diagnoses in this pattern, for example, Confusion and Impaired Thought Process. However, this diagnosis relates specifically to memory problems.

EXPECTED OUTCOMES

1. Will exhibit no memory deficit problem by (date) and/or
2. Will restate measures to avoid further memory impairment by (date)

TARGET DATES

For some patients, this may be a permanent problem, so dates would be stated in terms of weeks and months. For other patients, it would be appropriate to check for progress within 3 days.

NURSING ACTIONS/INTERVENTIONS WITH RATIONALES

Adult Health

ACTIONS/INTERVENTIONS	RATIONALES
• Identify self and patient by name at each interaction.	Memory loss necessitates frequent orientation to person, time, and environment.
• Support and reinforce patient's efforts to remember bits of information or behavioral skills. However, do not place unrealistic expectations on patient in this area.	Reinforcing patient's efforts at remembering can decrease anxiety levels and perhaps help with further recovery. Placing unrealistic expectations on patient can increase anxiety, frustration, and feelings of helplessness.
• Observe for improvement or deterioration in memory based on the suspected or confirmed underlying medical diagnosis.	Memory impairment due to some reversible physiologic problem should improve as the condition becomes resolved. Memory impairment due to irreversible physiologic-physical problems generally will not improve and will likely deteriorate over time.
• Teach family about patient's condition and how to respond to patient's loss of memory.	Assists family in understanding underlying cause(s) for memory impairment. Increases family's sense of competency in relating to patient during periods of memory loss.

Child Health

Same as Adult Health within developmental capacity for infant or child and safety-mindedness in all aspects.

ACTIONS/INTERVENTIONS	RATIONALES
• Determine all who may need to be involved to best support infant or child in situations where actual known level of involvement may not be clear. • Offer 30 min each shift and as needed for parents to ventilate concerns. • Offer appropriate advocacy on behalf of infant or child when parents are unable to offer this component.	Ambiguous unknowns present frustration for all involved so it is best to establish most complete team to manage care to foster holistic approach. Ventilation reduces anxiety and offers insight into parental concerns. Child advocacy will best protect child's interests when parents cannot.

Women's Health

Same as Adult Health except for magnesium sulfate therapy specific to pregnancy-induced hypertension. See Adaptive Capacity, Intracranial, Decreased.

Mental Health

ACTIONS/INTERVENTIONS	RATIONALES
• Monitor client's level of anxiety, and refer to Anxiety, Chap. 8, for detailed interventions related to this diagnosis.	Anxiety can increase the client's confusion and disorganization.
• Speak to client in brief, clear sentences.	Too much information can increase the client's confusion and disorganization, increasing memory problems.
• Interact with client for (*number*) minutes every 30 min. Begin with 5-min interactions, and gradually increase the length of interactions.	Time of interaction should be guided by the client's attention span.
• Be consistent in all interactions with the client.	Facilitates the development of a trusting relationship and meets the client's safety needs.
• Initially, place client in an area with little stimulation.	Inappropriate levels of sensory stimuli can contribute to client's sense of disorganization and confusion, increasing memory problems.
• Orient client to the environment, and assign someone to provide one-on-one interaction while client orients to unit.	Promotes client's safety needs while promoting the development of a trusting relationship.
• Do not argue with client about inaccurate memory of situations, for example, client insisting that he or she has not eaten when he or she has just finished a meal. Inform client in a matter-of-fact manner that this is not your experience of the situation.	Communicates acceptance of the client and promotes self-esteem.
• Provide orientation information to client as needed. Specify here what information this client needs, e.g., name on room, calendar, clock, written daily schedule, or information provided in written form in a notebook.	Facilitates maintenance of self-esteem and memory.
• Utilize reflection of the last statement made by client in conversations.	Facilitates memory within conversation.
• Establish a daily schedule for the client, and provide a written copy to him or her. Note client's specific schedule here.	Decreases anxiety and promotes consistency.
• Spend (*number*) minutes (*number*) times a day reviewing with client concerns about memory and developing memory techniques. These could include visual imagery, mnemonic devices, memory games, association techniques, making lists, rehearsing information, or keeping a journal about activities.	Associating information from various senses enhances memory by providing meaningful links. Written material provides prompts.

ACTIONS/INTERVENTIONS	RATIONALES
• Practice memory techniques with client (*number*) minutes 2 times a day. Note specific techniques to be practiced.	Practice improves performance and integrates behavior into client's coping strategies.
• Spend (*number*) minutes following an activity discussing the activity to provide the client with an opportunity to practice remembering.	Opportunities to use memory enhance memory.
• Provide positive verbal reinforcement to client for making progress toward accomplishing task.	Positive feedback encourages behavior.
• Sit with client each morning and develop a list of the day's activities. Review this list each evening.	Provides practice with memory techniques.
• Schedule client for groups that provide opportunities to utilize memory. These could be current event groups, reminiscence groups, or life review groups. Note client's group(s) schedule here with the assistance needed from staff to get client to the group.	Provides opportunities for client to practice using memory, which enhances memory.
• Spend (*number*) minutes each week discussing client's coping strategies with support system. Note here person responsible and time for this discussion.	Support system reactions impact the client.

Gerontic Health

ACTIONS/INTERVENTIONS	RATIONALES
• Introduce self with each client contact.	Promotes comfort for client to identify caregiver.
• Use client's preferred name in course of conversations.	Provides orienting cue to client's identity.
• Request photos and names of significant others from family or caregiver.	Provides information about the client and point of reference while providing care.
• Maintain sameness of environment.	Decreases need to cope with change on a frequent basis.
• Document any appliances client requires (prostheses, glasses, hearing aids, cane, or walker).	Provides a record of needed equipment that client may not be able to recall.
• Ensure permanent identification of all appliances required by client.	Assists in keeping equipment available to client and eliminates potential of using incorrect assistive devices.
• Maintain consistent routine for care.	Provides sense of the familiar.
• Avoid arguments over forgetful behavior.	Promotes client self-esteem, and decreases potential for escalating anxiety related to the memory loss.
• Omit statements or questions that emphasize memory loss such as "Don't you remember eating breakfast?" or "Do you know who came to see you this morning?"	Promotes client self-esteem, and decreases potential for escalating anxiety related to the memory loss.
• In congregate social or living situations, introduce clients prior to group activities.	Fosters social skills and interactions.
• Monitor solid and liquid intake on a daily basis.	Memory loss may prevent client from obtaining adequate nutrition or fluid intake.
• Document responses to medications, and note any changes in memory associated with medications.	Some medications may have side effects that in the older client promote amnesia. (This problem can occur especially with long-acting benzodiazepines and hypnotics.)
• Administer mental status exam on a semiannual basis unless client is receiving medication to enhance memory.	Monitors memory function and may assist in identifying changing strengths. Increased frequency recommended if client is taking memory-improving medication.
• Monitor for changes in ADL ability and for performance of ADLs without prompting.	If memory loss is progressive, ADL skills will decrease over time and increased assistance will be needed.
• Use distraction techniques if memory-impaired client becomes increasingly agitated or aggressive in the care setting.	Distraction can allow time for client to forget cause of agitation.
• Educate caregiver to recognize signs of personal stress when caring for client with impaired memory.	Decreases potential for caregiver burnout.
• Provide caregiver information on respite services in community.	Decreases potential for caregiver burnout.
• Monitor patient for changes in elimination patterns.	Memory-impaired client may not be able to report changes in bowel or bladder function.

Home Health

NOTE: If this is an acute development, immediate referral is required.

ACTIONS/INTERVENTIONS	RATIONALES
• Assist client and family in lifestyle adjustments that may be necessary: ○ Provide safe environment. ○ Provide frequent orientation to person, place, and time. ○ Structure teaching methods and interventions to person's ability. ○ Explain to the family the changes from their usual roles required in caring for the patient.	Home-based care requires involvement of the family. Impaired memory can disrupt family schedules and role relationships. Adjustments in family activities and roles may be required.
• Assist family in setting criteria to help them determine when additional intervention is required, for example, explain how to recognize change in baseline behavior.	Provides family background knowledge to seek appropriate assistance as need arises.
• Refer patient to appropriate assistive resources as indicated.	Additional assistance may be required for family to care for person with impaired memory. Use of readily available resources is cost-effective.
• Teach client and family memory involvement tasks, such as reminiscence and memory practice exercises.	Structured memory tasks can increase the client's functional ability.
• Teach client and family about compensation strategies, e.g., daily planner or checklists.	Compensation strategies can increase the client's functional ability.

Memory, Impaired

FLOWCHART EVALUATION: EXPECTED OUTCOME 1

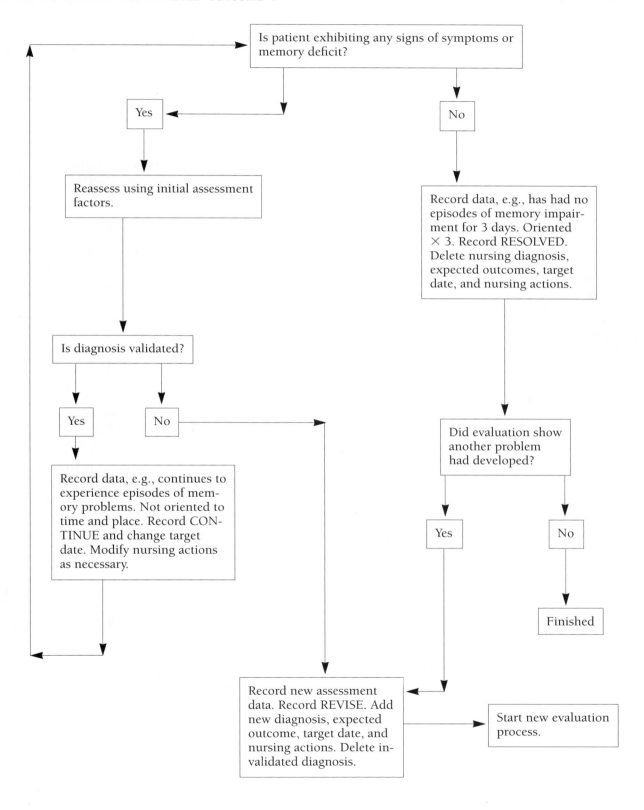

Memory, Impaired

FLOWCHART EVALUATION: EXPECTED OUTCOME 2

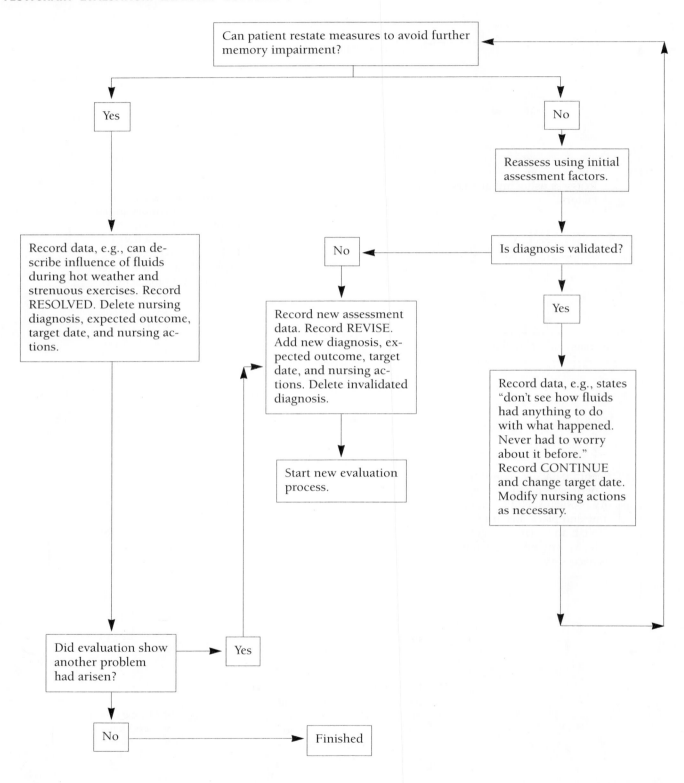

Pain

DEFINITION

NOTE: The 1994 Preconference Workgroup for this diagnosis suggested Pain as an umbrella diagnostic label with subcategories of Acute Pain and Chronic Pain.

PAIN An unpleasant sensory and emotional experience arising from actual or potential tissue damage or described in terms of such damage (International Association for the Study of Pain).

ACUTE PAIN Sudden or slow onset of any intensity from mild to severe with an anticipated or predictable end and a duration of less than 6 months.[2]

CHRONIC PAIN Sudden or slow onset of any intensity from mild to severe, constant or recurring without anticipated or predictable and a duration of greater than 6 months.[2]

NANDA TAXONOMY: FEELING 9.1.1

DEFINING CHARACTERISTICS[2]

1. Acute Pain
   a. Major defining characteristics:
      (1) Verbal or coded report
      (2) Observed evidence
      (3) Antalgic position
      (4) Protective behavior
      (5) Guarding behavior
      (6) Antalgic gestures
      (7) Facial mask
      (8) Sleep disturbance (eyes lack luster, "hecohe look," fixed or scattered movement, or grimace)
   b. Minor defining characteristics
      (1) Self-focus
      (2) Narrowed focus (altered time perception, impaired thought process, or reduced interaction with people and environment)
      (3) Distraction behavior (pacing, seeking out other people and/or activities, or repetitive activities)
      (4) Autonomic alteration in muscle tone (may span from listless to rigid)
      (5) Autonomic responses (diaphoresis, blood pressure, respiration, pulse change, or pupillary dilation)

      (6) Expressive behavior (restlessness, moaning, crying, vigilance, irritability, or sighing)
      (7) Changes in appetite and eating
2. Chronic Pain
   a. Major defining characteristics (verbal or coded report or observed evidence of)
      (1) Protective behavior
      (2) Guarding behavior
      (3) Facial mask
      (4) Irritability
      (5) Self-focusing
      (6) Restlessness
      (7) Depression
   b. Minor defining characteristics
      (1) Atrophy of involved muscle group
      (2) Changes in sleep pattern
      (3) Weight changes
      (4) Fatigue
      (5) Fear of reinjury
      (6) Reduced interaction with people
      (7) Altered ability to continue previous activities
      (8) Sympathetic mediated responses (temperature, cold, changes of body position, or hypersensitivity)
      (9) Anorexia

RELATED FACTORS[2]

1. Pain
   a. Injury agents (biologic, chemical, physical, psychologic)
2. Chronic Pain
   a. Chronic physical or psychosocial disability

RELATED CLINICAL CONCERNS

1. Any surgical diagnosis
2. Any condition labeled chronic, for example, rheumatoid arthritis
3. Any traumatic injury
4. Any infection
5. Anxiety or stress
6. Fatigue

HAVE YOU SELECTED THE CORRECT DIAGNOSIS?

There are no other nursing diagnoses that are easily confused with this diagnosis. Many of the other nursing diagnoses will serve as companion diagnoses and may have pain as a contributing factor to that diagnosis; for example, an individual with chronic pain may be exhausted from trying to deal with the pain and have a companion diagnosis of Fatigue or may be using alcohol or street drugs in an attempt to ease the pain and would have the companion diagnosis of Ineffective Individual Coping.

EXPECTED OUTCOMES

1. Will verbalize a decreased number of complaints of pain by (date) and/or
2. Will require no more than 1 medication for pain per 24 hours by (date)

TARGET DATES

For the majority of health disruptions, pain will begin to resolve within 72 hours after the patient has sought health care assistance. Thus, the suggested target date is 3 days after the date of diagnosis.

NURSING ACTIONS/INTERVENTIONS WITH RATIONALES
Adult Health

ACTIONS/INTERVENTIONS	RATIONALES
• Monitor for pain at least every 2 h on the (even/odd) hour. Have patient rank pain on a scale of 0–10 at each incidence of pain. Review and have patient review activity engaged in prior to each pain episode and document. Request patient to share thoughts and feelings prior to onset of painful episode.	Pain is subjective in nature, and only the patient can fully describe it.
• Teach patient to report pain as soon as it starts. Allow patient to talk about pain experience in as much detail as desired.	Initiates a preventive approach before the pain gets too severe.
• Administer pain medication as ordered. Monitor and record amount of pain relief within 30 min after administration. Have patient rerank pain (0–10). If pain is not relieved, collaborate with physician regarding change in medication.	Response to pain and pain medication is unique to each patient.
• Give massage immediately following administration of each pain medication and after each turning.	Assists in muscle relaxation and improves action of pain medication by stimulating peripheral nerve fibers to close the transmission gate.
• Turn at least every 2 h on (even/odd) hour. Maintain anatomic alignment with pillows or other padded support.	Helps to stimulate circulation. Alignment helps to prevent pain from malposition and enhances comfort.
• Provide calm, quiet environment. Limit activity for at least 2 h following pain medication administration.	Promotes action and effect of medication by providing decreased stimuli.
• Monitor vital signs at least every 4 h while awake at (times).	Detects early changes that might indicate pain.
• Monitor sleep-rest pattern. Promote rest periods during day and at least 8 h sleep each night (see nursing actions for Sleep Pattern Disturbance, Chap. 6).	Fatigue may contribute to an increased pain response, or pain can contribute to interrupted sleep.
• Offer 2–3 oz of wine before each meal and at bedtime.	Promotes relaxation and assists in decreasing pain response.
• Promote activity and exercise to extent possible (i.e., as long as it does not result in pain). Provide ROM exercises at least every 4 h while awake at (times).	Promotes release of natural endorphins and stimulates circulation. Prevents complications of immobility secondary to limitation of movement due to pain.
• Apply heat or cold (on 2 h, off 2 h). Select heat, cold, dry, or moist according to what patient states provides the best pain relief.	Causes vasoconstriction or vasodilation, either of which, depending on the individual patient's response, will assist in decreasing swelling, promote healing, and inhibit the transmission of the pain impulse.
• Check bowel elimination at least once per shift.	Immobility caused by pain may decrease the parasympathetic stimulation to the bowel.
• Encourage fluid intake every 2 h while awake on (even/odd) hour. Encourage up to 3000 mL per day.	Maintains hydration. Patient may limit intake because seeking fluids stimulates pain.
• Provide oral hygiene every 4 h while awake at (times).	Basic comfort measure.

• Allow time for patient to discuss fears and anxieties related to pain by scheduling at least 15 min once per shift to visit with patient on one-to-one basis. Provide accurate information to patient regarding:
  ○ Pain threshold
  ○ Pain tolerance
  ○ Addiction
  ○ Medication effectiveness and ineffectiveness
  ○ Expressing pain
	Just as pain is unique to the individual, so is the pain control intervention. Discussions with the patient provide collaboration and increase patient's compliance. Decreases feeling of powerlessness and initiates basic teaching regarding control of pain.

• Apply mentholated or aspirin ointment to affected area every 4 h while awake at (times) and when needed.	Provides topical relief for pain. Dulls peripheral nerve endings that carry pain impulse.

• Use noninvasive pain relief techniques as appropriate:
  ○ Biofeedback
  ○ Progressive relaxation
	Provides diversion from pain. Decreases anxiety and muscle tension. Increases comfort and empowers patient.

- ○ Guided imagery
- ○ Rhythmic breathing
- ○ Distraction
- ○ Contralateral stimulation
- ○ Stress reduction techniques
- ○ Self-hypnosis
- Collaborate with physician regarding use of transcutaneous electrical nerve stimulation (TENS).
- Teach patient and significant others:
  - ○ Cause of pain
  - ○ Self-administration of pain medication
  - ○ Avoiding and minimizing pain
  - ○ Splinting
  - ○ Gradual increase in activities
  - ○ Use of alternate noninvasive techniques (see nursing action above)
  - ○ Combining techniques, e.g., medication with relaxation technique
  - ○ To try various pain relief measures and to alternate pain relief measures
  - ○ To express anger, frustration, and grief with pain management and change in lifestyle
  - ○ To be more active in his or her own pain arrangement program and to note successes and minimize failure.
  - ○ Value of adequate rest and maintaining weight within normal range
- Refer patient to or collaborate with other health professionals.

Collaboration promotes the best approach to pain management.
Knowledge assists the patient in feeling like an active participant on the health team. Decreases sense of powerlessness.

Collaboration promotes the best long-range plan for management of pain.

Additional Information

Keep current on comparative doses of analgesics, true effect of so-called potentiators, and non-invasive means of pain relief. Do not worry about a patient's becoming addicted. Within the average length of hospital stay of 3 to 5 days, it is doubtful that addiction could occur. Current research in this area shows an extremely low rate of addiction due to medication administration in a health care setting. The same research indicates that we undermedicate, rather than over-medicate, for pain. Undermedication is particularly true in the case of infants, children, and older adults. See the Department of Health and Human Services Guidelines[51] for a discussion of this research as well as further information on pain control.

Child Health

ACTIONS/INTERVENTIONS	RATIONALES
<ul><li>Monitor for contributory factors to pain at least every 8 h or as required:<ul><li>○ Physical injury or surgical incision</li><li>○ Stressors</li><li>○ Fears</li><li>○ Knowledge deficit</li><li>○ Anxieties</li><li>○ Fatigue</li><li>○ Description of exact nature of pain whether per McGill or Elkind tools</li><li>○ Vital signs</li><li>○ Response to medication</li><li>○ Meaning of pain to child and family</li></ul></li></ul>	Provides the essential database for planning and modification of planning.
<ul><li>Provide appropriate support in management of pain for the patient and significant others by:<ul><li>○ Validation of the pain</li><li>○ Maintaining self-control to extent feasible</li></ul></li></ul>	Validation and support of the patient and family will serve to show value and respect for the individual's health need. Maintains basic standards of care. Ventilation reduces anxiety, and parental involvement enhances coping skills.

Continued

ACTIONS/INTERVENTIONS	RATIONALES

- Maintaining self-control to extent feasible
- Providing education to deal with specifics applicable; assisting patient and family to talk about the pain experience by allowing at least 30 min per shift for such ventilation at (times)
- Allowing parents to be present and participate in comforting of patient; assisting child and parents to develop a plan of care that addresses individual needs and is likely to result in a better coping pattern (particularly for chronic pain)
- Appropriate diversional activities for age and developmental level
- Attention to controlling external stimuli such as noise and light
- Use of relaxation techniques appropriate for child's capacity
- Appropriate follow-up of pain tolerance and response to medication as ordered
- Encourage pain medication route to be oral if there is no IV.
- If IV route is utilized, monitor for respiratory and blood pressure depression every 10 min × 6 at (times).
- Monitor intake and output for decrease due to hypomotility or spasm.
- Give appropriate emotional support during painful procedures or experiences:
  - Explain procedures at child's level of openness and honesty.
  - Use puppets to demonstrate procedure.
  - Explain to parents that even if child cries excessively, their presence is encouraged.
  - Comfort child before, during, and after the procedure.
  - Reward the child for positive behavior according to developmental need; e.g., place stars on a chart.
  - Discuss and encourage parents and child to share feelings about the painful experience.
- Collaborate with or refer patient to appropriate health care team members.
- Teach patient and family ways to follow up at home or school with needed pain regimen:
  - Appropriate timing of medication
  - Appropriate administration of medication
  - Not to substitute acetaminophen for aspirin in arthritis
- Monitor for stomach alterations or other complications, especially respiratory depression, secondary to administration of pain medication.
- Develop daily plans for pain management to determine those that might be suited for patient to use on a regular basis.
- Identify need to have several alternate plans to deal with pain.

NOTE: Chronic pain is going to recur; therefore, there is a need for long-term follow-up. This follow-up is especially critical since chronic pain places the patient at risk for developmental delays.

Women's Health

Gynecologic Pain

NOTE: A significant amount of the pain experienced by women is associated with the pelvic area and the reproductive organs. Determining the origin of the pain is one of the most difficult tasks facing nurses dealing with the gynecologic patient. An organic explanation for pain is never found in approximately 25 percent of women. Because of the close association with the reproductive organs, gynecologic pain can be extremely frightening, can connote social stigma, affect the perception of the feminine role, cause anger and guilt, and totally dominate the woman's existence. "Pain is culturally more acceptable in certain parts of the body and may elicit more sympathy than pain in other sites."[52]

ACTIONS/INTERVENTIONS	RATIONALES
• Identify factors in patient's lifestyle that could be contributing to pain. • Record accurate menstrual cycle and obstetric, gynecologic, and sexual history, being certain to note problems, previous pregnancies, descriptions of previous labors, previous infections or gynecologic problems, and any infections as a result of sexual activities. • Assist the client to describe her perception of pain as it relates to her. • Include dysmenorrhea pain pattern, being certain to determine if the pain occurs before, during, or after menstruation. • Monitor disturbance of client's daily routine as a result of pain. Have patient describe the location of the pain, e.g., lower abdomen, legs, breast, or back. • Have patient describe any edema, especially "bloating" at specific times during the month. • Have the patient describe the onset and character of the pain, e.g., mild or severe cramping. • Ascertain if pain is associated with nausea, vomiting, or diarrhea. • Identify any precipitating factors associated with pain, e.g., emotional upsets, exercise, or medication. • Assist patient in identifying various methods of pain relief, including exercise (pelvic rock), biofeedback, relaxation, and medication (analgesics or antiprostaglandins).	Provides the database to adequately assess pain and determine the underlying cause. This information can assist in pinpointing source of pain and devising a plan of care. Individualizes pain control and provides options for patient.

Women's Health

Labor Pain and Nursing

ACTIONS/INTERVENTIONS	RATIONALES
LABOR • Encourage patient to describe her perception of labor pain related to her previous laboring experiences.[53] • Provide factual information about the laboring process. • Refer patient to childbirth preparation group, e.g., Lamaze groups. • Describe methods of coping with labor pain, e.g., relaxation, imaging, breathing, medication, hydrotherapy, or ambulation.	Providing information about the laboring process helps the patient cope with the pain of labor.

Continued

ACTIONS/INTERVENTIONS	RATIONALES
• Provide support during labor. • Encourage involvement of significant others as support during labor process. **POSTPARTUM** • Encourage patient to describe her perception of pain associated with postpartum. • Provide information for pain relief, e.g., Kegel exercises, sitz baths, or medications. • Explain etiology of "afterbirth pains" to involution of uterus. • Explain relationship of breast-feeding to involution and uterine contractions. • Assist patient in putting on supportive bra. • Encourage early, frequent breast-feedings to enhance let-down reflex. • Support patient and provide information on correct breast-feeding techniques such as changing positions from one feeding to the next to distribute sucking pressure and prevent sore nipples. • Check baby's position on breast; be certain areola is in mouth and not just the nipple. • Provide warm, moist heat for relief of engorged breasts. • Provide analgesics for discomfort of engorged breasts. • Pump after infant nurses until breast is emptied. • Encourage patient to nurse on least sore side first to encourage let-down reflex. • Apply ice to nipple just before nursing to decrease pain.	Knowing the source of pain increases the patient's sense of control. Knowledge of how to lessen discomfort during breast-feeding contributes to successful or effective breast-feeding. Demonstrates to patient various pain relief methods.

Psychiatric Health

ACTIONS/INTERVENTIONS	RATIONALES
• Monitor nurse's response to the client's perception of pain. If the nurse has difficulty understanding or coping with the client's expression of pain, he or she should discuss his or her feelings with a colleague in an attempt to resolve the concerns. • Note any recurring patterns in the pain experience such as time of day, recent social interactions, or physical activity. If a pattern is present, begin a discussion of this observation with the client. • Determine effects pain has had on client's life, including role responsibilities, financial impact, cognitive and emotional functioning, and family interactions. • Review client's beliefs and attitudes about the role pain is assuming in client's life. If pain is very important to client's definition of self, assure client that you are not requiring him or her to give up the pain by indicating that you are only interested in the pain that causes undue discomfort or by indicating that you recognize that this client's pain is special and that it would be difficult, if not impossible, for the health care team to get rid of it. • Spend brief, goal-directed time with the client when he or she is focusing conversation on pain or pain-related activities.	The nurse's response to the client can be communicated and have an effect on the client's level of anxiety, which can then affect the pain response. Initiates client's awareness of this pattern and allows the nurse to assess the client's perception of this observation. Assesses meaning of pain to the client's amount of anxiety associated with the pain and possible benefits of pain in the client's life. If pain is assuming an important role, then it might be difficult for the client to "give up" all of the pain, and this should be considered in all further interventions.[45,46]

- Schedule time with the client when he or she is not complaining about pain. List this schedule here. Focus on special activities in which the client is involved or follow up on a non-pain-related conversation the client seemed to enjoy.

Provides positive feedback to the client about an aspect of himself or herself that is not pain related.

- Find at least one non-pain-related activity the client enjoys that can be the source of positive interaction between client and others, and encourage client participation in this activity with positive reinforcement (list client-specific positive reinforcers here along with the activity).

Reinforcement encourages positive behavior and improves self-esteem.

- Discuss with client alternatives for meeting personal need currently being met by pain. You may need to refer client to another, more specialized care provider if this is a problem of long standing or if client demonstrates difficulty in discussing these concerns. Refer to the self-esteem diagnoses, Chap. 8, for specific interventions related to perceptions of self.

- Develop with the client a plan to alter those factors that intensify the pain experience. For example, if the pain increases at 4 p.m. each day and the client associates this with his boss's daily visit at 5 p.m., then the plan might include limiting the visits from the boss or having another person present when the boss visits. List specific interventions here.

The social milieu can change the basic quality of the pain experience.

- Develop with client plan for learning relaxation techniques, and have client practice technique 30 min 2 times a day at (times). Remain with client during practice session to provide verbal cues and encouragement as necessary. These techniques can include:
  - Meditation
  - Progressive deep muscle relaxation
  - Visualization techniques that require the client to visualize scenes that enhance the relaxation response (such as being on the beach or having the sun warm the body)
  - Biofeedback
  - Prayer
  - Autogenic training

These techniques decrease anxiety.

- Monitor interaction of analgesic with other medications the client is receiving, especially antianxiety, antipsychotic, and hypnotic drugs.

These medications may potentiate one another.

- Review client's history for indication of illicit drug use and the effects this may have on client's tolerance to analgesics.

Client may have developed a cross tolerance for these drugs.

- If client is to be withdrawn from the analgesic, discuss the alternative coping methods and how they will assist client with the process. Assure client that support will be provided during this process. Help client identify those situations that will be most difficult, and schedule one-to-one time with client during these times.

Promotes perception of control and decreases anxiety.

- If client demonstrates altered mood, refer to Ineffective Individual Coping, Chap. 11, for interventions.

- Consult with occupational therapy to assist client in developing diversional activities. Note time for these activities here as well as a list of special equipment that may be necessary for the activity.

Decreases conscious awareness of pain, thus decreasing the pain experience.

- Involve client in group activities by sitting with him or her during a group activity such as a game, or assign client a responsibility for preparing one part of a unit meal. Begin with activities that require little concentration, and then gradually increase the task complexity.

Alters client's perception of the pain.

Continued

ACTIONS/INTERVENTIONS	RATIONALES
• Consult with physician for possible referral for use of hypnosis in pain management.	
• Sit with the client and the family during at least 2 visits to assess family interactions with the client and the role pain plays in family interaction.	
• Discuss with the client the role of distraction in pain management, and develop a list of those activities the client finds distracting and enjoyable. These could include listening to music, watching TV or special movies, or physical activity. Develop with the client a plan for including these activities in the pain management program, and list that plan here.	Provides other pain relief options for the client.
• Discuss with the client the role that exercise can play in pain management, and develop an exercise program with the client. This should begin at or below the client's capabilities and could include a 15-min walk twice a day or 10 min on a stationary bicycle. Note the plan here with the type of activity, length of time, and time of day it is to be implemented.	Exercise encourages release of natural endorphins.
• Provide positive reinforcement to the client for implementing the exercise program by spending time with the client during the exercise, providing verbal feedback, and allowing client the rewards that have been developed. These rewards are developed with the client.	Reinforcement encourages positive behavior and enhances self-esteem.
• Monitor family and support system's understanding of the pain and perceptions of the client. If they demonstrate the attitude that the client is closely perceived with the pain, then develop a plan to include them in the experiences described above. List that plan here. Consider referral to a clinical specialist in mental health nursing or a family therapist to assist family in developing non-pain-related interaction patterns.	Assists family in normalizing and in moving away from a pain-focused identity.
• Provide ongoing feedback on progress to client or support system.	
• Refer client to outpatient support systems, and assist with making arrangements for the client to contact these before discharge.	Long-term support enhances the likelihood of effective home management.

Gerontic Health

ACTIONS/INTERVENTIONS	RATIONALES
ACUTE PAIN	
• Medicate every 4–6 h rather than PRN for the first 48–72 h, especially postoperatively.[54]	Enhances pain control and thus promotes early mobility, which decreases the potential for postoperative complications.
• Encourage physician to prescribe morphine versus meperidine if a narcotic analgesic is required.	Meperidine is more likely to cause confusion and psychotic behavior when given to the older adult.[5]
• Investigate patient's beliefs regarding pain. Does he or she consider pain a punishment for prior misdeeds? Does he or she think that having to take pain medication signals severe illness or a potential for dying?[56]	May be a barrier to seeking pain relief.

- Encourage patient to report pain especially if medication order is PRN.
- Avoid presenting self in a hurried manner.

CHRONIC PAIN

- Explore with patient how he or she has managed chronic pain in the past.
- Determine use of distraction in helping patient cope with chronic pain.[54]
- Monitor skin status when thermal interventions are used such as ice or heat packs.
- In the presence of chronic pain, depression may also exist. Screen for depression.

Patient may not realize that medication won't be given on a scheduled basis.
Older adults are less likely to report pain if caregiver is rushed.[56]

Assists in determining what measures were of significant or of little help.
Music, humor, and relaxation techniques can provide temporary respite from discomfort.
Changes in sensation may result in thermal injury if not closely monitored.
Chronic pain is exhausting physically and mentally.

Home Health

ACTIONS/INTERVENTIONS	RATIONALES

• Teach client and family measures to promote comfort:
  ◦ Proper positioning
  ◦ Appropriate use of medications, e.g., narcotics as ordered if pain is severe, nonnarcotic analgesics, anti-inflammatories
  ◦ Knowledge regarding source of pain or of disease process
  ◦ Self-management of pain and of care as much as is appropriate
  ◦ Relaxation techniques
  ◦ Therapeutic touch
  ◦ Massage (if not contraindicated)
  ◦ Meaningful activities
  ◦ Distraction
  ◦ Breathing techniques
  ◦ Heat or cold treatments (if not contraindicated)
  ◦ Regular activity and exercise
  ◦ Planning and goal setting
  ◦ Biofeedback
  ◦ Yoga or tai chi
  ◦ Imagery or hypnosis
  ◦ Group or family therapy
	Involvement of the client and family promotes comfort and decreases self-reported pain and analgesic use.[51]

• Teach client and family factors that decrease tolerance to pain and methods for decreasing these factors:
  ◦ Lack of knowledge regarding disease process or pain control methods
  ◦ Lack of support from significant others regarding the severity of the pain
  ◦ Fear of addiction or fear of loss of control
  ◦ Fatigue
  ◦ Boredom
  ◦ Improper positioning
	Reducing these factors can increase the tolerance to pain.[41]

• Involve client and family in planning, implementing, and promoting reduction in pain:
  ◦ Family conference
  ◦ Mutual goal setting
  ◦ Communication
  ◦ Support for caregiver
	Involvement improves motivation and improves outcome.

Continued

ACTIONS/INTERVENTIONS	RATIONALES

• Assist client and family in lifestyle adjustments that may be required:
  ◦ Occupational changes
  ◦ Family role alterations
  ◦ Comfort measures for chronic pain
  ◦ Financial situation
  ◦ Responses to pain (mood, concentration, or ability to complete activities of daily living)
  ◦ Coping with disability or dependency
  ◦ Mechanism for altering need for assistance
  ◦ Providing appropriate balance of dependence and independence.
  ◦ Stress management
  ◦ Time management
  ◦ Obtaining and using assistive equipment, e.g., for arthritis
  ◦ Regular, rather than as-needed, schedule of pain medication
	Lifestyle changes require changes in behavior.

• Teach client and family purposes, side effects, and proper administration techniques of medications.	Provides necessary information for safe self-care.
• Consult with or refer patient to appropriate assistive resources as indicated.	Use of the existing community services network provides effective utilization of resources.

Pain

FLOWCHART EVALUATION: EXPECTED OUTCOME 1

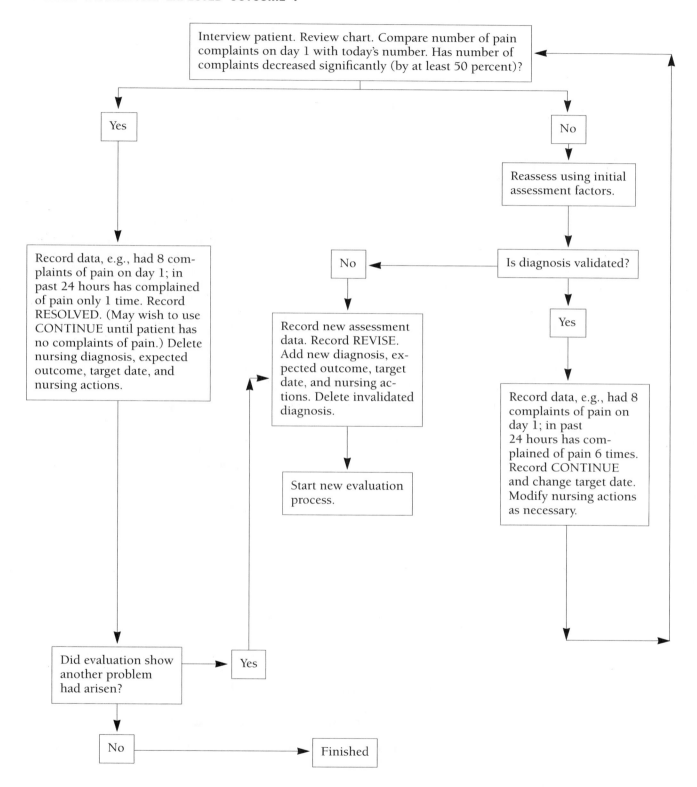

Pain

FLOWCHART EVALUATION: EXPECTED OUTCOME 2

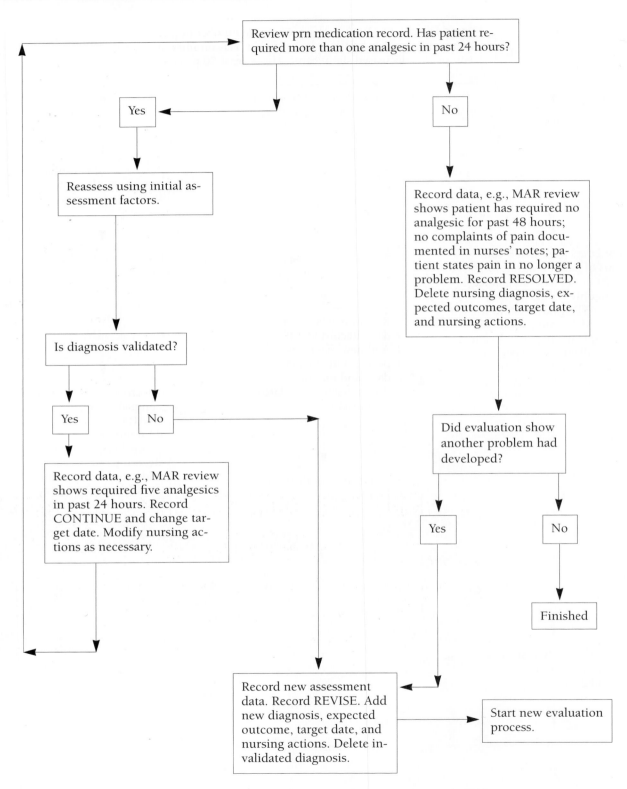

Sensory-Perceptual Alterations (Specify: Visual, Auditory, Kinesthetic, Gustatory, Tactile, Olfactory)

DEFINITION

A state in which an individual experiences a change in the amount or patterning of oncoming stimuli accompanied by a diminished, exaggerated, distorted, or impaired response to such stimuli.[2]

NANDA TAXONOMY: PERCEIVING 7.2

DEFINING CHARACTERISTICS[2]

1. Major defining characteristics
   a. Distorted in time, in place, or with persons
   b. Altered abstraction
   c. Altered conceptualization
   d. Change in problem-solving abilities
   e. Reported or measured change in sensory acuity
   f. Change in behavior pattern
   g. Anxiety
   h. Apathy
   i. Change in usual response to stimuli
   j. Indication of body image alteration
   k. Restlessness
   l. Irritability
   m. Altered communication patterns
2. Other possible characteristics
   a. Complaints of fatigue
   b. Alterations in posture
   c. Change in muscular tension
   d. Inappropriate responses
   e. Hallucinations

RELATED FACTORS[2]

1. Altered environmental stimuli (excessive or insufficient)
2. Altered sensory reception, transmission, and/or integration
3. Chemical alterations, endogenous (electrolyte) or exogenous (drugs, etc.)
4. Psychological stress

RELATED CLINICAL CONCERNS

1. Any neurological diagnosis
2. Glaucoma or cataracts
3. Intensive care unit patient
4. Psychosis
5. Substance abuse
6. Toxemia

HAVE YOU SELECTED THE CORRECT DIAGNOSIS?

Impaired Thought Process   Impaired Thought Process refers to a patient's cognitive abilities while sensory-perceptual relates to just the sensory input-output.

Self-Care Deficit   Certainly sensory-perceptual problems could result in self-care deficits, but remember, one diagnosis is speaking about ability to care for the self while the other focuses on response to sensory input.

EXPECTED OUTCOMES

1. Will identify and initiate at least two adaptive ways to compensate for (specific sensory deficit) by (date) and/or
2. Will verbalize fewer problems with (specific sensory deficit) by (date)

TARGET DATES

Assisting the patient in dealing with an uncompensated sensory deficit is a long-term process. Also, the patient may never accept the deficit but can be helped to adapt to the deficit. Therefore, an appropriate target date would be no sooner than 5 to 7 days from the date of diagnosis.

NURSING ACTIONS/INTERVENTIONS WITH RATIONALES

Adult Health

ACTIONS/INTERVENTIONS	RATIONALES
• Provide patient with appropriate prosthesis if the deficit has been previously diagnosed and a prosthesis provided.	Provides immediate assistance with sensory deficit to decrease deficit.
• Maintain prosthesis to ensure optimal functioning.	Prostheses that do not fit or function well lead to nonuse.
• Provide calm, nonthreatening environment.	Reinforces reality.
• Orient to room.	

Continued

ACTIONS/INTERVENTIONS	RATIONALES

• Check safety factors frequently:
  ○ Siderails
  ○ Uncluttered room
  ○ Lighting: Dim at night, increased during day, and nonglare
  ○ Environment arranged to assist in compensating for specific deficit
	Basic safety measures.

• Place bedside table, over-the-bed table in same position each time and within easy reach. Ascertain which items patient wants on these tables and where the items are to be placed. Place items in same place each time.	Maintains consistency of environment, which facilitates patient's comfort and decreases anxiety.
• Have significant others bring familiar items from home. • Promote consistency in care, e.g., same nurse, as near same routine as possible. • Follow patient's own routine as much as possible, e.g., bath, bedtime, meals, and grooming. Pace activities to patient's preference.	Enhances physical and psychologic comfort. Decreases unessential stimuli. Inspires trust. Reinforces patient's own routine. Promotes comfort and empowers patient.

• Provide reality orientation as necessary:
  ○ Keep clock and calendar in room.
  ○ Touch patient frequently.
  ○ Check orientation to person, time, and place at least once per shift.
  ○ Listen carefully.
	Reinforces reality.

• Monitor, at least once per shift:
  ○ Intake and output
  ○ Vital signs
  ○ Circulatory status
  ○ Neurologic status
  ○ Sleep-rest amounts
  ○ Mental status
	Basic monitoring for signs and symptoms of sensory overload or sensory deficit.

• Encourage activity and exercise to extent possible, and interspace with rest periods. Do ROM at least every 4 h while awake at (times).	Provides stimulation and prevents complications from immobility.
• Collaborate with occupational therapist regarding appropriate diversionary activity.	Provides stimuli.

AUDITORY DEFICITS

• Clean ear with wet washcloth over finger.	Assists in removal of ear wax without damaging inner ear structure.
• If eardrops are ordered, warm to body temperature before instilling into the ear.	Warm eardrops assist in removal of ear wax and are less likely to cause vertigo problems. Increases comfort.
• Speak in low tones when interacting with patient.	Allows for alteration in hearing high-frequency sounds. High-frequency tones are lost first.
• Allow patient extended time to respond to verbal messages.	Allows for understanding and interpretation of message.
• Decrease background noise as much as possible when talking with the patient.	Avoids confusion and increases the patient's ability to localize sounds.
• Do not shout when talking with client.	Shouting only accentuates vowel sounds while decreasing consonant sounds.
• Use visual cues as much as possible to enhance verbal messages.	Improves communication.
• Provide message board to use with patient. • Replace batteries in hearing aids as necessary.	A common problem in hearing deficits.
• Clean ear wax from ear mold of hearing aid as necessary.	Improves functioning of hearing aid.
• Stand where the patient can watch your lips when you are speaking to him or her.	
• Make lips visible to the patient by clipping moustaches away from lips (males) or wearing lipstick that highlights lips (females).	Provides added cues to what is being said.

- Teach patient and family proper care of ears, e.g., use of ear plugs when in an environment with loud noises, protecting the ear from water while swimming, blowing the nose with mouth and both nostrils open.

Protects the eardrum from trauma.

- Teach patient to turn better ear toward speaker. Note here patient's better ear so staff can stand on that side when speaking to patient.

Improves communication.

- Teach patient and family proper maintenance of hearing aid.

Promotes proper functioning of hearing aid.

VISUAL DEFICIT

- Provide patient with his or her eyeglasses or contact lenses during waking hours. Note here where they are to be kept when patient is not using them and place them in that place when patient removes them.

Facilitates patient's use of equipment and assists in preventing damage or loss of equipment.

- Provide written information in large-print or audio recorded format.
- Provide telephone dials and other equipment necessary that has large numbers on nonglare surfaces. List here special equipment that is necessary for this patient and when the patient may need it so it can be provided at appropriate times.
- Identify patient's room with large numbers or patient's name in large print.
- Provide large-screen TV and pictures with large, colorful images.

Larger images are easier for patient to interpret.

- Place patient in social or group situations so they are not looking directly into an open window.

Glare from window will decrease visual acuity.

- Provide nonglare work surfaces.
- Identify stairs and door frames with contrasting tape or paint.

Increases visual acuity. Basic safety measure.

- Verbally address patient when entering patient's proximity and approach patient from the front.

Makes patient aware of presence.

- Do not alter the patient's physical environment without telling him or her of the changes.

Promotes consistency in environment that improves safety.

- Address patient by name.

Clearly identifies who you are talking to.

- Ask patient about special environmental adaptations he or she prefers or uses (list those here).

Promotes familiarity of environment while in hospital.

- Provide patient with talking books and large-print periodicals.

Provides diversionary activity.

- Enter patient's environment every hour on the (hour/half-hour).

Frequent contact provides assurance that the patient is a matter of concern to the nursing staff.

- Teach patient and family proper maintenance of eyeglasses and other prostheses.

Assures proper functioning and prevents scratching of lenses.

- Teach patient and family methods to improve environmental safety.
- Assist patient with activities of daily living as necessary. List the activities that require assistance here along with the type of assistance that is needed, e.g., assisting patient to eat to the extent necessary (feed totally or cut up food and open packages).

Allows patient to be as indifferent as possible.

TOUCH AND KINESTHESIA DEFICIT

- Remove sharp objects from the patient's environment.

Basic safety measure.

- Protect patient from exposure to excessive heat and cold by:

Basic safety measures to prevent accidental burns.

  ○ Checking temperature of heat and cold packs carefully before application
  ○ Teaching patient to check with a thermometer the temperature of bath and other water to be placed on the skin
  ○ Checking temperature of bathwater for patient while he or she is on the nursing unit

Continued

ACTIONS/INTERVENTIONS	RATIONALES
◦ Teaching patient to wear protective clothing whenever he or she goes outdoors in the winter ◦ Teaching patient not to use heating pads or hot-water bottles. • Have patient and family lower the setting on the hot-water heater in the home to 124°F. • Instruct patient not to smoke unless someone is with him or her. • Have patient change position every 2 h on the (odd/even) hour. • Monitor condition of skin every 4 h at (times). Note any alteration in integrity. Teach patient to visually inspect skin on a daily basis. • Have patient wear well-fitting shoes when walking. • Trim toenails and fingernails for patient. Maintain these at a safe length. • Assist patient in determining if clothing is fitting properly without abrading the skin. • Perform foot care on a daily basis to include: ◦ Bathing feet in warm water ◦ Applying moisturizing lotion ◦ Trimming nails as needed ◦ Checking skin for abrasions or reddened areas • Note time for foot care here. This process should be taught to the patient, and the patient should be assuming primary responsibility for this care before discharge. This should be done with nursing supervision. • Provide patient with assistance with movement in the environment until he or she is able to make the necessary adaptations to alterations in sensations. • Consult with physical therapist regarding teaching patient appropriate adaptations for safe and effective movement. • Assist patient with care of affected body parts. • Assist patient with ADL (note type and amount of assistance needed here). • Refer patient to occupational therapy for assisting with learning new self-care behavior. SMELL DEFICIT • Assess for extent of neurologic dysfunction on admission. • Determine effect the smell deficit has on patient's appetite and work with dietitian to make meals visually appealing. • Provide for appropriate follow-up appointments before dismissal.	Promotes circulation and relieves pressure on bony prominences. Guards against skin breakdown. Prevents blisters and infection. Demonstrates and promotes safe care of extremities for patient. Prevents unilateral neglect and provides cues for patient. Promotes self-care through demonstrating care to patient. Determines what intervention can be planned. Assists to compensate for loss of smell. Providing specific appointments lessens the confusion about the specifics of appointments and increases the likelihood of subsequent follow-through.

Child Health

ACTIONS/INTERVENTIONS	RATIONALES
• Determine how the parent and child perceive the deficit addressed by setting aside adequate time (30 min) each shift for discussion and listening.	Appropriate attention to both subjective as well as objective data is required to best plan care.

- Stress the importance of follow-up evaluation for any suspected sensory deficits or infants and young children.
- Allow for extra anticipatory safety needs according to sensory deficit and child's developmental capacity.
- Initiate plans for home dismissal at least 4 days before discharge to allow time for instilling confidence in performance of necessary tasks according to deficit.

- Provide attention to family coping as it may relate to the deficit:
  ○ Assessment of usual dynamics
  ○ Identification of impact on parents and siblings
  ○ Presence of mental deficits
  ○ Values regarding the deficit
  ○ Support systems
- Review for appropriate immunization, especially rubella, mumps, and measles.

- In presence of ear infections, exercise caution regarding use of ototoxic medications such as gentamicin.

- Correlate medical history for potential risk factors such as chronic middle ear infections, upper respiratory infections, or allergies.
- Provide appropriate sensory stimulation for age, beginning slowly so as not to overload child.
- Deal with other contributory factors such as nutrition, illness.
- Include parents in plans for rehabilitation whenever possible by:
  ○ Using basic plan for care
  ○ Adapting intervention as required for child
  ○ Supporting them in their role
  ○ Pointing out opportune times for interaction
  ○ Informing them of appropriate safety precautions for age and situation
  ○ Encouraging gentle handling and comforting of infant
- Provide continuity in staffing for nursing care of child and family.
- In instances of handicapped child, provide appropriate attention to developing sequencing to best actualize potential offered.
- Especially note, on follow-up, the home environment for nurturing aspects and support systems.

Preventing or minimizing secondary and tertiary deficits is enhanced by appropriate attention to sensory-perceptual follow-up.

Sensory deficits and developmental capacity increase the risk of accidents.

Adequate practice time in a nonjudgmental situation allows positive feedback and corrective action. Lessens anxiety and performance pressures. Increases confidence in giving care at home.

A child with sensory-perceptual problems and the interventions necessary to deal with this problem place strain on the family. Promoting coping will lessen strain for the family while increasing the likelihood that the child's needs will be met.

In the event of early deficits, the likelihood exists for the need to modify the schedule of immunization. This is too often overlooked and will then place the infant or child at unnecessary risk for infectious diseases.

Treatment for chronic infections with antibiotics by several practitioners must be carried out with precaution for potential side effects.

Contributory factors to the pattern of health must be pursued with openness to all possible causes.

Appropriate sensory stimulation will favor gradual progress in development.

Related factors must be considered in total health of infant or child with altered sensory-perceptual pattern.

Inclusion of parents provides an opportunity for learning essential skills and enhances security of the infant or child. All efforts contribute to empowerment and potential growth of the family unit.

Continuity provides trust and opportunities for reinforcement of learning.

Appropriate introduction of new skills or reinforcement of existent patterns will favor progress.

The home to which the infant or child will go may require reasonable adaptation to foster appropriate resources.

Women's Health

ACTIONS/INTERVENTIONS	RATIONALES
VISION - Monitor patient for signs of pregnancy-induced hypertension (PIH). - Monitor for signs and symptoms of preeclampsia, e.g., headaches, visual changes such as blurred vision, increased edema of face, oliguria, hyperreflexia, nausea or vomiting, and epigastric pain.	Knowledge of signs of visual disturbances being associated with PIH can assist the patient in seeking early treatment.

Continued

ACTIONS/INTERVENTIONS	RATIONALES
• Teach patient the importance of reporting the above signs and symptoms, as they can be precursors to eclampsia.	

SMELL

• Be aware of patient's tendency during early pregnancy to experience morning sickness, i.e., nausea and vomiting.
 • In collaboration with dietitian:
  ○ Obtain dietary history.
  ○ Assist patient in planning diet that will provide adequate nutrition for her and her fetus's needs.
 • Teach methods for coping with gastric upset, nausea, and vomiting:
  ○ Eating bland, low-fat foods
  ○ Increasing carbohydrate intake
  ○ Eating small, frequent meals
  ○ Having dry crackers or toast before getting out of bed
  ○ Taking vitamins and iron with snack before going to bed
  ○ Supplementing diet with high-protein liquids, e.g., soups or eggnog
	Knowledge can assist patient in planning actions to decrease incidences of nausea and vomiting and assist in preventing dehydration and possibly hospitalization.

TOUCH DURING PREGNANCY

• Be aware of expectant mother's sensitivity to extraneous touching:
  ○ Shyness
  ○ Protectiveness of unborn child
  ○ Uterine sensitivity during pregnancy and particularly during labor
	Assists mother to know her feelings are normal.

MATERNAL TOUCH

• Encourage visual and tactile contact between mother and infant as soon as possible. • Provide conducive atmosphere for continual mother-infant contact. • Delay newborn eye treatment for 1 h, so that baby can see mother's face.	Provides time for beginning attachment process between mother and infant.

KINESTHESIA

• Be aware of expectant mother's increased vulnerability related to physical size of body in third trimester:
  ○ Protectiveness of unborn child
  ○ Heavy movement
  ○ Possible slowed reflexes
  ○ Tires easily
 • Assist in and out of furniture that is too low and difficult to get out of.
 • Encourage correct body mechanics when lying down or sitting up.
 • Encourage to wear seat belt when traveling in auto (shoulder belt best).
	Reassures mothers that this is a temporary state.
	
	 Provides for safety measures for mother and fetus.

Psychiatric Health

ACTIONS/INTERVENTIONS	RATIONALES
• Monitor client's neurologic status as indicated by current condition and history of deficit; e.g., if deficit is recent, assessment would be conducted on a schedule that could range from every 15 min to every 8 h. Note frequency and times of checks here. If checks are to be very frequent, then it might be useful to keep a record of these checks on a flow sheet.	Client safety is of primary importance. Early recognition and intervention can prevent serious alterations.
• If deficit is determined to result from a psychologic rather than a physiologic dysfunction, refer to Ineffective Individual Coping, Body Image Disturbance, Anxiety, and Self-Esteem Disturbance for detailed nursing actions.	Client safety is of primary importance.

NOTE: A comprehensive physical examination and other diagnostic evaluations should be completed before this determination is made. Each of these deficits can be symptoms of severe physiologic or neurologic dysfunction and should be approached with this understanding, especially in a mental health environment where the clients may be assigned without careful assessment. This is a great risk for the client who has a history of mental health problems.

ACTIONS/INTERVENTIONS	RATIONALES
• If deficit is related to a physiologic dysfunction, attend to needs resulting from the identified sensory deficit in a matter-of-fact manner, providing basic care and having client do the majority of the care.	Provides positive reinforcement for adaptive coping behaviors.
• If deficit is related to a psychologic dysfunction, spend 15 min every hour with the client in an activity that is not related to the sensory deficit. If the client begins to focus on the deficit, terminate the interaction.	Promotes client's sense of control and increases self-esteem.
• Spend 1 h twice a day discussing with the client the effects the deficit will have on his or her life and developing alternative coping behavior. Note times for conversations here. If family is involved in the client's care, they should be included in a planned number of these interactions.	
• Refer to appropriate mental health professional if client is going to require long-term assistance in adapting to the deficit or if current emotional adaptation becomes complicated.	
• Discuss with client and support system the necessary alterations that may be necessary in the home environment to facilitate daily living activities.	Promotes client's sense of control.

AUDITORY OR VISUAL ALTERATIONS[57–60]

ACTIONS/INTERVENTIONS	RATIONALES
• Observe for signs of hallucinations (intent listening for no apparent reason, talking to someone when no one is present, muttering to self, stopping in midsentence, or unusual posturing). When these symptoms are noted, engage client in here-and-now, reality-oriented conversation or involve client in here-and-now activity.	Interrupts patterns of hallucinations.
• Initiate touch only after warning client that you are going to touch him or her.	Client may perceive touch as a threat and respond in an aggressive manner.
• Communicate acceptance to the client to encourage the sharing of the content of the hallucination.	Provides information on the content of the hallucination so early intervention can be initiated when content suggests harm to client or others.

Continued

ACTIONS/INTERVENTIONS	RATIONALES
• If hallucinations place client at risk for self-harm or harm to others, place client on one-on-one observation or in seclusion.	Client and staff safety are of primary importance.
• If client is placed in seclusion, interact with client at least every 15 min.	Provides reality orientation and assists client in controlling the hallucinations.
• Have client tell staff when hallucinations are present or when they are interfering with client's ability to interact with others.	Early intervention promotes client's sense of safety and control.
• Maintain environment in a manner that does not enhance hallucinations, e.g., television programs that validate client's hallucinations, abstract art on the walls, wallpaper with abstract designs, or designs that enhance imagination.	High levels of environmental stimuli can increase the client's disorganization and confusion.

• Teach client to control hallucinations by:
  ○ Checking ideas out with trusted others
  ○ Practicing thought stopping by singing to self, telling the voices to go away (this can be done quietly to self, or asking the voices to come back later, but not to talk now)
	Promotes client's sense of control and enhances self-esteem.

• Talk with client about ways to distract himself or herself from the hallucinations, such as physical exercise or playing a game or a craft that takes a great deal of concentration. (Note those activities preferred by client here.)	
• When signs of client's hallucinating are present, assist client in initiating those activities or other control behaviors that have been identified by the client as useful.	Reinforces new coping behaviors and increases client's perceived control.
• As client's condition improves, primary nurse will assist client to identify onset of hallucinations and situations that facilitate their onset.	Facilitates the development of alternative coping behaviors.
• As difficult situations are identified, primary nurse can begin working with client on alternative ways of coping with these situations. (Note alternative coping behaviors selected by client here.)	Promotes client's sense of control and self-esteem.
• Refer client and support system to appropriate support systems in the community, e.g., Compeer. (Contact local mental health association for the program in your community also.)	

Gerontic Health

The nursing actions for the gerontic patient with this diagnosis are the same as those for the adult health patient.

Home Health

ACTIONS/INTERVENTIONS	RATIONALES

• Teach client and family measures to prevent sensory deficit:
  ○ Use of protective gear, e.g., goggles, sunglasses, earplugs, or special clothing in hazardous conditions to prevent radiation, sun, or chemical burns
  ○ Avoidance of sharp or projectile toys
  ○ Prevention of injuries to eyes, ears, skin, nose, and tongue
	Family and client involvement in basic safety measures enhances the effectiveness of preventive measures.

ACTIONS/INTERVENTIONS	RATIONALES
○ Prevention of nutritional deficiencies ○ Close monitoring of medications that may be toxic to the eighth cranial nerve ○ Correct usage of contact lenses ○ Prevention of fluid and electrolyte imbalances	
• Involve client and family in planning, implementing, and promoting correction or compensation for sensory deficit (specify) by (date): ○ Family conference ○ Mutual goal setting ○ Communication, e.g., use of memorabilia and audio or videotapes provided by family members to stimulate in cases of impaired communication.[61]	Involvement improves motivation. Communication and mutual goals increase the probability of positive outcomes.
• Assist patient and family in lifestyle adjustments that may be required: ○ Assistance with activities of daily living ○ Adjustment to and usage of assistive devices, e.g., hearing aid, corrective lenses, or magnifying glass ○ Providing safe environment, e.g., protecting kinesthetically impaired from burns ○ Stopping substance abuse ○ Changes in family and work role relationships ○ Techniques of communicating with individual with auditory or visual impairment ○ Providing meaningful stimulation ○ Special transportation needs ○ Special education needs	Lifestyle changes require change in behavior. Self-evaluation and support facilitate these changes.
• Consult with or refer patient to appropriate assistive resources as indicated.	Use of the network of existing community services provides for effective utilization of resources.

Sensory-Perceptual Alterations (Specify: Visual, Auditory, Kinesthetic, Gustatory, Tactile, Olfactory)

FLOWCHART EVALUATION: EXPECTED OUTCOME 1

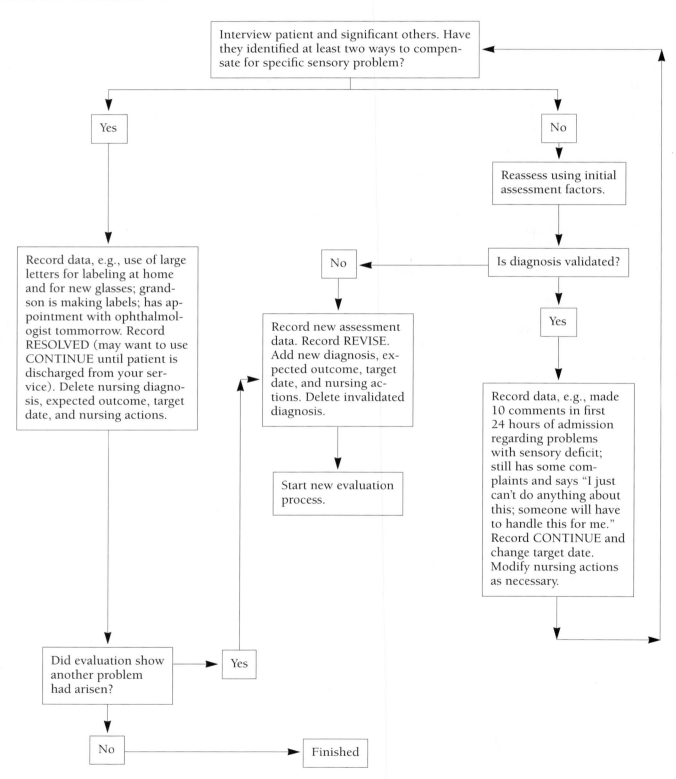

Sensory-Perceptual Alterations (Specify: Visual, Auditory, Kinesthetic, Gustatory, Tactile, Olfactory)

FLOWCHART EVALUATION: EXPECTED OUTCOME 2

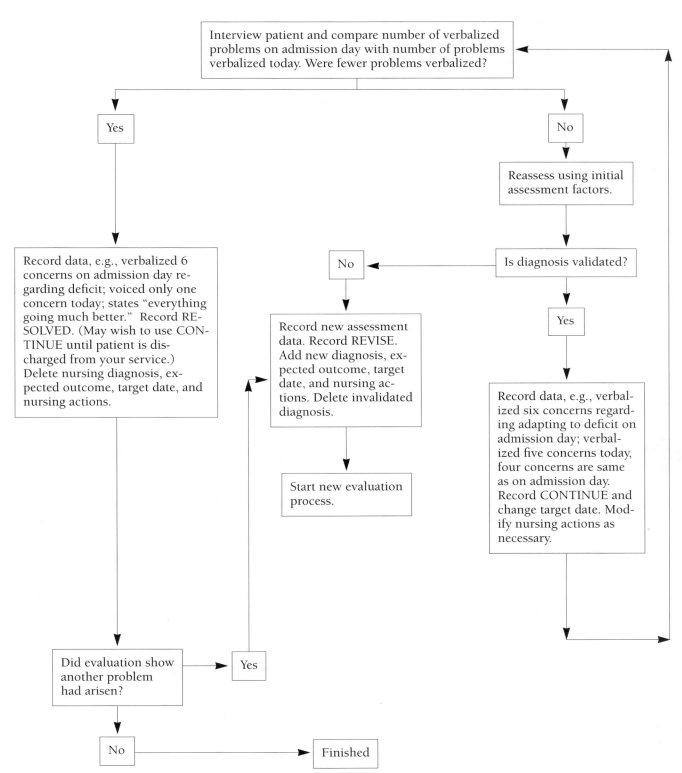

Thought Process, Altered

DEFINITION

A state in which an individual experiences a disruption in cognitive operations and activities.[2]

NANDA TAXONOMY: KNOWING 8.3

NOTE: The 1994 Preconference Workgroup for this diagnosis suggested expansion of this diagnosis into Distorted Thought, Impaired Cognition, Altered Level of Consciousness, and Acute Confusion. Subcategories under Distorted Thought include Altered Thought Content, Altered Thought Form, and Thought Insertion. Subcategories under Impaired Cognition include Attention, Memory, Learning, Sensory Reception, Perception, Language, and Problem Solving. Under the heading Altered Level of Consciousness are the subcategories of Altered Awareness, Coma and Persistent Vegetative State. The category of Acute Confusion was developed as a separate diagnosis. Rather than expanding this content, at this time, the authors have chosen to remain with the diagnoses accepted, and the reader is referred to the latest edition of the taxonomy for further details.

DEFINING CHARACTERISTICS[2]

1. Major defining characteristics
   a. Inaccurate interpretation of environment
   b. Cognitive dissonance
   c. Distractibility
   d. Memory deficit or problems
   e. Egocentricity
   f. Hyper- or Hypovigilance
2. Other possible characteristics
   a. Inappropriate, nonreality-based thinking

RELATED FACTORS[2]

To be developed.

RELATED CLINICAL CONCERNS

1. Dementia
2. Neurologic diseases impacting the brain
3. Head injuries
4. Medication overdose, for example, digitalis, sedatives, or narcotics
5. Major depression
6. Bipolar disorder, manic or depressive or mixed
7. Schizophrenic disorders
8. Dissociative disorders
9. Obsessive-compulsive disorders
10. Paranoid disorder
11. Delirium
12. Eating disorders

HAVE YOU SELECTED THE CORRECT DIAGNOSIS?

Sensory-Perceptual Alterations   This diagnosis refers to deficits or overloads in sensory inputs. If the patient is having difficulty with sight, hearing, or any of the other senses, then a confused patient might well be the result. Double-check the pattern assessment to be sure sensory deficit is not the primary problem.

Altered Health Maintenance   The diagnosis of Altered Thought Process might well contribute to Altered Health Maintenance. In this case, Altered Thought Process and Altered Health Maintenance would be companion diagnoses.

EXPECTED OUTCOMES

1. Will have at least a (number) percent decrease in signs and symptoms of Altered Thought Process by (date) and/or
2. Will be oriented to time, person, and place by (date)

TARGET DATES

A target date of 5 days would be acceptable since this can be a very long range problem.

NURSING ACTIONS/INTERVENTIONS WITH RATIONALES

Adult Health

ACTIONS/INTERVENTIONS	RATIONALES

• Monitor, at least every 4 h while awake:
  ○ Vital signs
  ○ Neurologic status, particularly for signs and symptoms of ICP
  ○ Mental status
  ○ Laboratory values for metabolic alkalosis, hypokalemia, increased ammonia levels, or infection
	Assists in determining pathophysiologic causes for altered thought process.

• Collaborate with psychiatric nurse clinician and rehabilitation nurse specialist.	Collaboration provides the best plan of care.

• Consistently provide a safe, calm environment:
  ○ Provide siderails on bed.
  ○ Keep room uncluttered.
  ○ Reorient client at each contact.
  ○ Reduce extraneous stimuli; e.g., limit noise and visitors, and reduce bright lighting.
  ○ Use touch judiciously.
  ○ Prepare patient for all procedures by explaining simply and concisely.
  ○ Provide good, but not intensely bright, lighting.
  ○ Have family bring clock, calendar, and familiar objects from home.
	Basic safety measures and reinforcement of reality.

• Design communications according to patient's best means of communication, e.g., writing, visuals, or sound:
  ○ Give simple, concise directions.
  ○ Listen carefully.
  ○ Present reality consistently.
  ○ Do not challenge illogical thinking.
	Enhances communication and quality of care.

• Encourage patient to use prosthetic or assistive devices, e.g., glasses, dentures, hearing aid, or walker.	Increases sensory input and reinforces reality.
• Provide frequent rest periods.	Reduces environmental stimuli that could contribute to confusion and helps to avoid sensory overload.
• Provide consistent approach in nursing care and routine.	Inspires trust, reinforces reality, decreases sensory stimuli, and provides memory cues.
• Encourage self-care to the extent possible.	Increases self-esteem, forces reality check, decreases powerlessness, and provides a means of evaluating patient's status.
• Involve significant others in care, and include them in teaching sessions.	Provides social support and consistency in management.
• Refer patient to and collaborate with appropriate assistive resources	Provides for long-term support and a more holistic approach to care.

Child Health

ACTIONS/INTERVENTIONS	RATIONALES
• Monitor cognitive capacity according to age and developmental capacity. • Note discrepancies in chronologic age and mastery of developmental milestones.	Basic data needed to plan individualized care.

Continued

ACTIONS/INTERVENTIONS	RATIONALES
• Provide ongoing reality orientation for the patient by encouraging his or her family to visit and by emphasizing time, personal awareness, and gradual resumption of daily routine to degree possible.	As the patient attempts to reorient, it is helpful that date, time, and specific concrete planning, hour by hour, are offered. The infant should be reintroduced to data, in a calm manner, that will assist him or her in regaining some control over the environment and in regaining the previous functioning level so that he or she can, hopefully, continue to progress.
• Provide anticipatory safety to reflect greater range of potentials according to psychomotor capacity.	Altered thought process serves as a high-risk factor for all involved. It would be a reasonable standard of care to increase all anticipatory safety efforts.
• Encourage family members to express concerns for child's condition by allowing 30 min each shift for discussion.	Promotes ventilation, which helps reduce anxiety and offers insight into thoughts about patient's condition.
• Provide for primary health needs, including administration of medications, comfort measures, and control of environment to aid in child's adaptation.	Attention to regular health needs must also be considered as the whole person is considered.
• Structure the room in a manner that befits the child's needs.	Keeping the environment adapted to personal needs will facilitate care, minimize the chance for accidents, and demonstrate the needed structure.
• Allow for ample rest periods according to sleep patterns during health and within parameters for age-related sleep needs.	Rest is a key and essential consideration to provide optimal potential for cognitive-perceptual functioning.
• Monitor for existence of other patterns, especially altered coping and role performance.	All contributing factors must be explored to ensure meeting the patient's needs.
• Assist family in dismissal plans by utilization of appropriate state and community resources.	Improves family adjustment and coping by assisting in preparing for home needs. Empowerment hopefully then permits them the opportunity for growth in coping skills and parenting.
• If institutionalization is required, assist family in learning about related issues such as visitations, medical records maintenance, prognosis, and risk factors.	Planning provides the means for coping and adjusting to the move with an opportunity for clarification. Provides advocacy for patient and family.
• Maintain ethical and legal confidentiality on patient's behalf.	Standard practice must include safeguarding the patient's needs for confidentiality and legal rights.
• Allow for culturally unique aspects in management of care, e.g., respect for visitation on religious holidays, family wishes for diet, and bathing.	Increases individuation and satisfaction with care. Shows respect for family's values. Enhances nurse-patient relationship.
• Provide for appropriate follow-up by making appointments for next clinic visits.	Follow-up arrangements for clinic visits enhances the likelihood of follow-up and demonstrates the importance of follow-up care.
• Allow family members opportunities for learning necessary care and mastery of content for long-term needs such as resolution of conflicts related to institutionalization or respite care and prognosis.	Anticipatory learning serves to minimize crises related to the child's condition.

Women's Health

This nursing diagnosis will pertain to the woman the same as any other adult.

Psychiatric Health

ACTIONS/INTERVENTIONS	RATIONALES
• Monitor client's level of anxiety and refer to Anxiety, Chap. 8, for detailed interventions related to this diagnosis. • Speak to client in brief, clear sentences.	Too much information can increase the client's confusion and disorganization. The amount of time devoted to interaction should be guided by the client's attention span.[62]

- Keep initial interactions short but frequent. Interact with client for (number) minutes every 30 min. Begin with 5-min interactions, and gradually increase the times of interactions.
- Assign the client a primary care nurse on each shift to assume responsibility for gaining a relationship of trust with the client.
- Be consistent in all interactions with the client.

- Set limits on inappropriate behavior that increase the risk of the client's or others' being harmed. Note the limits here as well as revisions to the limits.
- Initially place client in an area with little stimulation.

- Orient client to the environment, and assign someone to provide one-on-one interaction while client orients to unit.
- Do not make promises that cannot be kept.
- Inform client of your availability to talk with him or her; do not pry or ask many questions.
- Do not argue with client about delusions; inform client in a matter-of-fact way that this is not your experience of the situation, e.g., "I do not think I am angry with you."
- Recognize and support client's feelings, e.g., "You sound frightened."
- Respond to the feelings being expressed in delusions or hallucinations.
- Initially have client involved in one-to-one activities; as condition improves, gradually increase the size of the interaction group. Note current level of functioning here.
- Have client clarify those thoughts you do not understand. Do not pretend to understand that which you do not.
- Do not attempt to change delusional thinking with rational explanations.
- After listening to delusion once, do not engage in conversations related to this material or focus conversations on this material.
- Focus conversations on here-and-now content related to real things in the environment or to activities on the units.
- Do not belittle or be judgmental about the client's delusional beliefs.
- Avoid nonverbal behavior that indicates agreeing with delusional beliefs.
- When client's behavior and anxiety level indicate readiness, place client in small-group situations. Client will spend (number) minutes in group activities (number) times a day. (Time and frequency will increase as client's ability to cope with these situations improves.)
- Develop a daily schedule for the client that encourages focus on "here and now" and is adapted to client's level of functioning so that success can be experienced. Note daily schedule here.
- Assign client meaningful roles in unit activities. Provide roles that can be easily accomplished by client to provide successful experiences. Note client responsibilities here.
- Primary nurse will spend (amount) minutes with client twice a day to discuss client's feelings and the effects of the delusions on the client's life. (Number of minutes and the degree of exploration of client's feelings will increase as client develops relationship with nurse.)

Facilitates the development of a trusting relationship.

Facilitates the development of a trusting relationship.

Facilitates the development of a trusting relationship and meets the client's safety needs.
Client and staff safety are of primary importance.

Inappropriate levels of sensory stimuli can contribute to client's sense of disorganization and confusion.
Promotes client's safety needs while facilitating the development of a trusting relationship.

Facilitates the development of a trusting relationship.
Communicates acceptance of the client, which facilitates the development of trust and self-esteem.
May reinforce client's need to maintain the delusional system and interferes with the development of a trusting relationship.
Focuses on client's real feelings and concerns.

High levels of environmental stimuli may increase confusion and disorganization.

Facilitates the development of a trusting relationship and prevents inadvertent support of the delusional thinking.

This may encourage client to cling to these thoughts.

Decreases the possibility of supporting or reinforcing the delusion.

Facilitates the client's contact with reality.[58]

Protects the client's self-esteem.

Decreases the possibility of supporting or reinforcing the delusion.
Provides feedback about delusional beliefs from peers.

Facilitates client's contact with reality. Promotes positive self-image.

Facilitates client's contact with reality. Promotes positive self-image.

Assists in the development of alternative coping behaviors.

ACTIONS/INTERVENTIONS	RATIONALES
• Provide rewards to client for accomplishing task progress on the daily schedule. These rewards should be meaningful to the client.	Positive feedback encourages productive behavior.
• Spend (number) minutes twice a day walking with client. This should start at 10-min intervals and gradually increase. This can be replaced by any physical activity the client finds enjoyable. A staff member should be with the client during this activity to provide social reinforcement to the client for accomplishing the activity.	Facilitates the development of a trusting relationship. Social interaction provides positive reinforcement. Helps to increase daytime wakefulness, promoting a normal sleep-wakefulness cycle.
• Arrange a consultation with the occupational therapist to assist client in developing or continuing special interests.	Increases daytime wakefulness, maintaining a normal sleep-rest cycle.
• Monitor delusional beliefs for potential of harming self or others.	Patient and staff safety are of primary concern.
• Note any change in behavior that would indicate a change in the delusional beliefs that could signal a risk for violence.	Patient and staff safety are of primary concern.
• If client is placed in seclusion, interact with client at least once every 15 min.	Provides reality orientation and assists client with controlling hallucinations and delusions.
• Maintain environment that does not stimulate client's delusions; e.g., if client has delusions related to religion, limit discussions of religion and religious activity on unit to very concrete terms. Limit interaction with persons who stimulate delusional thinking.	Excessive environmental stimuli can increase confusion and disorganization.
• Primary nurse will assist client in identifying signs and symptoms of increasing thought disorganization and in developing a plan to cope with these situations before they get out of control. This will be done in the regular scheduled interaction times between the primary nurse and client.	Promotes client's sense of control and enhances self-esteem.
• As client's condition improves, primary nurse will assist client to identify onset delusions with periods of increasing anxiety.	Facilitates client's developing alternative coping behaviors.
• As connection is made between thought disorder and anxiety, client will be assisted to identify specific anxiety-producing situations and learn alternative coping behaviors. See Anxiety for specific interventions.	Promotes client's sense of control and enhances self-esteem.
• Refer client to outpatient support systems and assist him or her with making arrangements for contacting these sources before discharge.	Facilitates client's reintegration into the community.

Gerontic Health

NOTE: Problems related to Altered Thought Process with older adults may present themselves in various ways. Two conditions, dementia and delirium (acute confused state), are considered here. Irreversible dementia, such as Alzheimer's or multi-infarct dementia, is usually progressive, gradual in onset, of long duration, and has a steady downward course. Delirium, or acute confusional state, presents with acute onset, is of short duration, has a fluctuating course, and is often reversible with treatment.[63] Nursing interventions vary, depending on the course of the Altered Thought Process.

ACTIONS/INTERVENTIONS	RATIONALES

Dementia

- Maintain safe environment. Avoid leaving solutions, equipment, or medications near the patient that could result in injury through misuse or ingestion.
- Monitor environment to prevent overstimulating the patient with light, sounds, and frequent activity.
- Schedule activities that are of short duration (usually 20-min sessions).
- Use short sentences and clear directions when communicating with the patient.
- Determine self-care abilities that are intact, and encourage continued participation in these activities.
- Monitor food and fluid intake to determine that nutritional status is adequate.
- Provide consistent staff.
- Refer family to local Alzheimer's and related diseases support group.

Patient is unable to determine the harmful consequences of misuse.

With dementia, the patient has a reduced threshold for stress.
Prevents stresses on an individual already suffering from attention deficits and anxiety.
Allows processing of basic information without distraction.
Provides stimulation and sense of pride. Promotes physical activity.

Reduces anxiety.
Provides long-term support.

Delirium

- Monitor for conditions that can induce delirium.

Certain factors such as electrolyte imbalance, preoperative dehydration, unanticipated surgery, intraoperative hypotension, postoperative hypothermia, and a large number of medications have been found to be associated with acute confusional states in older adults.[64,65]

- Provide orienting information to the patient as often as necessary.
- Ensure that sensory deficits are corrected to extent possible.
- Provide consistent staff
- Provide sensory stimulation such as bathing, touching, and back massages.

Provides information to the patient about the current situation and assists in reducing anxiety and confusion.
Correcting sensory deficits enhances the patient's ability to use available cues to person, place, and time.
Avoids adding to confusion and promotes patient's security.
Assists in restoring the patient's sense of body image.[66]

Home Health

ACTIONS/INTERVENTIONS	RATIONALES

- Teach client and family to monitor for signs and symptoms of impaired thought process:
  - Poor hygiene
  - Poor decision making or judgment
  - Regression in behavior
  - Delusions
  - Hallucinations
  - Changes in interpersonal relationship
  - Distractibility
- Involve client and family in planning, implementing, and promoting appropriate thought processing:
  - Family conference
  - Mutual goal setting
  - Communication
- Assist client and family in lifestyle adjustments that may be necessary:
  - Providing safety and prevention of injury
  - Providing frequent orientation to person, place, and time
  - Providing reality testing and patient verification

Basic monitoring that allows for early intervention

Involvement improves cooperation and motivation, thereby increasing the probability of an improved outcome.

Continued

ACTIONS/INTERVENTIONS	RATIONALES
○ Providing reality testing and patient verification ○ Assisting in working through alterations in role functions in family or at work ○ Stopping substance abuse ○ Facilitating family communication ○ Setting limits ○ Learning new skills ○ Decreasing risk for violence ○ Preventing suicide ○ Explaining possible chronicity of disorder ○ Referring client to community resources for financial assistance ○ Reducing sensory overload ○ Teaching stress management ○ Teaching relaxation techniques ○ Referring client and family to support groups • Assist client and family to set criteria to help them to determine when professional intervention is required. • Teach client and family purposes, side effects, and proper administration techniques for medications. • Consult with or refer patient to appropriate assistive resources as required.	Early identification of issues requiring professional evaluation will increase the probability of successful interventions. Provides necessary information for client and family that promotes safe self-care. Efficient and cost-effective use of community resources.

Thought Process, Altered

FLOWCHART EVALUATION: EXPECTED OUTCOME 1

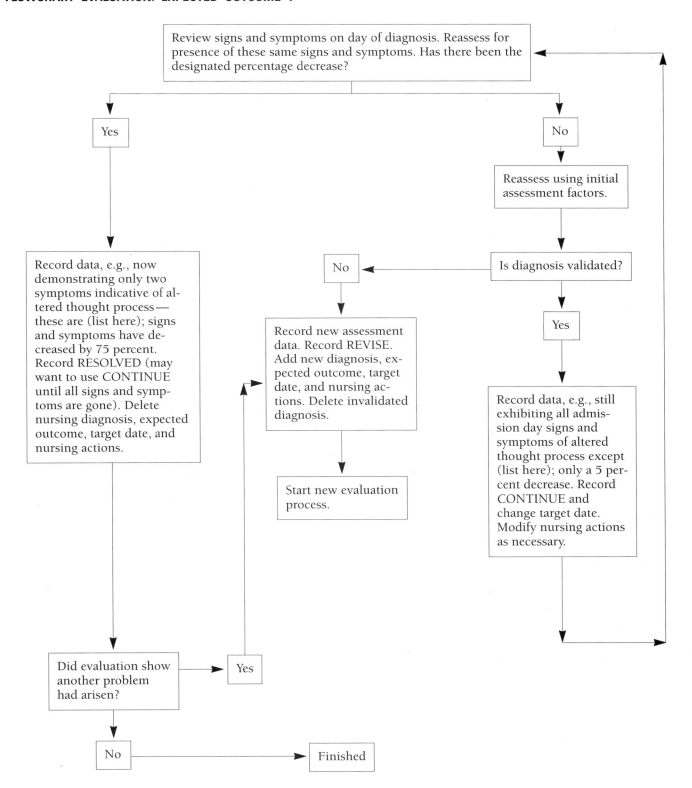

Thought Process, Altered

FLOWCHART EVALUATION: EXPECTED OUTCOME 2

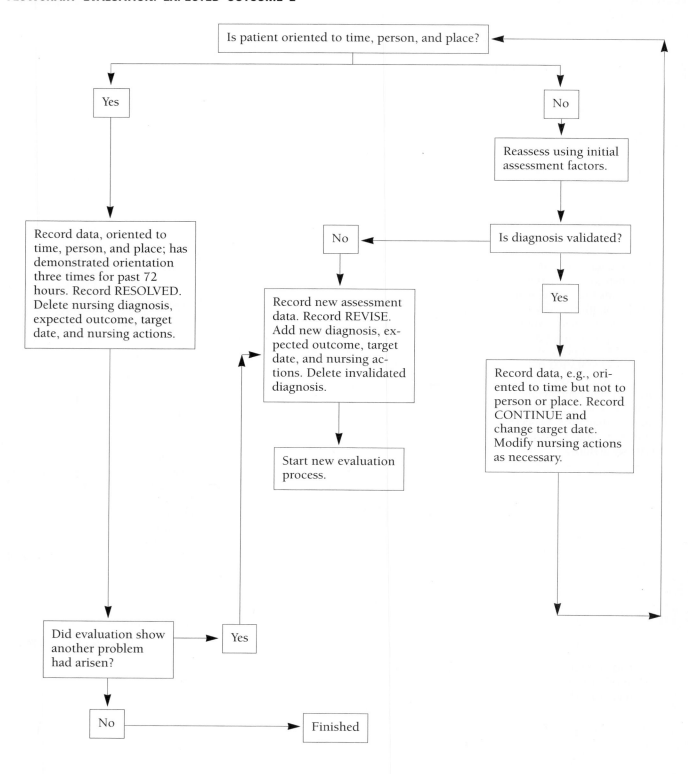

Unilateral Neglect

DEFINITION

A state in which an individual is perceptually unaware of, and inattentive to, one side of the body.[2]

NANDA TAXONOMY: PERCEIVING 7.2.1.1

DEFINING CHARACTERISTICS[2]

1. Major defining characteristics
   a. Consistent inattention to stimuli on an affected side
2. Minor defining characteristics
   a. Inadequate self-care
   b. Positioning and/or safety precautions in regard to the affected side

c. Does not look toward affected side
d. Leaves food on plate on the affected side

RELATED FACTORS[2]

1. Effects of disturbed perceptual abilities, for example, hemianopsia
2. One-sided blindness
3. Neurologic illness or trauma

RELATED CLINICAL CONCERNS

1. Cerebrovascular accident
2. Glaucoma
3. Blindness secondary to diabetes mellitus
4. Spinal cord injury
5. Amputation
6. Ruptured cerebral aneurysm
7. Brain trauma

HAVE YOU SELECTED THE CORRECT DIAGNOSIS?

Sensory-Perceptual Alterations This diagnosis refers to a problem with receiving sensory input and interpretation of this input. Unilateral Neglect could be, as indicated by the related factors, an outcome of this disturbance in sensory input and/or perception of this input.

EXPECTED OUTCOMES

1. Will return-demonstrate at least (number) measures to reduce the effect of unilateral neglect by (date) and/or
2. Will have decreased signs and symptoms of unilateral neglect by (date)

TARGET DATES

A target date between 5 and 7 days would be appropriate to evaluate initial progress.

NURSING ACTIONS/INTERVENTIONS WITH RATIONALES

Adult Health

ACTIONS/INTERVENTIONS	RATIONALES
• Frequently remind patient to attend to both sides of his or her body.	Repetition improves brain processing
• Assist patient to touch and feel neglected side of body. Help patient, by providing a variety of sensations (warm, cool, soft, harsh, etc.), to become more aware of and articulate sensations on neglected side.	Increases brain's awareness of neglected side.
• Assist patient with ROM exercises to neglected side of body every 4 h while awake at (times). Teach extent of movement of each joint on neglected side of body.	Increases brain's awareness of neglected side and maintains muscle tone and joint mobility.
• Help patient to position neglected side of body in a similar way as attended side of body whenever position is changed.	
• Remind patient to turn plate during each meal.	Assists patient to notice all of food and increases cues to brain.
• Turn every 2 h on the (odd/even) hours. Monitor skin condition on each turning.	Improves circulation. Relieves pressure areas. Avoids skin breakdown on affected side.
• Refer to rehabilitation nurse clinician.	Collaboration provides a more holistic plan of care and rehabilitation nurse will have most up-to-date knowledge regarding this diagnosis.

Child Health

NOTE: See nursing actions under Sensory-Perceptual Alterations in addition to those listed here.

ACTIONS/INTERVENTIONS	RATIONALES
• Allow 30 min every shift for patient and family to express how they perceive the unilateral neglect.	Ventilation of feelings is paramount in understanding the effect the problem has on the patient and the family; it is also critical as a means of evaluating needs.
• Determine how the unilateral neglect affects the usual expected behavior or development for the child.	Previous and/or current developmental capacity may be affected by the unilateral neglect depending on the degree of severity. To be able to judge the best means of therapy requires these data to be considered, e.g., does the child use the affected hand as a helper or not try to use it at all?
• Monitor for presence of secondary or tertiary deficits.	Identification of primary deficits should alert all to monitor for possible secondary and tertiary deficits to minimize further sequelae, which can be treated early.
• Establish, with family input, appropriate anticipatory safety guidelines that are based on the unilateral neglect and the developmental capacity of the child.	Safety needs and measures must reflect the developmental capacity of the child and slightly beyond it. There is a special need to structure the environment to allow for appropriate exploratory behavior while maintaining safety without overprotection.
• Stress appropriate follow-up prior to dismissal from hospital with workable time frame for family.	Arrangement for follow-up increases the likelihood of compliance and shows the importance of follow-up.

Women's Health

This nursing diagnosis will pertain to women the same as any other adult.

Psychiatric Health

Nursing interventions for this diagnosis are those described in Adult Health.

Gerontic Health

The nursing orders for the older adult with this diagnosis are the same as those for adults.

Home Health

ACTIONS/INTERVENTIONS	RATIONALES
• Monitor for factors contributing to unilateral neglect, e.g., disturbed perceptual abilities, neurologic disease, or trauma.	This action provides the database needed to identify interventions that will prevent or diminish unilateral neglect.
• Involve client and family in planning, implementing, and promoting reduction in effects of unilateral neglect:	Family involvement is important to ensure success. Communication and mutual goals improve the outcome.
○ Schedule family conferences, e.g., to discuss concerns family members have.	
○ Encourage the family's ideas for addressing the concern.	
○ Set mutual goals, e.g., establish two measures to offset the effect of unilateral neglect. Be sure roles for the participants are identified.	
○ Maintain communication.	
○ Provide support for caregiver, e.g., plan respite time for primary caregiver. Alternate caregivers are identified and trained.	
• Teach client and family measures to decrease effects of unilateral neglect:	These actions diminish the negative effects of unilateral neglect.
○ Active and passive ROM exercises	

- ○ Ambulation with assistive devices (canes, walkers, or crutches)
- ○ Objects placed within field of vision and reach
- ○ Assistive eating utensils
- ○ Assistive dressing utensils
- ○ Safe environment, e.g., objects removed from area outside field of vision
- Assist family and client to identify lifestyle changes that may be required:
  - ○ Change in role functions
  - ○ Coping with disability or dependency
  - ○ Obtaining and using assistive equipment
  - ○ Coping with assistive equipment
  - ○ Maintaining safe environment
- Consult with appropriate assistive resources as indicated.

Lifestyle changes require changes in behavior. Self-evaluation and support facilitate these changes.

Appropriate use of existing community services is effective use of resources.

Unilateral Neglect

FLOWCHART EVALUATION: EXPECTED OUTCOME 1

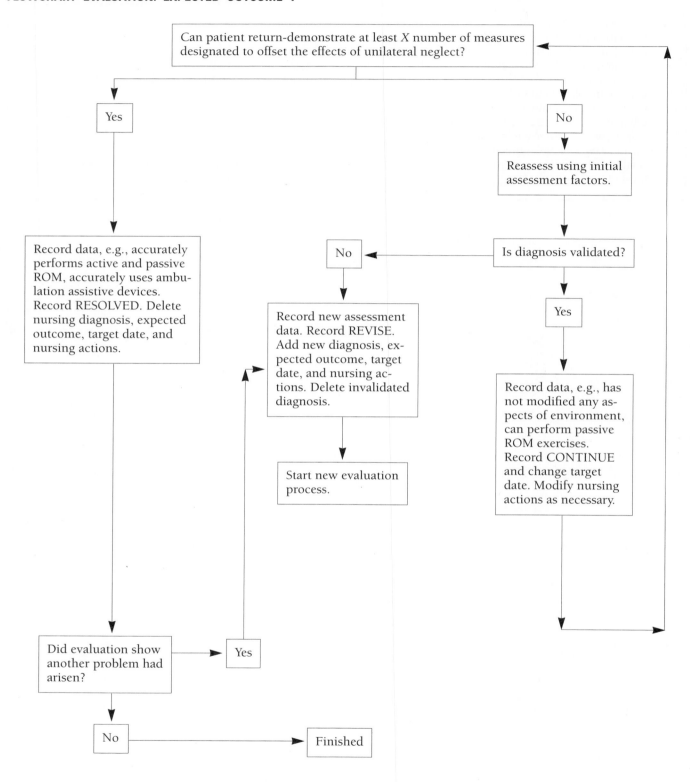

Unilateral Neglect

FLOWCHART EVALUATION: EXPECTED OUTCOME 2

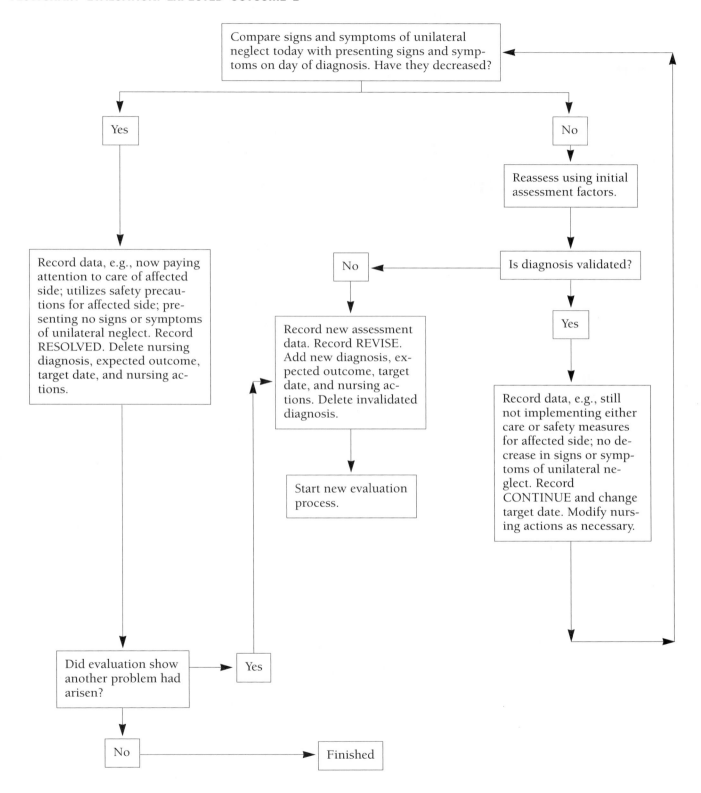

8

Self-Perception and Self-Concept Pattern

Pattern Description

As the nurse interacts with the client, the most important knowledge the client contributes is self-knowledge. It is this knowledge that determines the individual's manner of interaction with others. This knowledge base is most often labeled "self-concept." One's self-concept is composed of beliefs and attitudes about the self, body image, self-esteem, and information about abilities. The individual's behavior is not only affected by those experiences prior to interactions with the health care system but also by interactions with the health care system.

Pattern Assessment

1. Does the patient express concern regarding the current situation?
   a. Yes (Anxiety or Fear)
   b. No
2. Can the patient identify source of concern?
   a. Yes (Fear)
   b. No (Anxiety)
3. Is the patient going to have, as a result of this admission, a change in body structure or function?
   a. Yes (Body Image Disturbance)
   b. No
4. Does the patient verbalize a change in lifestyle as a result of this admission?
   a. Yes (Body Image Disturbance)
   b. No
5. Does the patient verbalize a negative view of self?
   a. Yes (Self-Esteem Disturbance)
   b. No
6. Does the patient believe he or she can deal with the current problem that led to this admission?
   a. Yes
   b. No (Self-Esteem Disturbance)
7. Does the patient or his or her family indicate that the self-negating impression is a long-standing (several years) problem?
   a. Yes (Chronic Low Self-Esteem)
   b. No (Situational Low Self-Esteem)
8. Does the patient question who he or she is or verbalize lack of an understanding regarding his or her role in life?
   a. Yes (Personal Identity Disturbance)
   b. No
9. Does the patient appear passive or verbalize passivity?
   a. Yes (Hopelessness)
   b. No
10. Does the patient demonstrate decreased verbalization and/or flat affect?
    a. Yes (Hopelessness)
    b. No
11. Does the patient have a problem with physical or social isolation?
    a. Yes (Risk for Loneliness)
    b. No
12. Has the patient recently suffered the loss of a significant other?
    a. Yes (Risk for Loneliness)
    b. No
13. Does the patient verbalize lack of control?
    a. Yes (Powerlessness)
    b. No
14. Is the patient participating in care and decision making regarding care?
    a. Yes
    b. No (Powerlessness)

Conceptual Information

Definition of the self and of a self-concept has been an issue of debate in philosophy, sociology, and psychology for many years, and many publications are available on this topic.[1] The complexity of the problem of defining self is compounded by the knowledge that external observation provides only a superficial glimpse of the self and introspection requires that the "knower" know himself or herself so that information actually gained is self-referential. In spite of these problems, the concept continues to be pervasive in the literature and in the universal experience of "self" or "not self." Intuitively one would say, of course, "There is a self because I have experiences separate from those around me, and I know where I end and they begin." The importance of self is also emphasized by the language in the multitude of self-referential terms such as self-actualization, self-affirmation, ego involvement, and self-concept.

Turner[2] addresses society's need for the individual to conceptualize the self-as-object. Recognizing the self-as-object allows society to place responsibility, which becomes a very valuable asset in maintaining social control and social order. This returns us to the initial problem of what the self is and how we can understand ourselves and others' selves.[3]

In this section the assumption is made that "self-concept" refers to the individual's subjective cognitions and evaluations of self; thus, it is a highly personal experience. This indicates that the self is a personal construct and not a fact or hard reality. It is further assumed that the individual will act, as stated earlier, in congruence with the self-concept. This conceptualization is consistent with the authors that will be discussed and with the assumptions utilized in psychological research.[3] It is also important to recognize that language assists in developing a concept. This becomes crucial when thinking about the concept of self in English because the English language comes from a tradition of Cartesian dualism that does not express integrated concepts well. Often it will appear that the information presented is separating the individual into various parts when, in fact, an integrated whole is being addressed. For example, James[4] talks about an I and Me. If these terms were taken at face value, it would appear that the individual is being divided into multiple parts when, in fact, an integrated whole is being discussed and the words describe patterns of the whole person. Unless otherwise stated, it can be assumed that the concepts presented in this book reflect on the individual as an integrated whole.

Symbolic interaction theory provides a basis for understanding the self. The foundation for the self in this theoretical model was developed by James[4] and Mead.[5] James outlines the internal working of the self with his concepts of "I" and "Me." "I" is the thinker or the state of consciousness.

"Me" is what the "I" is conscious of and includes all of what people consider theirs. This "me" contains three aspects: the "material me," the "social me," and the "spiritual me."[4] The self-construction outlined by Mead[5] indicates that there is the "knower" part of the self and that which the "knower" knows. Mead conceptualizes the thoughts themselves as the "knower" to resolve the metaphysical problem of who the "I" is. In Mead's writings, the consciousness of self is a stream of thought in which the "I" can remember what came before and continues to know what was known. The development of these memories and how they affect one's behavior is expressly addressed by Mead.[5]

Mead[5] describes the self-concept as evolving out of interactions with others in social contexts. This process begins at the moment of birth and continues throughout a lifetime. The definition of self can occur only in social interactions, for one's self exists only in relation to other selves. The individual is continually processing the reactions of others to his or her actions and reactions. This processing is taking place in a highly personalized manner, for the information is experienced through the individual's selective attention, which is guided by the current needs that are struggling to be expressed. This results in an environment that is constructed by one's perceptions. Mead's conceptualization leads to an interesting feedback process in that we can perceive self only as we perceive others perceive us. This continues to reinforce the idea that the self-concept is highly personalized.

Many authors[2,4,5] have addressed the process of developing a concept of self. The model developed by Harry Stack Sullivan[6] will be presented here because it is consistent with the information presented in the symbolic interaction literature and is used as the theoretical base in much of the nursing literature.

Sullivan[6] describes the self-concept as developing in interactions with significant others. Development of the self-concept is seen by Sullivan as a dynamic process resulting from interpersonal interactions that are directed toward meeting physiologic needs. This process has its most obvious beginnings with the infant and becomes more complex as the individual develops. This increasing complexity results from the layering of experiences that occurs in the developing individual. The biologic processes become less and less important in directing the individual the further away from birth one is, and as the importance of interpersonal interactions increases. The initial interpersonal interaction is between the infant and the primary caregivers. An infant expresses discomfort with a cry and the "parenting one" responds. This response, whether it be tender or harsh, begins to influence the infant's beliefs about herself or himself and the world in general. If the interaction does not provide the infant with a feeling of security, anxiety results and interferes with the progress toward other life goals. Sullivan makes a distinction between the inner experience and the outer event and describes three modes of understanding experience.

The first developmental experience is the *prototaxic mode*. In this mode the small child experiences self and the universe as an undifferentiated whole. At 3 to 4 months the child moves into the parataxic mode. The *parataxic mode* presents experiences as separated but without recognition of a connectedness or logical sequence. Finally, the individual enters the *syntaxic mode*, in which consensual validation is possible. This allows for events and experiences to be compared with others' experiences and for establishing mutually understandable communication instead of the autistic thinking that has characterized the previous stages.[7,8]

As one experiences the environment through these three modes of thought, the self system or self-concept is developed. Sullivan conceptualized three parts of the self. The part of the self that is associated with security and approval becomes the "good me." That which is within one's awareness but is disapproved of becomes the "bad me." The "bad me" could include those feelings, needs, or desires that stimulate anxiety. Those feelings and understandings that are out of awareness are experienced as "not me." These "not me" experiences are not nonexistent but are expressed in indirect ways that can interfere with the conduct of the individual's life.[6,7]

As the social sciences adopted a cybernetic worldview, this theoretical perspective has been applied to developing a concept of self. Glaserfeld[9] spoke of the self as a relational entity that is given life through the continuity of relating. This relating provides the intuitive knowledge that our experience is truly ours. This reflects the perspective of knowing presented at the beginning of this section.

Watts[10] describes what many authors feel is the self as it can be understood through a cybernetic worldview. Self is the whole, for it is part of the energy that is the universe and cannot be separated. "At this level of existence 'I' am immeasurably old; my forms are infinite and their comings and goings are simply the pulses or vibrations of a single and eternal flow of energy" (p. 12). Within this view, an individual is connected to every other living being in the universe. This places the self in a unique position of responsibility. The self then becomes responsible to everything because it is everything. This conceptual model resolves the issue of responsibility to society without relying on an individual self to which responsibility is assigned.

Although the conceptual model represented here by Watts[10] fits with current theoretical models being utilized in nursing and the social sciences, it is not congruent with the experience of most people in Western society. This limits its usefulness when working with clients in a clinical setting. It is presented here to provide practitioners with an alternative model for themselves.

Sidney Jourard[11] provides direction for interventions related to an individual's self-concept. The healthy self-concept allows individuals to play roles they have satisfactorily played while gaining personal satisfaction from this role enactment. This person also continues to develop and maintain a high level of physical wellness. This high level of wellness is achieved by gaining knowledge of oneself through a process of self-disclosure. Jourard[11] states:

> If self-disclosure is one of the means by which healthy personality is both achieved and maintained, we can also note that such activities as loving, psychotherapy, counseling, teaching and nursing, all are impossible—without the disclosure of the client. (p. 427)

Elaboration of this thought reveals that for the nurse to effectively meet the needs of the client, an understanding of the client's self must be achieved. This understanding must go beyond the interpretation of overt behavior, which is an indirect method of understanding, and access the client's understanding of self through the process of self-disclosure.

Default and Martocchio[12] present a conceptual model for hope that also provides a useful perspective for nursing intervention. Hope is defined as multidimensional and process oriented. Hopelessness is not the absence of hope but is the product of an environment that does not activate the process of hoping. Vaillot[13] supports the view presented by Default and Martocchio with the existential philosophical perspective that hope arises from relationships and the beliefs about these relationships. One believes that help can come from the outside of oneself when all internal resources are exhausted. Hopelessness arises in an environment where hope is not communicated. This model supports nursing interventions from a systems theory perspective because it validates the ever-interacting system, the whole. In this perspective the nurse, as well as the client, contributes to the "hopelessness," and thus the responsibility of nurturing hope is shared.[12–16]

Developmental Considerations

INFANT

In general the sources of anxiety begin in a very narrow scope with the infant and broaden out as he or she matures. Initially the relationship with the primary caregiver is the source of gratification for the infant, and disruptions in this relationship result in anxiety. As one matures, needs are met from multiple sources, and therefore the sources of anxiety expand. Specific developmental considerations are as follows.

The primary source of anxiety for the infant appears to be a sense of "being left." This response begins at about 3 months. Sullivan,[6] as indicated earlier, would contend that the infant could experience anxiety even earlier with any disruption in having needs met by the primary caregiver. At age 8 to 10 months, separation anxiety peaks for the first time. At 5 to 6 months the infant begins to demonstrate stranger anxiety. Primary symptoms include disruptions in physiologic functioning and could include colic, sleep disorders, failure to thrive syndrome, and constipation with early toilet training. Stranger anxiety and separation anxiety may be demonstrated with screaming, attempting to withdraw, and refusing to cooperate. Both stranger anxiety and separation anxiety are normal developmental responses and should not be considered pathologic as long as they are not severe or prolonged and the parental response is appropriately supportive of the infant's need.

Fear is a normal protective response to external threats and will be present at all ages. It becomes dysfunctional at the point that it is attached to situations that do not present a threat or when it prevents the individual from responding appropriately to a situation. Thus, it is important that children have certain fears to protect them from harm. The hot stove, for example, should produce a fear response to the extent that it prevents the child from touching the stove and being injured. Fear is a learned response to situations, and children learn this response from their caregivers. Thus, it becomes the caregivers' responsibility to model and teach appropriate fear. If a mother cannot tolerate being left alone in the house at night with her children, her children will learn to fear being in this situation. When this home is located in a low-crime area with supportive neighbors and appropriate locks, fear becomes an inappropriate response, and the children may be affected by it for a lifetime.

Various developmental stages have characteristic fears associated with them. In the mind of the child these characteristic fears present threats so the fears can be seen both as a source of fear and as a source of anxiety. The characteristic fears result from strong or noxious environmental stimuli such as loud noises, bright lights, or sharp objects against the skin. The response to fears produces physiologic symptoms. The most immediate and obvious response is crying and pulling away from the stressful object or situations.

Erickson[16,17] indicated that he thought hope evolved out of the successful resolution of this first developmental stage, basic trust versus mistrust. Hope was perceived by Erickson to be a basic human virtue. The type of environment that has been identified as prompting the development of this basic trust is warm and loving where there is respect and acceptance for personal interests, ideas, needs, and talents.[14] Several environmental conditions have been associated with early childhood and are seen as increasing the perceptions consistent with hopelessness. These conditions are economic deprivation, poor physical health, being raised in a broken home or a home where parents have a high degree of conflict, having a negative perception of parents, or having parents who are not mentally healthy. From an existential perspective, Lynch[18] identified five areas of human existence that can produce hopelessness. If these areas are not acknowledged in the developmental process, the individual is at greater risk of frustration and hopelessness because hope is being intermingled with a known area of hopelessness. The five areas that Lynch identified are death, personal imperfections, imperfect emotional control, inability to trust all people, and personal areas of incompetence. This supports Erickson's contention that hope evolves out of the first developmental stage, because these basic areas of hopelessness are issues primarily related to the resolution of trust and mistrust. It should be remembered that previously resolved or unresolved developmental issues must be renegotiated throughout life.

Each developmental stage has a set of specific etiologies and symptom clusters related to hopelessness. Since the relationship between self-concept strength and degree of hopefulness seen as a positive link, many of the etiologies and symptoms of hopelessness at the various developmental stages are similar to those of Self-Esteem Disturbance.[15]

As conceptualized by Erickson,[17] infancy is the primary age for developing a hopeful attitude about life. If the infant does not experience a situation in which trust in another can be developed, then the base of hopelessness has begun. Thus, if the infant experiences frequent changes in caregivers or has a caregiver who does not meet the basic needs in a consistent and warm manner, the infant will become hopeless. Research[18] has indicated that children who have been raised in an environment of despair are at greater risk for experiencing hopelessness. Symptoms of hopelessness in infants resemble infant depression or failure to thrive. Since symptoms in infants are a general response, the diagnosis of Hopelessness must be considered equally with other diagnoses that produce similar symptom clusters such as Powerlessness and Ineffective Coping.

One's perceptions of place in the larger system and of influence in this system begin at birth. These perceptions are developed through interactions with those in the immediate environment and continue throughout life with each new interaction in each new experience. Thus, the child learns from primary caregivers that his or her expressions of need may or may not have an effect on those around him or her and also learns what he or she must do to have an effect. If the caregiver responds to the earliest cries of the infant, a sense of personal influence has begun. The two areas that consistently influence one's perceptions of influence are discipline and communication styles.

Implementation of discipline in a manner that provides the child with a sense of control over the environment while teaching appropriate behavior can produce a perception of mutual system influence. Harsh, overcontrolling methods can produce the perception that the child does not have any influence in the system if acting in a direct manner. This produces an indirect influencing style. An example of indirect influence is the child who always becomes ill just before his parents leave for an evening on the town. The parents, out of concern for the child, decide to remain at home and thus never have time together as a couple. Authoritarian styles of interaction can also produce perceptions of powerlessness in adults in unfamiliar environments. If the hospital staff acts in an authoritarian manner, the client may develop perceptions of powerlessness.

Double-bind communication can place the individual in a position of feeling that "no matter what action I take, it appears to be wrong," and also can produce a perception of powerlessness. They are "damned if they do and damned if they don't." If the individual cannot influence this system in a direct manner, again, indirect behavior patterns are chosen. Bateson[19] proposes that this is the process behind the symptom cluster identified as schizophrenia. This suggests that if the child is continually placed in the position of being wrong no matter what he or she has done, the child could develop the perception that his or her position is one of powerlessness and carry this attitude with him or her throughout life.

Infants have a need for consistent response to having physiologic needs met, and the most important relationship becomes that with the "parenting one." If this relationship is disrupted and needs are not met, symptoms related to infant depression or failure to thrive could communicate a perception related to powerlessness.

It is important to remember that self-concept, including body image, is developed throughout life. For the infant, the primary source of developing self-concept and body image is physical interaction with the environment. This includes both the environment's response to physical needs and the body's response to environmental stimuli.

TODDLER AND PRESCHOOLER

The basic sources of anxiety remain the same as with the infant. Separation anxiety appears to peak again at 18 to 24 months, and stranger anxiety peaks again at 12 to 18 months. Loss of significant others is the primary source of anxiety at this age. In addition to the physiologic responses mentioned above, the child may demonstrate anxiety by motor restlessness and regressive behavior. The preschooler can begin to tolerate longer periods away from the parenting one and enjoys having the opportunity to test his or her new

abilities. Lack of opportunity to practice independent skills can increase the discomfort of this age group. Increased anxiety can be seen in regressive behavior, motor restlessness, and physiologic response.

Sources of anxiety can include concerns about the body and body mutilation, concerns about death, and concerns about loss of self-control. These concerns can be expressed in the ways discussed above as well as with language and dramatic play as language abilities increase. This could include playing out anxiety-producing situations with dolls or other toys. This play can assume a very aggressive nature. The anxieties of the day can also be expressed in dreams and result in nightmares or other sleep disturbance.

In this age group fears evolve from real environmental stimuli and from imagined situations. Fears typical within specific age groups are fear of sudden loud noise (2 years), fear of animals (3 to 4 years), fear of the dark (4 to 5 years), and fear of the dark and of being lost (6 years). Symptoms of fears include regressive behavior, physical and verbal cruelty, restlessness, irritability, sleep disturbance, dramatic play around issues related to the fear, and increased physical closeness to the caregiver.

Alterations to the body or its functioning place a child at this age at the greatest risk of experiencing hopelessness. If the child experiences a difference between self and other or is ashamed about body functioning, in a nonsupportive environment, hopelessness can develop. A specific issue encountered at this stage is toilet training. If the child is placed in a position of being required to gain control over bowel and bladder functions before the ability to physically master these functions has developed, the child can experience hopelessness in that he or she truly cannot make his or her body function in the required manner. Peer interactions are also important at this time because they foster the beginnings of trust in someone other than the "mothering" one, thus understanding that hope can be gained elsewhere.

Struggle between self-control and control by others becomes the primary psychosocial issue. If appropriate expansion of self-control is encouraged, the child will develop perceptions related to mutual systemic influence. This appropriate support is crucial if the child is to develop a perception of a personal role in the social system. If this struggle for self-control is thwarted, the child can express themes of overcontrol in play or become overly dependent on the primary caregiver and withdraw completely from new situations and learning.

For the preschooler there is a continuation and refinement of a sense of personal influence. Varying approaches are explored, and a greater sense of what can be achieved is developed. One of the primary sources of anxiety during this stage is loss of self-control. Symptoms of difficulties in this area include playing out situations with personal influence as a theme and aggressive play.

Sources of the self-concept perceptions are the responses of significant others to exploration of new physical abilities and to the toddler's place in these relationships. The primary concept of self is related to physical qualities, motor skills, sex type, and age. A concept of physical differences and of physical integrity is developed. Thus, situations that threaten the toddler's perception of physical wholeness can pose a threat. This would include physical injury. Toilet training poses a potential threat to the successful development of a positive self-concept or body image. Failure at training could produce feelings of personal incompetence or of the body being shameful.

In the preschooler, physical qualities, motor skills, sex type, and age continue to be the primary concepts of self-concept. Peers begin to assume greater importance in self-perceptions. Physical integrity continues to be important, and physical difference can have a profound effect on the preschool child.

SCHOOL-AGE CHILD

Typically, fears are aroused by strange noises; ghosts and imagined phantoms; natural elements such as fire, drowning, or thunder (6 years); not being liked or being late for school (7 years); and personal failure or inadequacy (8 to 10 years). Symptoms of these fears include physical symptoms of autonomic stimulation, increased verbalization, withdrawal, aggression, sleep disturbance, or needing to repeat a specific task many times.

Concerns about imagined future events produce the anxieties of the school-age child. The specific concern varies with the developmental age. Early school age children demonstrate concerns related to the unknowns in their environment such as dark rooms and natural elements such as fire or tornadoes. Middle school age children have anxieties related to personal inadequacies. Late school age brings increasing concerns about the valuation of peers and concerns about the acceptance of peers. Expression of anxiety can occur in the ways discussed in the previous level, with the addition of increased verbalization and compulsive behavior such as repeating a specific task many times.

Peers' perceptions of the individual assume a role in the development of attitudes related to personal hopelessness and influence within the larger social system. This is built on the perceptions achieved during earlier stages of development. The sense of a strong peer group can produce perceptions of help coming from the outside as long as the child thinks and believes along with the group but can produce perceptions of exaggerated personal influence. Problems at this developmental stage can be demonstrated by withdrawal, daydreaming, increased verbalizations of helplessness and hopelessness, angry outbursts, aggressive behavior, irritability, and frustration.

Self-perception expands to include ethnic awareness, ambition, ideal self, ordinal position, and conscience. There is increasing awareness of self as different from peers. Peers become increasingly important in developing a concept of self, and there is increased comparison of real to ideal self.

ADOLESCENT

The developmental theme that elicits anxiety in this age group revolves around the development of a personal identity. This is facilitated by peer relationships, which can also be the source of anxiety. Expression of this anxiety can occur in any of the ways previously discussed and with aggressive behavior. This aggression can take both verbal and physical forms. A certain amount of "normal" anxiety is experienced as the adolescent moves from the family into the adult world. Anxiety would be considered abnormal only if it violated societal norms and was severe or prolonged.

Parental education and support during this developmental crisis can be crucial.

Peer relationships, independence, authority figures, and changing roles and relations can contribute to fears for adolescents. Expression of these fears produces cognitive and affective symptoms. These symptoms could include difficulties with attention and concentration, poor judgment, and alterations in mood and thought content.

The cognitive development of adolescents would suggest that their perceptions of situations are guided by hypothetical-deductive thought, and as a result they could develop reasonable models of hopefulness. This cognitive process occurs in conjunction with a lack of a variety of life experience and self-discipline and with a heightened state of emotionality. This can result in a situation in which the immediate goal can overshadow future consequences or possibilities. An adolescent who appears very hopeful when cognitive functioning is not overwhelmed by emotions can be filled with despair when involved in a very emotional situation. Consideration of this ability is important when caring for this age group. It is important to distinguish problem behavior from normal behavior and mood swings. Kinds of behavior that could indicate problems in this area include withdrawal and increased or amplified testing of limits. Situations that affect the peer group hope can place the adolescent at great risk.

Again, issues of dependence-independence assume a primary role. The focus of this struggle is dependence on peers and independence from family. The challenge for the adolescent becomes achieving what Erickson et al.[20] refer to as "affiliated individuation." This requires that they learn how to be dependent on support systems while maintaining their independence from these same support systems and feeling accepted in both positions.

Body image becomes a crucial area of self-evaluation due to changing physical appearance and heightened sexual awareness. This evaluation is based on the cultural ideal as well as that of the peer group. Perceived personal failures are often attributed to physical differences.

ADULT

Changes in role and relationship patterns generate the fears specific to these age groups. These could include parenthood, marriage, divorce, retirement, or death of a spouse. Fear expression in these age groups produces cognitive and affective symptoms similar to those described under Adolescent.

A specific developmental crisis can produce a perception of hopelessness and powerlessness. The situations that place the adult at risk are marriage, pregnancy, parenthood, and divorce.

Concerns about role performance assume an important role in self-perceptions. Perceived failures in meeting role expectations can produce negative self-evaluation. The number of roles a person has assumed and the personal, cultural, and support system value placed on the identified roles determine the threat that negative evaluation of performance can be to self-perception. Cultural value and personal identity formation determine the degree to which body image remains important in providing a positive evaluation of self. The adult endows unique significance to various body parts. This valuing process is personal and is often not in personal awareness until there is a threat to the part.

OLDER ADULT

As the older adult continues to age, he or she faces numerous challenges to self-perception and self-concept. Roles may change secondary to retirement or loss of significant others, such as a spouse or child. Financial resources may become limited or fixed due to illness, retirement, or loss of spouse.[21] Chronic illness that necessitates a decrease in social interactions or increased dependence on others and the resulting loss of control have a negative impact on self-esteem for some elderly.[22]

Negative societal feedback, such as ageism, sends a message to older adults that they are somehow no longer valuable to the society. In the face of these decremental losses, it is necessary to consider what health care professionals can do to assist the older adult in maintaining a positive regard for self.

APPLICABLE NURSING DIAGNOSES

Anxiety

DEFINITION

A vague uneasy feeling whose source is often nonspecific or unknown to the individual.[23]

NANDA TAXONOMY: FEELING 9.3.1

DEFINING CHARACTERISTICS[23]

1. Subjective
   a. Increased tension
   b. Apprehension
   c. Painful and persistent increased helplessness
   d. Uncertainty
   e. Fearful
   f. Scared
   g. Regretful
   h. Overexcited
   i. Rattled
   j. Distressed
   k. Jittery
   l. Feelings of inadequacy
   m. Shakiness
   n. Fear of unspecific consequences
   o. Expressed concerns about change in life events
   p. Worried
   q. Anxious
2. Objective
   a. Sympathetic stimulation: Cardiovascular excitation, superficial vasoconstriction, or pupil dilation (critical)
   b. Restlessness
   c. Insomnia
   d. Glancing about
   e. Poor eye contact
   f. Trembling or hand tremors
   g. Extraneous movement (foot shuffling, or hand or arm movements)
   h. Facial tension
   i. Voice quivering
   j. Focus on self
   k. Increased wariness
   l. Increased perspiration

RELATED FACTORS[23]

1. Unconscious conflict about essential values or goals of life
2. Threat to self-concept
3. Threat of death
4. Threat to, or change in, health status
5. Threat to, or change in, role functioning
6. Threat to, or change in, environment
7. Threat to, or change in, interaction patterns
8. Situational or maturational crises
9. Interpersonal transmission or contagion
10. Unmet needs

RELATED CLINICAL CONCERNS

1. Any hospital admission
2. Failure to thrive
3. Cancer or other terminal illnesses
4. Crohn's disease
5. Impending surgery
6. Hyperthyroidism
7. Substance abuse
8. Mental health disorders

STOP

HAVE YOU SELECTED THE CORRECT DIAGNOSIS?

Fear Fear is the response to an identified threat, while Anxiety is the response to a threat that cannot be easily identified. Fear is probably the diagnosis that is most often confused with Anxiety. An example of a situation in which Fear would be an appropriate diagnosis is: After being released from jail, the prisoner threatened to kill the judge who placed him or her in jail. The judge, if experiencing psychologic stress due to this threat and knowing the prisoner was out of jail, would receive the diagnosis of Fear.

Personal Identity Disturbance This diagnosis is the most appropriate diagnosis if the individual's symptoms are related to a general disturbance in the perception of self. Anxiety would be used when the discomfort was related to other areas.

Dysfunctional Grieving This diagnosis would be considered appropriate if the loss was real, whereas the diagnosis of Anxiety would be used when the loss is a threat that is not necessarily real such as a perceived loss of esteem from others.

Ineffective Individual Coping This diagnosis would be appropriate if the individual is not making the necessary adaptations to deal with daily life. This may or may not occur with Anxiety as a companion diagnosis.

Spiritual Distress This diagnosis occurs if the individual experiences a threat to his or her value or belief systems. This threat may or may not produce Anxiety. If the primary expressed concerns are related to the individual's value or belief system, then the appropriate diagnosis would be Spiritual Distress.

EXPECTED OUTCOMES

1. Will design and implement a plan to reduce anxiety by (date) and/or
2. Will demonstrate, verbally or behaviorally, at least a (number) percent decrease in anxiety by (date)

TARGET DATES

A target date of 3 days would be realistic to start evaluating progress. The sooner anxiety is reduced, the sooner other problems can be dealt with.

NURSING ACTIONS/INTERVENTIONS WITH RATIONALES

Adult Health

ACTIONS/INTERVENTIONS	RATIONALES
• Obtain a thorough history upon admission.	Allows identification of all possible factors contributing to anxiety.
• Monitor anxiety behavior and relationship to activity, events, people, etc., every 2 h on the (odd/even) hour.	When anxiety increases, the ability to follow instruction or cooperate in plan of care decreases. Identification of the behavior and causative factors enhances intervention plans.
• Reassure patient that anxiety is normal. Assist patient to learn to recognize and identify the signs and symptoms of anxiety, e.g., hyperventilation, rapid heartbeat, sweaty palms, inability to concentrate, and restlessness.	Helps to identify connection between the precipitating cause and the anxiety experience; reassures the patient that he or she is not "going crazy."
• Provide calm, nonthreatening environment: ○ Explain all procedures and rationale for procedure in clear, concise, simple terms. ○ Decrease sensory input and distraction, e.g., lighting or noise. ○ Encourage significant other(s) to stay with patient but not force conversation, etc.	Conveys calm and helps the patient focus on conversation or activity.
• Monitor vital signs at least every 4 h while awake at (times).	Assists in determining the effects of anxiety. Helps to determine pathologic effects of anxiety.
• Attend to primary physical needs promptly.	Conserves patient's energy and allows patient to focus on coping with and reducing anxiety. Failure to attend to physical needs would serve to increase anxiety.
• Administer antianxiety medications as ordered. Monitor and document effects of medication within 30 min of administration.	Effectiveness of medication is determined so that modification can be provided if needed. Medication helps to reduce anxiety to a manageable level.
• Assist patient to develop coping skills: ○ Review past coping behaviors and success or lack of success.	Determines what has helped in the past and determines if the measures are still useful.

Continued

ACTIONS/INTERVENTIONS	RATIONALES
○ Help identify and practice new coping strategies such as progressive relaxation, guided imagery, rhythmic breathing, balancing exercise and rest, appropriate food and fluid intake, e.g., reducing caffeine intake, and using distraction.	Methods that can be used successfully to decrease anxiety. Allows patient to practice and become comfortable with skills in a supporting environment.
○ Challenge unrealistic assumptions or goals.	Assists patient to avoid placing extra stress on himself or herself.
○ Place limits on maladaptive behavior, e.g., alcohol or fighting.	Promotes use of appropriate techniques for reducing anxiety while avoiding harm to self and others.
• Provide at least 20–30 min every 4 h while awake for focus on anxiety reduction. List times here.	Provides opportunity for practice of technique and expression of anxiety-provoking experiences.
○ Encourage client to express feelings verbally and through activity.	
○ Answer questions truthfully.	
○ Offer realistic reassurance and positive feedback.	
• Collaborate with psychiatric nurse clinician regarding care (see Psychiatric Health nursing actions).	Collaboration helps to provide holistic care. Specialist may help discover underlying events for anxiety and assist in designing an alternate plan of care.
• Refer patient to and collaborate with appropriate community resources.	Support groups can provide ongoing assistance after discharge.

Child Health

ACTIONS/INTERVENTIONS	RATIONALES
• Review, with the child and parents, coping measures used for daily changes and crises.	The identification of coping strategies will provide essential information to deal with anxiety. Once identified, the nurse can begin to evaluate those strategies that are effective.
• Identify ways parents can assist child to cope with anxiety, e.g., set realistic explanations or demands and avoid bribing or not telling the truth.	A major starting point is to describe the feelings and attempt to create a sense of control, which is more likely in certain developmental capacity patients, e.g., those capable of abstract thinking. In younger infants rocking can provide soothing repetitious motion when all other measures seem not to have calmed infant.
• Adapt routine to best help child regain control, e.g., use of speech according to situation and simple but firm speech pattern.	Allowing the child to plan for meals or snacks with choices when possible or structuring the room to offer a sense of self is conducive to empowerment.
• Modify procedures, as possible, to help reduce anxiety, e.g., do not use intramuscular injection when an oral route is possible.	Unnecessary pain or invasive procedures make overwhelming demands on the already stressed hospitalized child.
• Use child's developmental needs as a basis for care, especially for ventilation of anxiety, e.g., use of toys.	The developmental level of the patient serves to guide the nurse in care. A holistic approach is more likely to meet holistic health needs.
• Allow child and parents adequate time and opportunities to handle required care issues and thus reduce anxiety, e.g., when painful treatments must be done, prepare all involved according to an agreed-upon plan.	Appropriate time in preparation offers structure and allows focused attention, which empowers and helps reduce anxiety as efforts are directed to what is known.
• Encourage family to assist with care as appropriate, including feeding, comfort measures, and stories.	Family involvement provides a sense of empowerment and growth in coping, thereby reducing anxiety and promoting a sense of security in the child.
• Offer sufficient opportunities for rest according to age and sleep requirements.	Proper attention to rest for each individual child will best foster coping capacities by conserving energy for coping.
• Identify knowledge needs, and address these by having family explain what they understand about treatments, procedures, needs, etc.	Allows teaching opportunity that increases patient's and family's knowledge about situation, which assists in reducing anxiety.

- Point out and reinforce successes in conquering anxiety.
- Assist patient and family to apply coping in future potential anxiety-producing situations by presenting possible scenarios that would call for utilization of the new skills, e.g., someone pushes ahead of you in line, or a salesperson is rude to you.

Positive reinforcement assists in learning.
Allows practice in a non-anxiety-producing environment. Increases skill in using coping strategy. Empowers patient and family.

Women's Health

ACTIONS/INTERVENTIONS	RATIONALES

ACUTE ANXIETY ATTACK

- Provide a realistic, tranquil atmosphere, e.g., close door, sit with patient, remind patient you are there to help:
  - Do not leave the patient alone.
  - Speak softly using short, simple commands.
  - Be firm but kind.
  - Be prepared to make decisions for the patient.
  - Decrease external stimuli, and provide a "safe" atmosphere.
- Administer antianxiety medication as ordered, and monitor effectiveness of medication within 30 min to 1 h of administration.

Provides an atmosphere that assists in calming patient and promotes the initiation of coping by the patient.

MILD OR MODERATE ANXIETY

- Guide the patient through problem solving related to the anxiety:
  - Assist the patient to verbalize and describe what she thinks is going to happen.
  - Describe to the patient what will happen (to the best of your ability), and compare it with her expectations.
  - Assist the patient in describing ways she can more clearly express her needs.
- Assist the patient in changing unrealistic expectations, by explaining procedures, e.g., labor process or sensations during a pelvic exam.
- Encourage the patient to participate in assertiveness training.

By providing factual information, clarification of misconceptions, and emotional support, the patient's coping can be enhanced.[24]

PREGNANCY AND CHILDBIRTH

- Provide the patient and significant others with factual information about the physical and emotional changes experienced during pregnancy.
- Review daily schedule with the patient and significant other. Assist them to identify lifestyle adjustments that may be needed for coping with pregnancy.
  - Practicing relaxation techniques when stress begins to build
  - Establishing a routine for relaxing after work
  - Developing a plan to provide frequent rest breaks throughout the day (particularly in the last trimester)
- Refer to a support group, e.g., childbirth education classes or MCH nurses in the community.
- Provide the patient and significant other with factual information about sexual changes during pregnancy:
  - Answer questions promptly and factually.
  - Meet people who have had similar experiences.
  - Discuss fears about sexual changes.
  - Discuss aspects of sexuality and intercourse during pregnancy:

Helps reduce anxiety about financial concerns due to having to quit work. Good planning and working with patient and partner to establish a realistic work schedule to present to employer can assist patient to reduce edema and fatigue and thus remain on job longer.

Factual information provides the family with the essential knowledge needed in planning for the pregnancy, accomplishing the task of pregnancy, and adapting to a new infant.

ACTIONS/INTERVENTIONS	RATIONALES

(1) Positions for intercourse during different stages of pregnancy
(2) Frequency of intercourse
(3) Effect of intercourse on pregnancy or fetus
  ◦ Describe healing process postpartum and timing of resumption of intercourse.
• Provide patient support during birthing process, e.g., Montrice, support person, or coach.

Assists in reducing anxiety. Increases coping.

• Provide support for significant other(s) during this process:
  ◦ Encourage verbalization of fears.
  ◦ Answer questions factually.
  ◦ Demonstrate equipment.
  ◦ Explain procedures.

Support of significant others leads to more support for patient.

POSTPARTUM (EARLY DISCHARGE)

• Provide support for new parents during the first few days of the postpartum period. Provide new parents with telephone number to call with questions and concerns. Call new parents 36–48 h after discharge:
  ◦ Formulate questions to receive simple one- or two-word answers.
  ◦ Allow new parents time to ask questions and voice concerns.

Provides support and information from an "expert," helping to reduce anxiety of being new parents.

• Give new mother appointment before discharge from hospital to return to follow-up clinic or schedule home visit by nurse for herself and her infant.
  ◦ Assess mother and baby for appropriate physical recovery from the birth:
    (1) Maternal: Episiotomy, C/S incision, breasts (lactating and nonlactating), involution of uterus, lochia flow, fatigue level, etc.
    (2) Infant: Number of wet diapers in 24-h period, number of stools in 24-h period, color and consistency of stools, feeding patterns, bilirubin check.
  ◦ Discuss with mother and partner or family, psychosocial aspects of being new parents.
  ◦ Assist in developing and planning coping skills for new roles.

Provides a continuity of services and support and education for new family during time between discharge and follow-up visit to primary health care provider.

• Provide appropriate education. (May have to repeat all education done on postpartum unit in acute care setting.)
• Monitor infant and parents for attachment behaviors.
• Refer parents to appropriate resources for support and further follow-up:
  ◦ Lactation consultants
  ◦ Primary care provider (obstetrician, pediatrician, certified nurse midwife, family practitioner, or nurse practitioner)
  ◦ Public health nurse
  ◦ Visiting nursing services
• Provide documentation of follow-up to the patient's primary care provider.

Psychiatric Health

ACTIONS/INTERVENTIONS	RATIONALES
• Provide a quiet, nonstimulating environment. For the client experiencing severe or panic anxiety, this may be a seclusion setting.	Inappropriate levels of sensory stimuli can contribute to the client's sense of disorganization and confusion.
• Provide frequent, brief interactions that assist the client with orientation. Verbal information should be provided in simple, brief sentences.	Appropriate levels of sensory stimuli promote the client's sense of control.
• If the client is experiencing severe or panic anxiety, provide support in a nondemanding atmosphere.	Communicates acceptance of the client, which facilitates the development of trust and self-esteem.
• If the client is experiencing severe or panic anxiety, provide a here-and-now focus.	High levels of anxiety decrease the client's ability to process information.
• Provide the client with a simple repetitive activity until anxiety decreases to the level at which learning can begin.	High levels of anxiety decrease the client's ability to problem solve. Promotes client's sense of control.
• If the client is hyperventilating, guide him or her in taking slow, deep breaths. If necessary, breathe along with the client, and provide ongoing, positive reinforcement.	Reestablishes a normal breathing pattern and promotes the client's sense of control.
• Approach the client in a calm, reassuring manner, assessing the caregiver's level of anxiety and keeping this to a minimum.	Anxiety is contagious and can be communicated from the social network to the client.
• Provide a constant, one-on-one interaction for the client experiencing severe or panic anxiety. This should preclude use of physical restraints, which tend to increase the client's anxiety.	Presence of a calm trusted individual can promote a sense of control and calm in the client.
• Provide the client with alernative outlets for physical tension. This should be stated specifically and could include walking, running, talking with a staff member, using a punching bag, listening to music, doing a deep muscle relaxation sequence (number) times per day at (state specific times). The outlet should be selected with the client's input.	Promotes the client's sense of control and begins the development of alternative, more adaptive coping behaviors.
• Sit with the client (number) times per day at (times) for (number) minutes to discuss feelings and complaints. As the client expresses these openly, the nurse can then explore the onset of the anxiety with the purpose of identifying the sources of the anxiety.	Identification of precipitating factors is the first step in developing alternative coping behaviors and promoting client's sense of control.
• After the source of the anxiety has been identified, the time set aside above can be utilized to assist the client in developing alternative coping styles.	Promotes the client's sense of control.
• Provide (number) times per day to discuss with the client interests in the external environment (especially with those clients who tend to focus strongly on nonspecific physical complaints).	Provides positive reinforcement through the nurse's attention for improved coping behaviors.
• Talk with the client about the advantages and disadvantages of the current condition. (Help the client to identify secondary gain from the symptoms.) This would be done in the individual discussion sessions or in group therapy when a trusting relationship has been developed.	Identification of contributing factors is the first step in developing alternative coping behaviors.
• Provide the client with feedback on how his or her behavior affects others (this could be done in an individual or group situation).	Assists client with consensual validation.
• Provide positive feedback as appropriate on changed behavior. (The target behavior and goals should be listed here.)	Positive feedback encourages behavior and enhances self-esteem.
	Client safety is of primary importance.

Continued

ACTIONS/INTERVENTIONS	RATIONALES
• Provide appropriate behavioral limits to control the expression of aggression or anger. These limits should be specific to the client and listed here on the care plan, e.g., client will be asked to go to seclusion room for 15 min when he raises his voice to another client. The client should be informed of these limits, and the limits should not exceed the client's capability. The client should be informed of the limits of the limits, e.g., the time limit of the limit for raising his voice is 15 min. No limit should be set for an indefinite time. All staff should be aware of the limits so they can be enforced consistently with consistent consequences.	Client safety is of primary importance.
• Provide the client with an opportunity to discuss the situation after the consequences have been met.	Assists client with an opportunity to review behavioral limits and provides the staff with an opportunity to communicate to the client that limit setting is not a punishment. Promotes the development of a trusting relationship.
• Interact with the client in social activities (number) times per day for (number) minutes. This will provide the client with staff time other than that which is used to set limits. The activities selected should be done with the client's input and stated here in the care plan.	
• Provide medication as ordered, and observe patient for appropriate side effects (these should be listed here).	
• Inform the client of community resources that provide assistance with crisis situations, and provide a phone number before the client leaves the unit.	Promotes the client's sense of control and self-esteem.
• Develop a list of alternative coping strategies that the client can use at home, and have the client practice them before leaving the unit.	Repeated practice of a behavior internalizes and personalizes the behavior.
• Provide the client with a written list of appointments that have been scheduled for outpatient follow-up.	Provides visible documentation of the importance of follow-up. Increases likelihood that appointments will be kept.

Gerontic Health

ACTIONS/INTERVENTIONS	RATIONALES
• Daily monitor for side effects of antianxiety agents if prescribed.	The potential for side effects and drug interactions are increased with older adults due to the decreased metabolism of drugs.
• Identifiy environmental factors that may increase anxiety such as noise level, harsh lighting, and high traffic flow.	The environmental factors mentioned, if not addressed, induce more stress in the older individual.
• Provide direct, basic information on usual routines and procedures.	May help decrease autonomic nervous system activity and feelings of anxiety.

Home Health

ACTIONS/INTERVENTIONS	RATIONALES
• Teach the client and family appropriate monitoring of signs and symptoms of anxiety: 　○ Increased pulse 　○ Sleep disturbance 　○ Fatigue 　○ Restlessness 　○ Increased respiratory rate 　○ Inability to concentrate 　○ Short attention span 　○ Feeling of dread 　○ Faintness 　○ Forgetfulness	Provides baseline data for early recognition and intervention.
• Involve the client and family in planning and implementing strategies to reduce and cope with anxiety: 　○ Family conference: Identification of sources of anxiety and interventions designed to decrease anxiety 　○ Mutual goal setting: Specific ways to decrease anxiety, and identification of role of each family member 　○ Communication	Family and client involvement enhances effectiveness of intervention.
• Assist the client and family in lifestyle adjustments that may be required: 　○ Relaxation techniques, e.g., yoga, biofeedback, hypnosis, breathing techniques, or imagery 　○ Problem-solving techniques 　○ Crisis intervention 　○ Maintaining the treatment plan of health care professionals who are guiding the therapy 　○ Redirecting energy to meaningful or productive activities, e.g., active games and hobbies, walking, or sports 　○ Decreasing sensory stimulation	Lifestyle changes require changes in behavior. Self-evaluation and support facilitate these changes.
• Assist the client and family to set criteria to help them determine when the intervention of a health care professional is required, e.g., inability to perform activities of daily living or threat to self or others.	Early identification of issues requiring professional evaluation will increase the probability of successful interventions.
• Teach the client and family purposes, side effects, and proper administration techniques of medications.	Provides necessary information for self-care.
• Consult with or refer patient to assistive resources as indicated.	Provides for effective use of existing community services and resources.

Anxiety

FLOWCHART EVALUATION: EXPECTED OUTCOME 1

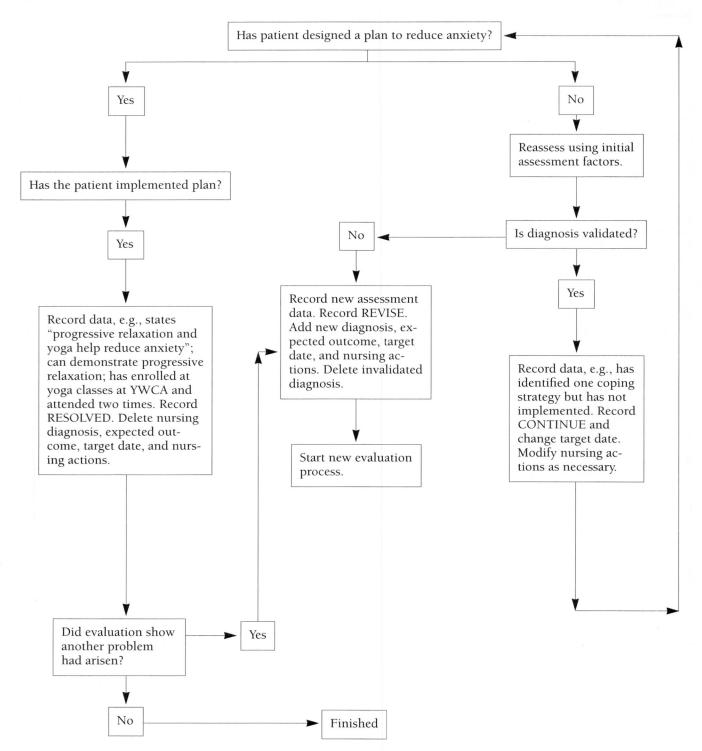

Anxiety

FLOWCHART EVALUATION: EXPECTED OUTCOME 2

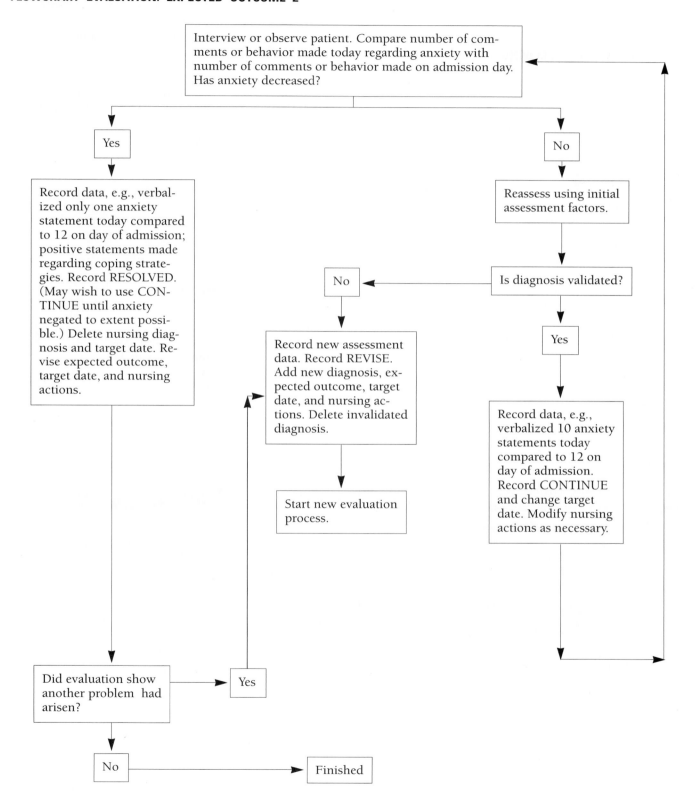

Body Image Disturbance

DEFINITION

Disruption in the way one perceives one's body image.[23]

NANDA TAXONOMY: PERCEIVING 7.1.1

DEFINING CHARACTERISTICS[23]

A *or* B must be present to justify the diagnosis of Body Image Disturbance. A is a verbal response to actual or perceived change in structure and/or function; B is a nonverbal response to actual or perceived change in structure and/or function. (Note that both A and B are considered critical.) The following clinical manifestations may be used to validate the presence of A *or* B:

1. Objective
   a. Missing body part
   b. Actual change in structure and/or function
   c. Not looking at body part
   d. Not touching body part
   e. Hiding or overexposing body part (intentional or unintentional)
   f. Trauma to nonfunctioning part
   g. Change in social involvement
   h. Change in ability to estimate spatial relationship of body to environment
2. Subjective—verbalization of:
   a. Change in lifestyle
   b. Fear of rejection or of reaction by others

c. Focus on past strength, function, or appearance
d. Negative feelings about body
e. Feelings of helplessness, hopelessness, or powerlessness
f. Preoccupation with change or loss
g. Emphasis on remaining strengths or heightened achievement
h. Extension of body boundary to incorporate environmental objects
i. Personalization of part or loss by name
j. Depersonalization of part or loss by impersonal pronouns
k. Refusal to verify actual change

RELATED FACTORS[23]

1. Biophysical
2. Cognitive or perceptual
3. Psychosocial
4. Cultural
5. Spiritual

RELATED CLINICAL CONCERNS

1. Amputation
2. Mastectomy
3. Acne or other visible skin disorders
4. Visible scarring from surgery or burns
5. Obesity
6. Anorexia nervosa

HAVE YOU SELECTED THE CORRECT DIAGNOSIS?

Self-Esteem Disturbance This diagnosis addresses a lack of confidence in one's self and is characterized by negative self-statements, lack of concern about personal appearance, and withdrawal from others not related to physical problems or attributes. Body Image Disturbance relates to alterations in the perceptions of self due to actual or perceived alterations in body structure or function.

Personal Identity Disturbance Personal Identity Disturbance is defined as the inability to distinguish between self and nonself. This diagnosis is more involved in the mental health arena. Body Image Disturbance is a reaction to an actual or perceived change in the body structure or function and incorporates the adult health area as well as mental health.

EXPECTED OUTCOMES

1. Will verbalize at least (number) of positive body image statements by (date) and/or
2. Will identify at least (number) measures to overcome body part loss by (date)

TARGET DATES

A target date of 3 to 5 days would be acceptable to use for initial evaluation of progress.

NURSING ACTIONS/INTERVENTIONS WITH RATIONALES
Adult Health

ACTIONS/INTERVENTIONS	RATIONALES
• Monitor for pain every 2 h on the (odd/even) hour. Administer analgesics. Monitor effectiveness of analgesic within 30 min of administration, and use noninvasive techniques to keep pain under control.	Uncontrolled pain contributes significantly to problems with body functioning, thus promoting the development and continuation of body image disturbance.
• Use anxiety-reducing techniques as often as needed.	Assist the patient in adapting to the changed body image.
• Stay in frequent contact with the patient:	Promotes verbalization of feelings and allows consistent intervention.
○ Be honest with patient.	Any dishonesty in terms of recovery, return of function, or rehabilitation needs causes patient to distrust caregivers and promotes maintenance of body image disturbance.
○ Point out and limit self-negation statements.	Self-negating statements prolong the problem and interfere with the rehabilitation potential.
○ Do not support denial. Focus on reality and adaptation (not necessarily acceptance).	The patient does not have to accept the problem, but he or she does have to, and can, adapt to the problem.
○ Set limits on maladaptive behavior.	Maladaptive behavior supports the continuation of body image disturbance.
○ Focus on realistic goals.	Supports continued progress. Allows positive feedback for achievement and permits patient to see progress.
○ Be aware of own nonverbal communication and behavior.	Any avoidance behavior or nonverbal communication that indicates dismay would support the patient's idea of his or her unacceptability as a damaged person.
○ Avoid moral, value judgments.	
• Assist and encourage patient to look at and use affected body part during activities of daily living.	Helps patient to attend to altered body image constructively and assists patient to accept self.
• Promote calm, safe environment throughout hospitalization.	When using adaptive equipment, the patient's safety must be foremost. A calm environment allows the patient to focus on working with the equipment or techniques without undue pressure.
• Collaborate with psychiatric nurse clinician regarding care as needed. (See Psychiatric Health nursing actions.)	Collaboration promotes a holistic care plan and hastens solving of the patient's problem.
• Teach patient, and significant others, self-care requirements.	Helps patient to adapt to body change and improves self-care management. Provides support for self-care and assists significant others to adapt also.
• Encourage patient to use available resources:	Facilitates adaptation and decreases isolation. Provides long-term support.
○ Prosthetic devices	
○ Assistive devices	
○ Reconstructive and corrective surgery	
○ Occupational therapy	
○ Physical therapy	
○ Rehabilitation services	
• Refer patient to and collaborate with community resources.	Provides long-term support. Cost-effective use of already available support.

Child Health

ACTIONS/INTERVENTIONS	RATIONALES
• Monitor for contributory factors for Body Image Disturbance, e.g., disfigurement or perceived disfigurement. (Family may perceive such on behalf of the young infant or child.)	Provides database needed to plan interventions more accurately.

Continued

ACTIONS/INTERVENTIONS	RATIONALES
• Utilize developmentally appropriate communication to assess and determine exact expression of Body Image Disturbance, e.g., use puppet play or constructive dialogue for the toddler.	Developmental capacity has to guide the interaction to gain accurate information.
• Provide factual information to assist in dealing with Body Image Disturbance, e.g., availability of assistive devices or surgery.	Knowledge serves to reduce anxiety and assists patient to cope. Provides options to assist in decision making.
• Include other specialists such as occupational, physical, and speech therapists, as required.	Promotes a more accurate and holistic plan of care.
• Monitor, on a daily basis, for attitude toward body.	Allows daily evaluation, which promotes changes in plan of care to best meet patient's current status.

NOTE: In some instances, such as an infant or child with an anomaly or a condition offering no hope of resolution, this alteration may accompany other disturbances such as self-esteem, parental coping, and loss.

Women's Health

ACTIONS/INTERVENTIONS	RATIONALES
BODY IMAGE: SURGERY	
• Assist the patient to identify lifestyle adjustments that may be needed, e.g., recuperation time or prosthesis as necessary (mastectomy).	Initiates discharge planning.
• Monitor the patient's anxiety level and discuss, preoperatively:	
○ Routines related to surgery, e.g., anesthesia, pain, length of surgery, or postoperative care.	
○ Physical changes, e.g., cessation of menstruation or menopausal symptoms.	
• Allow the patient to grieve loss of body image, e.g., no longer able to have children, and provide an empathetic atmosphere that will allow the patient to ventilate concerns about appearance or reaction of significant other.	
• Dispel "old wives' tales" (usually connected to hysterectomy) such as:	Provides factual information, allowing patient to ask further questions and be realistic about her status and goals.
○ You will no longer feel like a woman. (Reassure patient there will be no more pregnancies or menstruation, but hysterectomy does not affect sexual performance, enjoyment, or response.)	
○ There will be masculinization. (There is no basis for this belief, and it does not occur.)	
○ There will be weight gain. (Weight gain will not occur if patient follows former lifestyle, participates in an exercise routine, and follows proper diet.)	
• Involve significant others in discussion and problem-solving activities regarding life cycle changes that might affect self-esteem and interpersonal relationships, e.g., hot flashes, appearance, sexual relationships, or ability to have children.	Provides basic information and allows early intervention for anxiety. Provides opportunity for teaching and clarification of misinformation.[25]
• In collaboration with physician, provide factual information on estrogen replacement therapy.	Assists patient in making decision regarding use or nonuse of estrogen therapy.

BODY IMAGE: PREGNANCY

• Assist the patient in identifying lifestyle adjustments due to physiologic, physical, and emotional changes that will occur throughout pregnancy and postpartum.	Knowledge that body changes in pregnancy are normal and temporary encourages patient to follow through on care. Assists the patient to cope with the pregnancy and adapt to the changing images.
• Review with patient the body changes that occur during pregnancy and the effect on body image (particularly for teenagers): ○ Weight gain ○ Breast tenderness and enlargement ○ Enlargement of abdomen ○ Change in gait ○ Chloasma (mask of pregnancy) ○ Striations (stretch marks) from pregnancy	
• Consider the patient's age and preparation for pregnancy, including (particularly for teenagers): ○ Stress that weight loss after delivery usually takes 1 or 2 wk. ○ Discuss physical development. ○ Evaluate patient's attitude toward health care providers. ○ Discuss self-esteem. ○ Provide emotional support. ○ Prepare patient for lifestyle interruptions. ○ Encourage the patient to bring an attractive, loose-fitting dress to wear home. ○ Caution breast-feeding women against purposeful weight loss while lactating. ○ Encourage non-breast-feeding mothers to follow low-calorie, high-protein diet for weight loss. ○ Encourage exercise (begin slowly and work up to desired plan). ○ Caution patient to avoid fatigue.	Continued home care planning that encourages patient to better apply good health practices and thus increase maternal and fetal well-being.

Psychiatric Health

ACTIONS/INTERVENTIONS	RATIONALES
• Spend (number) minutes with the client at (times) discussing perception of disruption in lifestyle necessitated by change. • Discuss with the client meaning of loss or change from a personal and cultural perspective. • Discuss with the client significant other's reaction to loss or change. • Set an appointment to discuss with the client and significant others effects of the loss or change on their relationships. (Time and date of appointment and all follow-up appointments should be listed here.) • Spend (number) minutes with the client at (times) to assist with efforts to enhance appearance. • Provide physical activities 2 times per day at (times) that provide the client opportunities to define boundaries of body. These activities should be ones the client identifies as enjoyable and that are easily accomplished by the client. Those activities that are selected should be listed here. If this diagnosis is in conjunction with an eating disorder, adjust exercise to appropriate levels for the client.	Promotes client's sense of control and provides information that can be utilized in developing a plan of care that will fit within the client's perception of self. Expression of feelings in an accepting environment can facilitate the client's problem solving. Support system understanding can facilitate the client's adjustment. Expression of feelings and concerns in an accepting environment can facilitate problem solving. Promotes client's sense of control and enhances self-esteem. Assists client in developing a new perception of body.

Continued

ACTIONS/INTERVENTIONS	RATIONALES
• Discuss with the client the difference between the cultural ideal of physical appearance and the population norm based on the realities of physiology. This activity should be done by the primary care nurse who has developed a relationship with the client.	Helps to promote reality orientation by contrasting real with ideal and confronts irrational goals.
• Have the client draw a picture of self before and after body change, and discuss this picture with him or her. This activity can also be done with clay models constructed by the client. This activity should be done by the primary care nurse who has developed a relationship with the client.	Assists client in contrasting and externalizing perceptions of self to facilitate development of congruence between real and ideal.
• Have the eating disorder client draw a life-size picture of self on paper hung on the wall; then have the client stand against the picture and trace the real outline and discuss the differences. This activity should be done by the primary care nurse who has developed a relationship with the client.	Assists client in confronting the difference between his or her perception of his or her body and his or her real body size and shape.
• When the client has begun to discuss issues related to body change with the primary care nurse, the client can then be asked to discuss reactions to image of self in a mirror. One hour should be allowed for this activity. This activity should be done by the primary care nurse who has developed a relationship with the client.	Facilitates the development of a congruence between real and perceived self.
• Discuss with the client the mental images held of what the altered body is like and what life will be like. One hour should be allowed for this activity, and it should be implemented by the primary care nurse after a relationship has been established.	Discussion of concerns in a safe environment facilitates the development of strategies of coping.

Gerontic Health

The nursing actions for the older adult with this diagnosis are the same as those for the adult.

Home Health

ACTIONS/INTERVENTIONS	RATIONALES
• Involve client and family in planning and implementing strategies to reduce and cope with disturbance in body image: ○ Family conference: Discuss meaning of loss or change from family perspective and from perspective of individual members. Discuss the effects of the loss on family relationships roles. ○ Mutual goal setting: Establish realistic goals, and identify specific activities for each family member, e.g., assisting with activities as required or attending support groups as needed. ○ Communication: Clarify responses to Body Image Disturbance.	Family involvement enhances effectiveness of interventions.
• Assist the client and family in lifestyle adjustments that may be required: ○ Obtaining and providing accurate information regarding specific Body Image Disturbance and potential for rehabilitation ○ Maintaining safe environment	Rehabilitation is a long-term process. Permanent changes in behavior and family roles require evaluation and support.

- ○ Encouraging appropriate self-care without encouraging dependence or expecting unrealistic independence
- ○ Maintaining the treatment plan of the health care professional's guiding therapy
- ○ Altering family roles as required
- Consult with or refer patient to assistive resources as indicated.

Utilization of existing services is efficient use of resources. Rehabilitation therapists and support groups can enhance the treatment plan.

Body Image Disturbance

FLOWCHART EVALUATION: EXPECTED OUTCOME 1

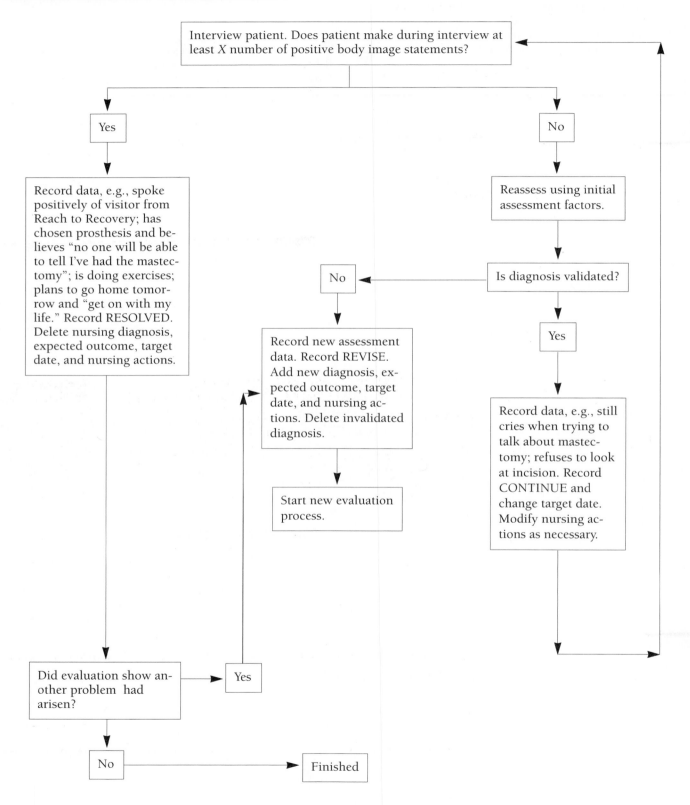

Body Image Disturbance

FLOWCHART EVALUATION: EXPECTED OUTCOME 2

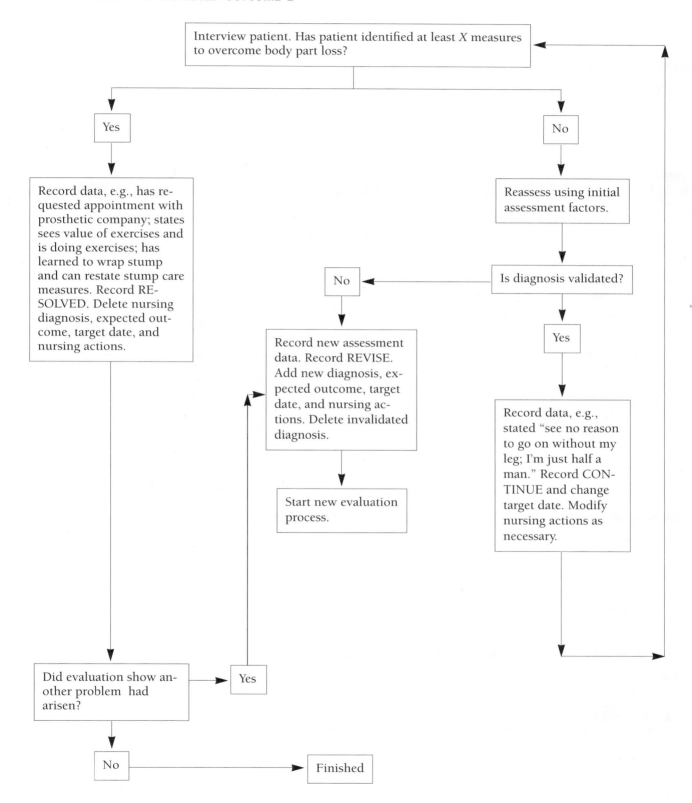

Fear

DEFINITION

Feeling of dread related to an identifiable source that the person validates.[23]

NANDA TAXONOMY: FEELING 9.3.2

DEFINING CHARACTERISTICS[23]

1. Major defining characteristics
   a. Ability to identify object of fear

2. Minor defining characteristics
   None given

RELATED FACTORS[23]

To be developed.

RELATED CLINICAL CONCERNS

1. Any hospitalization
2. Any threat to loss of a body part, loss of functioning, or loss of life

HAVE YOU SELECTED THE CORRECT DIAGNOSIS?

Anxiety   Anxiety is the response to a threat that cannot be easily identified, while Fear is the response to an identified threat. Thus, if the individual was responding to the thought of a bear in the woods or actually confronting the bear, the diagnosis would be Fear. If the threat could not be directly identified or attached to a specific situation, the diagnosis would be Anxiety.

Altered Parenting   This diagnosis should be considered as the appropriate diagnosis when the child's fears result from the parent's modeling or reinforcing of a child's fear or when the parent is not providing the appropriate support for the developmental fears. An example might be the child who becomes uncontrollable in the clinic each time an injection is indicated. During the assessment the nurse discovers that the parents tell their children that if they do not behave, the nurse or doctor will give them a shot as a reinforcer to discipline at home. In this situation the parent's inappropriate use of the threat of the injection produced a fear in the child.

Knowledge Deficit   If the patient indicates that he or she is afraid of not being able to care for himself or herself, then the most appropriate diagnosis would be Knowledge Deficit. Providing the patient with information, teaching, and reinforcement of self-care ability will overcome this diagnosis.

EXPECTED OUTCOMES

1. Will design and implement a plan to reduce fear by (date) and/or
2. Will be able to identify specific source of fear by (date)

TARGET DATES

A target date of 2 to 3 days would be acceptable since the sooner the fear can be reduced, the sooner other problems can be resolved.

NURSING ACTIONS/INTERVENTIONS WITH RATIONALES

Adult Health

ACTIONS/INTERVENTIONS	RATIONALES
• Assist patient to correct any sensory deficits.	Inability to correctly sense and perceive stimuli may increase fear.
• Maintain calm, safe environment throughout the hospitalization: ○ Use frequent reassurance. ○ Touch patient frequently. ○ Have someone remain with patient.	A nonthreatening environment decreases fear.

- Administer antianxiety medications as ordered. Observe and record response to medication within 30 min after administration.

Determines effectiveness of medication and allows changing of medication as needed.

- Monitor, at least every 4 h while awake:
  - Vital signs
  - Degree of confusion
  - Degree of reality orientation

Determines physiologic changes due to fear. Assists in determining if physiologic changes are causing pathology.

- Provide information to patient in both written and verbal forms.

Fear interferes with interpretation of verbal input. Written forms provide reinforcement and assist patient to focus and attend to activities.

- Sit down and visit with patient at least 15–20 min every 4 h while awake:
  - Listen carefully.
  - Support positive coping.
  - Give clear, concise, straightforward information.

Provides an opportunity for patient to ask questions and verbalize fears.

- Assist patient to increase development of decision-making skills:
  - Review decision-making process with patient.
  - Provide opportunity for decision making regarding care.
  - Assist patient in developing a list of potential solutions to the threatening situation.
  - Review the developed list of solutions with the patient, and assist him or her in evaluating the benefits and costs of each solution.
  - Rehearse with the patient, if necessary, the solution selected, or have patient practice a new response to the threatening situation.
  - Give positive feedback regarding decision making.
  - Involve significant others in promoting patient's decision making.

Helps patient to practice, in a nonthreatening environment, the problem-solving process. Increases feeling of personal control of situation.

- Collaborate with psychiatric nurse clinician regarding care. (See Psychiatric Health nursing actions.)

Collaboration promotes a holistic and thorough plan of care.

- Teach patient and significant others:
  - Use of progressive relaxation and guided imagery
  - Use of exercise balanced with rest
  - Proper food and fluid intake

Gives additional methods that are successful in dealing with fear.

- Refer patient to appropriate community resources for assistance.

Provides support resources for follow-up on plan after discharge from the hospital.

Child Health

ACTIONS/INTERVENTIONS	RATIONALES
• Offer brief interactions that assist the patient and family with orientation, e.g., hospital unit, procedures, and aspects of care.	Brief explanations and factual information serve to empower the patient and family as the unknown is made known. The patient and family can then focus of dealing with the identified fear rather than dealing with added fears.

• In instances of severe fear:
  ○ Provide support in a nondemanding atmosphere.
  ○ Provide a here-and-now focus.
  ○ Provide one-on-one care.
  ○ Offer simple, direct, repetitive tasks.
	Avoids overwhelming patient. Promotes a sense of trust.

• Provide patient and family with alternative outlets for physical tension. These outlets should be stated specifically and could include walking, talking, etc., at least (number) times per day at (times). These outlets should be designed with input from patient.	Providing such outlets promotes release of tension.

Continued

ACTIONS/INTERVENTIONS	RATIONALES
• Sit with the patient and parents (number) times per day at (times) for (number) minutes to discuss feelings and complaints.	As the patient or parents express these factors openly, the nurse can explore the possible onset of fear with the purpose of individualizing the plan according to patient's needs. The subjective verbalization of fears helps to reduce the preoccupation of the patient with the fear. Reflection on an ongoing basis demonstrates a sensitivity to need.
• Provide feedback to patient and parents to clarify and reexplore changes regarding feelings about fear.	
• Provide appropriate behavioral limits to control the expression of aggression or anger. These limits should be specific in time, expected behavior, and consequences.	Structured rules regarding behavioral consequences create a sense of limits, which provide security for the child.
• Provide the patient and parents with opportunities to discuss the situation after consequences have been met.	Rediscussing and clarification of events serves to update needs and provides feedback for evaluation. Valuing of the patient is also shown.
• Provide opportunities for socialization appropriate for patient and family.	Socialization is vital as the individual or family assumes coping behaviors and learns new coping skills.
• Develop a list of alternative coping strategies to be practiced by patient and family before dismissal, e.g., communication or progressive relaxation.	Allow practice in a nonthreatening environment. Increases skills.
• Ensure follow-up appointments by scheduling them for patient before dismissal.	Follow-up appointments help ensure follow-up care.
• Assist patient and family to view situation represented as something that can be managed. Encourage positive reinforcement of desired behavior patterns.	Validation of success in coping will provide a sense of empowerment.

Women's Health

NOTE: Phobias affect approximately 2 to 3 percent of the adult population, and 80 percent of the affected group are female. The most common phobias among women are agoraphobia, fear of animals, and fear of social situations.[26,27]

ACTIONS/INTERVENTIONS	RATIONALES
• Obtain a detailed history of patient's fears: ○ Encourage patient to discuss signs and symptoms or precipitating event. ○ Ascertain how often problem occurs. ○ Have patient describe her reaction. ○ Identify coping mechanisms that have previously helped. ○ Identify those factors or coping mechanisms that do not help.	Provides essential database for planning appropriate interventions.

DOMESTIC VIOLENCE

• Provide a nonjudgmental, safe environment for the patient to verbalize her fears. In childbirth and parenting classes, discuss family violence. Obtain a good history that can identify high-risk families. Be alert to subtle clues in patient's history or physical exam that hint at physical abuse.

- Patiently explain all procedures and their purpose to patient before performing them. Be aware that procedures in labor and delivery can trigger unpleasant fears and anxieties in patient with possible flashbacks to an abusive situation or rape. Perform necessary procedures as quickly as possible and with empathy, allowing patient to direct as much of the care as possible. Encourage patient to verbalize her fears and verbally relive the birth experience in a nonjudgmental environment.
- Inform patients of services and shelters for the battered woman. Post telephone numbers in conspicuous places. Post telephone numbers in women's bathroom (unavailable to men, so they cannot see partner getting number). Tell women to memorize number, never write it down.

It is important to provide information about resources to these women in an unobtrusive manner, so they can access the resources when *they are ready*.

BIRTHING PROCESS

- Provide a comfortable, nonjudging atmosphere to encourage the patient and her significant other to verbalize their fears of:
  ○ The unknown
  ○ Safety for herself and her baby
  ○ Pain during the birthing process
  ○ Mutilation during the birthing process
  ○ "Losing control" during the birthing process
- Refer patient to appropriate support groups for information:
  ○ Childbirth education classes in the community
  ○ Schools of nursing (students in obstetrics that have follow-through of families of pregnant women)
  ○ Special national organizations
- Monitor patient's level of confidence using prepared childbirth techniques during labor:
  ○ Encourage use of relaxation and prepared childbirth techniques during labor.
  ○ Provide ongoing and accurate information, during the labor and birth process, to both the patient and her significant other.
  ○ Assist patient in using "imagery" to overcome fears during the birthing process.
- Provide continuity of care by remaining with and providing comfort for the laboring woman throughout the birthing process:
  ○ Provide clear answers to patient's questions.
  ○ Keep patient informed of her progress in the birthing process.
- Provide the patient and significant others with as many opportunities as possible to make decisions about her care during the birthing process.

Assists in decreasing fear through promotion of verbalization.

Provides effective use of existing resources and long-range support.

Use of relaxation techniques and provision of information regarding progress facilitate the labor process by easing anxiety and promoting comfort.[25]

Encourages involvement in process, which enhances coping.

Psychiatric Health

ACTIONS/INTERVENTIONS	RATIONALES
• Provide a quiet, nonstimulating environment for the client. This would include removing persons and objects that the person perceives as threatening. If the person is experiencing a thought disorder with delusions and hallucinations, attention should be paid to the details of the environment that could be misinterpreted. At times a same-sex caregiver can increase fear in the client.	Inappropriate levels of environmental stimuli can increase disorientation and confusion.
• Obtain the client's understanding of the threat.	Facilitates the development of interventions that directly address the client's concerns.
• Provide a one-on-one relationship for the client with a member of the nursing staff. This should be maintained until the symptoms return to normal levels.	Promotes a trusting relationship and enhances the client's self-esteem.
• Provide clear answers to client's questions.	Inappropriate amounts of sensory stimuli can increase the client's confusion and disorganization.
• Carry on conversations in the client's presence or vision in a voice that the client can hear.	Meets safety needs of client by eliminating stimuli that could be misinterpreted in a personalized manner.
• Inform the client of plans related to care before the plans are implemented. If possible, discuss these with the client (e.g., if it is necessary to move the client to another room or institution, the client should be informed of this change before it takes place).	Promotes the client's sense of control and enhances self-esteem.
• Orient the client to the environment.	Promotes safety needs by increasing the client's familiarity with the environment in the accompaniment of a trusted individual.
• Maintain a consistent environment and routine. Record client's daily routine here along with notes about client's special reactions to visitors and staff members.	Promotes the client's sense of safety and trust by maintaining consistency in the environment.
• Provide a primary care nurse for the client on each shift.	Promotes the development of a trusting relationship.
• Sit with the client (number) minutes (number) times per shift. (Initially the times should reflect short, frequent contact. This can change with the client's needs.)	Promotes the development of a trusting relationship. Interaction with the nurse can provide positive reinforcement and enhance self-esteem.
• Provide the client with objects in the environment that promote security. These may be symbolic items from home or religious objects. List significant items here.	Meets the need for affiliation by providing meaningful objects to which the client is attached.[20]
• Note the client's desired personal space, and respect these limits (the general guidelines should be stated here).	Communicates respect for the client while decreasing the client's anxiety by maintaining a comfortable personal space.

• Assist the client with sorting out the fearful situation by:
  ○ Recognizing that the experience is real for the client even though that is not your experience of the situation: "I can see that you are very upset. I can understand how those thoughts could make you fearful."
  ○ Providing feedback about distorted thoughts: "No, I am not going to punish you. I am here to talk with you about your concerns."
  ○ Encouraging client to develop an understanding of the threat by talking about it in specific terms and not vague generalizations: "When you say your family is out to get you, who and what do you mean?"
  ○ Focusing conversations in the here and now: This would include information about the effects of the client's behavior on those around him or her, your experience of the client, and your perceptions of the environment.
	Communicates respect for the client while encouraging reality testing.

- Not arguing about client's perceptions: Instead, provide feedback in the here and now with your perceptions of the situation. The client tells you that you must be angry with him or her because of the look you had on your face while reviewing the client's chart. Your response is, "I am not angry with you. When I was looking at your chart, I was thinking about the conversation we had this morning about your job."
- Provide the client with as many opportunities as possible to make decisions about his or her care and current situation.

Promotes the client's sense of control and enhances self-esteem.

- Assist the client in developing a list of potential solutions to the threatening situation.
- Review developed list of solutions with the client, and assist him or her in evaluating the benefits and costs of each solution.

Teaches client problem-solving skills while promoting the client's sense of control and strengths.
Facilitates the client's decision-making process.

- Rehearse with the client, if necessary, the solution selected, or have client practice a new response to the threatening situation.
- Provide positive feedback to the client about his or her efforts to resolve the threatening situation.
- Assist the client in developing alternative outlets for the feelings generated by the threatening situation, and provide the opportunity for the use of these outlets. These would be noted in the chart so other staff members would be aware of them and could encourage their use when they notice the client's discomfort increasing.

Behavioral rehearsal helps to facilitate the client's learning new skills through the use of feedback and modeling by the nurse.[28]
Positive feedback encourages behavior and enhances self-esteem.
Planned coping strategies facilitate the enactment of new behaviors when the client is experiencing stress.

- Assist the client in identifying early behavioral cues that indicate fear or that he or she is entering a fearful situation.

Early recognition and intervention enhance the opportunities for new coping behaviors to be effective.

- Encourage the client in alternative coping strategies developed by:
  - Providing the necessary environment
  - Providing the appropriate equipment
  - Spending time with the client doing the activity
  - Providing positive reinforcement for the use of the strategy (this could be verbal as well as with special privileges)

Promotes client's perception of control. Positive reinforcement encourages behavior.

- If fear is related to a specific object or situation, teach the client to use deep muscle relaxation, and then teach this along with progressively real mental images of the threatening situation. This is for those situations that will not cause the client harm if he or she is approached, such as riding in elevators. This could also include other methods of relaxation such as music, deep breathing, thought stopping, fantasy, assertiveness training, audiotapes with relaxation images or sequences, yoga, hypnosis, and meditation.

The relaxation response inhibits the activation of the autonomic nervous system's fight-or-flight response.

- Explore ways to increase client's feeling of control in threatening situation; e.g., a fear of elevators could be altered by the client's only riding in elevators with emergency phones and only riding when he or she can stand near the phone. The fear may also indicate that the client is feeling out of control in an unrelated area of his or her life. If this is suspected, this should be explored, and ways of increasing control should be explored; e.g., a woman's fear of driving could indicate that she feels out of control in her marriage, and increased assertive behavior with her husband removes the fear.

Continued

ACTIONS/INTERVENTIONS	RATIONALES
• If the method to increase control involves interactions with the health care team, these should be noted in specific terms on the client's chart.	Promotes the client's sense of control and enhances self-esteem.
• Assist the client in developing strategies to be used in the community after discharge, and role-play various situations with the client for at least 1 h for at least 2 days.	Behavioral rehearsal provides opportunities for feedback and modeling from the nurse.

Gerontic Health

ACTIONS/INTERVENTIONS	RATIONALES
• Assist patient in identifying the source of fear—e.g., pain, death, or loss of function—by scheduling at least 30 min twice a day at (times) to confer with patient about fear.	Identifying the source of fear enables the patient to develop a specific plan of action to reduce the fear.
• Assist the patient in determining what resources are available to enhance his or her coping skills.	Knowledge and use of appropriate resources aids in reducing fear-provoking experiences by increasing the patient's inventory of skills to deal with fear.

Home Health

ACTIONS/INTERVENTIONS	RATIONALES
• Teach the client and family appropriate monitoring of signs and symptoms of fear: ○ Increased pulse ○ Flushed face ○ Sweaty palms ○ Shortness of breath ○ Muscle tightness ○ Nausea, vomiting, or diarrhea ○ Sleep disturbance ○ Fainting ○ Sweating ○ Urinary frequency or urgency ○ Crying	Provides baseline data for early recognition and intervention.
• Involve the client and family in planning and implementing strategies to reduce and cope with fear.	Family involvement is important to ensure success. Communication and mutual goal setting will increase the probability of a positive outcome.
• Assist the client and family in making lifestyle adjustments that may be required: ○ Relaxation techniques: Yoga, biofeedback, hypnosis, breathing techniques, or imagery ○ Providing a secure environment: Familiar objects and familiar people or predictable events with surprises ○ Communication techniques: Responses that reflect reality; orienting to person, time, and place; explaining activities; providing predictable and consistent situations; and maintaining visual, auditory, and tactile contact ○ Problem-solving strategies	Lifestyle changes require changes in behavior. Self-evaluation and support facilitate these changes.
• Provide a sense of mastery (i.e., accomplishable goals in secure environment).	

- Maintain the treatment plan of the health care professional guiding the therapy.
- Assist the patient and family to set criteria to help them to determine when the intervention of a health care professional is required, e.g., prolonged nausea, vomiting or diarrhea, or uncontrolled crying.
- Consult with or refer patient to assistive resources as indicated.

Early identification of situations requiring professional evaluation will increase the probability of successful interventions.

Provides efficient and cost-effective use of already available resources.

Fear

FLOWCHART EVALUATION: EXPECTED OUTCOME 1

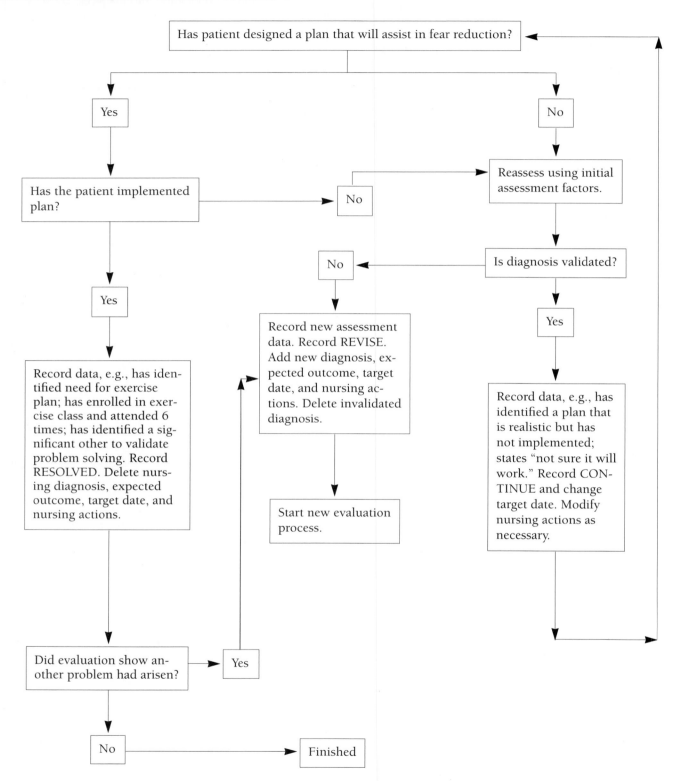

Fear

FLOWCHART EVALUATION: EXPECTED OUTCOME 2

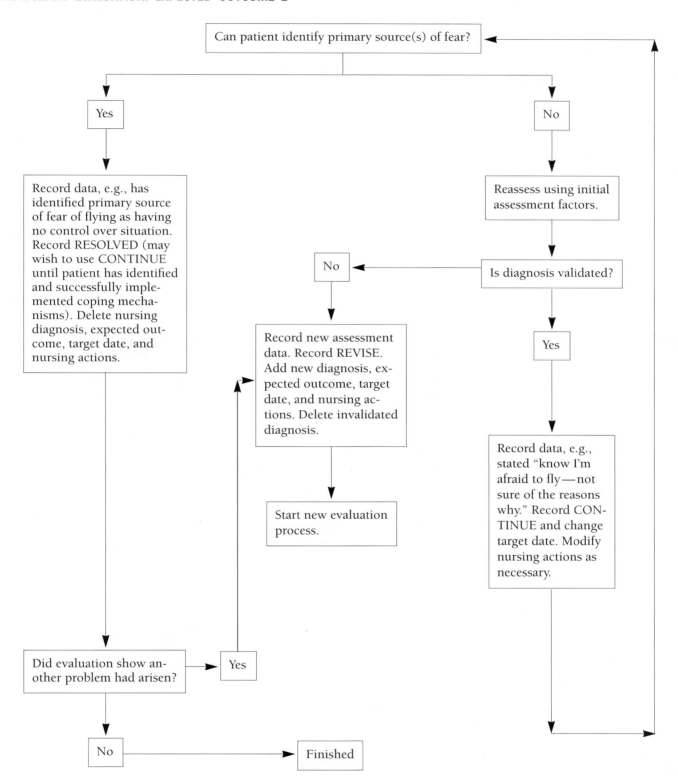

Hopelessness

DEFINITION

A subjective state in which an individual sees limited or no alternatives or personal choices available and is unable to mobilize energy on own behalf.[23]

NANDA TAXONOMY: PERCEIVING 7.3.1

DEFINING CHARACTERISTICS[23]

1. Major defining characteristics
   a. Passivity, or decreased verbalization
   b. Decreased affect
   c. Verbal cues (despondent content, "I can't," sighing)
2. Minor defining characteristics
   a. Lack of initiative
   b. Decreased response to stimuli
   c. Decreased affect
   d. Turning away from speaker
   e. Closing eyes
   f. Shrugging in response to speaker
   g. Decreased appetite
   h. Increased or decreased sleep
   i. Lack of involvement in care or passivity allowing care

RELATED FACTORS[23]

1. Prolonged activity restriction creating isolation
2. Failing or deteriorating physiologic condition
3. Long-term stress
4. Abandonment
5. Lost belief in transcendent values or God

RELATED CLINICAL CONCERNS

1. Any disease of a chronic nature
2. Any disease with a terminal diagnosis
3. Any condition where a diagnosis cannot be definitely established

HAVE YOU SELECTED THE CORRECT DIAGNOSIS?

Powerlessness   This diagnosis is present when the individual perceives that his or her actions will not change a situation regardless of the options that the person may see in a situation. Hopelessness occurs when the individual perceives that there are few or limited choices in a situation. Powerlessness may evolve out of Hopelessness. Powerlessness is the perception that one's actions will not make a difference, while Hoplessness is the perception that there are not options to act upon. The decision about which is the most appropriate diagnosis is based on the clinical judgment of the nurse about which symptoms predominate.

Anxiety   Anxiety may have as a component a perception of Hopelessness. This could evolve out of the narrowed perception of the anxious client. Hopelessness may have as a component Anxiety. This situation could develop when the client is feeling overwhelmed with the perception that there are no alternatives in a difficult situation. The primary diagnosis evolves from the symptoms sequence. If Anxiety is the predominant symptom cluster, it should be the primary diagnosis because of the strong influence it has on the client's perceptions.

Altered Thought Process   If the individual cannot accurately assess the situation, then a sense of Hopelessness might occur. In this instance Hopelessness would be a companion diagnosis.

Fear   If the client is fearful in a situation, perception can be narrowed and alternative options may be overlooked. When Fear and Hopelessness occur together, Fear should be the primary diagnosis.

EXPECTED OUTCOMES

1. Will initiate a realistic plan to reduce perception of hopelessness by (date) and/or
2. Will verbalize a decrease in complaints regarding hopelessness by (date)

TARGET DATES

A target date ranging between 3 and 5 days would be appropriate for initial evaluation. A target date over 5 days might lead to increased complications such as potential for self-injury. A target date sooner than 3 days would not provide a sufficient length of time for realizing the effects of intervention.

NURSING ACTIONS/INTERVENTIONS WITH RATIONALES

Adult Health

ACTIONS/INTERVENTIONS	RATIONALES
• Establish a therapeutic and trusting relationship with patient and family by actively listening, being nonjudgmental, sitting with patient, touching (as welcomed by patient), etc.	Promotes a safe environment to encourage the patient and/or family to verbalize concerns. Promotes empathetic environment.
• Identify other primary nursing needs, and deal with them as needed.	Inattention to basic needs increases feelings of hopelessness and of being of no value.
• Support patient's efforts at objectively describing feelings of hopelessness when interacting with patient.	Assists patient in releasing tension. Allows patient to validate reality.
• Assist the patient to find alternatives to feelings of hopelessness as patient expresses them.	Validates reality and encourages use of coping techniques. Points out the variety of solutions available.
• Assist the patient to engage in social interaction at least once per shift.	Provides diversion and decreases sense of isolation.
• As health status permits, increase activity level. Have patient participate in self-care management by adding an activity such as washing face one day, washing face and arms the next day, etc., or have patient walk to bathroom first day and ambulate 30 ft down the hall the next day.	Encourages patient to regain control in small increments. Decreases the idea that the personal self is responsible for the situation.
• Encourage food and fluid intake to at least 1500 calories per day and at least 2000 mL per day.	Hopelessness may prompt unhealthy eating patterns.
• Moderate sleep-wake cycles: ○ Provide diversional activities during the day. ○ **Do not** let patient take naps during the day. ○ Provide massage at bedtime. ○ Darken the room, but provide a night light for sleep. ○ Give sleep medication as ordered, and monitor effects.	Maintains diurnal rhythm and promotes rest.
• Encourage active participation in activities of daily living. Allow for preferences in day-to-day decisions, e.g., establishing a bath time. Provide explanations and appropriate teaching for procedures and treatments.	Helps restore sense of being in control.
• Refer patient to psychiatric nurse clinician as needed (see Psychiatric Health nursing actions).	Collaboration promotes a more holistic and complete plan of care.
• Identify religious, cultural, or community support groups prior to discharge. Provide appointments for follow-up.	Support groups can provide advocacy for the patient and continued monitoring and support of patient after discharge from the hospital.

Child Health

ACTIONS/INTERVENTIONS	RATIONALES
• Monitor for the etiologic components contributing to hopelessness pattern.	Provides database that results in a more accurate and complete plan of care.
• Encourage patient and family to verbalize feelings about current status with 30 min set aside each shift at (times) for this purpose.	Verbalization helps reduce anxiety and assigns value to the patient's concerns. Allows ongoing assessment.
• Assist patient and family to explore growth potential afforded by this specific experience.	Opportunity for growth may be overlooked in times of crisis.
• Allow for opportunities for child to "play out" feelings under appropriate supervision if possible: ○ Play with dolls for toddler ○ Art and puppets for preschooler ○ Peer discussions for adolescents	Play and the acting out of feelings provide insight into coping and perceptions of the child in a noninvasive mode. Provides valuable data to monitor feelings, concerns, etc.

Women's Health

> **NOTE:** The following nursing actions for the couple (husband or wife) who have been unable to conceive a child. See Chapter 10 for detailed information on infertility. Provide a nonjudgmental atmosphere to allow the infertile couple to express their feelings such as anger, denial, inadequacy, guilt, depression, or grief.

ACTIONS/INTERVENTIONS	RATIONALES
INFERTILITY	
• Support and allow couple to work through grieving process for loss of fertility, for loss of children, for loss of idealized lifestyle, and for the loss of feminine life experiences such as pregnancy, birth, and breast-feeding.	Provision of support for and encouragement of discussion regarding emotions allows the couple to begin to deal with emotions and lays groundwork for future decision making.[25]
• Encourage couple to talk honestly with one another about feelings.	
• Encourage couple to seek professional help if necessary to deal with feelings related to sexual relationship, conflicts, anxieties, parenting, and coping mechanisms used for dealing with loss of fertility (their expectations, relatives' expectations, and society's expectations).	
• Be alert for signs of depression, anger, frustration, and impending crisis.	Allows early intervention and avoidance of complications.
• Provide the infertile couples with accurate information on adoption and living without children.	Provides informational support for decision making.
POSTPARTUM DEPRESSION	
NOTE: The majority of patients who experience hopelessness leading to postpartum depression have been found to have underlying psychiatric disorders or life experiences other than pregnancy that accounted for the depression.[29]	

• Provide factual information to patient and partner on postpartum depression. Describe difference between baby blues and depression. Identify potential psychosocial triggers in patient's environment that could lead to postpartum depression, such as:
  ○ Feelings of ambivalence
  ○ Feelings of inadequacy
  ○ Marital discord
  ○ Guilt and irritability
	Give the patient and partner realistic guidelines to when they might need to seek professional help for depression beyond baby blues.

DOMESTIC VIOLENCE	
• Provide nonjudgmental atmosphere that allows patient to express anger, fears, and feelings of hopelessness. Refer patient to appropriate agency for assistance to find shelter and psychologic counseling. Assist patient in developing a plan of action in the event of a situation that could threaten her or her children's safety.	
• Place telephone numbers for assistance in women's bathroom and other places women can see and memorize them without fear of reprisal from partner.	Provides resources and information to patients without putting them or their children in further danger.

Psychiatric Health

ACTIONS/INTERVENTIONS	RATIONALES
• Monitor health care team's interactions with client for behavior (verbal and nonverbal) that would encourage the client not to be hopeful. If situations are identified, they should be noted here and the team should discuss alternative ways of behaving in the situation. The actions that are determined to be needed to support the client's hope should be noted on the client's chart.	Negative attitudes from staff can be communicated to the client.
• Sit with client (number) times per day at (times) for 30 min to discuss feelings and perceptions the client has about the identified situation. These times should also include discussions about the client's significant others, times the client has enjoyed with these persons, the projects or activities the client was planning with or for these persons that have not been accomplished, client's values and beliefs about health and illness, and his or her attitudes about the current situation.	Promotes positive orientation by assisting the client in remembering past successes and important aspects of life that make it important that they succeed this time.[30]
• Identify with client's significant others the times that they can talk with the staff about the current situation. Themes that should be explored during this interaction should be their thoughts and feelings about the current situation, ways in which they can support the client, the importance of their support for the client, questions they may have about the client's situation, and possible outcomes. (Note the time for this interaction here as well as the name of the person who will be talking with the significant others.)	Negative expectations from the support system can be communicated to the client.
• Note times when significant others will be visiting, and schedule this time so that there will be a private time for them to interact with the client. (Note these times here, and designate those times that are scheduled as private visitation times.) Inform client and significant others of those places on the unit where they can have privacy to visit.	Assists the client in maintaining connections with the support systems and increases awareness of contributions the client has made in the past and can make in the future to this system.
• Identify with client preferences for daily routine, and place this information on the chart to be implemented by the staff. It is vital to this client to have the information shared with all staff so that it will not appear that the time spent in providing information was wasted.	Promotes client's sense of control.
• Provide answers to questions in an open, direct manner.	Promotes client's sense of control while building a trusting relationship.
• Provide information on all procedures at a time when the client can ask questions and think about the situation.	
• Allow client to participate in decision making at the level at which he or she is capable of doing so. The client who has never made an independent decision would be overwhelmed by the complexity of the decisions made daily by the corporation executive. If necessary, offer decision situation in portions that the client can master successfully (the amount of information that the client can handle should be noted here as well as a list of decisions the client has been presented with).	Promotes the client's sense of control in a manner that increases the opportunities for success. This success serves as positive reinforcement.
• Provide positive reinforcement for behavior changed and decisions made. Those things that are reinforcing for this client should be listed here along with the reward system that has been established with the client; e.g., play one game of cards with the client when a decision about ways to cope with a specific problem has been made.	Positive reinforcement encourages behavior while enhancing self-esteem.

Continued

ACTIONS/INTERVENTIONS	RATIONALES
• Provide verbal social reinforcements along with behavioral reinforcements.	Promotes the development of a trusting relationship.
• Keep promises (specific promises should be listed on the chart so that all staff will be aware of this information).	
• Accept client's decision if the decision was given to the client to make. These decisions should be noted on the chart.	Promotes the client's sense of control while enhancing self-esteem.
• Provide ongoing feedback to client on progress.	Provides positive reinforcement for accomplishments.
• Spend 30 min a day talking with client about current coping strategies and exploring alternative coping methods. Note time for this discussion here as well as the person responsible for this interaction. When alternative coping styles have been identified, this time should be used to assist client with necessary practice. The alternative styles that the client has selected should be noted on the chart, and the staff should assist the client in implementing the strategy when appropriate. These could include deep muscle relaxation, visual imagery, prayer, or talking about alternative ways of coping with stressful events.	Interaction with the nurse can provide positive reinforcement. Behavioral rehearsal provides opportunities for feedback and modeling of new behaviors from the nurse.
• Allow client to express anger and assist with discovering constructive ways of expressing this feeling (e.g., talking about this feeling, using a punching bag, playing Ping-Pong, or throwing or hitting a pillow). Talk with client about signs of progress, and assist him or her in recognizing these as they occur with verbal reminders or by keeping a record of steps taken toward progress.	Promotes the development of a positive orientation.
• Assist client in establishing realistic goals and realistic expectations for situations. The goals should be short term and be stated in measurable behavioral terms. Usually, dividing the goal set by the client in half provides an achievable goal. This could involve dividing one goal into several smaller goals. Note goals and evaluation dates here.	Goals that are achieved serve as positive reinforcement for behavior change and enhance self-esteem and a positive expectational set.
• Determine times with the client to evaluate progress toward these goals and to discuss their observations about this progress. These specific times should be listed here with the name of the person responsible for this activity. Initially this may need to be done on a daily basis until the client develops competency in making realistic assessments.	Provides positive reinforcement for movement toward goal and provides opportunity for the nurse to provide positive verbal reinforcement.
• Assist client in developing a list of contingencies for possible blocks to the goals. These would be "what-if" and "if-then" discussions. This would be done in the goal-setting session, and a record of the alternatives discussed would be made in the chart for future reference.	Provides direction for the client with an opportunity to mentally rehearse situations that could require alteration of goals. This protects the client from all-or-none situations.
• Discuss with client values and beliefs about life, and assess importance of formal religion in the client's life. If client requires contact with a person of his or her belief system, arrange this, and note necessary information for contacting this person here. Provide client with the time necessary to perform those religious rituals that are important to him or her. Note the rituals here with the times scheduled and any assistance that is required from the nursing staff.	Spirituality can provide hope-giving experiences.

• Provide the client with opportunities to enjoy aesthetic experiences that have been identified as important such as listening to favorite music, having favorite pictures placed in the room, enjoying favorite foods, or having special flowers in the room. Spend 5 min 3 times a day discussing these experiences and assisting the client in becoming involved in the enjoyment of them. Note here those activities that have been identified by the client as important and times when they will be discussed with the client.	Promotes the client's interest in the positive aspect of life, promoting a positive orientation.
• Assist client in developing an awareness and an appreciation for the here and now by helping him or her focus attention in the present by pointing out to him or her the beauty in the flowers in the room, the warmth of the sunshine as it comes through the window, the calmness or aliveness of a piece of music, the taste and smell of a special food item, the odor of flowers, etc.	Provides the client with an opportunity to access past positive experiences in the present, thus promoting a positive orientation.
• Establish a time to talk with client about maximizing potential at his or her current level of functioning. Note date and time for this discussion here. This may need to be done in several stages during more than one time depending on the client's level of denial. Note here the person responsible for these discussions.	Promotes the client's sense of control. Enhances self-esteem.

Gerontic Health

The nursing actions for the older adult with this diagnosis are the same as for the adult health and mental health patient.

Home Health

ACTIONS/INTERVENTIONS	RATIONALES
• Monitor for factors contributing to the hopelessness, e.g., psychologic, social, economic, spiritual, or environmental factors.	Provides database for earlier recognition and intervention.

• Involve client and family in planning, implementing, and promoting reduction or elimination of hopelessness:
  ○ Family conference: To identify and discuss factors contributing to hopelessness
  ○ Mutual goal setting: Setting goals with roles of each family member identified
  ○ Communication
  ○ Support for the caregiver
	Clarifies roles. Personal involvement in planning, etc., increases the likelihood of success in resolving problem.

• Assist client and family in making lifestyle adjustments that may be required:
  ○ Use relaxation techniques: Yoga, biofeedback, hypnosis, breathing techniques, or imagery.
  ○ Provide assertiveness training.
  ○ Provide opportunities for individual to exert control over situation. Give choice when possible, and support and encourage self-care efforts.
  ○ Provide sense of mastery by setting accomplishable and meaningful goals in secure environment.
  ○ Look for meaning in situation, e.g., what can be learned from the situation.
  ○ Provide treatment for physiologic condition.
  ○ Provide grief counseling.
  ○ Provide spiritual counseling.
  ○ Prevent suicide.
	Lifestyle changes require significant behavior change. Self-evaluation and support can assist in ensuring that changes are not transient.

• Consult with or refer patient to assistive resources as indicated.	Effective use of existing community resources.

Hopelessness

FLOWCHART EVALUATION: EXPECTED OUTCOME 1

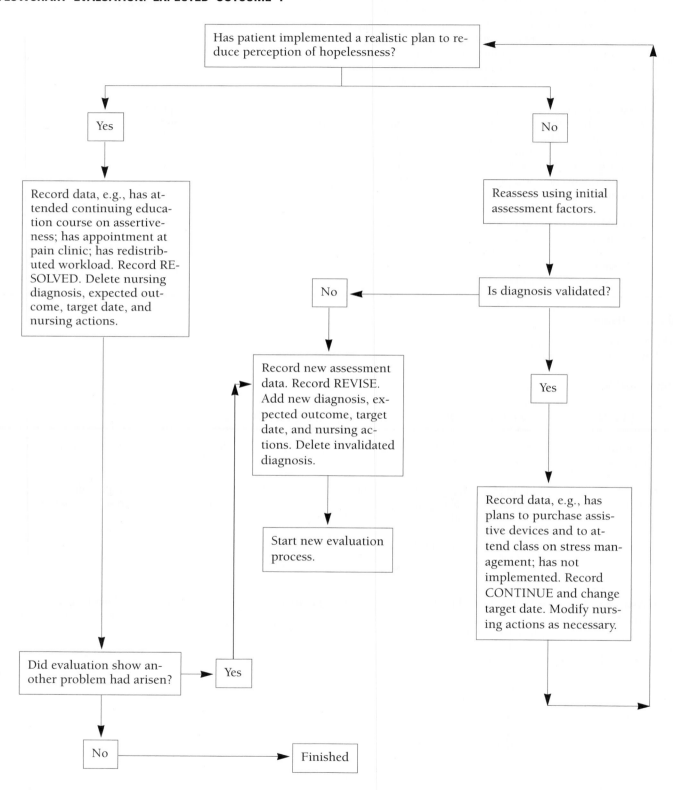

Hopelessness

FLOWCHART EVALUATION: EXPECTED OUTCOME 2

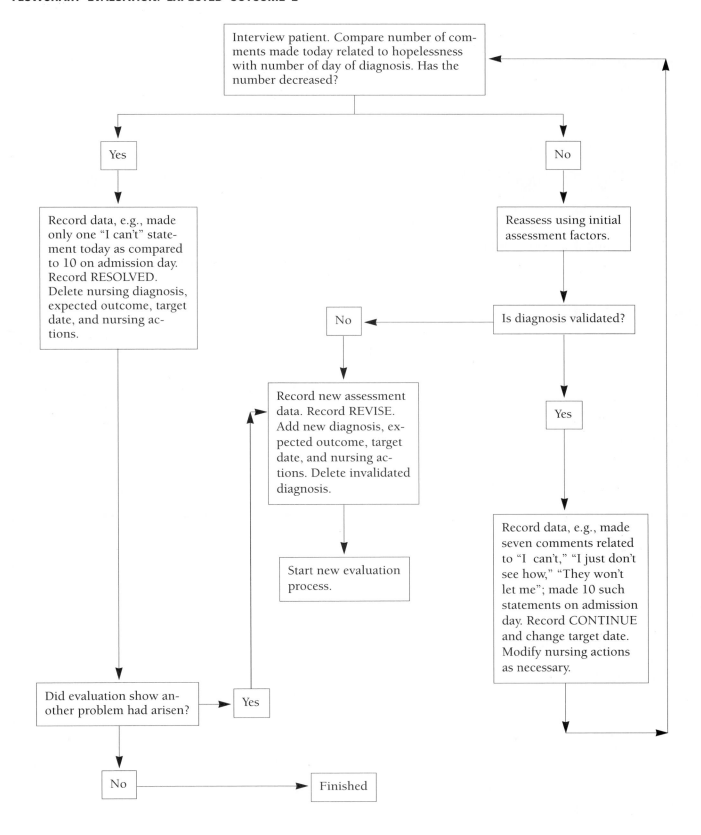

Loneliness, Risk for

DEFINITION

A subjective state in which an individual is at risk of experiencing vague dysphoria.[23]

NANDA TAXONOMY: RELATING 3.1.3

RISK FACTORS[23]

1. Affectional deprivation
2. Physical isolation
3. Cathectic deprivation
4. Social isolation

RELATED CLINICAL CONCERNS

1. Any chronic illness
2. AIDS
3. Mental health diagnoses
4. Cancer
5. Any condition causing impaired mobility

HAVE YOU SELECTED THE CORRECT DIAGNOSIS?

Social Isolation   Social isolation is an actual diagnosis. Loneliness is a risk diagnosis. Social isolation is a risk factor for the diagnosis of loneliness.

Impaired Social Interaction   This diagnosis is also an actual diagnosis. In Impaired Social Interaction, the problem can be insufficient or excessive quantity of social activity.

EXPECTED OUTCOMES

1. Will implement a plan to reduce risk for loneliness by (date) and/or
2. Will demonstrate a (number) percentage decrease in risk factors for loneliness by (date)

TARGET DATES

This is a fairly long term diagnosis and will require much support to offset. Therefore, an appropriate initial target date would be 10 to 14 days.

NURSING ACTIONS/INTERVENTIONS WITH RATIONALES
Adult Health

ACTIONS/INTERVENTIONS	RATIONALES
• Monitor for symptoms of loneliness. Symptoms are often hidden or disguised: expressed through withdrawal, depression, or a profound sense of hopelessness, or vague physical symptoms such as headache, hostility, anger toward those around him or her or with life in general. Prolonged internal conflicts may manifest as inappropriate coping such as overeating, excessive drinking or smoking, drug use, or other self-destructive behaviors.	Helps to develop a database on which planning can take place.
• Note significant other(s) who visit or call patient. Assess the degree of support and the availability of significant other(s).	The separation from significant other(s) and from previously established support systems may contribute to loneliness.[31]
• Help to identify beliefs, values, hobbies, and areas of interest.	
• Encourage to join a group with common interests. Age-related groups may be helpful for the older patient. Group process should focus on realistic, relevant issues.	Older adult is not as easily accepted into social interactions or relationships because of social bias toward the aged.[32] The use of groups and group process has been most successful in treating loneliness.[33]
• Encourage patient to be involved in his or her care.	Involving the patient in care directly influences movement away from loneliness.[34] It also reduces feelings of powerlessness and fosters interest in self-care.[31]

• Discuss body image, hygiene, visible signs of illness, function loss, and his or her perceptions of how he or she can change things.	The person becomes isolated either because of rejection of others or because he or she seeks little interaction as a result of the self-consciousness he or she feels.[32] Negative ways of viewing self arising from physical or emotional disabilities can confound problems, lower self-esteem, and lead to loneliness.[33]
• Assist patient to find alternate support systems, even short, quality interactions with the nurse.	Patients perceive that nurses can offer psychological support with even short visits.[33]
• Assign a primary nurse to care for patient.	Provides consistency in care.
• Use multidisciplinary approach to patient care.	Ensures continuity in care.
• Assist patient to establish relationship with one other patient.	Decreases social isolation.

Child Health

Same as for Adult Health, with attention to developmentally appropriate approach for all interventions. When other diagnoses, e.g., Grief or Loss, Parent-Infant Separation, Coping, also contribute to this pattern, seek follow-up with concurrent plan for loneliness as well.

ACTIONS/INTERVENTIONS	RATIONALES
• If anaclitic depression is to be considered, stage appropriately for current or ongoing status, i.e., protest, despair, or withdrawal.	In separation anxiety, the infant or child may have different needs, but all will help direct caregivers to support client in regaining bonds with others.

• Determine best how to support the infant, child, or adolescent coping with loneliness as applicable:
  ○ Play therapy or counseling
  ○ Consideration of developmental capacity
  ○ Access to activities within the local community
  ○ Assessment of physical or emotional readiness, for both the individual and the family
  ○ Allowance for regression due to illness
  ○ Support services, foster grandparents, volunteers, CPS, or college interest groups
	Holistic planning according to realistic capacity of infant, child, or adolescent will provide appropriate chance to reestablish sense of belonging.

• Involve all who have input in establishing consistent long-term goals.	Often underlying dynamics may require long-range planning.
• When necessary, advocate for infant or child.	Loneliness may be related to abuse on part of parents and must be considered appropriately.
• Ensure allowance for counseling for appropriate valuing of family needs.	Loneliness will undermine family dynamics if left unrecognized.
• Offer 30 min each shift for client or parents to ventilate feelings about loneliness.	Frequent verbalization will offer cues to suggest insight into how loneliness is being perceived and provide basis for most appropriate treatment.

Women's Health

ACTIONS/INTERVENTIONS	RATIONALES
POSTPARTUM	
• Provide patient with access to support by providing phone number and name of available support person she can call with questions.	
• Encourage new parents to attend parenting support groups and participate in parent education programs in the acute care setting and in the community after discharge. Suggest to parents: ○ YWCA	Provides new parents support and guidance during the first days of the postpartum period and assists in the transition to parenthood.

Continued

ACTIONS/INTERVENTIONS	RATIONALES

- Churches
- Neighborhood groups
- Friends who have had babies
- State-funded follow-up programs

SINGLE PARENTS

- Assist new mother to develop a plan for coordinating activities of daily living with new infant.
- Assist patient in identifying available resources:
  - Family
  - Significant others
  - Community agencies
  - Peer groups
- Assist patient in identifying and developing intrapersonal skills.
- Encourage attendance at parenting classes or support groups. Learn about baby cues and how to provide for psychological needs of new infant. Identify others with similar concerns and needs. Identify new sources of support and contact opportunities for developing new friendships.
- Encourage patient to identify friends or acquaintances who have recently had new babies and to begin:
  - discussing similar concerns and problems with caring for a new baby;
  - sharing "babysitting activities" to reduce costs and increase opportunities for new mom to get away for a while.

Provides support and guidance during the transition to parenthood, as well as additional resources specific to assisting the single parent.

DIVORCE AND WIDOWHOOD

- Provide a relaxed atmosphere that will encourage patient to express feelings, identify concerns, and allow for grieving.
- Evaluate need for professional assistance and/or family support.
- Identify and clarify with patient feelings of abandonment, anger, and loss of previous lifestyle.
- Assist patient in identifying new opportunities for involvement with others, e.g., church groups, community volunteer groups, or social groups (ski club, travel clubs, etc.) for people with similar interests, returning to college, cultural events, etc.
- Provide opportunities for new interactions in a supportive atmosphere, e.g., identify friend to accompany patient to social events or identify friend she can talk to.
- Provide referrals to appropriate professional resources for assistance if necessary.

Provides support and guidance during a time of crisis for patient. Assists client to find and utilize available resources.

Psychiatric Health

ACTIONS/INTERVENTIONS	RATIONALES
• Spend (*number*) minutes (*number*) times a day discussing with client his or her perception of the source of the loneliness, and discuss how he or she has tried to resolve the situation.	Assists in understanding the client's worldview, which facilitates the development of client-specific interventions. Increases the client's sense of involvement and empowerment.[35]
• Have client list those persons in the environment who are considered family, friends, and acquaintances. Then have client note how many interactions per week occur with each person. Have client identify what interferes with feeling connected with these persons. Note here the person responsible and schedule for this interaction.	Facilitates the client's reality testing of perception of being alone.

• When contributing factors have been identified, develop a plan to alter them. This plan could include:
  ○ Assertiveness training
  ○ Role-playing difficult situations
  ○ Teaching client relaxation techniques to reduce anxiety in social situations
  ○ Providing clients with aids to compensate for sensory deficits
	Facilitates the development of alternative coping behaviors and improves social skills, which improves role performance and social confidence.

○ Providing client with special clothing or prosthetic devices to enhance physical appearance ○ Teaching client personal hygiene necessary to maintain aesthetic appearance (ostomy care, incontinence care, or wound care)	Positive reinforcement encourages behavior and enhances self-esteem. Increases the client's competence and thus enhances role performance and self-esteem.
• Note here the specific interventions and schedule necessary for this client with person responsible for the activity. For example, the primary nurse will interact with client 30 min 2 times a day to teach assertive skills or client will attend social skills group at (time).	
• Develop a list of those things the client finds rewarding, and provide these rewards as client successfully completes progressive steps in treatment plan. This schedule should be developed with the client. Note here the schedule for rewards and the kinds of behavior to be rewarded.	
• Consult with occupational therapist if client needs to learn specific skills to facilitate social interactions, such as cooking skills so that friends can be invited to dinner, craft skills, or dancing so that client can join others in these social activities.	
• Include client in groups on the unit. Assign client activities that can be accomplished easily and that will provide positive social reinforcement from other persons involved in the activities. Note here the group and activity schedule.	Successful accomplishment of a valued task can provide positive reinforcement, which encourages social behavior. Provides opportunities for client to practice social interaction skills.
• If lack of activities contributes to the loneliness, refer to Diversional Activity Deficit (Chap. 5) for detailed interventions.	Decreased activities can increase the sense of time passing slowly, which perceptually increases the time spent alone, increasing the sense of loneliness.[35]
• Consult with social services if transportation or financial resource problems contribute to social isolation.	Decreased mobility can decrease social interaction and sense of aloneness.
• Discuss with clients those times it would be appropriate to be alone, and develop a plan for coping with these times in a positive manner. For example, client will develop a list of books to read and music to listen to or call a friend.[36]	Promotes client's sense of control while facilitating the development of alternative coping behaviors.

Continued

ACTIONS/INTERVENTIONS	RATIONALES
• When client is demonstrating socially inappropriate behavior, keep interactions to a minimum, inform client that the behavior is inappropriate, and escort him or her to a place away from group activities. Note here the target behaviors for this client here.	Lack of positive reinforcement decreases a behavior.
• When inappropriate behaviors stop, discuss the behavior with the client and develop a list of alternative kinds of behavior for the client to use in situations in which the inappropriate behavior is elicted. Note here those behaviors that are considered problematic, with the action to be taken if they are demonstrated. For example, client will spend time out in seclusion or sleeping area.	Promotes client's sense of control while promoting the development of alternative coping behaviors.
• Primary nurse will spend 30 min once a day with client at (time) discussing client's reactions to social interactions and assisting client with reality testing of social interactions, for example, what others might mean by silence or various nonverbal and common verbal expressions. This time can also be used to discuss role relationships and client's specific concerns about relationships.	Provides positive reinforcement for appropriate problem solving.
• Assign client a room near areas with high activity.	Facilitates client's participation in unit activities.
• Assign one staff person to the client each shift, and have this person interact with client every 30 min while awake.	Decreases the client's opportunities for socially isolating self.
• Have client identify those activities in the community that are of interest and would provide opportunities for interactions with others. List client's interests here.	
• Develop with the client a plan for making contact with the identified community activities before discharge.	Promotes the client's sense of control and begins the development of adaptive coping behaviors.
• Arrange at least 1 h a week for client to interact with support system in the presence of the primary nurse. This will allow the nurse to assess and facilitate these interactions. Note here the schedule and responsible person.	Support system understanding facilitates the maintenance of new behaviors after discharge.
• Discuss with the support system the ways in which they can facilitate client interaction, for example, frequent phone calls, teaching the client to use public transportation, meals-on-wheels, or community phone call check-in services.	
• Model for support system and for client those kinds of behavior that facilitate communication.	
• Limit the amount of time client can spend alone in room. This should be a gradual alteration and should be done in steps that can easily be accomplished by client. Note specific schedule for client here. For example, client will spend 5 min per hour in day area. Have staff person remain with client during these times until client demonstrates an ability to interact with others.[35]	Provides opportunities for client to practice new role behaviors in a safe, supportive environment.
• Refer client to appropriate community agencies.	

Gerontic Health

See actions and interventions under Psychiatric Health. The older adult who is experiencing losses associated with aging, such as loss of a spouse, decline in physical health, and changes in role, is especially vulnerable to loneliness.

Home Health

ACTIONS/INTERVENTIONS	RATIONALES

• Teach client and family to identify and prevent risk factors of loneliness:
  ○ Physical and social isolation
  ○ Deprivation
	Early recognition and intervention can interrupt development of loneliness.

• Assist client and family in lifestyle adjustments that may be necessary:
  ○ Develop a plan for increased involvement; e.g., begin with social contacts that are least threatening.
  ○ Provide for personal hygiene
  ○ Provide supportive environment.
	Home-based care requires involvement of the family. Loneliness can disrupt family schedules and role relationships. Adjustments in family activities and roles may be required.

• Assist family to set criteria to help them determine when additional intervention is required, for example, inability of client or family to care for client.	Provides family with background knowledge to seek appropriate assistance as need arises.
• Refer patient to appropriate assistive resources as indicated.	Additional assistance may be required for the family to care for the family member with loneliness.

Loneliness, Risk for

FLOWCHART EVALUATION: EXPECTED OUTCOME 1

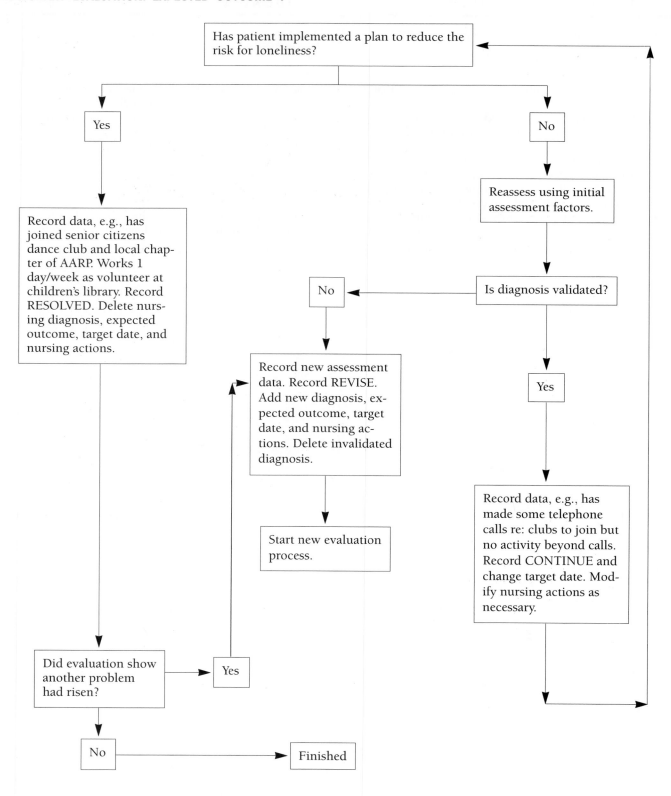

Has patient implemented a plan to reduce the risk for loneliness?

Yes

Record data, e.g., has joined senior citizens dance club and local chapter of AARP. Works 1 day/week as volunteer at children's library. Record RESOLVED. Delete nursing diagnosis, expected outcome, target date, and nursing actions.

Did evaluation show another problem had risen?

Yes

No → Finished

Record new assessment data. Record REVISE. Add new diagnosis, expected outcome, target date, and nursing actions. Delete invalidated diagnosis.

Start new evaluation process.

No

Reassess using initial assessment factors.

Is diagnosis validated?

No

Yes

Record data, e.g., has made some telephone calls re: clubs to join but no activity beyond calls. Record CONTINUE and change target date. Modify nursing actions as necessary.

Loneliness, Risk for

FLOWCHART EVALUATION: EXPECTED OUTCOME 2

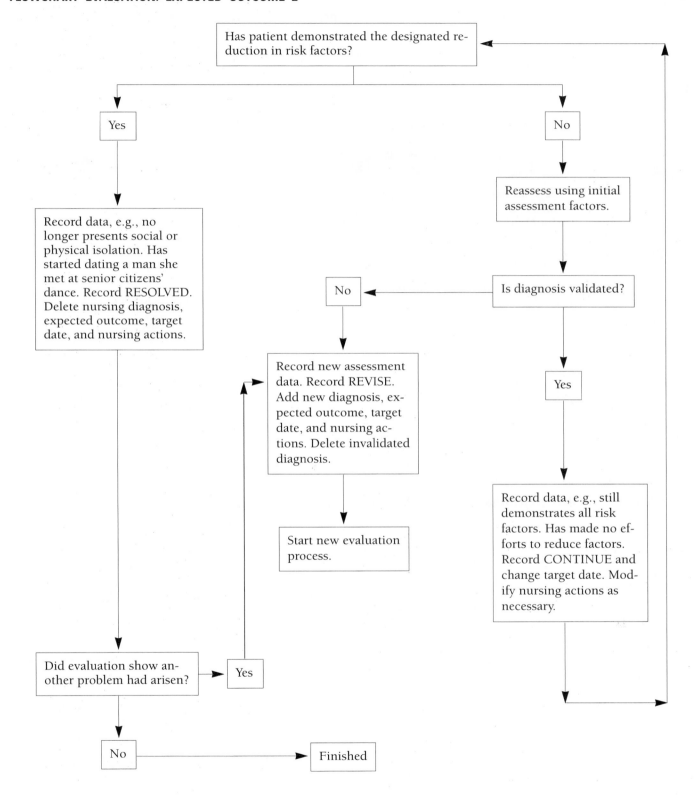

Personal Identity Disturbance

DEFINITION

Inability to distinguish between self and nonself.[23]

NANDA TAXONOMY: PERCEIVING 7.1.3

DEFINING CHARACTERISTICS[23]

To be developed.

RELATED FACTORS[23]

None given.

RELATED CLINICAL CONCERNS

1. Autism
2. Mental retardation
3. Dissociative disorders, for example, psychogenic amnesia, psychogenic fugue, multiple personality, depersonalization disorder
4. Borderline personality disorder

HAVE YOU SELECTED THE CORRECT DIAGNOSIS?

Self-Esteem Disturbance This diagnosis addresses the lack of confidence in one's self and is characterized by negative self-statements, lack of concern about personal appearance, and withdrawal from others not related to physical problems or attributes. The self is defined. If the client demonstrates an inability to differentiate self from the environment, then the most appropriate diagnosis is Personal Identity Disturbance. An example would be the client who perceives a life-support machine as part of the self.

Body Image Disturbance This diagnosis relates to alterations in perceptions of self in conjunction with actual or perceived alterations in body structure or function. Again, the self is known with this diagnosis.

EXPECTED OUTCOMES

1. Will verbalize differentiation of self from environment by (date) and/or
2. Will list at least (number) of characteristics of self versus nonself by (date)

TARGET DATES

A target date of 5 days would be acceptable for initial evaluation of progress toward expected outcomes.

NURSING ACTIONS/INTERVENTIONS WITH RATIONALES

Adult Health

Should the patient develop this nursing diagnosis on an adult health care unit, referral should be made immediately to a mental health nurse clinician. See nursing actions under Psychiatric Health.

Child Health

ACTIONS/INTERVENTIONS	RATIONALES

• Monitor for contributing factors that might predispose the development of a Personal Identity Disturbance:
  ○ Risk indicating an altered maternal or infant attachment, e.g., parents' overprotection or ignoring of infant
  ○ Altered development norms related to independent functioning, e.g., following commands (Check for organic or sensory-perceptual deficits.)
  ○ Preference for solitary play
  ○ Display of self-stimulation and/or self-mutilation behaviors
  ○ History of altered identity problems in family
	Provides the database needed to more accurately and completely plan care.

- Provide basis care for other needs with prioritization for safety needs. Close observation is mandatory.

- Administer medications as ordered with attention to hydration and nutritional concerns.
- Provide appropriate follow-up and collaboration with family.

- Assist family in decision making regarding long-term care, e.g., institutionalization versus daycare.

In anticipatory safety planning, standards must be in accord with both the known as well as the unknown self-injury potential of the patient.
The patient is prone to dehydration and malnutrition due to inability to rely on usual thirst or appetite regulators.
Appropriate use of specialists will offer a more individualized plan of care with greater likelihood of meeting needs.
Assistance and support in identification of options assist in decision making, reducing stress, and empowering the family.

Women's Health

The nursing actions for the woman with this nursing diagnosis would be the same as those for the mental health client. Also see Risk for Loneliness.

Psychiatric Health

ACTIONS/INTERVENTIONS	RATIONALES
• Provide a quiet, nonstimulating environment.	Inappropriate levels of sensory stimuli can increase confusion and sense of disorganization.
• Provide frequent interactions that assist the client with orientation.	Promotes the development of a trusting relationship within the client's attention span.
• Verbal information should be provided in simple, brief sentences.	Interactions with others also assist in reestablishing weak ego boundaries.
• Sit with the client (number) minutes (number) times per day at (times) to provide the client with an opportunity to discuss feelings and thoughts.	Promotes the development of a trusting relationship. Provides positive reinforcement for the client's meeting needs in a more constructive way.
• Provide the client with honest, direct feedback in all interactions.	Promotes the development of a trusting relationship.

• Utilize constructive confrontation if necessary to include:
  ◦ I statements
  ◦ Relationship statements that reflect nurse's reaction to the interaction
  ◦ Responses that will assist the client in understanding such as paraphrasing and validation of perceptions
	Assists client in establishing ego boundaries while supporting self-esteem.

• Discuss with the client the source of the threat.	Assists client in developing more adaptive coping behaviors.
• Develop with the client alternative coping strategies. Those activities, items, or verbal responses that are rewarding for the client should be listed here.	Promotes client's sense of control and positive expectational set by providing a concrete plan for responding to stressful situations.
• When the client is presented with a threat, assist him or her by progressing through one of the alternative coping methods, or practice with the client the alternative coping methods, (number) minutes twice a day.	Behavioral rehearsal provides opportunities for feedback and modeling from the nurse.
• Develop achievable goals with the client. (The goals that are appropriate for this client should be listed here.)	Goal achievement enhances self-esteem and promotes a positive expectational set, which motivates client to move on to more complex goals and behavior change.
• As the client masters the first set of goals, develop increasingly complex goals and problems.	Moves client toward health goals in a manner that promotes self-esteem.
• Provide positive reinforcement for accomplishments at any level. (Those activities, items, or verbal responses that are rewarding for the client should be listed here.)	Positive reinforcement encourages behavior while enhancing self-esteem.
• Do not argue with the client who is experiencing an alteration in thought process. (Refer to Chap. 7 for nursing actions related to Altered Thought Process.)	Arguing with the belief interferes with the development of a trusting relationship and does not serve to change the perceptions.

Continued

ACTIONS/INTERVENTIONS	RATIONALES
• Monitor the client's mental status before attempting learning or confrontation. If the client is disoriented, orient to reality as needed.	Alterations in mental status can interfere with the client's ability to process information, and teaching at this point could increase stimuli to a level that would only increase the client's confusion and disorganization.
• If disorientation is present related to organic brain dysfunction, distract client from those disorientations that are not correct with a brief, simple explanation.	Short-term memory loss will assist with changing the client's orientation without getting into a strong confrontation.

Gerontic Health

In the event that the patient is unable to distinguish between self and nonself, it is necessary to contact a mental health clinician to further assess and devise the plan of care. Please see Psychiatric Health nursing actions.

Home Health

ACTIONS/INTERVENTIONS	RATIONALES

• Involve client and family in planning and implementing strategies to reduce and cope with disturbance in personal identity:
  ○ Family conference: Discuss feelings related to disturbance in personal identity of client.
  ○ Mutual goal setting: Establish realistic goals, and identify roles of each family member, e.g., provide a quiet environment and provide client with honest and direct feedback.
  ○ Communication: Clear and honest communication among family members is essential. If organic brain dysfunction is present, nurse may need to use distraction techniques.
	Family involvement enhances effectiveness of interventions.

• Assist the client and family in lifestyle adjustments that may be required:
  ○ Maintaining a safe environment
  ○ Altering roles as necessary
  ○ Maintaining the treatment plan of the health care professionals' guiding therapy
	Personal identity disturbance can be a chronic condition that alters family relationships. Permanent changes in behavior and family roles require evaluation and support.

• Consult with or refer patient to assistive resources as indicated.	Utilization of existing services is efficient use of resources. Psychiatric nurse clinicians and support groups can enhance the treatment plan.

Personal Identity Disturbance

FLOWCHART EVALUATION: EXPECTED OUTCOME 1

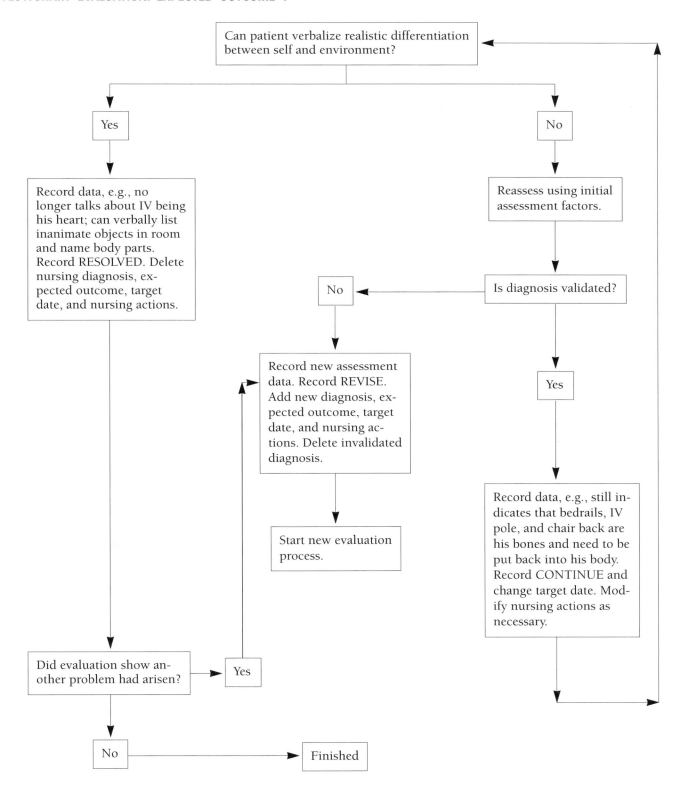

Personal Identity Disturbance

FLOWCHART EVALUATION: EXPECTED OUTCOME 2

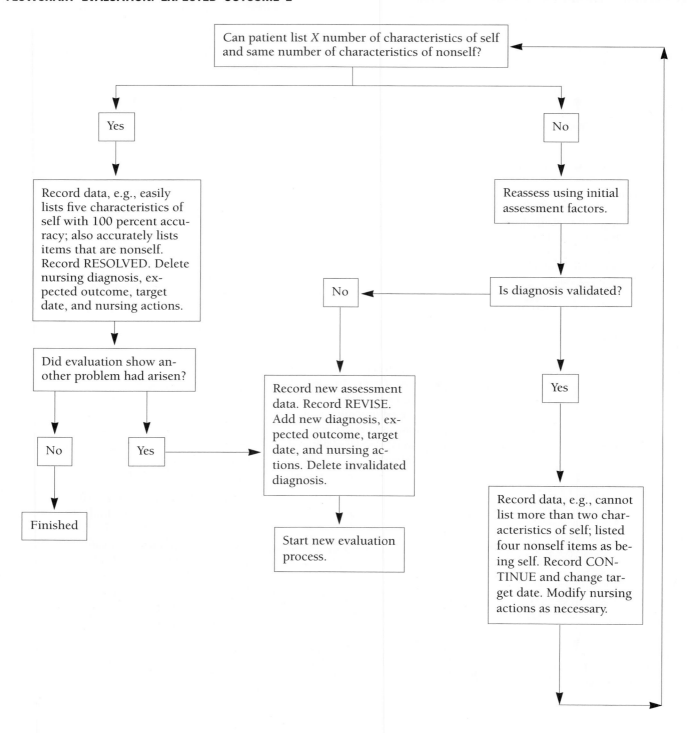

Powerlessness

DEFINITION

Perception that one's own action will not significantly affect an outcome; a perceived lack of control over a current situation, or immediate happening.[23]

NANDA TAXONOMY: PERCEIVING 7.3.2

DEFINING CHARACTERISTICS[23]

1. Severe
   a. Verbal expressions of having no control or influence over situation
   b. Verbal expressions of having no control or influence over outcome
   c. Verbal expressions of having no control over self-care
   d. Depression over physical deterioration that occurs despite patient compliance with regimens
   e. Apathy
2. Moderate
   a. Nonparticipation in care or decision making when opportunities are provided
   b. Expressions of dissatisfaction and frustration over inability to perform previous tasks and/or activities
   c. Does not monitor progress
   d. Expression of doubt regarding role performance
   e. Reluctance to express true feelings
   f. Fearing alienation from caregivers
   g. Passivity
   h. Inability to seek information regarding care
   i. Dependence on others that may result in irritability, resentment, anger, and guilt
   j. Does not defend self-care practices when challenged
3. Low
   a. Expressions of uncertainty about fluctuation of energy levels
   b. Passivity

RELATED FACTORS[23]

1. Health care environment
2. Interpersonal interaction
3. Illness-related regimen
4. Lifestyle of helplessness

RELATED CLINICAL CONCERNS

1. Any diagnosis that is unexpected or new to the patient
2. Any diagnosis resulting from a sudden, traumatic event
3. Any diagnosis of a chronic nature
4. Any diagnosis with a terminal prognosis

HAVE YOU SELECTED THE CORRECT DIAGNOSIS?

Anxiety Anxiety may have as a component a perception of Powerlessness. This would evolve into a situation where the anxious client would not attempt to resolve the situation. Powerlessness can also have as a component anxiety. Deciding on the primary diagnosis is based on the clinical judgment of the nurse about which symptoms predominate.

Ineffective Individual Coping A perception of Powerlessness can produce Ineffective Individual Coping because if one perceives that one's own actions cannot influence a situation, appropriate actions may not be taken. If Ineffective Individual Coping is determined to result from a perceived lack of influence, then Powerlessness would be the primary diagnosis.

Impaired Thought Process This diagnosis can produce a sense of Powerlessness because of the individual's inability to accurately assess the situation. Thus, the most appropriate diagnosis would be Altered Thought Process.

Fear Fear can produce a sense of Powerlessness just as Powerlessness can produce Fear. Differentiation is based on the predominant symptom sequence.

Knowledge Deficit If the client lacks sufficient knowledge about a situation, a perception of Powerlessness may result. Therefore, Knowledge Deficit would be the primary diagnosis.

EXPECTED OUTCOMES

1. Will describe at least (number) of areas of control over self by (date) and/or
2. Will initiate a plan to deal with feelings of powerlessness by (date)

TARGET DATES

A target date of 3 days would be realistic to check for progress toward reduced feeling of powerlessness.

ADDITIONAL INFORMATION

The paradox of the metaphor of power has been presented in the literature. Systems theorists and cyberneticians have presented the most useful information when one is planning intervention strategies. Keeney[37] presents a summary of the debate over the power metaphor. In sum, most cyberneticians find this to be an invalid metaphor when discussing systems of interaction. The process of a system involves mutual interactions, and within a system each member exerts influence over the other members. Therefore, the individual who acts as if he or she is powerless is exerting "power" over the other parts of the system to act in a manner that would increase this "lost" personal power. The "powerless" one is then actually exercising power to motivate other parts of the system to act in certain ways. Understanding this conceptual model provides the client with an opportunity to know how one's behavior affects the situation and provides nurses with an opportunity to understand their reactions to and feelings toward the client with the diagnosis of Powerlessness. If the power metaphor is not accepted, this affects the concept of internal versus external locus of control. The concepts of internal and external loci of control become metaphors for how a person perceives personal influence within an interactional system. Persons with an external locus of control do not understand their influence on the system, whereas persons with an internal locus of control have an understanding of personal influence.

NURSING ACTIONS/INTERVENTIONS WITH RATIONALES
Adult Health

ACTIONS/INTERVENTIONS	RATIONALES

• Plan care with patient on a daily basis:
  ○ Likes and dislikes
  ○ Where he or she wants personal items placed
  ○ Routines, to extent possible, according to patient's own pace and schedule
  ○ Diet selected by patient
• Encourage patient to provide as much self-care as possible.
	Allows patient to have control over environment and care attributes. Imparts to patient a sense of power.

• Avoid, when interacting with the patient:
  ○ Reinforcing manipulative behavior
  ○ Using negative feedback, e.g., arguing with patient
  ○ Overuse of health care terminology
• Do not ignore cultural and religious preferences.
	Sets limits on behavior. Facilitates a nonthreatening environment.

• Provide calm, safe environment throughout hospitalization:
  ○ Answer questions truthfully.
  ○ Explain all procedures and rationale for procedures.
  ○ Give positive reinforcement to extent possible.
  ○ Reduce sensory input. Balance high technology with high touch and appropriate attention.
  ○ Provide diversional activity.
  ○ Use same staff to degree possible.
	Allows for verbalization of feelings and acceptance of those feelings. Avoids overwhelming patient and increasing sensation of powerlessness.

• Involve significant others in care.
 	
• Monitor, at least once per shift:
  ○ Vital signs
  ○ Exercise
  ○ Sleep-rest periods
  ○ Food and fluid intake
	Promotes involvement in care and advocacy for patient, thus empowering both patient and significant others. Changes in these signs may signal dysfunctions in other patterns and deterioration of diagnosis to depression.

• Refer patient to appropriate community resources prior to discharge.	Support groups can encourage progress in building self-esteem, provide advocacy, and provide long-term support.

Child Health

ACTIONS/INTERVENTIONS	RATIONALES
• Perform a thorough assessment appropriate for patient's developmental needs to identify specific factors that are causing "powerlessness": ○ Use of art ○ Use of puppetry ○ Use of group therapy	Developmentally appropriate assessment will provide cues and reveal data to generate a more accurate and complete plan of care.
• Allow family to participate in care as they are able and choose to.	Family participation provides security to the child and empowerment for the parents with increased growth in coping skills.
• Adopt plan of care to best meet child's and family's needs by including them in voicing preferences whenever appropriate.	Valuing individual preferences is demonstrated by frequent encouragement to express choices. Promotes a sense of control.
• Identify and address educational needs that might be contributing to powerlessness.	Misinformation and inadequate knowledge are contributing factors that can be easily overcome by teaching.
• Refer to patient by preferred name or nickname. List that name here.	Promotes personalized communication. Points out individuality and serves to empower the patient.
• Allow for privacy and need to withdraw to family as a unit.	Demonstrates appropriate respect for family. Attaches value to the family unit.
• Keep patient and family informed as changes occur.	Frequent updates and provision of information help to clarify actions and reduce anxiety, which result in a greater sense of control.
• Provide opportunities for parents to demonstrate appropriate care for child to aid in feeling in control on dismissal from hospital.	Allows practice in a nonthreatening environment, which increases sense of control.

Women's Health

ACTIONS/INTERVENTIONS	RATIONALES
• Provide the prospective parents with factual information about the type of choices available for birth, and assist them to identify their preference: ○ Traditional obstetric services ○ Family-centered maternity care units ○ Single-room maternity care ○ Mother-baby care ○ Birthing center	Provides basic information that assists family in decision making, thus promoting empowerment of the family unit.[24]
• Provide answers to questions in an open, direct manner.	
• Provide information on all procedures so the patient can make informed choices: ○ Assist the patient and significant others in establishing realistic goals (list the goals with evaluation dates here). ○ Allow the patient and significant others to participate in decision making.	
• Allow the patient maximum control over the environment. This could include husband's staying in postpartum room to assist with infant care, keeping the newborn with the mother at all times, using different positions for birth, e.g., squatting or hand-knee position, or having grandparents and siblings in the room with mother and newborn.	Decreases perception of powerlessness and assists in transition to parenthood.

Continued

ACTIONS/INTERVENTIONS	RATIONALES
• Provide positive reinforcement for parenting tasks. • Assist the patient in identifying infant behavior patterns and understanding how they allow her infant to communicate with her. • Support the patient's decisions, e.g., to breast-feed or not to breast-feed or who she wants as significant others during the birthing process. • Reassure the new mother that it takes time to become acquainted with her infant. • Support and reassure the mother in learning infant care, e.g., breast-feeding, bathing, changing, holding a newborn, cord care, or bottle-feeding. • Allow the parents to verbalize fears and insecure feelings about their new roles as parents. • Assist the parents in identifying lifestyle adjustments that may be needed due to the incorporation of a newborn into the family structure. • Involve significant others in discussion and problem-solving activities regarding role changes within the family.	Promotes decision making and leaves decisions up to family by providing the guidance and support that are needed. Involvement enhances motivation to stay with plan, thus reinforcing decision-making capacity of new parents.[38]

DOMESTIC VIOLENCE (See Hopelessness also.)

- Provide patient with support, and assist patient in identifying actions she can take to begin helping herself.
- Provide safe atmosphere for identifying needs and making decisions.
- Provide information in an honest, clear manner to help with decision-making process.
- Assist patient in identifying resources available to her and her children.

Psychiatric Health

ACTIONS/INTERVENTIONS	RATIONALES
• Sit with the client (number) times per day at (times) for 30 min to discuss feelings and perceptions the client has about the identified situation. • Identify client preferences for daily routine, and place this information on the chart to be implemented by the staff. • Provide information to questions in an open, direct manner. • Provide information on all procedures at a time when the client can ask questions and think about the situation. • Allow the client to participate in decision making at the level to which he or she is capable. If necessary, offer decision situations in portions that the client can master successfully. (The amount of information that the client can handle should be noted here as well as a list of decisions the client has been presented with.)	Promotes the development of a trusting relationship and assists client in identifying factors contributing to the feelings of powerlessness. It is vital to this client to have the information shared with all staff so that it will not appear that the time spent in providing information was wasted. Promotes the client's perception of control. Facilitates the development of a trusting relationship. Facilitates the development of a trusting relationship and promotes the client's sense of control. The client who has never made an independent decision would be overwhelmed by the complexity of the decisions made daily by the corporation executive. Promotes the client's sense of control.

- Identify the client's needs and how these are currently being met. If these involve indirect methods of influence, discuss alternative direct methods of meeting these needs. (The client who requests medication for headache every 15 min is requesting attention and is encouraged to approach the nurse and ask to talk when the need for attention arises.)

Assertive direct communication increases the opportunity for the client's needs to be met. When the client is successful in getting needs met in a direct manner, his or her sense of control and self-esteem will increase.

- Provide positive reinforcement for behavior changed and decisions made. (Those things that are reinforcing for this client should be listed here along with the reward system that has been established with the client—e.g., play one game of cards with the client when a decision about what to eat for dinner is made or walk with client on hospital grounds when a decision is made about grooming.)

Positive reinforcement encourages behavior while enhancing self-esteem.

- Provide verbal social reinforcements along with behavioral reinforcements.

Promotes the development of a trusting relationship.

- Keep promises (specific promises should be listed here so that all staff will be aware of this information).

Promotes positive orientation by assisting client in identifying way in which they are already "powerful."

- Assist the client in identifying current methods of influence and in understanding that influence is always there by providing feedback on how influence is being used in the client's interactions with the nurse.

- Accept the client's decisions if the decisions were given to the client to be made—e.g., if the decision to take or not take medication was left with the client, the decision not to take this medication should be respected.

Promotes client's sense of control and enhances self-esteem.

- Allow the client maximum control over the environment. This could include where clothes are kept, how room is arranged, times for various activities. Note preferences here.

Promotes client's sense of control.

- Spend 30 min 2 times per day at (times) allowing the client to role-play interactions that are identified as problematic. (The specific situations as well as new behavior should be noted here.)

Promotes client's sense of control in a manner that increases opportunities for success. This success serves as positive reinforcement.

- Provide opportunities for significant others to be involved in care as appropriate. Careful assessment of the interactions between client and significant others must be made to determine best balance of influencing behavior between client and support system. Specific situations should be listed here.

Provides opportunities for support system and client to practice new ways of interacting while in a situation where they can receive feedback from the health care team.

- Monitor the health care team's interactions with the client for behavior patterns that would encourage the client to choose indirect methods of influence. This could include interactions that encourage the adult client to assume a childlike role. If situations are identified, they should be noted here.

The role of the nurse in the therapeutic milieu is to promote healthy interpersonal interactions.

- Provide ongoing feedback to the client on progress.
- Assist the client in establishing realistic goals. List goals with evaluation dates here. Usually dividing the goal set by the client in half provides an achievable goal; this could also involve dividing one goal into several smaller goals.

Positive reinforcement encourages behavior.
Realistic goals increase the client's opportunities for success, providing positive reinforcement and enhancing self-esteem.

- Refer the client to outpatient support systems, and assist him or her with making arrangements to contact these before discharge. These could be systems that would assist the client in maintaining a perception of influencing ability and could include assertiveness training groups, battered wives' programs, and legal aid.

Provides the client with support for continuing new behaviors in the community after discharge.

Gerontic Health

ACTIONS/INTERVENTIONS	RATIONALES
• Ensure access to call light, telephone, personal care items, and television control.[22] • Advocate for patient, ensuring that health care professionals are not leaving patient out of the decision loop due to the patient's chronological age.	Increases patient's ability to take control of some aspects of care. Stereotyping of older adults is problematic in health care professions.[39]

Home Health

ACTIONS/INTERVENTIONS	RATIONALES

• Involve the client and family in planning and implementing strategies to reduce powerlessness:
  ○ Family conference: Identify and discuss strategies.
  ○ Mutual goal setting: Agree on goals to reduce Powerlessness. Identify roles of all participants.
  ○ Discuss effective communication techniques.
• Assist the client and family in lifestyle adjustments that may be required:
  ○ Relaxation techniques: Yoga, biofeedback, hypnosis, breathing techniques, imagery
  ○ Providing opportunities for individual to exert control over situation, giving choices when possible, supporting and encouraging self-care efforts
  ○ Problem solving and goal setting
  ○ Providing sense of mastery and accomplishable goals in secure environment
  ○ Maintaining the treatment plan of the health care professionals' guiding therapy
  ○ Obtaining and providing accurate information regarding condition
• Consult with or refer patient to assistive resources as indicated.
• Assist the client and family to set criteria to help them determine when the intervention of a health care professional is required—e.g., inability to perform activities of daily living, or condition beginning to decline rapidly.
	Personal involvement and goal setting according to personal wishes enhance the likelihood of success in resolving problem.
	
	Lifestyle adjustments require permanent changes in behavior. Self-evaluation and support facilitates the success of these lifestyle changes.
	
	Use of existing community resources provides for effective use of resources.
	Early identification of issues requiring professional evaluation will increase the probability of successful intervention.

Powerlessness

FLOWCHART EVALUATION: EXPECTED OUTCOME 1

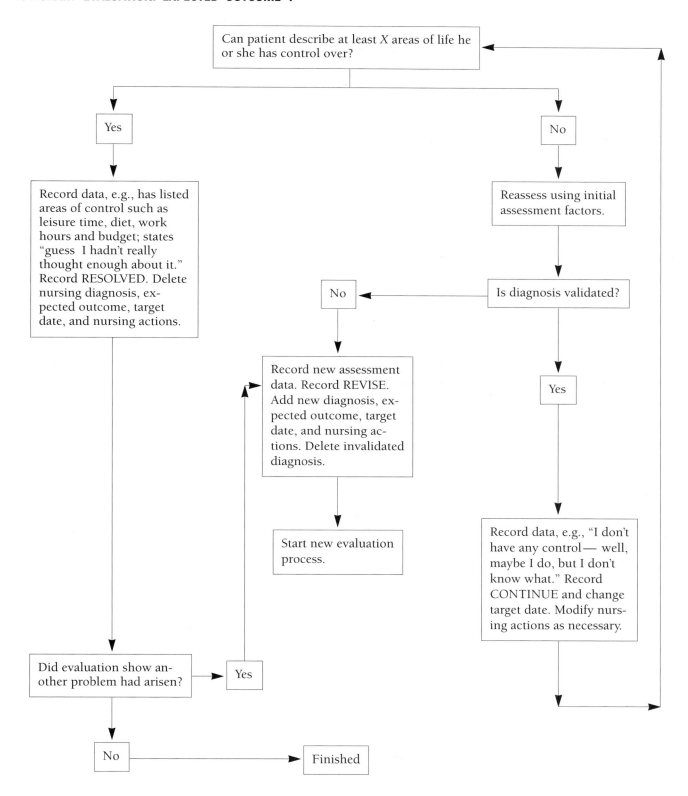

Powerlessness

FLOWCHART EVALUATION: EXPECTED OUTCOME 2

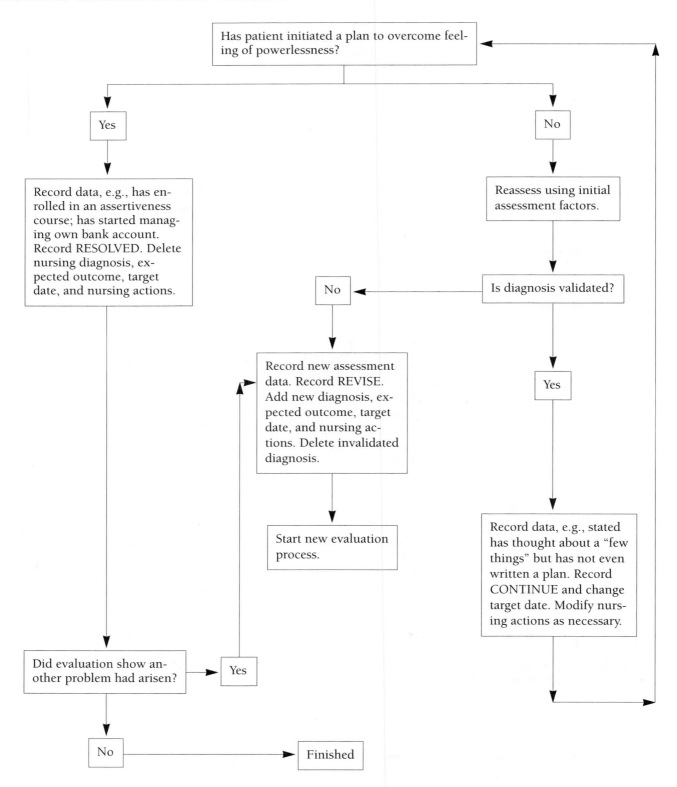

Self-Esteem Disturbance

DEFINITION

SELF-ESTEEM DISTURBANCE   Negative self-evaluation or feelings about self or self capabilities, which may be directly or indirectly expressed.[23]

> **NOTE:** The 1994 Preconference Group suggested that this diagnosis be renamed "low self-esteem" with the definition of "negative feelings based on negative appraisal about self or capabilities."

CHRONIC LOW SELF-ESTEEM   Long-standing negative feelings about self or capabilities.[23]

SITUATIONAL LOW SELF-ESTEEM   Episodic feelings about self or capabilities that develop in response to a loss or change.[23]

NANDA TAXONOMY: PERCEIVING 7.1.2., 7.1.2.1, AND 7.1.2.2

DEFINING CHARACTERISTICS[23]

1. Self-Esteem Disturbance
   a. Makes self-negating verbalizations
   b. Expresses shame or guilt
   c. Evaluates self as unable to deal with events
   d. Rationalizes away or rejects positive feedback and exaggerates negative feedback about self
   e. Hesitates to try new things or situations
   f. Denies problems obvious to others
   g. Projects blame or responsibility for problems
   h. Rationalizes personal failures
   i. Is hypersensitive to slight or criticism
   j. Is grandiose
2. Chronic Low Self-Esteem
   a. Major defining characteristics
      Observations or self-reports of:
      (1) Self-negation
      (2) Shame
      (3) Guilt
      (4) Evaluating self as unable to deal with events
      (5) Rationalizing away or rejecting positive feedback about self
      (6) Exaggerating negative feedback
      (7) Hesitant to try new things or situations
   b. Minor defining characteristics
      Observations or self-reports of:
      (1) Frequent lack of success in work or other life events
      (2) Being overly conforming or dependent on others' opinions
      (3) Does not make culturally appropriate eye contact
      (4) Nonassertion
      (5) Passivity
      (6) Indecisiveness
      (7) Excessively seeking reassurance
3. Situational Low Self-Esteem
   a. Major defining characteristics
      Self-reports of:
      (1) Significant recent loss or change
      (2) Negative feelings about self
   b. Minor defining characteristics
      Observations or self-reports of:
      (1) Self-negation
      (2) Shame
      (3) Guilt
      (4) Inability to handle situations or events
      (5) Difficulty making decisions

RELATED FACTORS[23]

To be developed.

RELATED CLINICAL CONCERNS

1. Pervasive developmental disorders
2. Disruptive behavior disorders
3. Eating disorders
4. Organic mental disorders
5. Substance use or dependence or abuse disorders
6. Mood disorders
7. Adjustment disorders
8. Personality disorders
9. Trauma
10. Surgery
11. Medical problems that contribute to the loss of body functions

HAVE YOU SELECTED THE CORRECT DIAGNOSIS?

Body Image Disturbance   This diagnosis relates to alterations in the perception of self when there is an actual or perceived change in body structure or function. If interviewing reveals that the patient perceives a potential change in body structure or function, then Body Image Disturbance is the most appropriate diagnosis.

Personal Identity Disturbance   When the patient cannot differentiate self from nonself, there probably also exists some self-esteem problems; however, the primary diagnosis would be Personal Identity Disturbance. Working with the Personal Identity Disturbance will take care of the self-esteem problem.

Ineffective Individual Coping   This diagnosis results from the client's inability to appropriately cope with stress. If the client demonstrates a decreased ability to cope appropriately, he or she may also have some defining characteristics related to self-esteem disturbance. Teaching and supporting coping will also assist in correcting the self-esteem problem.

EXPECTED OUTCOMES

1. Will verbalize an increased number of positive self-statements by (date) and/or
2. Will list at least (number) positive aspects about self by (date)

TARGET DATES

A target date of 3 to 5 days would be acceptable to begin monitoring progress.

NURSING ACTIONS/INTERVENTIONS WITH RATIONALES

NOTE: An attitude of genuine warmth, acceptance of clients, and respect for uniqueness are characteristics required for successful nursing interventions.[38]

Adult Health

ACTIONS/INTERVENTIONS	RATIONALES
• Collaborate with psychiatric nurse clinician regarding care (see Psychiatric Health nursing actions).	Collaboration promotes a more holistic plan of care.
• Teach the patient and significant others the patient's self-care requirements as needed. Support patient's self-care management activities.	Participation in own care increases confidence and self-esteem.
• Control pain with medication, stress management techniques, and diversional activities.	Conserves energy to focus on adaptive coping strategies.
• Encourage patient to use anxiety-reducing techniques, e.g., progressive muscle relaxation, deep breathing, yoga, meditation, assertiveness, or guided imagery.	Assists patient to reduce anxiety and regain self-control, thus increasing self-esteem.
• Encourage assertive behavior in interacting with patient. Assist patient to review passive and aggressive behavior.	Helps patient avoid vacillating from one behavior to another. Promotes self-control and a "win-win" situation, which increases self-esteem.
• Promote calm, safe environment by avoiding judgmental attitude, actively listening, using reflection, being consistent in approach, and setting boundaries.	Decreases anxiety and promotes a trusting relationship.
• Allow patient to progress at own rate. Start with simple, concrete tasks. Reward success.	Helps patient have sense of mastering of tasks and promotes self-esteem.
• Use frequent contact, 15 min every 2 h on the (odd/even) hour, with patient to encourage verbalization of feelings: ○ Be honest with patient. ○ Point out and limit self-negating statements. ○ Do not support denial. ○ Focus on reality and adaptation (not necessarily acceptance). ○ Set limits on maladaptive behavior. ○ Focus on realistic goals. ○ Be aware of own nonverbal communication and behavior. ○ Avoid moral, value judgments. ○ Encourage patient to try to note differences in situations and events.	Assists in self-understanding and facilitates self-acceptance.
• Help patient to ascertain why he or she can maintain self-esteem in one situation and not in another situation.	
• Build on coping mechanisms or interpretations that maintain or increase self-esteem. Assist to find alternative coping mechanisms.	Supports adaptive coping and helps to broaden inventory of coping strategies.
• Encourage patient to use available resources: ○ Prosthetic devices ○ Assistive devices ○ Reconstructive and corrective surgery	Decreases feelings of loss and increases self-esteem when patient does not feel "different" from previous self.
• Refer patient to and collaborate with community resources.	Provides ongoing and long-term support.

Child Health

ACTIONS/INTERVENTIONS	RATIONALES
• Monitor for contributory factors related to poor self-esteem, including: 　◦ Family crisis 　◦ Lack of adequate parenting 　◦ Lack of sensory stimulation 　◦ Physical scars, malformation, or disfigurement 　◦ Altered role performance 　◦ Social isolation 　◦ Developmental crisis	Generates the database needed to more accurately and completely plan care.
• Identify ways patient can formulate or reestablish a positive self-esteem according to developmental needs: 　◦ Coping skills 　◦ Communication skills 　◦ Role expectations 　◦ Self-care 　◦ Activities of daily living 　◦ Basic physiologic needs; primary health care 　◦ Expression of self 　◦ Peer and social relationships 　◦ Feelings of self-worth 　◦ Decision making 　◦ Validation of self, e.g., setting developmentally appropriate expectations	Developmental norms serve as the conceptual framework for assisting the child to increase self-esteem.
• Praise and reinforce positive behavior.	Reinforcement of desired behavior serves to enhance permanence of behavior.
• Explore value conflicts and their resolution.	Values must be clarified as one strives to find one's identity. A healthy sense of self contributes to a positive self-image.
• Collaborate with other health care team members as needed.	Collaboration promotes a more holistic plan of care.
• Meet primary health needs in an expedient manner.	Conserves energy, minimizes stress, and enhances trust.
• Provide appropriate attention to other alterations, especially those directly affecting this diagnosis such as Risk for Violence or Ineffective Parenting.	Related issues must be considered as contributing factors to the diagnosis. Inattention to these factors means resolution of problem will not occur.
• Provide for follow-up before child is dismissed from hospital.	Attaches value to follow-up and promotes likelihood of compliance.
• Use developmentally appropriate strategies in care of these children: 　◦ Infant and toddlers: Play therapy or puppets 　◦ Preschoolers: Art 　◦ School-agers: Art or role-playing 　◦ Adolescents: Discussion or role-playing	Developmentally based strategies are most likely to not frighten the child or parent unnecessarily.
• Carry out teaching of appropriate health maintenance. This could be the appropriate way of dealing with crisis related to shyness or poor communication skills.	Personal hygiene and self-care will enhance self-esteem as the patient copes with daily living.
• Monitor for contributory factors related to poor self-esteem, including: 　◦ Family crisis 　◦ Lack of adequate parenting 　◦ Lack of sensory stimulation 　◦ Physical scars, malformation, or disfigurement 　◦ Altered role performance 　◦ Social isolation 　◦ Developmental crisis	Generates the database needed to more accurately and completely plan care.
• Identify ways patient can formulate or reestablish a positive self-esteem according to developmental needs: 　◦ Coping skills 　◦ Communication skills 　◦ Role expectations	Developmental norms serve as the conceptual framework for assisting the child to increase self-esteem.

Continued

ACTIONS/INTERVENTIONS	RATIONALES
○ Self-care ○ Activities of daily living ○ Basic physiologic needs; primary health care ○ Expression of self ○ Peer and social relationships ○ Feelings of self-worth ○ Decision making ○ Validation of self, e.g., setting developmentally appropriate expectations	
• Praise and reinforce positive behavior.	Reinforcement of desired behavior serves to enhance permanence of behavior.
• Explore value conflicts and their resolution.	Values must be clarified as one strives to find one's identity. A healthy sense of self contributes to a positive self-image.
• Collaborate with other health care team members as needed.	Collaboration promotes a more holistic plan of care.
• Meet primary health needs in an expedient manner.	Conserves energy, minimizes stress, and enhances trust.
• Provide appropriate attention to other alterations, especially those directly affecting this diagnosis such as Risk for Violence or Ineffective Parenting.	Related issues must be considered as contributing factors to the diagnosis. Inattention to these factors means resolution of problem will not occur.
• Provide for follow-up before child is dismissed from hospital.	Attaches value to follow-up and promotes likelihood of compliance.
• Use developmentally appropriate strategies in care of these children: ○ Infant and toddlers: Play therapy or puppets ○ Preschoolers: Art ○ School-agers: Art or role-playing ○ Adolescents: Discussion or role-playing	Developmentally based strategies are most likely to not frighten the child or parent unnecessarily.
• Carry out teaching of appropriate health maintenance. This could be the appropriate way of dealing with crisis related to shyness or poor communication skills.	Personal hygiene and self-care will enhance self-esteem as the patient copes with daily living.

Women's Health

ACTIONS/INTERVENTIONS	RATIONALES
POSTPARTUM AND PARENTING ROLES	
• Allow the patient to "relive" birthing experience by listening gently to her perception of the birthing experience.	Promotes ventilation of feelings and provides a database for intervention.
• Encourage the patient to express her concerns about her physical appearance.	
• List here the activities in which the patient can engage to gain positive feelings about herself.	
• Join friends or an exercise group with the same goals as the patient.	Provides a support system that demonstrates adaptive behaviors.
• Encourage participation in activities outside the home as appropriate—e.g., parenting support groups or women's groups.	Support and positive activities assist in adaptation to new parental role and increase sense of self-worth.
• Encourage networking with other women with similar interests.	
• Encourage the patient to "do something for herself": ○ Buy a new dress. ○ Fix her hair differently. ○ Find some time for herself during the day. ○ Take a walk.	

- ○ Take a long bath.
- ○ Rest quietly.
- ○ Do a favorite thing, e.g., reading, sewing, or some hobby.
- ○ Spend time with spouse, without the children.
- Encourage the patient to engage in positive thinking.
- Encourage the patient to engage in assertiveness training.

NOTE: Pregnant teenagers, single mothers, and battered women have similar needs in building or rebuilding their self-esteem.

- Provide a safe, nonjudgmental atmosphere that will encourage patient to verbalize her needs and concerns.
- Assist patient in identifying support groups with similar concerns and available community resources.
- Encourage teen mothers to take advantage of opportunities provided by various school systems to finish their education.

Psychiatric Health

ACTIONS/INTERVENTIONS	RATIONALES
• Sit with client (number) minutes (number) times per shift to discuss client's feelings about self. • Answer questions honestly. • Provide feedback to client about the nurse's perceptions of the client's abilities and appearance by: 　○ Using I statements 　○ Using references related to the nurse's relationship to the client 　○ Describing the client's behavior in situations 　○ Describing the nurse's feelings in relationship	Expression of feelings and concerns in an accepting environment can facilitate problem solving. Promotes the development of a trusting relationship. Assists client with reality testing in a safe, trusting relationship.
• Provide positive reinforcement. List here those things that are reinforcing for the client and when they are to be used. Also list here those things that have been identified as nonreinforcers for this client, and include social rewards.	Positive reinforcement encourages behavior.
• Provide group interaction with (number) of persons (number) minutes 3 times a day at (times). This activity should be gradual and within client's ability—e.g., on admission client may tolerate 1 person for 5 min. If the interactions are brief, the frequency should be high— i.e., 5-min interactions should occur at 30-min intervals.	Disconfirms the client's sense of aloneness and assists client to experience personal importance to others while enhancing interpersonal relationship skills. Increasing these competencies can enhance self-esteem and promote positive orientation.
• Protect client from harm by: 　○ Removing all sharp objects from environment 　○ Removing belts and strings from environment 　○ Providing a one-to-one constant interaction if risk for self-harm is high 　○ Checking on client's whereabouts every 15 min 　○ Removing glass objects from environment 　○ Removing locks from room and bathroom doors 　○ Providing a shower curtain that will not support weight 　○ Checking to see if client swallows medications	Client safety is of primary concern.
• In a supportive attitude and manner, reflect back to the client negative self-statements he or she makes.	Increases client's awareness of negative evaluations of self.

Continued

ACTIONS/INTERVENTIONS	RATIONALES
• Set achievable goals for client.	Goals that can be accomplished increase the client's perceptions of power and enhance self-esteem.
• Provide activities that the client can accomplish and that the client values.	Activities the client finds demeaning could reinforce the client's negative self-evaluation. Accomplishment of valued tasks provides positive reinforcement and enhances self-esteem.
• Provide verbal reinforcement for achievement of steps toward a goal.	Positive reinforcement encourages behavior while enhancing self-esteem.
• Have the client develop a list of strengths and potentials.	Promotes positive orientation and hope.
• Define the client's lack of goal achievement or failures as simple mistakes that are bound to occur when one attempts something new—e.g., learning comes with mistakes or if one does not make mistakes, one does not learn.	Promotes positive orientation.
• Make necessary items available for the client to groom self.	Physical grooming can facilitate positive self-esteem by encouraging positive feedback from others.
• Spend (number) minutes at (time) assisting the client with grooming, providing necessary assistance and positive reinforcement for accomplishments.	Presence of the nurse can serve as a positive reinforcement. Reinforcement encourages positive behavior while enhancing self-esteem.
• Reflect back to the client those statements that discount the positive evaluations of others.	Raises the client's awareness of this behavior, which facilitates change.
• Focus the client's attention on the here and now.	Past happenings are difficult for the nurse to provide feedback on.
• Present the client with opportunities to make decisions about care, and record these decisions in the chart.	Promotes the client's sense of control.
• Develop with the client alternative coping strategies.	Promotes client's sense of control and enhances opportunities for positive outcome when stressful events are encountered.
• Practice new coping behavior with client (number) minutes at (times).	Behavioral rehearsal provides opportunities for feedback and modeling of new behaviors from the nurse.
• Place the client in a therapy group for (number) minutes once a day where the focus is mutual sharing of feelings and support of each other.	Facilitates the client's awareness of others' thoughts about themselves and him or her.
• Identify with the client those situations that are perceived as most threatening to self-esteem.	Facilitates developing alternative coping behavior.
• Assist the client in identifying alternative methods of coping with the identified situations. These should be developed by the client and listed here.	Increases the client's opportunities for success, and each success enhances self-esteem.
• Role-play with the client once per day for 45 min those high-risk situations that were identified and the alternative coping methods.	Behavioral rehearsal provides opportunities for feedback and modeling of new behaviors from the nurse.
• Establish an appointment with the client and significant others to discuss their perceptions of the client's situation (the time of this and follow-up appointments should be listed here).	Support system understanding facilitates the maintenance of new behaviors after discharge.[40]
• Discuss with the client current behavior and reactions of others to this behavior.	Provides opportunities for feedback on new behaviors in a safe, trusting environment.
• Practice with client (number) minutes twice a day making positive I statements.	Promotes the development of a positive orientation.

Gerontic Health

ACTIONS/INTERVENTIONS	RATIONALES
• Assist patient in developing self-care skills needed for managing the current illness.[41]	Enhances perception of control over the situation.
• Assist patient in identifying his or her unique abilities, and relate the benefits you as a nurse receive from your interactions with the patient.[41]	Increases recognition of successes that come from the use of personal strengths.
• Review patient's current abilities and how they may require role modification.[41]	Increases perception of functional ability in preferred life roles.
• Assist with personal grooming needs such as removal of excess facial hair and use of cosmetics where applicable.[42]	Attention to personal appearance can have a positive influence on self-esteem and thus perception of the individual.

Home Health

ACTIONS/INTERVENTIONS	RATIONALES
• Involve the client and family in planning and implementing strategies to reduce and cope with disturbance in self-esteem: ○ Family conference: Discuss perceptions of client's situations and identify realistic strategies. ○ Mutual goal setting: Establish goals and identify roles of each family member—e.g., provide safe environment, assist with grooming, or focus on here and now. ○ Communication.	Family involvement improves effectiveness of implementation.
• Assist the client and family in lifestyle adjustments that may be required[43]: ○ Obtaining and providing accurate information ○ Clarifying misconceptions ○ Maintaining safe environment ○ Encouraging appropriate self-care without encouraging dependence or expecting unrealistic independence ○ Providing opportunity for expressing feelings ○ Realistic goal setting ○ Providing sense of mastery and accomplishable goals in secure environment ○ Maintaining the treatment plan of the health care professionals' guiding therapy ○ Relaxation techniques: Yoga, biofeedback, hypnosis, breathing techniques, or imagery ○ Altering roles	Lifestyle changes require long-term changes in behavior. Such changes in behavior require support.
• Consult with or refer patient to assistive resources as indicated.	Utilization of existing services is efficient use of resources. Psychiatric nurse clinician and support groups can enhance the treatment plan.

Self-Esteem Disturbance

FLOWCHART EVALUATION: EXPECTED OUTCOME 1

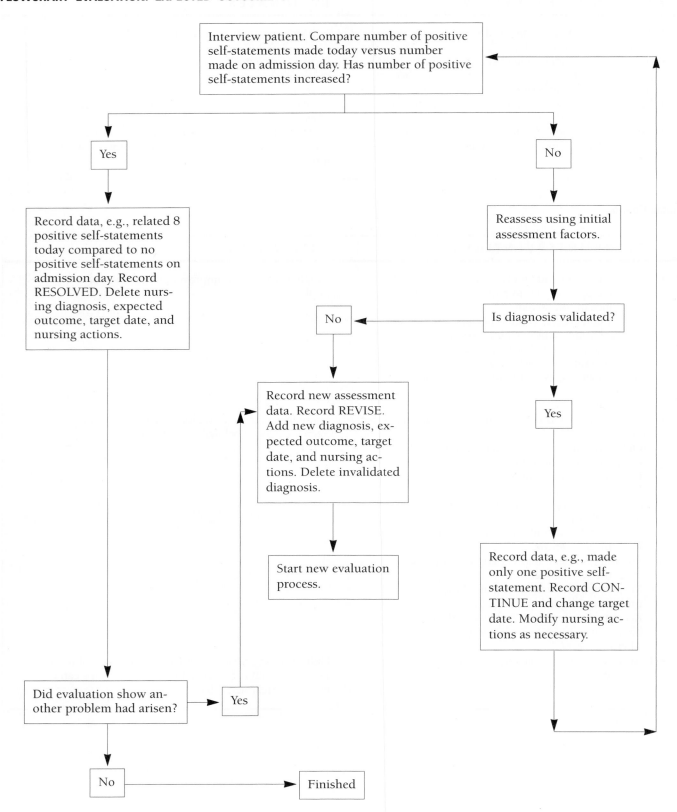

Self-Esteem Disturbance

FLOWCHART EVALUATION: EXPECTED OUTCOME 2

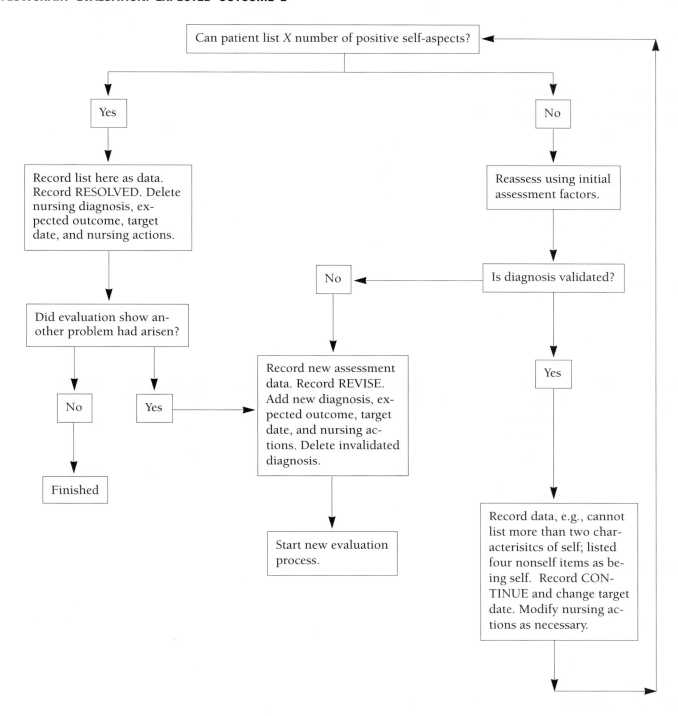

Self-Mutilation, Risk for

DEFINITION

A state in which an individual is at risk to perform an act upon the self with the intent to injure, not kill, which produces immediate tissue damage to the body and tension relief.[23]

NANDA TAXONOMY: FEELING 9.2.2.1

DEFINING CHARACTERISTICS[23]

1. Inability to cope with increased psychological or physiological tension in a healthy manner
2. Feelings of depression, rejection, self-hatred, separation anxiety, guilt, and depersonalization
3. Fluctuating emotions
4. Command hallucinations
5. Need for sensory stimuli
6. Parental emotional deprivation
7. Dysfunctional family

RISK FACTORS[23]

1. Groups at risk
   a. Clients with borderline personality disorder, especially females 16 to 25 years of age
   b. Clients in psychotic state—frequently males in young adulthood
   c. Emotionally disturbed and/or battered children
   d. Mentally retarded and autistic children
   e. Clients with a history of self-injury
   f. History of physical, emotional, or sexual abuse

RELATED FACTORS[23]

The risk factors serve as the related factors.

RELATED CLINICAL CONCERNS

1. Borderline personality disorder
2. Organic mental disorders
3. Autism
4. Schizophrenia
5. Major depression
6. Multiple personality disorder
7. Sexual masochism
8. Affective disorder or mania

HAVE YOU SELECTED THE CORRECT DIAGNOSIS?

Potential for Violence   This diagnosis is very similar to the Risk for Self-Mutilation. However, self-mutilation speaks only to the intent to injure self and specifically exempts suicide.

Ineffective Individual Coping   Certainly self-mutilation would be indicative of ineffective coping. These could be companion diagnoses with priority being given to the self-mutilation problem to decrease the life-threatening aspects before working with the client to increase coping abilities.

EXPECTED OUTCOMES

1. Will demonstrate no self-mutilation attempts by (date) and/or
2. Will verbalize reasons behind self-mutilation threats by (date)

TARGET DATES

Initially progress should be evaluated on a daily basis due to the danger involved for the patient. After stabilization has been demonstrated, the target date could be moved to 5- to 7-day intervals.

NURSING ACTIONS/INTERVENTIONS WITH RATIONALES

Adult Health

Should this diagnosis be made for an adult health patient, immediately refer him or her to a mental health practitioner. See Psychiatric Health nursing actions.

Child Health

Refer patient to a mental health practitioner. See Psychiatric Health nursing actions related to this diagnosis.

Women's Health

The nursing actions for the woman with this diagnosis would be the same as those given for the mental health patient.

Psychiatric Health

ACTIONS/INTERVENTIONS	RATIONALES
• Sit with client (number) minutes (number) times per shift at (times) to assess the client's mood, distress, needs, and feelings.	Promotes the development of a trusting relationship in a nonintrusive manner.[44]
• Place the client on a frequent observation schedule. Note that schedule here. This observation should take place in a nonintrusive manner.	Client safety is of primary importance. Increased attention may inadvertently reinforce injury if it occurs in relation to self-injury episodes.[44] Client safety is of primary importance.
• Remove from the environment any objects that could be used to harm self.	
• Use 1:1 observation to protect the client during periods of risk for self-harming behavior.	Physical and chemical restraints have been demonstrated to escalate behavior. At times clients may escalate their behavior to be placed in restraints.[45]
• Develop a baseline assessment of the self-injury patterns. This should include frequency of behavior, type of behavior, factors related to self-harm, and effects of self-harm on client and other clients. Note this information here.	Provides baseline information on which to base criteria for behavioral change. Provides positive reinforcement.
• Answer client's questions honestly.	Promotes the development of a trusting relationship.
• Reframe the client's self-harming behavior as habitual behavior that can be changed as any habit. While doing this, do not diminish the client's experience of pain and discomfort.	Promotes a positive orientation and supports the client's strengths.[46]
• Identify, with the client, goals that are reasonable. Note those goals here—e.g., client will contact staff when feeling need to harm self.	Assists client in gaining internal control of problematic behaviors.[46] Achieving goals provides reinforcement of positive behavior and enhances self-esteem.
• Provide positive verbal reinforcement for desired behavior change.	Reinforcement encourages positive behavior and enhances self-esteem.
• Have client develop a list of "feel-good" reinforcers. Note those reinforcers here.[45]	Promotes the client's sense of control while supporting a positive orientation.
• Provide feel-good reinforcers according to the reinforcement plan developed. Note the plan here.	Provides consistency in behavioral rewards. Positive reinforcement encourages behavior and enhances self-esteem.
• Identify with the client those situations and feelings that trigger self-injury.[45]	Promotes client's perception of control by paring self-injurious behavior to specific situations and decreasing cognitive exaggerations.[47]
• Identify with the client strategies that can be utilized to cope with these situations. Note the identified strategies here.	Promotes the client's sense of control and assists the client with cognitive preparation for coping with these situations.[47]
• Select 1 identified strategy and spend 30 min a day at (times) practicing this with the client. This practice could be in the form of a role-play. Note here the person responsible for this practice.	Behavioral rehearsal provides opportunities for feedback and modeling from the nurse.
• Meet with the client just prior to and after trigger situations to assist with planning coping strategies and processing outcome to revise plans for future situations.[45]	Promotes the client's sense of control and provides an opportunity for the nurse to provide positive reinforcement for client's use of adaptive coping mechanisms.
• Initiate the client's coping strategy or provide distraction, such as physical activity, when the client identifies that the urge to harm self is strong. Acknowledge that the distraction will not increase comfort as much as self-harm would at the present time, but the feelings of mastery will be satisfying.[46]	Provides opportunity for the client to practice new behaviors in a supportive environment where positive feedback can be provided. Promotes the client's sense of control and enhances self-esteem. Promotes positive orientation.

Continued

ACTIONS/INTERVENTIONS	RATIONALES
• Identify, with the client, areas of social skill deficits, and develop a plan for improving these areas. This could include assertiveness training, communication skills training, and/or relaxation training to reduce anxiety in trigger situations. Note plan and schedule for implementation here. This should be progressive plan with rewards for accomplishment of each step.[45–47]	Enhances interpersonal skills by providing the client with more adaptive ways of achieving interpersonal goals.
• Develop a schedule for the client to attend group therapies. Note this schedule here.	Provides an opportunity for the client to practice interpersonal skills in a supportive environment and to observe peers modeling interpersonal skills.
• Meet with the client and the client's support system to plan coping strategies that can be used at home. Assist system in obtaining resources necessary to implement this plan.	

Gerontic Health

The nursing actions for the gerontic patient with this diagnosis would be the same as those given for the mental health patient.

Home Health

NOTE: See Psychiatric Health nursing actions for additional interventions.

ACTIONS/INTERVENTIONS	RATIONALES
• Monitor for factors contributing to risk for self-mutilation.	Provides database for early recognition and intervention.

• Involve client and family in planning, implementing, and promoting reduction or elimination of risk for self-mutilation:
  ○ Family conference: Discuss perspective of each family member.
  ○ Mutual goal setting: Develop short- and long-term goals with evaluative criteria. Tasks and roles of each family member should be specified.
  ○ Communication: Use open, direct, reality-oriented communication.
	Family involvement enhances effectiveness of interventions.

• Assist client and family in lifestyle adjustments that may be required:
  ○ Development and use of support networks
  ○ Provision of safe environment
  ○ Protection of client from harm
  ○ Long-term care necessity
	Adjustments in lifestyle require long-term behavioral changes. Such changes are enhanced by education and support.

• Consult with or refer patient to assistive resources as indicated.	Utilization of existing services is efficient use of resources. A psychiatric nurse clinician, support group, and mental health–mental retardation expert can enhance the treatment plan.

Self-Mutilation, Risk for

FLOWCHART EVALUATION: EXPECTED OUTCOME 1

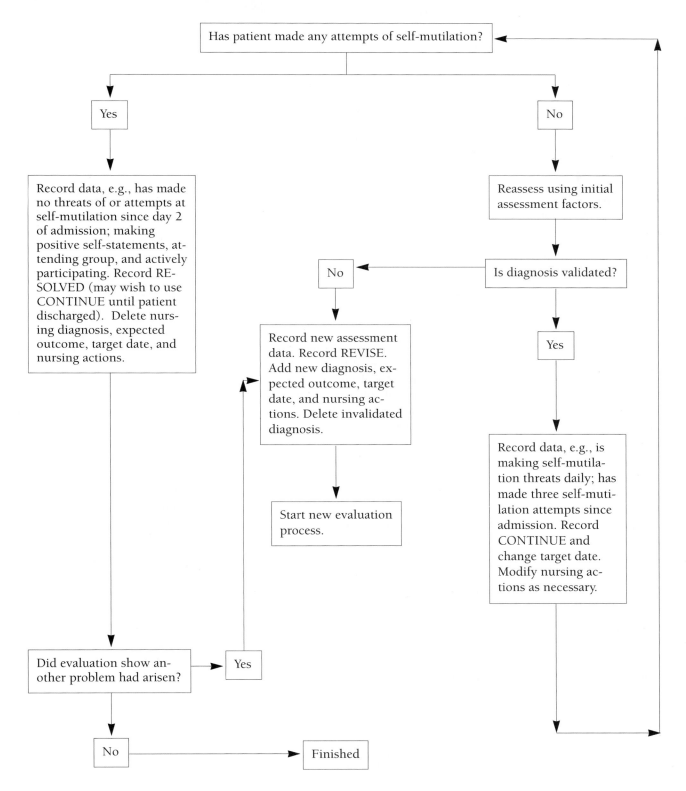

Self-Mutilation, Risk for

FLOWCHART EVALUATION: EXPECTED OUTCOME 2

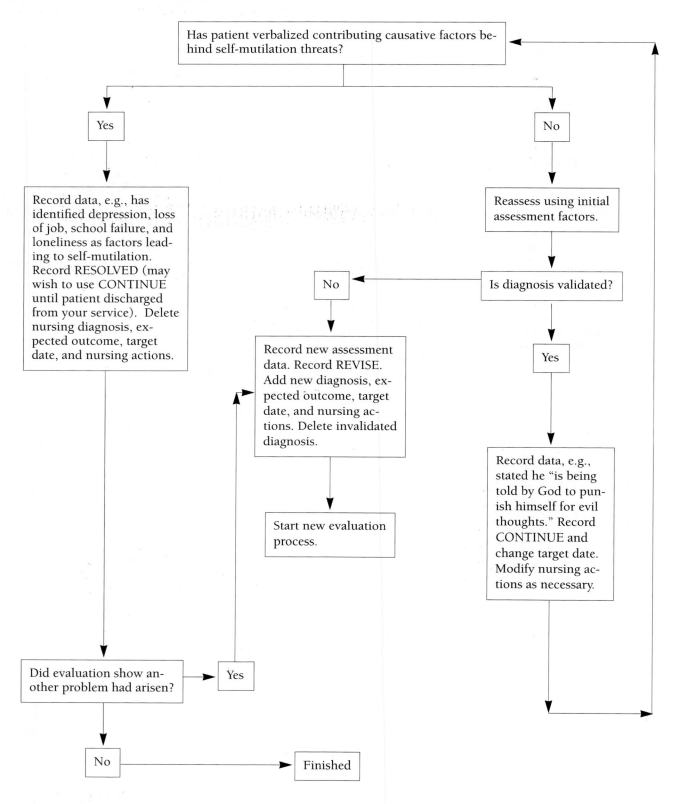

Role-Relationship Pattern

Pattern Description

The role-relationship pattern is concerned with how a person feels he or she is performing the expected behavior delineated by the self and others. Each of us has several roles we fulfill during our daily life, and with these roles come related responsibilities. Included in our roles are family, work, and social relationships. Disruption in these roles, relationships, and responsibilities can lead a patient to seek assistance from the health care system. Likewise, satisfaction with the roles, relationships, and responsibilities is patient strength that can be used in planning care for other health problem areas.

Pattern Assessment

1. Is the client exhibiting distress over a potential loss?
   a. Yes (Anticipatory Grieving)
   b. No
2. Is the client denying a potential loss?
   a. Yes (Anticipatory Grieving)
   b. No
3. Is the client exhibiting distress over an actual loss?
   a. Yes (Dysfunctional Grieving)
   b. No
4. Is the client denying an actual loss?
   a. Yes (Dysfunctional Grieving)
   b. No
5. Is the client making verbal threats against others?
   a. Yes (Risk for Violence)
   b. No
6. Is the client exhibiting increased motor activity?
   a. Yes (Risk for Violence)
   b. No
7. Can the patient speak English?
   a. Yes
   b. No (Impaired Verbal Communication)
8. Does the patient demonstrate any difficulty in talking?
   a. Yes (Impaired Verbal Communication)
   b. No
9. Does the client verbalize difficulty with social situations?
   a. Yes (Impaired Social Interaction)
   b. No
10. Does the client indicate strained relationships with his or her family or others?
    a. Yes (Impaired Social Interaction)
    b. No
11. Does the patient have family or significant others visiting or calling?
    a. Yes
    b. No (Social Isolation)
12. Is the patient uncommunicative, withdrawn, or not making eye contact?
    a. Yes (Social Isolation)
    b. No
13. Does the client indicate admission might impact role (family, work, or leisure)?
    a. Yes (Altered Role Performance)
    b. No
14. Does the family or do significant others verbalize that admission might impact the patient's role (family, work, or leisure)?
    a. Yes (Altered Role Performance)
    b. No
15. Does the child show signs or symptoms of physical or emotional abuse?
    a. Yes (Altered Parenting)
    b. No
16. Do the parents indicate difficulty in controlling the child?
    a. Yes (Altered Parenting)
    b. No
17. Do the parents demonstrate attachment behaviors?
    a. Yes

    b. No (Risk for Altered Parenting, Risk for Altered Parent, Infant, or Child Attachment)
18. Do the parents make negative comments about the child?
    a. Yes (Risk for Altered Parenting)
    b. No
19. Does the family demonstrate capability to meet the child's physical needs?
    a. Yes
    b. No (Altered Family Process)
20. Does the family demonstrate capability to meet the child's emotional needs?
    a. Yes
    b. No (Altered Family Process)
21. Does a family member exhibit signs and symptoms of alcoholism?
    a. Yes (Altered Family Process, Alcoholism)
    b. No
22. Do the parents express concern about their ability to meet child's physical or emotional needs?
    a. Yes (Parental Role Conflict)
    b. No
23. Are the parents frequently questioning decisions about the child's care?
    a. Yes (Parental Role Conflict)
    b. No
24. Was the infant premature?
    a. Yes (Risk for Altered Parent, Infant, or Child Attachment)
    b. No
25. Do the parents express anxiety regarding the parental role?
    a. Yes (Risk for Altered Parent, Infant, or Child Attachment)
    b. No

Conceptual Information

The social connotation for role performance and relationships is a major premise for the intended use of this pattern. A *role* is a comprehensive pattern of behavior that is socially recognized and that provides a means of identifying and placing an individual in a society. Role is the interaction point between the individual and society. It also serves as a means of coping with recurrent situations. The term "role" is a borrowed theatrical noun that emphasizes the distinction of the actor and the part. A role remains relatively stable even though there may be a variety of persons occupying the position or role; however, the expectations of the script, other players, and the audience all influence role enaction.[1] The importance of each of these factors varies with the context. In our personal roles the script is equivalent to the societal "norms" and our audience can be real or imagined. Uniqueness of style may exist within the boundaries of the role as determined by society.

Because our roles are such an integral part of our lives, we seldom analyze them until they become a problem to our internal or external adaptation to life's demands. Roles that are often associated with stages of development serve as society's guides for meaningful and satisfying relationships in life by facilitating an orderly method for transferring knowledge, responsibility, and authority from one generation to the next.

During the childhood years, an individual will have numerous contacts with different individuals who have different sets of values. The child learns to internalize the values of those significant in his or her life as personal goals are actualized. When the goals are realistic, consistent, and attainable, the individual is assisted in developing a sense of self-esteem as these various roles are mastered. Each new role carries with it the potential for gratification and increased ego identity if the role is acquired. If the role is not mastered, poor self-esteem and role confusion may ensue. The potential for successful role mastery is diminished with multiple role demands and the absence of suitable role models. Additionally, role acquisition depends on adequate patterns of cognitive-perceptual ability and a healthy sense of self.

Although all roles are learned within the context of one's culture, specific roles are delineated in two ways: acquired and achieved. *Acquired roles* are those roles with variables over which the individual has no choice such as gender or race. *Role achievement* allows for some choice by the individual with the result of purposefully earning a role such as choosing to become a professional nurse.

Many roles are not clearly defined as being either acquired or achieved but rather are a combination of the two. Roles are not mutually exclusive but are interdependent. The roles an individual assumes usually blend well; however, the roles that a person achieves or acquires may not always make for a harmonious blend. Role conflicts may occur from the most internalized personal level to a generalized societal level.

Roles may be influenced by a multitude of factors, including economics, family dynamics, changing roles of institutions, and gender role expectations. Roles can be mediated through role-playing skills and self-conceptions. It is hoped that with the increased demands on the individual, society will continue to value human dignity with respect for life itself. Roles should allow for self-actualization.

One of the more recent eclectic theories of personality development encompassing role theory is that of *symbolic interaction*. In this orientation, social interaction has symbolic meaning to the participants in relation to the roles assigned by society. (For further related conceptual information, refer to Chapter 8, Self-Perception and Self-Concept Pattern.)

Symbolic interaction encompasses the roles assumed by humans in their constant interaction with other humans, communicating symbolically in almost all they do. This interaction has meaning to both the giver and the receiver of the action, thus requiring both persons to interact symbolically with themselves as they interact with each other. Symbolic interaction involves *interpretation*, that is, the ascertaining of the meaning of the actions or remarks of the other person, and *definition*, that is, the conveying of an indication to another person as to how he or she is to act. Human association consists of a process of such interpretation and definition. Through this process the participants fit their own acts to the ongoing acts of one another and guide others in doing so.[2]

To explore further how relationships develop, a brief overview of kinship is offered. A *kinship system* is a structured system of relationships in which individuals are bound one to another by complex, interlocking relationships. These relationships are commonly referred to as *families*. It is not so much the family form in which one lives as how that family form functions that defines whether or not there is a cohesive family structure:

An ideal family environment consists of a family that has many routines and traditions, provides for quality time between adults and children, has regular contact with relatives and neighbors, lives in a supportive and safe neighborhood, has contact with the work world and has adult members who model a harmonious and problem-solving relationship. (pp. 505–507)[3]

The 1980s saw great change in family structures with an explosion of individualized living arrangements and lifestyles requiring new definitions of the "family."[3-6] Fewer nuclear families consisting of husband, wife, and children exist today, and this is no longer the only acceptable form for family life. Some of the different family forms identified in today's society are[3-6]:

Nuclear family: Husband, wife, and children living in a common household, sanctioned by marriage

Nuclear dyad: Husband and wife alone; childless or children have left home

Single-parent family: One head of household, mother or father, as a result of divorce, abandonment, or separation

Single adult alone: Either by choice, divorce, or death of a spouse

Three-generation family: Three generations or more in a single household

Kin network: Nuclear households or unmarried members living in close geographical proximity

Institutional family: Children in orphanages or residential schools

Homosexual family: Homosexual couples with or without children

Despite the differences in family forms and cultural differences, primary relationships within various family structures reveal markedly similar characteristics in all societies. These relationships were described in 1949[7] and still exist in the various family forms cited today:

Husband and wife: Economic specialization and cooperation, sexual cohabitation; joint responsibility for support, care, and upbringing of children; well-defined reciprocal rights with respect to property, divorce, spheres of authority

Father and son: Economic cooperation in masculine activities under leadership of the father; obligation of material support vested in father during childhood of son and in son during old age of father; responsibility of father for instruction and discipline of son; duty of obedience and respect on part of son; tempered by some measure of comradeship

Mother and daughter: Relationship parallel to that between father and son but with more emphasis on child care and economic cooperation and less on authority and material support (However, strong relationships in the development of mothering skills and parenting techniques lead to obligations of emotional support and caretaking activities vested in the mother during the childhood of daughter and in daughter during old age of mother.)

Father and daughter: Responsibility of father for protection and material support prior to marriage of daughter; economic cooperation, instruction, and discipline appreciably less prominent than in father-son relationship; playfulness common in infancy of daughter but normally yields to a measure of reserve with the development of a strong incest taboo

Mother and son: Relationship parallel to mother and daughter but with more emphasis on financial and emotional support in later life of mother

Elder and younger brothers: Relationship of playmates, developing into that of comrades; economic cooperation under leadership of elder; moderate responsibility of elder for instruction and discipline of younger

Elder and younger sister: Relationship parallel to that between elder and younger brother but with more emphasis on physical care of the younger sister

Brother and sister: Early relationship of playmates, varying with relative age; gradual development of an incest taboo, commonly coupled with some measure of reserve; moderate economic cooperation; partial assumption of parental role, especially by the elder sibling

The nurse must exercise great caution in maintaining sensitivity to the individual meaning attached to various roles and the ways in which these roles are perceived and assumed. With the current societal and economic changes, the individual's roles are being impacted on a daily basis even without the added stress of a health problem.

Developmental Considerations

NEONATE AND INFANT

The newborn period is especially critical for the development of the first attachment that is so vital for all future human relationships. Attachment behavior includes crying, smiling, clinging, following, and cuddling. The infant is dependent on its mother and father for basic needs of survival. This is often demanding and requires parents to place self-needs secondary to the needs of the infant. This makes for a potential role-relationship alteration.

Although dependent on others, the infant is an active participant in the role-relationship pattern development from conception on. The infant is capable of influencing the interactions of those caring for him or her. Reciprocal interactions also influence the maternal-paternal-infant relationship. Positive interactions will be greatly influenced by infant-initiated behavior at well as maternal-paternal responses and the reciprocal interaction of all involved. The state of the infant as well as the state of the parent interacting with the infant must be considered as critical.

It is important to note than any alteration in the health status of the mother, the neonate, or both has the potential of interfering with the establishment of the maternal-infant relationship. This may not necessarily be the case, but it is often critical that the potential risk be acknowledged early so that residual, secondary problems can be prevented with appropriate nursing intervention. It is also important to keep in mind that the infant is taking in all situational experiences and that as learning occurs through interaction with the environment, a gradual evolution of role-relationship patterns occurs.

By approximately 12 months of age, the infant shows fear of being left alone and will search for the parents with his or her eyes. The infant will avoid and reject strangers. There is an obvious increasing interest in pleasing the parent. In protest the infant cries, screams, and searches for the parent. In despair the infant is listless, withdrawn, and disinterested with the environment. In detachment or resignation a superficial "adjustment" occurs in which the infant appears interested in surroundings, happy, and friendly for short periods of time. The infant is emotionally changeable from crying to laughing with a beginning awareness of separation from the environment. Still, the infant uses mother as a safe haven from which to explore the world. The infant will have a favorite toy, blanket, or other object that serves to comfort him or her in times of stress. (Sucking behavior may also serve to calm the infant, and eventually the infant will develop self-initiated ways of dealing with the stressors of life, such as thumbsucking versus the actual taking of formula or milk.)

This infant receives cues from significant others and primary caregivers regarding grief responses such as crying, with a preference for the other. Depending on age and situational status, the infant may protest by crying for mother. In a weakened state, the infant may make little response of preference for caregivers.

According to family structure, the neonate or infant will adapt to usual socialization routines within reasonable limits. Actual isolation for the infant would occur perhaps if the primary caregiver could not exercise usual role-taking behavior for socialization. If this behavior is arrested for marked periods of time, there is a potential for developmental delays secondary to the lack of appropriate social stimulation.

The newborn period is especially critical for the development of the neonate's first attachment for future human relationships. During this period the infant must depend on others for his or her care and basic needs. This is often a demanding situation for parents who must sacrifice their own needs to best meet the needs of others.

The infant is dependent on others for care ranging from required food for physical growth to appropriate sensory and social stimulation. In the absence of the stability usually afforded by the family in its usual functioning pattern, the infant may be at risk for failure to thrive or developmental delay. Ultimately, rather than developing a sense of trust and a feeling that the world is a place in which one's needs are met, the infant will doubt and mistrust others. This in turn places the infant at risk for an abnormal pattern of development.

Crying serves as the primitive verbal communication for the neonate and infant. As the infant begins to understand and respond to the spoken word, the world should be symbolized as comforting and safe. With time, basic attempts at verbalization are noted in imitation of what is heard. There is a correlation between parental speech stimulation and the actual development of speech in young children, suggesting a positive effect for early stimulation. *Echolalia* (the often pathologic repetition of what is said by other people as if echoing them) and attempts at making speech are most critical to note during this time.

The infant may be the recipient of violent behavior, and, all too often, it is because of crying. The attempt to quiet the infant can take the form of lashing out for those individuals unable to deal with the usual role-relationship patterns. The infant is unable to defend itself, and therefore is to be protected by reporting of any suspected abusive or negligent behavior. At particular risk would be infants with feeding or digestive disorders, premature or small-for-gestational-age infants who require feedings every 2 hours, or others perceived as "demanding" or "irritable." Also at risk would be infants who are born with congenital anomalies or disfigurements.

TODDLER AND PRESCHOOLER

The toddler has an increasing sense of identity and knows himself or herself as a separate person. The toddler treats other children as if they were objects and gradually becomes involved in parallel play, which then leads to a more interactive play with peers. The sharing of possessions is not yet to be expected for toddlers. The toddler begins to formulate a sense of right and wrong with the ability to conform to some social demand, as exemplified by the capacity for self-toileting. It is reasonable that a toddler would begin to work through problems of family relations with other children while playing.

The preschool child talks and plays with an imaginary playmate as a projection. What is offered may be what the child views as bad in himself or herself. The preschooler may have some friends of the same sex, and opportunities for socialization serve critical functions. The preschool child lives in the "here and now" and is capable of internalizing more and more of society's norms. There is a sense of morality and conscience by this age. A strong sense of family exists for the preschooler.

The toddler may be unusually dependent on mother, objects of security, and routines. He or she is capable of magical thinking and may believe in animation of inanimate objects, such as believing an x-ray machine is really a mean monster. Toddlers may be fearful of seeing blood. These fears may be unrelated to actual situations.

The preschooler may be critical of himself or herself and may blame himself or herself for a situation with some attempt at viewing the current situation as punishment for previous behavior or thoughts. He or she will tolerate brief separation from parents in usual functioning. Play or puppet therapy that is appropriate to the situation will help the preschooler in expressing feelings.

The toddler must have room to safely explore with a sense of autonomy evolving in the ideal situation. If social isolation limits these opportunities, the toddler will be limited in role-relationship exposure. This will often result in either social isolation or a form of forced precocious role-taking in which the toddler is perceived as being able to satisfy the companionship needs of adults. The toddler may misinterpret socialization opportunities as abandonment or punishment, so short intervals of parallel play with one peer, to begin with, would be appropriate. Toddlers who are denied opportunities for peer interaction would be at risk for role-relationship problems.

The child of the preschool age group may experience alteration in socialization attempts if overpowered by peers, if there are too many rigid or unrealistic rules, or if the situation places the child in a situation that presents values greatly different from those of the child and his or her family. If the child at this age experiences prolonged social isolation or rejection, there could be marked potential for difficulty in forming future relationships. If things do not go well

in his or her socialization, the child at this age may blame himself or herself.

The toddler will seek out opportunities to explore and interact with the environment, provided that there is a safe haven to return to as represented by the family. When this facilitative factor is not present, the toddler may regress and become dependent on primary caregivers or others or may manifest frustration via extremes in demanding behavior. The child's subsequent development may also be affected by family process alteration.

The preschool child is able to verbalize concerns regarding changes in family process but is unable to comprehend dynamics. It is critical to attempt to view the altered process through the eyes of the preschooler who could blame himself or herself for the change or crisis, or who may think magically and have fears that may be unrelated to the situation. Subsequent development may be altered by family process dysfunction, with regression often occurring.

At this age it is important to stress the need for ritualistic behavior as a means of mastering the environment with adequate anticipatory safety. This period allows for knowing "self" as a separate entity. The toddler is capable of attempting to conform to social demands but lacks ability of self-control.

The importance of setting limits must be stressed with regard to safety and disciplinary management. At this age the child begins to resist parental authority. Methods of dealing with differences or rules from one setting to another must be simple and appropriate to the situation.

For the toddler this time can prove frustrating with a need to be understood despite a limited vocabulary. Jargon and gestures may be misinterpreted with resultant frustration for child and parent. Patience and understanding go far with a child of this age. Pictures and the telling of stories serve as a means of enhancing speech as well as instilling an appreciation for reading and speech. Feelings come to be expressed by the spoken word also. The child is able to refer to self as "I," "me," or by name.

By preschool age, the child is able to count to 10, is able to define at least one word, and may name four or five colors. Speech now serves as a part of socialization in play with peers. Wants should be expressed freely as the child broadens his or her contact with persons other than primary family members. The preschooler enjoys stories and television programs and attempts to tell stories of his or her own creation.

If the toddler is unable to fulfill the expectations of parents or caregivers who demand unrealistic behavior, there is risk of abuse. Especially noteworthy would be a desire for the young toddler to be capable of self-toileting behavior when in fact it is not possible. This places the toddler in a target population for abuse also. At this age the toddler may be unable to express hostility or anger in the verbal mode, and so a common occurrence may be temper tantrums. At risk for violence would be the toddler who resists parental authority in discipline and cannot meet demands of the parents.

SCHOOL-AGE CHILD

Learning social roles as male or female is a major task for the school-age child with a preference for spending time with friends of the same sex rather than the family. The school-ager is capable of role-taking and values cooperation and fair play. There may be a strict moralism of "black and white" with no gray areas noted. The school-ager enjoys simple household chores, likes a reward system, and has the capacity for expressing feelings. Fear of disability and concern for missing school are typical concerns for this age group.

Illness may impose separation from the peer group. Although independent of parents in health, the school-ager may require close parental relationship in illness or crisis. Loss of control and fear of mutilation and death are real concerns. The school-age child may fear disgracing parents if loss of control such as crying occurs. He or she is aware of the severity of his or her prognosis and may even deal with reality better than parents or adults might. The school-age child may use art as a means of expressing his or her feelings.

This child is at risk of social isolation if a situation is different from previous socialization opportunities. He or she may experience value conflict and question the rules. He or she may also be afraid to express desires or concerns regarding socialization needs for fear of punishment. Peer involvement is a most vital component of assisting the school-ager to formulate views of acceptable social behavior.

The school-ager may try to assume the role of a parent if the dysfunction of the family relates to the parent of the same sex. This may be healthy with appropriate acknowledgment of limitations. At this age, the child is concerned with what other friends may think about the family with some stigma attached in certain cultures to divorce, homosexuality, and altered lifestyles. It would be critical for the school-ager to have a close friend who might share the cultural views of his or her own family to best endure the altered family process.

Allowance for increasing interests outside the home should be made with a sensitivity to parental approval or disapproval. The child may rebel against parental authority in an attempt to be like peers.

Confidence in self and a general sense of well-being will promote adequacy in communication development. The child of this age continues to learn vocabulary and takes pride in his or her ability to demonstrate appropriate use of words. At this age jokes and riddles serve as a means of encouraging peer interaction with speech. Reading is a leisure activity for the school-age child.

The child will usually enjoy school and consider peer interaction an enjoyable part of life. In instances in which the child feels inferior, there may be a risk for violence or abusive behavior as a cover-up for poor self-image or low self-esteem. Often there will be related role-relationship alterations as well. The family serves as a means of valuing the interaction, which should foster the appropriate enjoyment of friendships. At risk would be those children with learning disabilities or handicaps, parental conflicts, or related role-relationship alteration.

ADOLESCENT

Vacillation between dependence and independence is a common occurrence for the adolescent who is attempting to establish a sense of identity. The adolescent questions traditional values, especially those of parents. There is a gradual trend to independent functioning that allows the adolescent to assume roles of adulthood, including the development of intensive relationships with members of the opposite sex.

The adolescent will be constantly weighing self-identity versus perceived identity expressed via peers. He or she may be fearful of expressing true feelings or concern for fear of rejection by peers, parents, or significant others. Isolation from peers will place the adolescent at risk for altered self-identity as well as altered role-relationship patterns.

The adolescent is able to assist within the family during times of altered process. It is important to stress that in more and more dual-career or single-parent families, young adolescents spend more and more time alone. Nonetheless, adolescents should still have opportunities for peer interaction and socialization according to the family's needs.

There may be marked vacillations, as the adolescent strives to find self-identity, with dependence and independence issues. Even more marked rebellion against parental wishes may be manifest at this time as peer approval is sought.

Any factors that may interfere with usual speech patterns may prove especially difficult for the adolescent. Bracing of teeth may be common, with the potential for self-image alteration. Also, the eruption of 12-year molars could prove painful as might the possible impaction of wisdom teeth later. Expressed wit is valued in this age group, as might be special colloquial expressions to qualify group or peer identity. Difficulty in expression of self may prove most difficult for this individual. Respect for times of reflection and estrangement should be maintained.

The adolescent may be caught in a crossfire of strife for independence versus dependence. For this group it is paramount that self-control be attained to develop the meaningful relationships so critical for appropriate role-relationship patterns. Often those adolescents who have not acquired appropriate socialization skills resort to drugs or alcohol as a means of feeling better and escaping the reality of life. This may also foster loss of control as reality is distorted. In many instances there may be related juvenile delinquency with resultant records of lawbreaking.

Additionally, any adolescent who is assuming a role that stresses or negates the usual development of self-identity would be at risk for violence as a means of coping. An example of this would be two young teenagers attempting to parent when they themselves still require parenting.

YOUNG ADULT

Although biophysical and cognitive skills reach their peak during the adult years, the young adult is still in a period of growth and development. Striving for achievement of an education, job security, meaningful intimate relationships with others, and establishment of a family are the primary focuses of the young adult. While young adults usually have achieved independence, they find themselves learning socially relevant behavior and settling into specific acquired roles within a chosen profession or occupation. They begin to adopt some of the values of the group to which they belong and to assume assured roles such as marriage and parenting.

Cognitively, young adults have reached their peak level of intellectual efficiency, and they are able to think abstractly and to synthesize and integrate their ideas, experiences, and knowledge. Thinking for the adult usually involves reasoning, taking into consideration past experiences, education, and the possible outcomes of a situation more realistically and less egocentrically than the adolescent.

Young adulthood is still a time of great adjustment. The

individual is expected to look at self in relation to society, learning how to deal with personal needs and desires as opposed to the needs and desires of others, and managing the economic and physical needs of life. Sexual activity focuses toward the development of a single intimate, meaningful relationship and the establishment of a family. In developing the role of parenting, the young adult often falls back on the parenting patterns and behavior of his or her own parents.

The young adult begins to assume the responsibility of providing for a family. Most young adults are members of dual-career families and thus face the stresses of multiple roles. Many of these young adults become single parents, and the stresses of multiple responsibilities and roles are greater both at home and at work. Just as during adolescence, the negation of development of self-identity can lead to crises, role strain, conflict, and often failure in the young adult.

As the adult acquires full role responsibility, there may be difficulties related to role diffusion, role confusion, role strain, or related assumption of appropriate roles. Also, the ultimate developmental need for assumption of accountability for self may be unresolved. There may be a greater likelihood for the various demands of society on male and female roles to be experienced at this time as women assume the multiple roles of wife, mother, worker, housekeeper, and so on, just as men also have assumed more and more roles that were formerly assumed by females. This challenge also brings the potential for growth and fulfillment in self-actualizing individuals.

MIDDLE-AGE ADULT

Middle age, or middlescence, is often considered the most productive years for an individual. People in this age group are usually secure in a profession or career, are in the middle of raising a family, and often must assume responsibility for aging parents.

As biophysical changes occur, there is a concurrent adaptation of the cognitive and physical activities of the individual. The body ages in varying stages or degrees, and young middle-age adults usually retain the body structure and activity level they established as young adults. Middle-age adults, with more sedentary lifestyles, must establish exercise programs to retain their youthful figures. The greatest changes facing both men and women during this time are those associated with the climacteric and the loss of reproductive capabilities. These biologic and physical changes can affect sexual lifestyles either positively or negatively, depending on the perception and orientation of the individual.

Most middle-age adults function well and learn to gradually accept the changes of aging, and with proper nutrition, exercise, and a healthy lifestyle, they can experience excellent health and a productive middlescence. Middle-age people usually begin to face more accidents, illness, and death; they begin to deal with their own aging process and death, as well as that of their parents. There is often a role reversal with the middle-age adult assuming the role of parent.

This is the time of life when individuals usually review their goals and aspirations, sometimes to find that they did not reach the potential they once dreamed. Most middle-age adults begin to feel that there is not enough time to accomplish all they want to accomplish, and they begin to adjust to the fact that they may not reach all of the goals they set in their youth. This can result in a loss of self-esteem, or it can be a motivation to develop previously untapped reservoirs, which can lead to self-actualization and personal satisfaction.

OLDER ADULT

With aging, individuals may have fewer demands placed upon them, thus leaving more time and fewer potential opportunities for role performance. This may also be a time when one is able to fulfill volunteer roles and those of choice versus those of demand. A critical factor may be the freedom one feels as basic needs are met. If health is satisfactory and one has children or grandchildren to enjoy, financial stability, and the ability to pursue fulfillment via role engagement, this experience would be self-actualizing. On the other hand, if one's health fails, few meaningful family supports exist, and financial needs arise, self-actualizing role performance is potentially threatened.

The older adult must deal with decreasing function with resultant decreasing socialization potential. This is a time for retrospection and pondering the past with sincere concerns regarding the future and death. In some people full functional level is possible, whereas for others life is lived vicariously. Elder role-modeling opportunities, with respect for those who have lived life, still exist in many cultures. For these individuals the aging process is welcomed and enjoyed as the fullest potential is actualized for role-relationship patterning, namely, the generation of values to the young in society. In those instances where aging is accompanied by loss in whatever form, the potential exists for the individual to become dependent. This dependency may range from a minor form to a major form of total dependence on others. The onset of dependency may be gradual or sudden. In either instance the nurse must recognize the impact of the loss for the patient according to the values of the patient and family.

APPLICABLE NURSING DIAGNOSES

Caregiver Role Strain, Risk for and Actual

DEFINITION

RISK FOR A caregiver is vulnerable for the felt difficulty in performing the family caregiver role.[8]

ACTUAL A caregiver's felt difficulty in performing the family caregiver role.[8]

NANDA TAXONOMY: RELATING 3.2.2.1 AND 3.2.2.2

DEFINING CHARACTERISTICS[8]

1. Risk for Caregiver Role Strain
   a. The risk factors also serve as the defining characteristics.
2. Caregiver Role Strain—caregivers report that they:
   a. Do not have enough resources to provide the care needed

b. Find it hard to do specific caregiving activities
c. Worry about such things as the care receiver's health and emotional state, having to put the care receiver in an institution, and who will care for the care receiver if something should happen to the caregiver
d. Feel that caregiving interferes with other important roles in their lives
e. Feel loss because the care receiver is like a different person than before caregiving began or, in the case of a child, that the care receiver was never the child the caregiver expected
f. Feel family conflict around issues of providing care
g. Feel stress or nervousness in their relationship with the care receiver
h. Feel depressed

RELATED FACTORS[8]

1. Risk for Caregiver Role Strain—risk factors:
   a. Pathophysiological
      (1) Illness severity of the care receiver
      (2) Addiction or codependency
      (3) Premature birth or congenital defect
      (4) Discharge of family member with significant home care needs
      (5) Caregiver health impairment
      (6) Unpredictable illness course or instability in the care receiver's health
      (7) Caregiver is female
      (8) Psychological or cognitive problems in care receiver
   b. Developmental
      (1) Caregiver is not developmentally ready for caregiver role, for example, a young adult needing to provide care for middle-aged parent
      (2) Developmental delay or retardation of the care receiver or caregiver
   c. Psychological
      (1) Marginal family adaptation or dysfunction prior to the caregiving situation
      (2) Marginal caregiver's coping patterns
      (3) Past history of poor relationship between caregiver and care receiver
      (4) Caregiver is spouse
      (5) Care receiver exhibiting deviant or bizarre behavior
   d. Situational
      (1) Presence of abuse or violence
      (2) Presence of situational stressors that normally affect families, such as significant loss, disaster, or crisis, poverty or economic vulnerability, major life events, for example, birth, hospitalization, leaving home, returning home, marriage, divorce, employment, retirement, or death
      (3) Duration of caregiving required
      (4) Inadequate physical environment for providing care, for example, housing, transportation, community services, or equipment
      (5) Family or caregiver isolation
      (6) Lack of respite and recreation for caregiver
      (7) Inexperience with caregiving
      (8) Caregiver's competing role commitments
      (9) Complexity or amount of caregiving tasks
2. Caregiver Role Strain—the related factors for this diagnosis are exactly the same as the risk factors for the risk diagnosis.

RELATED CLINICAL CONCERNS

1. Any chronic, debilitating illness, for example, Alzheimer's disease, cancer, or rheumatoid arthritis
2. Severe mental retardation
3. Chemical abuse
4. Closed head injury
5. Schizophrenia
6. Personality disorders

HAVE YOU SELECTED THE CORRECT DIAGNOSIS?

Ineffective Individual Coping This diagnosis and Caregiver Role Strain are very close; however, the differentiating factor is whether or not the individual is involved in a caregiver role. If significant caregiving is a part of the individual's role, then initial interventions should be directed toward resolving the problems within the caregiving role.

Impaired Adjustment Certainly needing to assume a caregiver role would require some adjustment. However, this diagnosis relates to an individual adjusting to his or her own illness or health problem, not adjusting to someone else's illness or health problem.

Ineffective Family Coping (Compromised or Disabling) These diagnoses could be companion diagnoses to Caregiver Role Strain. If the family cannot adapt to a change in a family member's condition and assigns the caregiver role to just one family member, then both Ineffective Family Coping and Caregiver Role Strain are likely to develop.

EXPECTED OUTCOMES

1. The caregiver will implement a plan to reduce strain by (date) and/or
2. The caregiver will verbally describe decreased strain by (date)

TARGET DATES

A target date of 5 days would be the earliest date to begin evaluation of progress toward meeting the expected outcome.

NURSING ACTIONS/INTERVENTIONS WITH RATIONALES

Adult Health

ACTIONS/INTERVENTIONS	RATIONALES
• Encourage patient to talk about caregiver role by active listening, reflection, asking open-ended questions, and accepting his or her feelings for 15 min twice a day at (times).	Decreases anxiety when allowed to ventilate positive and negative feelings in nonthreatening, empathetic environment.
• Teach stress management techniques such as relaxation, meditation, or deep breathing.	
• Have patient return-demonstrate techniques for 5 min every 4 h while awake at (times).	Relieves stress, identifies alternative coping strategies, and decreases depression.
• Identify community support groups such as Mother's Day Out, daycare centers, housekeeping services, home health aids, hospice, or respite care prior to discharge. Also, cooperative arrangement could be made with friends and neighbors for release time from care activities.	Provides alternatives for coping and resources to support in short-term and long-term problems.
• Encourage family conferences to discuss role expectations, role conflict, role strain, and role negotiation for 1 h every other day.	Opens communication and promotes cooperative problem solving.
• Refer to psychiatric nurse specialist as needed (see Psychiatric Health nursing actions).	Collaboration promotes holistic health care. Interventions may require expertise of specialist.

Child Health

ACTIONS/INTERVENTIONS	RATIONALES
• Monitor for contributing factors with a focus on high-risk populations: ○ Excessive demands exist secondary to a child requiring extensive care, e.g., several small children in family with one child requiring extensive assistance with physical or mental problems ○ A patient who has a total self-care deficit ○ Caregiver indicating inability to carry out usual routines	Unrealistic demands of parenting or care provision increases the likelihood of role strain.
• Schedule a daily conference with caregiver of at least 30 min.	Allows identification of current perception of role strain by encouraging ventilation of feelings. Provides teaching opportunity. Assists in identification of referrals that are needed.
• Explore with parent or caregiver, during conference, options available to assist with the demands of the situation. Encourage caregiver to provide time for self on a daily basis through such means as seeking outside help—e.g., visiting nurse, housekeeping assistance, respite care, institutionalizations such as temporary per day or, if appropriate and desired, permanent.	Support from others serves as a means of preventing further demise of desired role-taking while also allowing for long-term needs. Time for self will enhance coping abilities and, ultimately, self-esteem.
• Identify, during conference, community resources, especially parenting support groups, that are available.	Provides long-term support and information. Encourages sharing of concerns with others in the same situation.

Continued

ACTIONS/INTERVENTIONS	RATIONALES
• Schedule family conference, as needed, to focus on family's willingness to provide assistance in caregiving.	Assists in delineating roles for each family member. Assists in providing relief for primary caregiver on a more regular basis. Unresolved conflict increases the likelihood of little change in behavior.
• Determine, via an ongoing assessment, any unresolved guilt regarding role demands, "less-than-perfect child," or related aspects of situation (see Dysfunctional Grieving).	
• Assist caregiver and significant other(s) to explore, during conference, inevitabilities and realities associated with the care situation.	Expectations may be unrealistic. Clarification of expectations and reality assist in problem solving.
• Preserve the effective functioning of the caregiver through teaching and support in conferences.	The likelihood of secondary and tertiary alterations for the caregiver increase when primary needs of rest and own physical self are not met.

Women's Health

ACTIONS/INTERVENTIONS	RATIONALES
NEW MOTHER OR PARENT ROLE	
• Assist new mother in developing realistic plans for infant care from hospital. Have mother review plans for self-care and plans for care of the infant in the home.	Provides time for assessment and planning for home care. Affords opportunity to teach and give realistic feedback regarding the impact a newborn makes on former lifestyle.
• Include significant other in plans for care of new mother and infant after discharge from the hospital. Encourage discussion by mother and significant other of various role changes in the family that will occur with the new infant being incorporated into the household—e.g., sibling's role, wife's role, husband's role, or grandparent's role.[9]	
• Encourage discussion of the "new" role of being a mother and father, as well as being husband and wife.	
• Assist with development of plan to save time such as learning to sleep when the infant sleeps, turning telephone off when trying to rest, or putting sign on front door when sleeping.[10]	Assist in reducing fatigue, which is a significant contributor to the development of caregiver role strain.
• Identify areas in which the significant other can assist the new mother and help reduce fatigue—e.g., if breast-feeding, let dad get the infant, change the diaper, and bring the infant to the mother for feeding during the night.[10,11]	
• Plan meals for the family before leaving for the hospital, cook them, and freeze them so that meals can be prepared easily during the first few weeks at home.[10]	
TEEN PARENTING	
NOTE: The nursing actions for the teenage parent will be the same as above with the following additions:	
• Refer the young couple or teenager to young parents' groups in the community for social and personal support.	Provides long-term support and a source of information.[11]
• Give the young couple telephone hotlines they can call for assistance and support—e.g., hospital nursery, young parent services, or the YWCA.	
• Assist the young parent to get into or stay in school by giving references for child care.	Promotes long-range planning and reduces the likelihood of strain for the young parents.
• Encourage the young couple to express their feelings about the new responsibilities they face.	

PARENT TO YOUR PARENTS

NOTE: Approximately 80 percent of women will become the primary care providers for their elderly parents.

- Provide supportive atmosphere for discussion of situation in order to:
  ○ Identify specific concerns and needs.
  ○ Explore the inevitabilities and realities of the situation.
  ○ Identify possible resources in the community (financial assistance, personal support, social work, or daycare).
  ○ Identify methods by which family members and siblings can share responsibilities.
  ○ Establish ties from primary caretaker to other family members to provide relief for each other.
  ○ Identify methods of sharing expenses associated with housing (keeping parent[s] in own home, nursing home or extended care, or assisted living).
  ○ Assist with development of plan to provide supervision for parent while working (neighbors of parents, family members, daycare, or home aide assistant).

Sharing responsibilities of elderly parents assists the entire family to lead better lives. Many women have entire burden of elderly parents while trying to maintain jobs and their own families. Often they will not speak of this; therefore, the nurse must patiently interview the women.

Psychiatric Health

NOTE: For information related to the caregivers of those clients with a medical diagnosis of dementia, refer to Gerontic Health. As used in this discussion "caregiver" can mean one person or an extended family system.

ACTIONS/INTERVENTIONS	RATIONALES
• Spend (number) minutes (number) times per week interacting with primary caregiver.	Promotes the development of a trusting relationship.
• Provide a role model for effective communication by: ○ Seeking clarification ○ Demonstrating respect for individual family members and the family system ○ Listening to expression of thoughts and feelings ○ Setting clear limits ○ Being consistent	Family problem solving is improved when family members can effectively communicate with one another and the health care team.[12]
• Include caregiver in weekly treatment planning meetings with the client. Note here the time for this meeting and persons responsible for providing the information.	Assists in providing information to the caregiving system so that they can better cope with the uncertainty of a psychiatric diagnosis.[12,13]
• Spend (number) minutes (number) times per week educating the primary caregiver about the client's diagnosis. Provide both written and verbal information.	Provides caregiver with an increased understanding of the diagnosis and assists in the development of a home care plan. When anxiety is high, caregivers may have difficulty remembering information provided only in verbal form. Increases the stability in the living environment by decreasing caregiver's anxiety.
• Communicate understanding of the difficulty of the caregiver role by: ○ Answering questions honestly ○ Providing time to interact with the caregiver when he or she visits ○ Inquiring about the caregiver's self-care activities ○ Encouraging the caregiver to use the time the client is in the hospital to rest and meet personal needs ○ Providing time for the caregiver to express feelings related to the client and the hospitalization	Promotes the development of a trusting relationship and assists the caregiver in the process of working through feelings related to the client.

Continued

ACTIONS/INTERVENTIONS	RATIONALES
• Normalize caregiver's feelings of guilt and/or ambivalence by informing him or her that these are normal feelings for anyone who assumes the level of responsibility he or she has assumed.	Promotes a positive orientation and enhances self-esteem.
• Have caregiver identify areas where he or she feels a need for support on a daily basis, and assist him or her in networking community resources to meet these needs. This should be a process that allows the nurse to teach the caregiver the skills necessary to accomplish this networking on his or her own after discharge.	Promotes caregiver's sense of control and provides positive reinforcement when he or she can accomplish the task, which enhances self-esteem.
• Spend (number) minutes (number) times per week discussing his or her self-care activities. This could include planning time away from the client, inviting friends to visit, going for a walk, or arranging to get uninterrupted sleep. Inform the caregiver that if he or she does not care for himself or herself, he or she will eventually not have the energy to care for the client. A specific plan should be developed and noted here.	Gives permission to the caregiver to care for self. Promotes the caregiver's strengths.

• Before the client is discharged, meet with the client and caregiver to:
  ○ Review information about the diagnosis and hospital course.
  ○ Review special treatments the client is to receive.
  ○ Explain the client's medications.
  ○ Anticipate problems that may arise upon discharge.
• A specific plan should be developed for coping with anticipated problems. This plan should be written down and given to both the client and the caregiver.
	Anxiety can decrease an individual's ability to process information during hospitalization. A specific coping plan provides direction during times of crisis and prevents the reliance on ineffective patterns of coping. These actions increase the caregiver's repertoire of strategies to deal with the problems.[14]

Gerontic Health

ACTIONS/INTERVENTIONS	RATIONALES
• Monitor for signs of increasing strain in caregiver, such as an increase in episodes of illness.	The stresses of caregiving have a negative effect on the caregiver's immune system.[15]
• Assist caregiver in discussing feelings about caregiving. For example, encourage sharing by use of statements such as "Often people in your situation say they feel angry, helpless, guilty, or depressed."	Provides opportunity for ventilation of feelings about caregiving, which assists in reducing stress.
• Determine caregiver's knowledge of support services in the community such as adult daycare, respite services, or family support groups.	Assists in identifying actual or potential resources based on the individual's current knowledge of services. Expands options available to caregiver.
• Discuss with caregiver stress management techniques such as imagery, deep breathing, or exercise. What has been tried? How helpful was it?	
• Encourage caregiver to use a journal to evaluate stresses, prioritizing stresses and noting his or her usual response. Are there specific times, days, or circumstances when stress is especially high?	Provides database to use in planning interventions to reduce stress.
• If needed, consult with social services for increased support in home care.	
• Discuss with caregiver, prior to patient discharge, his or her plan for maintaining self-health and coping abilities.[16]	Highlights attention to caregiver. Realistic planning serves to reduce stress.

Home Health

> **NOTE:** See Psychiatric Health section for additional interventions.

ACTIONS/INTERVENTIONS	RATIONALES

• Monitor for factors contributing to caregiver role strain.
• Involve client and family in planning, implementing, and promoting reduction or elimination of caregiver role strain:
  ◦ Family conference: Clarify expected role performance of all family members. Discuss each member's perception of the situation.
  ◦ Mutual goal setting: Set short-term goals to relieve caregiver strain. Specify tasks and roles for each member.
  ◦ Communication: Use open, direct communication, and provide positive feedback.
• Assist client and family in lifestyle adjustments that may be required:
  ◦ Institutionalization of care receiver
  ◦ Respite for care provider
  ◦ Family relationships
  ◦ Treatment of physical or emotional disability in caregiver and care receiver
  ◦ Stress management
  ◦ Development and use of support networks
  ◦ Requirements for redistribution of family tasks
  ◦ Education and practice if special treatments are required
  ◦ Safe and supportive environment
• Consult with assistive resources as indicated.
	Provides database for early recognition and intervention. Family involvement enhances effectiveness of intervention.
	
	Long-term changes in behavior require support and education.
	
	Utilization of existing services is efficient use of resources. A psychiatric nurse clinician, family therapist, daycare or respite center, and support groups can enhance the treatment plan.

Caregiver Role Strain, Risk for and Actual

FLOWCHART EVALUATION: EXPECTED OUTCOME 1

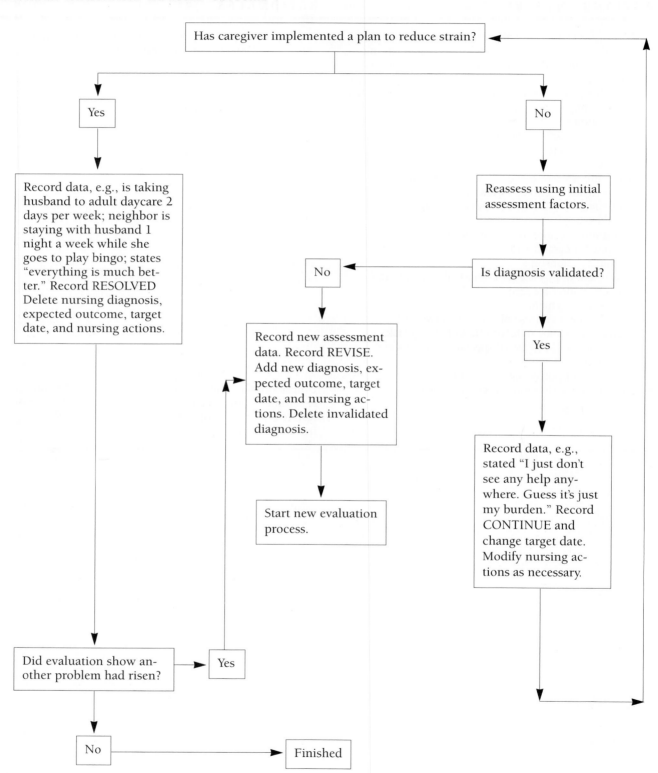

Has caregiver implemented a plan to reduce strain?

Yes

Record data, e.g., is taking husband to adult daycare 2 days per week; neighbor is staying with husband 1 night a week while she goes to play bingo; states "everything is much better." Record RESOLVED Delete nursing diagnosis, expected outcome, target date, and nursing actions.

Did evaluation show another problem had risen?

Yes

No

Finished

No

Record new assessment data. Record REVISE. Add new diagnosis, expected outcome, target date, and nursing actions. Delete invalidated diagnosis.

Start new evaluation process.

No

Reassess using initial assessment factors.

Is diagnosis validated?

Yes

Record data, e.g., stated "I just don't see any help anywhere. Guess it's just my burden." Record CONTINUE and change target date. Modify nursing actions as necessary.

Caregiver Role Strain, Risk for and Actual

FLOWCHART EVALUATION: EXPECTED OUTCOME 2

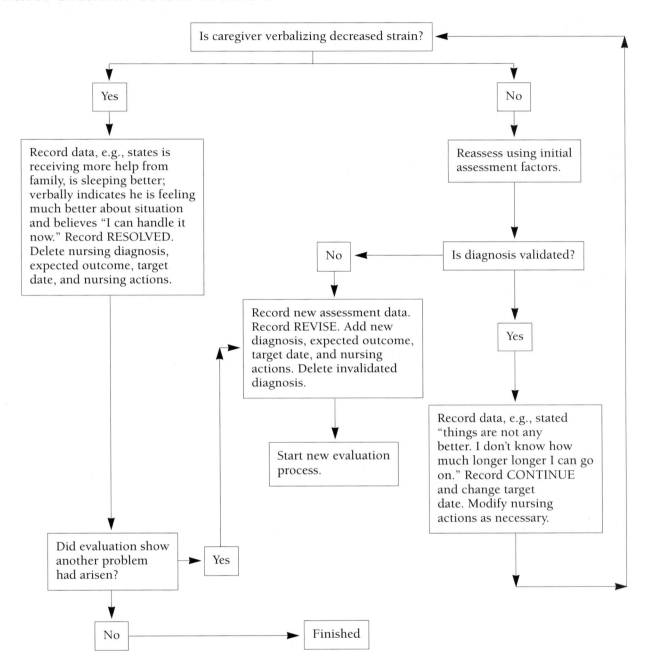

Is caregiver verbalizing decreased strain?

Yes

Record data, e.g., states is receiving more help from family, is sleeping better; verbally indicates he is feeling much better about situation and believes "I can handle it now." Record RESOLVED. Delete nursing diagnosis, expected outcome, target date, and nursing actions.

No

Reassess using initial assessment factors.

Is diagnosis validated?

No

Record new assessment data. Record REVISE. Add new diagnosis, expected outcome, target date, and nursing actions. Delete invalidated diagnosis.

Start new evaluation process.

Yes

Record data, e.g., stated "things are not any better. I don't know how much longer longer I can go on." Record CONTINUE and change target date. Modify nursing actions as necessary.

Did evaluation show another problem had arisen?

Yes

No

Finished

Family Processes, Altered, and Family Process, Altered, Alcoholism

DEFINITION

FAMILY PROCESS, ALTERED The state in which a family that normally functions effectively experiences a dysfunction.[8]

FAMILY PROCESS, ALTERED, ALCOHOLISM The state in which the psychosocial, spiritual, and physiologic functions of the family unit are chronically disorganized, leading to conflict, denial of problems, resistance to change, ineffective problem solving, and a series of self-perpetuating crises.[8]

NANDA TAXONOMY: RELATING 3.2.2 AND 3.2.2.3.1

DEFINING CHARACTERISTICS[8]

1. Family Processes, Altered
   a. Major defining characteristics
      (1) Family system unable to meet physical needs of its members
      (2) Family system unable to meet emotional needs of its members
      (3) Family system unable to meet spiritual needs of its members
      (4) Parents not demonstrating respect for each other's views on child-rearing practices
      (5) Inability to express or accept wide range of feelings
      (6) Inability to express or accept feelings of members
      (7) Family unable to meet security needs of its members
      (8) Inability of the family members to relate to each other for mutual growth and maturation
      (9) Family uninvolved in community activities
      (10) Inability to accept or receive help appropriately
      (11) Rigidity in function and roles
      (12) Family not demonstrating respect for individuality and autonomy of its members
      (13) Family unable to adapt to change or deal with traumatic experience constructively
      (14) Family failing to accomplish current or past developmental task
      (15) Unhealthy family decision-making process
      (16) Failure to send and receive clear messages
      (17) Inappropriate boundary maintenance
      (18) Inappropriate or poorly communicated family rules, rituals, or symbols
      (19) Unexamined family myths
      (20) Inappropriate level and direction of energy
   b. Minor defining characteristics
      None given
2. Family Processes, Altered, Alcoholism
   a. Major defining characteristics
      (1) Feelings:
         (a) Decreased self-esteem, or feelings of worthlessness
         (b) Anger or suppressed rage
         (c) Frustration
         (d) Powerlessness
         (e) Anxiety, tension, or distress
         (f) Insecurity
         (g) Repressed emotions
         (h) Feelings of responsibility for alcoholic's behavior
         (i) Lingering resentment
         (j) Shame or embarrassment
         (k) Hurt
         (l) Unhappiness
         (m) Guilt
         (n) Emotional isolation or loneliness
         (o) Vulnerability
         (p) Mistrust
         (q) Hopelessness
         (r) Rejection
      (2) Roles and relationships:
         (a) Deterioration in family relationships or disturbed family dynamics
         (b) Ineffective spouse communication or marital problems
         (c) Altered role function or disruption of family roles
         (d) Inconsistent parenting or low perception of parental support
         (e) Family denial
         (f) Intimacy dysfunction
         (g) Chronic family problems
         (h) Closed communication systems
      (3) Behaviors:
         (a) Anger expressed inappropriately
         (b) Difficulty with intimate relationships
         (c) Loss of control of drinking
         (d) Impaired communication
         (e) Ineffective problem-solving skills
         (f) Enabling to maintain drinking
         (g) Inability to meet emotional needs of family members
         (h) Manipulation
         (i) Dependency
         (j) Criticizing
         (k) Alcohol abuse
         (l) Broken promises
         (m) Rationalization or denial of problems
         (n) Refusal to get help or inability to accept and receive help appropriately
         (o) Blaming
         (p) Inadequate understanding or knowledge of alcoholism
   b. Minor defining characteristics
      (1) Feelings:
         (a) Being different from other people
         (b) Depression
         (c) Hostility
         (d) Fear
         (e) Emotional control by others
         (f) Confusion
         (g) Dissatisfaction
         (h) Loss
         (i) Misunderstood
         (j) Abandonment
         (k) Confused love and pity
         (l) Moodiness
         (m) Failure
         (n) Being unloved
         (o) Lack of identity
      (2) Roles and relationships:

(a) Triangulating family relationships
(b) Reduced ability of family members to relate to each other for mutual growth and maturation
(c) Lack of skills necessary for relationships
(d) Lack of cohesiveness
(e) Disrupted family rituals
(f) Family unable to meet security need of its members
(g) Family not demonstrating respect for individuality and autonomy of its members, or pattern of rejection
(h) Economic problems
(i) Neglect of family members' basic needs

(3) Behaviors:
(a) Inability to meet spiritual needs of its members
(b) Inability to express or accept wide range of feelings
(c) Orientation toward tension relief rather than achievement of goals
(d) Family special occasions are alcohol centered
(e) Escalating conflict
(f) Lying
(g) Contradictory, paradoxical communication
(h) Lack of dealing with conflict
(i) Harsh self-judgment
(j) Isolation
(k) Nicotine addiction
(l) Difficulty having fun
(m) Self-blaming
(n) Unresolved grief
(o) Controlling of communication or power struggles
(p) Inability to adapt to change
(q) Immaturity
(r) Stress-related physical illness
(s) Inability to deal with traumatic experiences
constructively
(t) Seeking approval and affirmation
(u) Lack of reliability
(v) Disturbances in academic performance in children
(w) Disturbances in concentration
(x) Chaos
(y) Substance abuse other than alcohol
(z) Failure to accomplish current or past developmental tasks or difficulty with life cycle transitions
(aa) Verbal abuse of spouse or parent
(bb) Agitation
(cc) Diminished physical contact

RELATED FACTORS[8]

1. Family Processes, Altered
   a. Situation transition and/or crisis
   b. Developmental transition and/or crisis
2. Family Processes, Altered, Alcoholism:
   a. Abuse of alcohol
   b. Family history of alcoholism or resistance to treatment
   c. Inadequate coping skills
   d. Genetic predisposition
   e. Addictive personality
   f. Lack of problem-solving skills
   g. Biochemical influences

RELATED CLINICAL CONCERNS

1. Surgery
2. Trauma
3. Mental retardation
4. Chronic illness
5. Alcoholism
6. Chemical abuse

HAVE YOU SELECTED THE CORRECT DIAGNOSIS?

Ineffective Family Coping   This diagnosis has a history of destructive patterns of behavior. For the diagnosis of Altered Family Processes to be applicable, there would be evidence that the usual adequacy in coping is altered in relation to a specific crisis.

EXPECTED OUTCOMES

1. Will verbalize increased satisfaction with family interactional pattern by (date) and/or
2. Will describe specific plan to cope with (specific stressor) by (date)

TARGET DATES

Five to 7 days would be the earliest acceptable target date. Even after the expected outcome has initially been met, there may be other precipitating events that will again alter family processes; therefore, a long-term date should be designated.

NURSING ACTIONS/INTERVENTIONS WITH RATIONALES

Adult Health

ACTIONS/INTERVENTIONS	RATIONALES
• Monitor interaction styles, communication patterns, and role behaviors in the family.[17]	Baseline information about family dynamics can assist the nurse with planning and developing family interventions. Provides comfort and aids in crisis resolution.
• Promote a trusting therapeutic relationship during interaction with patient and family by being empathetic, actively listening, accepting feelings and attitudes, and being nonjudgmental.	
• Promote open, honest communications among the family members by facilitating group interaction. Encourage the patient and family to express feelings regarding current family process by spending (specific time) each shift, while awake, for this purpose.	Promotes verbalization of feelings and shared understanding of problems. Assists the family to acknowledge and accept the problem. Promotes a common definition of the problem and assists in identifying ways to cope with the problem.
• Determine the family's level of recognition of problems within the family unit associated with patient's alcoholism.	Level of recognition may serve as an indicator of family's acceptance or denial of problems.
• Allow the family to grieve by providing time, giving permission, and referring them to clergy and/or a bereavement group.	Assists in crisis intervention and provides extra coping mechanisms.
• Support efforts of the family to deal with previously identified problems within the family unit associated with patient's alcoholism.	Family may already be involved in therapy for previously identified family unit problems. Hospitalization can cause regression and/or intensification of problems.
• Monitor readiness to learn; then teach family about the precipitating situation, its implications, and the expected response to treatment.	Provides knowledge base to assist in problem solving. Decreases anxiety.
• Allow family members to participate in patient care as possible.	
• Help the family to identify its strengths and weaknesses in dealing with the situation during family conference.	Identifies existing resources for crisis resolution and areas to strengthen. Provides positive feedback for strengths that already exist.
• Help family organize to continue usual family activities.	Decreases sense of overwhelming loss of everything. Adds stability to activities.
• Refer family to a health professional or organization specializing in substance abuse.	If family is not already involved in therapy, it is essential to provide resources for treatment or rehabilitation following discharge from the hospital. Provides long-term support and effective use of already available resources.
• See Psychiatric Health nursing actions for more detailed interventions.	Collaboration promotes more holistic care; many need specific interventions by a specialist.

Child Health

NOTE: Depending on the age of the infant or child, there may be a range of possible needs represented in the context of the family—all interventions should be developmentally appropriate. Include all children in family counseling as applicable.

ACTIONS/INTERVENTIONS	RATIONALES
• Promote sibling participation in patient's hospitalization and plans for discharge, e.g., allowing visitation during game time.	Inclusion of sibling(s) fosters a sense of family concern, and the need for support is met for all involved. Undue prolonged separations increase stress for the sibling(s) and family relationships.
• Provide for cultural preferences when possible, including diet, religious needs, and plans for health care.	Attention to preferences demonstrates valuing and sensitivity for the family.

• Provide reinforcement to appropriately value caretaking behavior.	Reinforcement of desired behaviors serves to offer positive learning with increased likelihood of compliance.
• Advocate on infant's or child's behalf to best offer management of alcohol or substance abuse impact on current or future development.	Infant, child, or adolescent may be unable to look after self-interests, and when this is so, it is legally and morally mandated that the client have an advocate.
• Determine child's or adolescent's feelings of family per ventilation about same for 30 min each shift.	Ventilation assists in anxiety reduction and values input of all individual family members. Also, data may be known for best treatment.

Women's Health

ACTIONS/INTERVENTIONS	RATIONALES
NEW PARENTS	
• Assist patient and significant others in establishing realistic goals related to changes in role due to newborn, e.g., sharing of tasks or parenting skills.	Assist family with role changes during a normal, but often unexpected, amount of role change event. Provides basis for planning necessary changes.
• Provide positive reinforcement for parenting tasks.	Provides motivation and enhances likelihood of effective parenting.
• Assist parents in identifying infant behavior patterns and understanding how they allow the infant to communicate with them, e.g., crying or fussing.	Assists in reducing stress and promotes positive parenting.
• Assist patient in verbalizing her perceptions of the infant's growth and development, individual and family needs, and the stresses of being a new parent.	Provides database that allows more effective teaching and planning for effective parenting.
• Identify support groups, e.g., formal groups such as Mother's Day Out, and informal groups such as parenting groups, family, or friends.	Promotes planning and allows early intervention for potential stress areas.
• Encourage open communication between mother and father on household tasks, discipline, fears, and anxieties, e.g., less-than-perfect baby.	
• Help develop a plan for sharing household tasks and child caretaking activities: ○ Bathing ○ Feeding ○ Care of siblings ○ Quality time with older children	Reduces stress-provoking events.
• Allow older children to assist with newborn care (even the smallest child can do this with parental supervision); ○ Bringing a diaper to parent ○ Pushing baby in stroller ○ Holding baby (while sitting on couch is best)	
• Follow up with home visits after discharge from hospital to physically monitor the infant, monitor family interactions, provide support, and provide referrals to the proper agencies.	Provides long-term support.
• Teach and reinforce methods of caring for and coping with the emotional and physiologic needs of the infant, siblings, parents, and other relatives such as grandparents.	Provides measures and preplanning to cope with potential stressful events.
PARENT TO YOUR PARENTS	
• Assist client and family to establish realistic goals related to increasing responsibilities in caring for elderly parents, e.g., sharing of tasks, time, and resources (financial and emotional).	
• Assist in identifying resources in the community: ○ Daycare for the elderly ○ Church groups	

Continued

ACTIONS/INTERVENTIONS	RATIONALES

- ○ YWCAs
- ○ Professional help in the home, such as home health aides
- Assist in exploring and identifying need for care of elderly parent outside of home, e.g., assisted living or skilled nursing care.

ALCOHOLISM

Diagnosis under Adult Mental Health will apply here, except for the following:

PERINATAL

- Check your state's laws. Because of the widespread drug use in this country, some states have mandatory screening for drug use during the perinatal period.[18,19]
- Screen clients for chemical use during pregnancy by means of interview at first visit. Provide a relaxed, secure atmosphere for the client when trying to obtain a substance-abuse history. Include the following in your questions:
  - ○ Use of nonprescription drugs
  - ○ Use of coffee
  - ○ Use of cigarettes
  - ○ Use of alcohol
  - ○ Use of prescription drugs
  - ○ Use of recreational drug use, such as marijuana
  - ○ Use of multiple drugs
  - ○ Problems encountered in trying to abstain from drug use
- Assure client of acceptance for her and her family but not for self-destructive behaviors.[20]
- Support and praise the client for health-seeking behaviors.[20]
- Thoroughly assess the woman and fetus who present with complications related to substance abuse in order to provide the best physiologic support for her and her fetal well-being.
- Obtain sample for toxicology screening:
  - ○ Maternal or neonatal urine toxicology screen
  - ○ Meconium and maternal or neonatal hair samples

Because of slow growth of hair and meconium produced by the second trimester, these methods provide the best analysis of long-term data on drug use.[20]

- Collaborate with physician to provide appropriate pain control during labor.
- Notify neonatal personnel of patient's labor and history of substance abuse.
- Support and guide maternal-infant interactions in order to encourage maternal-infant attachment.

Women with narcotic dependency problems have a high tolerance to analgesics and usually have a low pain threshold.[20]

For the addicted infant, see Child Health.

Psychiatric Health

ACTIONS/INTERVENTIONS	RATIONALES

• Provide a role model for effective communication by:
  ○ Seeking clarification
  ○ Demonstrating respect for individual family members and the family system
  ○ Listening to expression of thoughts and feelings
  ○ Setting clear limits
  ○ Being consistent
  ○ Communicating with the individual being addressed in a clear manner
  ○ Encouraging sharing of information among appropriate system subgroups
	Communication skills provide a framework for effective problem solving.

• Demonstrate an understanding of the complexity of system problems by:
  ○ Not taking side in family disagreements
  ○ Providing alternative explanations of behavior that recognize the contributions of all persons involved with the problem, including health care providers as appropriate
  ○ Requesting the perspective of multiple family members on a problem or stressor
	Outcome improves when psychosocial problems are treated from a systems perspective.[21]

• Include all family members in the first interview.	Provides opportunity to assess all family members' perception of the problem and in identification of problem-solving strategies that are acceptable to more family members.
• Have each member provide his or her perspective to the current difficulties.	Assist the family in defining a problem that can be resolved. For example, rather than defining the problem as "We don't love each other anymore," the problem can be defined as "We do not spend time together in family activities." This definition evolves from the family's description of what they mean by the more general problem description.

• Assist family in developing behavioral short-term goals by:
  ○ Asking what they would see happening in the family if the situation improved
  ○ Having them break the problem into several parts that combine to form the identified stressor
  ○ Asking them what they could do in a week to improve the situation (should include a response from each family member)
	Setting achievable goals increases the opportunities for success, which increases the motivation to continue to work toward problem resolution.

• Maintain the nurse's role of facilitator of family communication by:
  ○ Having family members discuss possible solutions among themselves
  ○ Having each family member talk about how he or she might contribute to both the problem and the problem's resolution
	Maintains a context that enhances and supports the family's problem-solving skills.

• Provide the family with the information necessary for appropriate problem solving.	
• Answer all questions in a open, direct manner.	Promotes a trusting relationship.

• Support the expression of affect by:
  ○ Having family members share feelings with one another
  ○ Normalizing the expression of emotion—e.g., "Most persons experience anger after they have experienced a loss."
  ○ Providing a private environment for this expression
	Promotes communication among family members while developing a positive expectational set.

Continued

ACTIONS/INTERVENTIONS	RATIONALES
• Maintain and support functional family role—e.g., allow parents private time alone, allow children to visit parents, and encourage the presenting of problems to the "family leader."	Provides positive reinforcement for functional interactions and serves to encourage this behavior while enhancing self-esteem.
• Schedule a time with the family to discuss how the current situation affects family roles and possible changes that may be necessary.	
• Have family identify those systems in the community that could support them during this time, and assist family in contacting these systems. Note here the systems to be contacted as well as how they will assist the family.	Promotes and develops family's strengths.
• Provide positive verbal reinforcement for the family's accomplishments.	Positive reinforcement encourages behavior and enhances self-esteem.
• Assist family in identifying patterns of interaction that interfere with successful problem resolution—e.g., the husband frequently asks his wife closed-ended questions, which discourages her from sharing her ideas; the children interrupt the patents when their level of conflict increases to a certain level; or the wife walks out of the room when the husband brings up issues related to finances.	Facilitates the development of more appropriate coping behaviors.
• Assist family in planning fun activities together. This could include time to play together, exercise together, or engage in a shared project.	Families in crisis often limit their emotional experience.
• Teach family methods of anxiety reduction, and establish a practice schedule and a schedule for discussing how this method could be used on a daily basis in the family. The selected method along with the schedule for discussion and practice should be listed here.	Relaxation response inhibits the activation of the autonomic nervous system's fight-or-flight response. Repeated practice of a behavior internalizes and personalizes the behavior.
• Include family in discussions related to planning care and sharing information about the client's condition.	Support system involvement in problem solving increases the opportunities for a more positive outcome.
• Assist family in developing a specific plan when the client is scheduled for a pass or discharge. Note that plan here with the assistance needed from the nursing staff for implementation.	Promotes client's sense of control. Planned coping strategies facilitate the enactment of new behaviors when stress is experienced. This increases the opportunities for successful coping and enhances self-esteem.

ALCOHOL

• Promote a trusting therapeutic relationship during interaction with client and family by being empathetic, listening actively, accepting feelings and attitudes, and being nonjudgmental.	Provides comfort and aids in the development of a context that supports expressions of emotions and risking change.[22]
• Establish a therapeutic relationship with whatever part of the family system initiates treatment.	Working with the nonalcoholic spouse and family members can facilitate the entry of the alcoholic family member into treatment.[23]
• Promote open, honest communications among the family members by facilitating group interaction. Promote the expression of feelings regarding current family process by spending (specific time) each shift, while awake, for this purpose.	Promotes verbalization of feelings and shared understanding of problems. Assists the family to acknowledge and accept the problem. Promotes a common definition of the problem and assists in identifying ways to cope.

• Schedule family for psychoeducational groups that explore basic information, family responses to alcoholism, family roles in intervention, and codependence. Included topics should be
  ○ Basic disease concepts
  ○ Family control behaviors
  ○ Anger
  ○ Threats
	Family involvement in early treatment improves outcome.[23]

- ○ Covering up for alcoholic or enabling
- ○ Personal responsibility
- ○ Self-care
- ○ Healthy communication
- Provide a role model for effective communication by:
  - ○ Seeking clarification
  - ○ Demonstrating respect for individual family members and the family system
  - ○ Listening to expression of thoughts and feelings
  - ○ Setting clear limits
  - ○ Being consistent
  - ○ Communicating clearly with the individual being addressed
- Demonstrate an understanding for the complexity of system problems by:
  - ○ Not taking sides in family disagreements
  - ○ Providing alternative explanations of behavior that recognize the contributions of all persons involved with the problem
  - ○ Requesting the perspective of multiple family members on a problem or stressor
- Assist family in defining a problem that can be resolved. For example, rather than defining the problem as "I want him to be more responsible around the house," try "I would like him to take responsibility for paying the bills by the first of the month."
- Assist the family in developing behavioral short-term goals by:
  - ○ Asking what they would see happening in the family if the situation improved
  - ○ Having them break the problem into several parts that can bring to fore the identified stressor
  - ○ Asking them what they could do in a week to improve the situation
- Maintain the nurse's role of facilitator of family communication by:
  - ○ Having family members discuss possible solutions among themselves
  - ○ Having each family member take responsibility for their own actions and not accept responsibility for others
- Support the expression of affect:
  - ○ Have family members share feelings with one another.
  - ○ Normalize the expressions of emotion—for example, "Most families experience anger as part of the recovery process."
  - ○ Provide a private environment for this expression.
- Schedule time with the family to discuss how the current situation affects family roles and possible changes that may be necessary. Note that schedule here with responsible person.
- Maintain and support functional family roles; for example, allow parents private time alone or allow children to visit parents.
- Have family identify those systems in the community that could support them in recovery, and assist them in contacting these systems (AA, Al-Anon, Al-Ateen). Note here the systems to be contacted and person responsible for this activity.
- Provide positive verbal reinforcement for family's accomplishments.

Communication skills provide a framework for effective problem solving.

Outcome improves when family communication problems are addressed.[23]

Setting achievable goals increases the opportunities for success, which increases the motivation to continue to work toward problem resolution.

Maintains a context that enhances and supports the family's problem-solving skills.

Expression of affect is one of the most difficult areas for these families. Promotes learning positive ways of communicating among family members while developing a positive expectational set.[24]

Provides positive reinforcement for functional interactions and serves to encourage this behavior while enhancing self-esteem.
Promotes and develops family's strengths and provides support systems for behavior changes.

Positive reinforcement encourages behavior and enhances self-esteem.

Continued

ACTIONS/INTERVENTIONS	RATIONALES
• Assist family in planning fun activities together. This could include time to play together, exercise together, or engage in a shared project.	Families in crisis often limit emotional experiences.
• Teach family methods of anxiety reduction. Establish a practice schedule and a schedule for discussing how this method could be used on a daily basis in the family. The selected method along with the schedule for discussion and practice should be listed here.	Relaxation response inhibits the activation of the autonomic nervous system's fight-or-flight response. Repeated practice of a behavior internalizes and personalizes the behavior.
• Assist family in developing a specific plan when the client is scheduled for a pass or discharge. Note that plan here, including the assistance needed from the nursing staff for implementation.	Promotes client's sense of control. Planned coping strategies facilitate the enactment of new behaviors when stress is experienced. This increases the opportunities for successful coping and enhances self-esteem.

Gerontic Health

The nursing actions for the gerontic patient with this diagnosis would be the same as those given for Adult Health and Psychiatric Health. The prevalence of alcoholism in older adults is reportedly lower than the general population; however, this may be due to the lack of age-specific screening instruments.[25] In older adults, there may be late-onset alcoholism due to an increase in the stresses associated with aging. Such things as the loss of a spouse, changes in health, and retirement may precipitate alcohol abuse.[26] Some researchers advocate programs that are connected to aging service programs, such as senior programs, to assist the older alcoholic and his or her family in dealing with aging issues as well as alcoholism.[27]

Home Health

NOTE: See Psychiatric Health nursing actions for detailed psychosocial interventions.

ACTIONS/INTERVENTIONS	RATIONALES

• Teach client and family appropriate information regarding the care of family members:
  ○ Discipline strategies appropriate for developmental level
  ○ Normal growth and development
  ○ Expected family life cycles, e.g., child rearing or grandparenting
  ○ Coping strategies for family growth
  ○ Care of health deviations
  ○ Developing and using support networks
  ○ Safe environment for family members
  ○ Anticipatory guidance regarding growth and development, discipline, family functioning, responses to illness, role changes, etc.
	Basic knowledge that contributes to successful family functioning.

• Involve client and family in planning and implementing strategies to decrease or prevent alterations in family process:
  ○ Family conference to ascertain perspective of members on current situation and to identify strategies to improve situation
  ○ Mutual goal setting to identify realistic goals with evaluation criteria and specific activities for each family member
  ○ Encourage clear, consistent, and honest communication with positive feedback
  ○ Distribution of family tasks so that all members are involved in maintaining family based on developmental capacity
	Family involvement enhances effectiveness of intervention.

- Assist client and family in lifestyle adjustments that may be required:
  - Separation or divorce
  - Temporary stay in community shelter
  - Family therapy
  - Communication of feelings
  - Stress reduction
  - Identification of potential for violence
  - Providing safe environment
  - Therapeutic use of anger
  - Seeking and providing support for family members
  - Coping with catastrophic or chronic illness
  - Requirements for redistributing family tasks
  - Changing role functions and relationships
  - Financial concerns

Permanent changes in behavior and family roles require support.

- Consult with or refer to assistive resources as required.

Utilization of existing services is efficient use of resources. Support groups, psychiatric nurse clinicians, and teachers can enhance the treatment plan.

Family Process, Altered, and Family Process, Altered, Alcoholism

FLOWCHART EVALUATION: EXPECTED OUTCOME 1

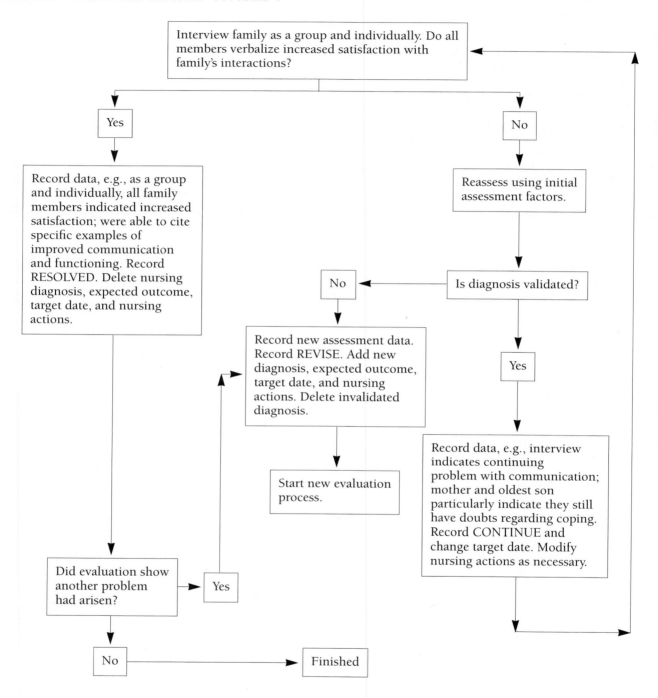

Family Process, Altered, and Family Process, Altered, Alcoholism

FLOWCHART EVALUATION: EXPECTED OUTCOME 2

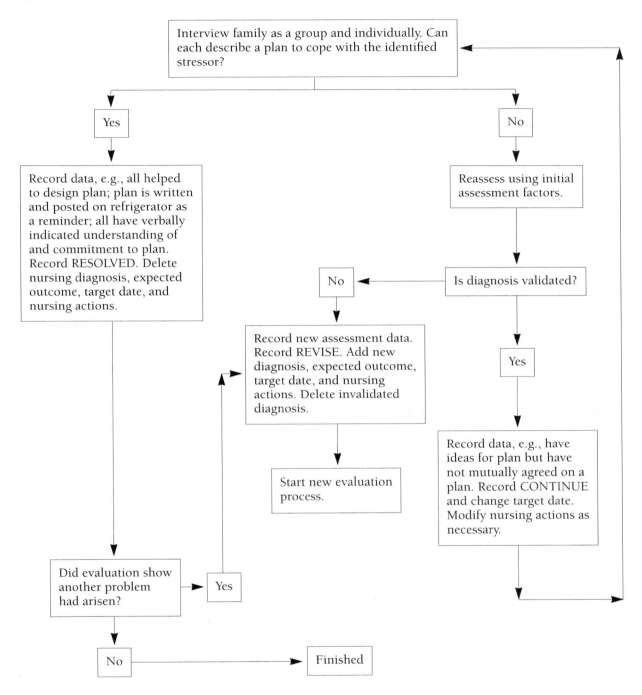

Grieving, Anticipatory

DEFINITION[8]

Intellectual and emotional responses and behaviors by which individuals (families or communities) work through the process of modifying self-concept based on the perception of potential loss.

NANDA TAXONOMY: FEELING 9.2.1.2

DEFINING CHARACTERISTICS[8]

1. Major defining characteristics
   a. Potential loss of significant object
   b. Expression of distress at potential loss
   c. Denial of potential loss
   d. Denial of the significance of the loss
   e. Guilt
   f. Anger
   g. Sorrow
   h. Bargaining
   i. Alteration in:
      (1) Eating habits
      (2) Sleep patterns
      (3) Dream patterns
      (4) Activity level
      (5) Libido
   j. Altered communication patterns
   k. Difficulty taking on new or different roles
   l. Resolution of grief prior to the reality of loss
2. Minor defining characteristics
   None given

RELATED FACTORS[8]

To be developed

RELATED CLINICAL CONCERNS

1. Cancer
2. Amputation
3. Spinal cord injury
4. Birth defects
5. Any diagnosis that family has been told has a terminal prognosis

HAVE YOU SELECTED THE CORRECT DIAGNOSIS?

Sensory-Perceptual Alteration This diagnosis will be identified according to the patient's change in capacity to exercise judgment or think critically with appropriate sensory-perceptual functioning. This may well be related to Anticipatory Grieving.

Anxiety or Fear Anxiety is the response the individual has to a threat that is for the most part unidentified. Fear is the response made by an individual to an identified threat. When the patient is faced with the thought of death, loss of a limb, loss of functioning, loss of a loved one, and so on, Anxiety and Fear may arise as parallel diagnoses with Anticipatory Grieving.

Ineffective Individual Coping This is the appropriate diagnosis if the individual is not making the necessary adaptations to deal with the threatened loss. This diagnosis can be a companion diagnosis to Anticipatory Grieving.

Spiritual Distress When faced with a devastating loss, the client may well express Spiritual Distress. This quite often is a companion diagnosis to Anticipatory Grieving.

EXPECTED OUTCOMES

1. Will verbalize feelings about impending loss by (date) and/or
2. Will identify at least two support systems by (date)

TARGET DATES

A target date ranging from 2 to 4 days would be appropriate in evaluating progress toward achievement of the expected outcome.

NURSING ACTIONS/INTERVENTIONS WITH RATIONALES

Adult Health

For this diagnosis, the Psychiatric Health nursing actions serve as the generic actions. Please see those actions.

Child Health

ACTIONS/INTERVENTIONS	RATIONALES

• Spend at least 30 min every 8 h (or as situation dictates) to address specific anticipated loss by:
  ○ Encouraging patient and family to express perception of current situation (may be facilitated by age and developmentally appropriate intervention such as drawing, play or puppet therapy)
  ○ Providing active listening in a quiet, private environment
  ○ Offering clarification of procedures, treatment, or plans for patient and family
  ○ Revising plan of care to honor preferences when possible
  ○ Discussing and identifying impact of anticipated loss
	A structured discussion places value on the importance of grieving and provides critical data for the plan of care.

• Collaborate with appropriate health care professional members to meet needs of patient and family in realistically anticipating loss.
 	
• Encourage patient and family to realistically develop coping strategies to best prepare for anticipated loss through:
  ○ Engaging in diversional activities of choice
  ○ Reminiscing of times spent with loved one or associated with anticipated loss
  ○ Identification of support groups
	Appropriate collaboration and the coordination of efforts result in holistic versus fragmented care at a time of special need. A sense of support remains long after the event itself.
	Fostering coping strategies provides an opportunity for growth with minimal support from others, thereby increasing empowerment for the family.

• Encourage optimal function for as long as possible with identification of need for proper attention to rest, diet, and health of all family members at this time of stress.
• Promote parental and sibling participation in care of infant or child according to situation:
  ○ Feedings and selection of menu
  ○ Comfort measures such as holding child or giving backrubs
  ○ Diversional activities, quiet games, or stories
  ○ Decisions regarding life-support measures and resuscitation
	Participation in usual daily activities provides a sense of normalcy despite impending loss and provides validation of life.
	Maintenance of family input and participation in care offer continuation of the family unit at a time when unity can serve to positively influence daily coping for all.

• Reassure infant or child that he or she is loved and cared for with ample opportunities to answer questions regarding specific anticipated loss whether related to self or others. According to age and developmental status, provide reassurance that cause for situation is not patient's own doing.	Reassurance lessens the likelihood of guilt while demonstrating that there is no need for assignment of blame to any member of the family.
• Remember that hearing is one of the last of the senses to remain functional. Exercise opportunities for loved ones and staff to continue to address patient even though patient may be unable to answer or respond.	Speaking can serve to reassure child of worth; urge caution in conversations that indicate child cannot hear.
• Provide for appropriate safety and maintenance related to physiologic care of patient.	Standard practice requires safety maintenance. Special attention is required when the infant or child is comatose or cannot respond regarding sensations, especially for pressure areas, heat, or cold.

Women's Health

ACTIONS/INTERVENTIONS	RATIONALES
• Obtain a thorough obstetric history, including previous occurrences of fetal demise.	Provides essential database needed to plan for effective interventions.
• Ascertain if there were any problems conceiving this pregnancy or any attempts to terminate this pregnancy.	
• Assess and record mother's perception of cessation of fetal movements.	
• Monitor and record fetal activity or lack of activity.	
• Inform mother and significant others of antepartal testing and why it is being ordered, and explain results:	
○ Nonstress testing	
○ Oxytocin (Pitocin) challenge test	
○ Ultrasound	
• Be considerate and honest in keeping patient and significant other(s) informed. Share information as soon as it becomes available.	Promotes trusting relationship and provides support during a very difficult time.
• Allow mother and family to express feelings and begin grieving process.	Provides support and care to patient and family, who are unable to begin real grieving because death is not yet real to them while they are going through a "normal" birthing process.
• With collaboration of physician, facilitate necessary laboratory tests and procedures, e.g., blood tests such as CBC, type, and crossmatch, DIC screening and coagulation studies, real time or ultrasound, or amniotomy.	
• Provide emotional support for the couple during labor and birth process.	
• Closely monitor physiologic process of labor.	
• Explain the procedure of induction of labor and the use of Pitocin, IVs, and the uterine contraction pattern.	In instances where fetal death has been ascertained, labor is induced to prevent further complications.
• Watch for nausea, vomiting, and diarrhea.	
• Provide comfort measures: analgesics, tranquilizers, and medications for side effects or prostaglandins as ordered.	
• Change patient's position at least every 2 h on the (odd/even) hour.	
• Observe for full bladder. Record intake and output every 8 h.	
• Provide ice chips for dry mouth and lip balm or petroleum jelly for dry lips.	
• Monitor vital signs every 2–4 h at (times).	
• Utilize breathing and relaxation techniques with patient for comfort.	
• Inform physician of mother's wishes for use of anesthetic for birth, e.g., awake and aware, sedated, or asleep.	
• Prepare infant for viewing by mother and significant others:	Initiates the grieving process in a supportive environment. Demonstrates respect for and understanding of the family's emotional state.
○ Clean infant as much as possible.	
○ Use clothing to hide gross defects, such as hat for head defects and a T-shirt or diapers for trunk defects.	
○ Wrap in soft, clean baby blanket (allow mother to unwrap infant if she desires).	
• Provide private, quiet place and time for parents and family to:	Provides essential support for family during time of grief. Provides reality by letting parents hold infant.
○ See and hold infant	
○ Take pictures	
• Provide a certificate with footprints, handprints, lock of hair, armbands, date and time of birth, weight of infant, and name of infant.	

- Contact religious or cultural leader as requested by mother or significant other. Provide for religious practices such as baptism.
- Provide references to supportive groups within community, such as Resolve with Sharing or Parents of Miscarried Children.
- Explain need for autopsy or genetic testing of infant.
- In instances of infertility, assist in realistic planning for future:
  - Possible extensive testing
  - Fear
  - Economics
  - Uncertainty
  - Embarrassment
  - Surgical procedures
  - Feelings of inadequacy
  - Life without children
  - Adoption

Provides database that can be used in assisting couple to cope with situation and initiate realistic planning for the future.

Psychiatric Health

NOTE: It may take clients anywhere from 6 months to a year to grieve a loss. This should be taken into consideration when developing evaluation dates. In a short-stay hospitalization, a reasonable set of goals would be to assist the client system in beginning a healthy grieving process. It is also important to note the anniversary date since grief reaction can be experienced past the 1-year period noted here.

ACTIONS/INTERVENTIONS	RATIONALES
• Assign client a primary care nurse and inform client of this decision. This nurse must have a degree of comfort in discussing issues related to loss and grief.	Promotes the development of a trusting relationship.
• Primary nurse will spend 30 min once a shift with client discussing his or her perceptions of the current situation. These discussions could include: ◦ His or her perceptions of the loss ◦ His or her values or beliefs about the lost "object" ◦ Client's past experiences with loss and how these were resolved ◦ Client's perceptions of the support system and possible support system responses to the loss	Promotes the development of a trusting relationship and provides a supportive environment for the expression of feelings, which facilitates a healthy resolution of the loss.
• Primary nurse will schedule 30-min interactions with client and support system to assist them in discussing issues related to the loss and answering any question they might have (note time and date of this interaction here).	
• Primary nurse will discuss with client and family role adjustments and other anticipated changes related to the loss.	Anticipatory planning facilitates adaptation.
• If necessary after the first interaction, primary nurse will schedule follow-up visits with the client and his or her support system (note schedule for these interactions here).	

Continued

ACTIONS/INTERVENTIONS	**RATIONALES**
• Spend (number) minutes (this should begin as 5-min times and can increase to 10 min as client needs and unit staffing permits) with client each hour. If client does not desire to talk during this time, the time can be used to give a massage (backrub) or sit with client in silence. Inform client of these times, and let him or her know if for some reason this schedule has to be altered and develop a new time for the visit. Inform client that the purpose of this time is for him or her to use as he or she sees fit. The nurse should be seated during this time if he or she is not providing a massage.	Promotes the development of a trusting relationship and client's sense of control.
• Provide positive verbal and nonverbal reinforcement to expressions of grief from both the client and the support system. This would include remaining with the client when he or she is expressing strong emotions.	Positive reinforcement encourages the behavior and enhances self-esteem.
• Once the client and the support system are discussing the loss, assist them in scheduling time when they can be alone with the client.	Facilitates healthy resolution of the loss.
• Answer questions in an open, honest manner.	Promotes the development of a trusting relationship and promotes the client's sense of control.

• If the client expresses anger toward the staff and this anger appears to be unrelated to the situation, accept it as part of the grieving process and support the client in its expression by:
  ○ Not responding in a defensive manner
  ○ Recognizing the feelings that are being expressed—e.g., "It sounds like you are very angry right now," or "It can be very frustrating to be in a situation where you feel you have little control."
	Expression of anger is a normal part of the grieving process and it is "safer" to be angry with members of the health care team than with the family.

• Recognize that the stages of grief can progress at individual rates and in various patterns. Do not "force" a client through stages or express expectations about what the "normal" next step should be.	Supports the client's perception of control and strengths.
• If the client is in denial related to the loss, allow this to happen and provide client with information about the loss at the client's pace. If client does not remember information given before, simply provide the information again.	Serves as a way of client's protecting self from information he or she is not ready to cope with. As coping behaviors are strengthened, the client will be able to accept and respond to this information.
• Allow client and support system to participate in decisions related to nursing care. Those areas in which client decision making is to be encouraged should be noted here along with the client's decisions.	Promotes the client's sense of control and enhances his or her strengths.
• Normalize client's and support system's experience of grief by telling client that his or her experience is normal and by discussing with him or her potential future responses to loss.	Promotes the client's sense of control and promotes a positive orientation that enhances self-esteem.
• Recognize that this is an emotionally painful time for the client and the support system, and share this understanding with the client system.	Encourages expression of feelings and facilitates progression through the grieving process.
• Assist client in obtaining the spiritual support needed.	
• Monitor the use of sedatives and tranquilizers. Consult with the physician if overuse is suspected.	Extensive use of these medications may delay the grieving process.
• Monitor the client system's use of alcohol and nonprescription drugs as a coping method. Refer to Ineffective Individual Coping (Chap. 11) if this is assessed as a problem.	These are symptoms of ineffective coping and interfere with the normal grieving process.
• Have client and support system develop a list of concerns and problems, and assist them in determining those they have the ability to change and those they do not.	Promotes the client's strengths.

• When they have a list of workable problems, have client system list all of the solutions they can think of for a problem; encourage him or her to include those solutions that he or she thinks are impossible or just fantasy solutions. Do this one problem at a time.	Facilitates creative problem solving by assisting the family to break the "more-of-the-same" problem-solving set.
• After solutions have been generated, assist client in evaluating solutions generated. Solutions can be combined, eliminated, or altered. From this list the best solution is needed. It is important that the solution selected is the client's solution.	Promotes the development of creative problem solutions.
• Assist client in developing a plan for implementing this solution. Note here any assistance needed from the nursing staff.	Planned coping strategies facilitate the enactment of new behaviors when the client is experiencing stress.
• Observe client for signs and symptoms of dysfunctional grieving.	Early intervention promotes positive outcome.
• Monitor client's nutritional pattern, and refer him or her to appropriate nursing diagnoses if a problem is identified.	Nutritional status impacts the individual's ability to cope.
• Develop an exercise plan for the client. Consult with physical therapist as needed. Develop a reward schedule for the accomplishment of this plan. Note schedule for plan here. This can also include the support system.	Exercise increases the production of endorphins, which contribute to feelings of well-being.
• Provide assistance for the support system by:	Support system reactions can impact the client.
◦ Having them develop a schedule for rest periods	
◦ Providing snacks for them and scheduling periods of high nursing involvement with the client at a time when support persons can obtain meals (This can reassure the support person that client will not be alone while he or she is gone.)	
◦ Assisting support system in finding cafeteria and transportation	
◦ Suggesting that support persons rest or walk outside or around hospital while client is napping	
◦ Helping support persons discuss with client their feelings	

Gerontic Health

ACTIONS/INTERVENTIONS	RATIONALES
• Provide information to patient regarding what is occurring and expected or anticipated changes.	This intervention is viewed by survivors as especially helpful during the dying process.[28]
• Discuss, with the individual, the grieving process, what can be anticipated, and how each person grieves in his or her own way.	Provides information on common responses to loss and what emotions are commonly experienced by grieving people. Promotes grieving process and reassures survivor that he or she is coping well.

Home Health

> **NOTE:** See Psychiatric Health nursing actions for detailed interventions.

ACTIONS/INTERVENTIONS	RATIONALES

• Teach client and family appropriate monitoring of signs and symptoms of anticipatory grief:
  ◦ Crying or sadness
  ◦ Alterations in eating and sleeping patterns
  ◦ Developmental regression
  ◦ Alterations in concentration
  ◦ Expressions of distress at loss
  ◦ Denial of loss
  ◦ Expressions of guilt
  ◦ Labile affect
  ◦ Grieving beyond expected time
  ◦ Preoccupation with loss
  ◦ Hallucinations
  ◦ Violence toward self or others
  ◦ Delusions
  ◦ Prolonged isolation
	Provides database for early recognition and intervention.

• Involve client and family in planning and implementing strategies to reduce or cope with anticipatory grieving:
  ◦ Family conference: Develop list of concerns and problems, and identify those concerns that family can control.
  ◦ Mutual goal setting: Set short-term realistic goals and evaluation criteria. Specify role of each member.
  ◦ Communication: Discuss loss in supportive environment.
	Family involvement in planning enhances effectiveness of plan.

• Assist client and family in lifestyle adjustments that may be required:
  ◦ Providing realistic hope
  ◦ Identifying expected grief pattern in response to loss
  ◦ Recognizing variety of accepted expressions of grief
  ◦ Developing and using support networks
  ◦ Communicating feelings
  ◦ Providing a safe environment
  ◦ Therapeutic use of denial
  ◦ Identifying suicidal potential or potential for violence
  ◦ Therapeutic use of anger
  ◦ Exploring meaning of situation
  ◦ Stress reduction
  ◦ Promoting expression of grief
  ◦ Decision making for future
  ◦ Promoting family cohesiveness
	Permanent changes in behavior and lifestyle are facilitated by knowledge and support.

• Assist client and family to set criteria to help them to determine when intervention of health care professional is required—e.g., if client is threat to self or others or if client in unable to perform activities of daily living.	Provides data for early intervention.
• Consult with and/or refer patient to assistive resources as indicated.	Utilization of existing services is efficient use of resources. Self-help groups, religious counselor, or psychiatric nurse clinician can enhance the treatment plan.

Grieving, Anticipatory

FLOWCHART EVALUATION: EXPECTED OUTCOME 1

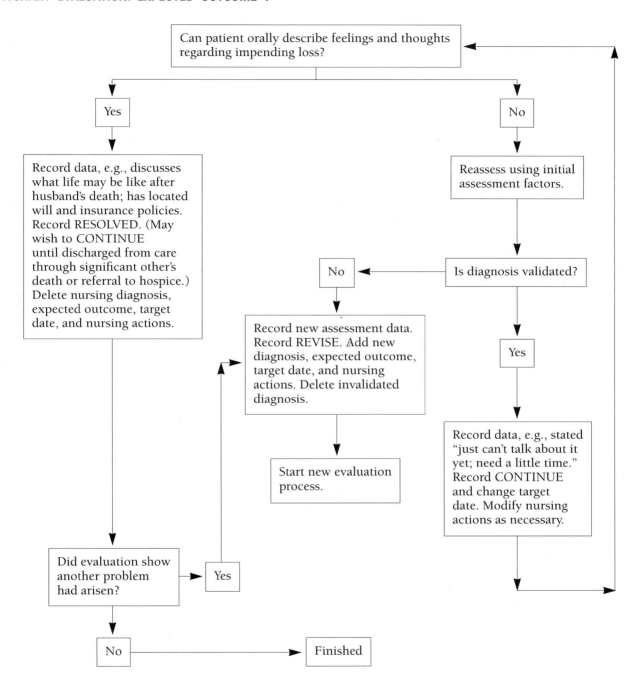

Can patient orally describe feelings and thoughts regarding impending loss?

Yes

No

Record data, e.g., discusses what life may be like after husband's death; has located will and insurance policies. Record RESOLVED. (May wish to CONTINUE until discharged from care through significant other's death or referral to hospice.) Delete nursing diagnosis, expected outcome, target date, and nursing actions.

Reassess using initial assessment factors.

Is diagnosis validated?

No

Yes

Record new assessment data. Record REVISE. Add new diagnosis, expected outcome, target date, and nursing actions. Delete invalidated diagnosis.

Record data, e.g., stated "just can't talk about it yet; need a little time." Record CONTINUE and change target date. Modify nursing actions as necessary.

Start new evaluation process.

Did evaluation show another problem had arisen?

Yes

No

Finished

Grieving, Anticipatory

FLOWCHART EVALUATION: EXPECTED OUTCOME 2

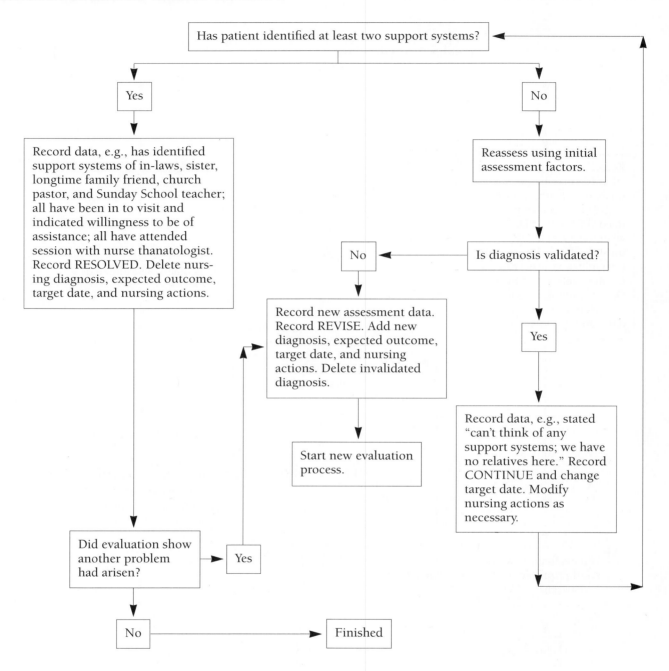

Grieving, Dysfunctional

DEFINITION[8]

Extended, unsuccessful use of intellectual and emotional responses by which individuals (families or communities) attempt to work through the process of modifying self-concept based upon the perception of potential loss.

NANDA TAXONOMY: FEELING 9.2.1.1

DEFINING CHARACTERISTICS[8]

1. Major defining characteristics
   a. Repetitive use of ineffectual behaviors associated with attempts to reinvest in relationships
   b. Reliving of past experiences with little or no reduction (diminishment) of intensity of the grief
   c. Prolonged interference with life functioning onset or exacerbation of somatic or psychosomatic responses
2. Minor defining characteristics
   Extended
   a. Expression of distress at loss
   b. Denial of loss
   c. Expression of guilt
   d. Expression of unresolved issues
   e. Anger
   f. Sadness
   g. Crying
   h. Difficulty in expressing loss
   i. Alterations in:
      (1) Eating habits
      (2) Sleep patterns
      (3) Dream patterns
      (4) Activity level
      (5) Libido
      (6) Concentration and/or pursuit of tasks
   j. Idealization of lost object
   k. Reliving of past experiences
   l. Interference with life functioning
   m. Developmental regression
   n. Labile affect

RELATED FACTORS[8]

1. Actual or perceived object loss ("object loss" is used in the broadest sense)—Objects may include people, possessions, a job, status, home, ideals, or parts and processes of the body.

RELATED CLINICAL CONCERNS

1. Cancer
2. Amputation
3. Spinal cord injury
4. Birth defects
5. Any diagnosis that family has been told has a terminal prognosis
6. Sudden infant death syndrome (SIDS)
7. Stillbirth
8. Infertility

HAVE YOU SELECTED THE CORRECT DIAGNOSIS?

Sensory-Perceptual Alteration This diagnosis will be identified according to the patient's change in capacity to exercise judgment or think critically with appropriate sensory-perceptual functioning. This may well be related to Dysfunctional Grieving.

Anxiety or Fear Anxiety is the response the individual has to a threat that is for the most part unidentified. Fear is the response made by an individual to an identified threat. When the patient has experienced a loss, it is not a threat but an actual event. Therefore, the diagnoses of Anxiety and Fear would not be appropriate.

Ineffective Individual Coping This can be an appropriate diagnosis if the individual is not making the necessary adaptations to deal with crises in his or her life; however, if a real loss has occurred, the most appropriate diagnosis is Dysfunctional Grieving.

Spiritual Distress When faced with a devastating loss, the client may well express Spiritual Distress. This quite often is a companion diagnosis to Dysfunctional Grieving.

EXPECTED OUTCOMES

1. Will verbalize grief feelings by (date) and/or
2. Will identify at least (number) ways to appropriately cope with grief by (date)

TARGET DATES

Grief work should begin within 1 to 2 days after the nurse has intervened; the complete process of grief may take 6 months to a year.

NURSING ACTIONS/INTERVENTIONS WITH RATIONALES

Adult Health

For this diagnosis, the Psychiatric Health nursing actions serve as the generic actions. Please see Psychiatric Health nursing actions.

Child Health

> **NOTE:** It is difficult to make general assumptions as to how each child views death, but according to previous patterns of behavior, including communication, it would be necessary to allow for developmental patterns previously attained. In young children there may be manifestations of obsessive, ritualistic behavior related to the loss or activities surrounding loss. For example, if a loved one died, young children may think that if they fall asleep they may also die. In the event of grieving, regardless of the precipitating event, the child must be allowed to respond in keeping with developmental capacity. At times when the child is in danger of self-injury or injuring others, the risk for violence must be considered.

ACTIONS/INTERVENTIONS	RATIONALES
• Provide opportunities for expression of feelings related to loss or grief according to developmental capacity, e.g., puppets or play therapy for toddlers.	Expression of feelings helps to deal with sense of loss and provides a database for intervention. Expression of grief reduces uncontrolled outbursts.
• In the event of a family member's death, offer support in understanding deceased family member's relationship to patient and status for family, with special attention to siblings and their reactions. Identify impact grief has for family dynamics via assessment of same.	Provides database for more accurate intervention in dealing with loss.
• Allow for cultural and religious input in plan of care, especially related to care of dying patient and care of patient at time of death.	Demonstrates valuing of these beliefs to family and decreases stress for family.
• Collaborate with professionals and paraprofessionals to aid in resolution of grief according to family preferences.	Collaboration offers the most comprehensive plan of care and avoids fragmentation of care.
• Identify support groups to assist in resolution of grief, such as Compassionate Friends Organization.	Support groups offer validation of feelings and a sense of hope as similar concerns are shared.
• Assist family members in identification of coping strategies needed for resultant role-relationship changes.	Provides for support during the adjustments that are required due to the loss of a loved one.
• Assist family members to resolve feelings of loss via reminiscing of loved one, positive aspects of situation, or personal growth potential presented. Remember that behavior often serves as the most effective communication for the child or young toddler.	Reminiscing and valuing past experiences will offer an opportunity to project the impact for the present and future.
• Allow family members time and space to face reality of situation and ponder meaning of loss for self and family.	Time and readiness promote the willingness to discuss feelings after the major emotional shock has diminished.
• Direct family to appropriate resources regarding positive methods of acknowledging loved one through memorials or related processes.	A sense of fulfillment may be derived from the sharing of time, talent, or money in the honor of the loved one. This affords some sense of resolve of the guilt or emptiness associated with the loss.
• Assist in referral to appropriate resources for funeral planning and arrangements if needed.	In times of emotional duress, objective decisions may be difficult. Providing assistance will offer empowerment and a sense of coping.
• In the event of SIDS, provide an opportunity, through a scheduled conference, for verbalization of: ○ How infant's death occurred ○ Police investigation ○ Sense of guilt ○ Feelings of powerlessness ○ Questions ○ Anger ○ Disbelief ○ Fears for future pregnancies and birth	
• Identify the impact the death or grief has on other family members, the relationship of the couple, and the couple's attitude toward having other children.	Provides the essential database that can assist in planning that will offset the development of dysfunctional grieving.

Women's Health

ACTIONS/INTERVENTIONS	RATIONALES
• Schedule a 30-min daily conference with couple and focus on: ○ Expression of grief, anger, guilt, or frustration ○ Exploring expectations regarding children, e.g., the couple's expectations, relative's expectations, and society's expectations	Initiates expression of emotions that allows gradual transference through the grief process. Allows clarification of issues related to a pregnancy that has not resulted in a healthy infant.
• Providing factual information (on whichever diagnosis is appropriate) regarding SIDS, stillbirth, or abortion. • Encouraging couple to honestly share feelings with each other. • During conference, encourage couple to ask questions through open-ended questions, reflection, etc. • Monitor, during hospitalization, for signs and symptoms of depression, anger, frustration, and impending crisis.	Provides the database necessary to permit early intervention and prevention of more serious problems during this crisis.
• Encourage couple to seek professional help, as necessary, to deal with continued concerns such as their sexual relationship, conflicts, anxieties, parenting, and coping mechanisms that can be used to deal with the loss of fertility.	Fetal demise, SIDS, the decision to have an abortion, etc. all have long-term effects; therefore, long-term support will be required.
• Assist couple, through teaching and provision of written information, to realize that grief may not be resolved for over a year.	Avoids unrealistic expectations regarding grief resolution.

Psychiatric Health

ACTIONS/INTERVENTIONS	RATIONALES
• Monitor source of the interference with the grieving process. • Monitor client's use of medications and the effects this may have on the grieving process. Consult with physician regarding necessary alterations in this area.	Early recognition and intervention can facilitate the grieving process. Sedatives and tranquilizers may delay the grieving process.
• Assign a primary care nurse to the client. • Provide a calm, reassuring environment.	Facilitates the development of a trusting relationship. Excessive environmental stimuli can increase the client's confusion and disorganization.
• When client is demonstrating an emotional response to the grief, provide privacy and remain with the client during this time.	Encourages appropriate expression of feelings.
• Primary nurse will spend 15 min twice a day with the client at (times). These interactions should begin as nonconfrontational interactions with the client. The goal is to develop a trusting relationship so the client can later discuss issues related to the grieving process.	Facilitates the development of a trusting relationship.
• Monitor level of dysfunction, and assist client with activities of daily living as necessary. Note type and amount of assistance here.	Facilitates the development of a trusting relationship.
• Monitor nutritional status, and refer to Altered Nutrition (Chap. 3) for detailed care plan.	Alterations in nutrition can impact coping abilities.
• Monitor significant others' response to the client, and have primary nurse set a schedule to meet with them and the client every other day to answer questions and facilitate discussion between the client and the support system. Note schedule for these meetings here.	Support system understanding facilitates the maintenance of new behaviors after discharge.

Continued

ACTIONS/INTERVENTIONS	RATIONALES
• Provide the spiritual support that the client indicates is necessary. Note here the type of assistance needed from the nursing staff.	Clients may find answers to their questions about life and loss through spiritual expression.
• Allow client to express anger, and assure him or her that you will not allow harm to come to anyone during this expression.	Violent behavior can evolve from unexpressed anger. Appropriate expression of anger promotes the client's sense of control and enhances self-esteem.
• Provide client with punching bags and other physical activity that assists with the expression of anger. Note tools preferred by this client here. Note here the specific activities that assist this client with this expression.	Assists client in developing appropriate coping behaviors enhancing self-esteem.
• Remind staff and support system that client's expressions of anger at this point should not be taken personally even though they may be directed at the persons.	Support system understanding facilitates the maintenance of new behaviors after discharge.
• Answer questions directly and openly.	Promotes the development of a trusting relationship.
• Provide time and opportunity for the client to participate in appropriate religious rituals. Note here the assistance needed from the nursing staff.	Rituals provide clarity and direction for the grieving process.
• Sit with client while he or she is talking about the lost object.	The presence of the nurse provides positive reinforcement. Positive reinforcement encourages the behavior.
• When client's verbal interactions increase with the primary nurse to the level that group interactions are possible, schedule client to participate in a group that allows expression of feelings and feedback from peers. Note schedule of group here.	Provides opportunities for peer feedback and for peer assistance for problem solving.
• Assign client appropriate tasks in unit activities. Note type of tasks assigned here. These should be based on the client's level of functioning and should be at a level that the client can accomplish. Note type of tasks to be assigned to client here.	Successful accomplishment of tasks enhances self-esteem.
• If delusions, hallucinations, phobias, or depression are present, refer to Ineffective Individual Coping (Chap. 11) and Altered Thought Process (Chap. 7).	
• Primary nurse will engage client and the support system in planning for lifestyle changes that might result from the loss. Note schedule for these interactions here along with the specific goals.	Planned coping strategies facilitate the enactment of new behaviors when the client is experiencing stress, which enhances self-esteem.

Gerontic Health

The nursing actions for the gerontic patient with this diagnosis are the same as those given in Psychiatric Health.

Home Health

NOTE: See Psychiatric Health nursing actions for detailed interventions.

ACTIONS/INTERVENTIONS	RATIONALES
• Teach client and family appropriate monitoring of signs and symptoms of dysfunctional grief: 　○ Crying or sadness 　○ Alterations in eating and sleeping patterns 　○ Developmental regression 　○ Alterations in concentration 　○ Expressions of distress at loss	Provides database for early recognition and intervention.

- ○ Denial of loss
- ○ Expressions of guilt
- ○ Labile affect
- ○ Grieving beyond expected time
- ○ Preoccupation with loss
- ○ Hallucinations
- ○ Violence toward self or others
- ○ Delusions
- ○ Prolonged isolation

- Involve client and family in planning and implementing strategies to reduce or cope with dysfunctional grieving:
  - ○ Family conference: Identify concerns.
  - ○ Mutual goal setting: Set realistic goals with evaluation criteria. Specify activities for each family member.
  - ○ Communication: Provide open and honest communication with positive feedback. Recognize that anger is common and should not be taken personally.

Family involvement in designing the plan of care enhances the effectiveness of the interventions.

- Assist client and family in lifestyle adjustments that may be required:
  - ○ Providing realistic hope
  - ○ Identifying expected grief pattern in response to loss
  - ○ Recognizing a variety of accepted expressions of grief
  - ○ Developing and using support networks
  - ○ Communicating feelings
  - ○ Providing a safe environment
  - ○ Therapeutic use of denial
  - ○ Identifying suicidal potential or potential for violence
  - ○ Therapeutic use of anger
  - ○ Exploring meaning of situation
  - ○ Stress reduction
  - ○ Promoting expression of grief
  - ○ Promoting family cohesiveness

Dysfunctional grieving can be a chronic condition. Permanent changes in behavior and family roles require support.

- Assist client and family to set criteria to help them to determine when intervention of health care professional is required, e.g., prolonged inability to complete activities of daily living or threat to self or others.

Provides for early recognition and intervention.

- Consult with or refer patient to assistive resources as indicated.

Psychiatric nurse clinician and support groups can enhance the treatment plan.

Grieving, Dysfunctional

FLOWCHART EVALUATION: EXPECTED OUTCOME 1

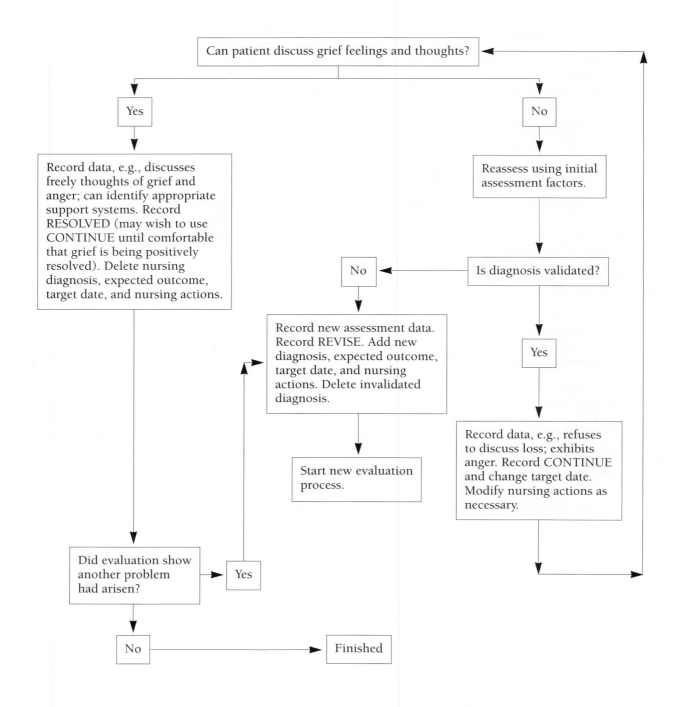

Grieving, Dysfunctional

FLOWCHART EVALUATION: EXPECTED OUTCOME 2

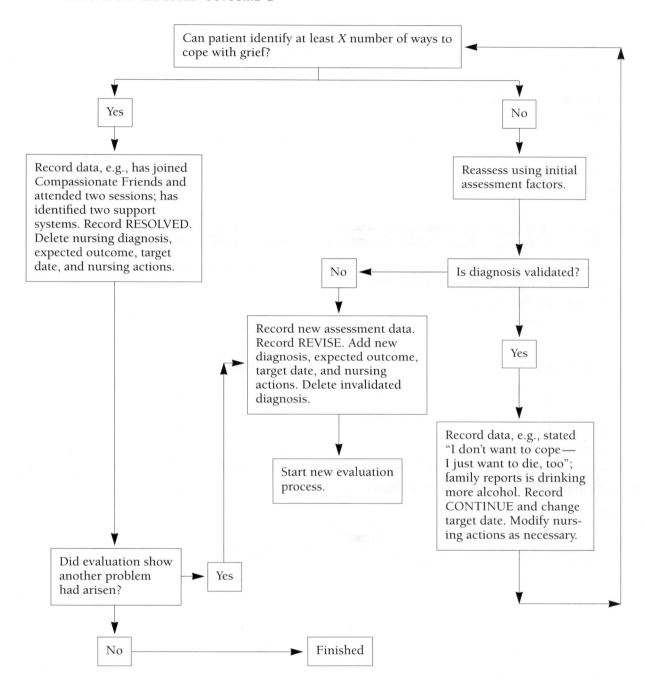

Parent, Infant, and Child Attachment, Risk for Altered

DEFINITION[8]

Disruption of the interactive process between parent or significant other and infant that fosters the development of a protective and nurturing reciprocal relationship.

NANDA TAXONOMY: RELATING 3.2.1.1.2.1

RISK FACTORS[8]

1. Inability of parents to meet the personal needs
2. Anxiety associated with the parent role
3. Substance abuse
4. Premature infant or ill infant or child who is unable to effectively initiate prenatal contact due to altered behavioral organization
5. Separation
6. Physical barriers
7. Lack of privacy

RELATED FACTORS

The risk factors also serve as the related factors.

RELATED CLINICAL CONCERNS

1. Premature infant
2. Chronically ill child
3. Chronically ill parent
4. Mental retardation

 HAVE YOU SELECTED THE CORRECT DIAGNOSIS?

Altered Family Process This diagnosis is an actual diagnosis and would be used if there were an actual problem with attachment.

Altered Parenting Again, this is an actual diagnosis. Risk for Altered Parenting occurs beyond the attachment phase.

EXPECTED OUTCOMES

1. Will verbally express more comfort with caring for infant by (date) and/or
2. Will show (number) percent decrease in risk factors by (date)

TARGET DATES

This diagnosis will require time periods that are longer than those for other diagnoses to reduce the risk factors. An appropriate initial target date would be 5 to 7 days.

NURSING ACTIONS/INTERVENTIONS WITH RATIONALES

Adult Health

ACTIONS/INTERVENTIONS	RATIONALES
• Make arrangement, when possible, for patient to interact with infant or child. Accompany patient to cafeteria, chapel, or visitor lounge. Provide protection for the infant or child. Provide privacy, but remain close at hand during parent-child interactions.	Gives opportunity to practice parenting skills and obtain feedback in a supportive environment.
• Encourage patient with substance-abuse problem to seek counseling, treatment, and support groups; initiate referrals as needed.	Provides long-term support and assistance.
• Encourage timeline planning to provide time for care of infant or child as well as time for self.	Helps patient not to get overwhelmed with activities needed to care for infant or child.
• Encourage patient to trade skills or barter for babysitting respite.	Provides time for self. Can increase patient's self-esteem knowing that he or she has skills that can be traded.
• Allow patient to talk about anxiety with parenting. Teach stress management and alternate coping strategies.	Provides alternate strategies for coping.
• Have child health clinical nurse specialist or pediatric FNP teach parenting skills and growth and development of premature infant.	Provides knowledge base and helps patient to know that some of the things they are experiencing are normal.

Child Health

ACTIONS/INTERVENTIONS	RATIONALES
• Monitor for factors regarding infant that contribute to or influence maternal or paternal parent or infant reciprocity: ○ Inability to send cues for needs ○ Inability of mother or father to attend to cues ○ Inability of mother or father to comfort infant ○ Mismatch of temperament of the infant to the mother or father ○ Parental verbalization of feelings about infant less than ideal for appropriate bonding • Explore actual parent-infant interactions, and note strengths and deficits	A thorough assessment of reciprocal behaviors will serve as a guide to specific needs of parental-infant dyad.
• Identify behaviors so unsafe as to suggest separation of infant from parent, e.g., physical or emotional abuse. (Involve CPS according to protocols for location; hotline available nationally.)	Safety and legal needs will help protect infant in an unsafe relationship.
• Offer role modeling and parenting teaching modules at readiness of parents and when deemed suitable to do so: ○ Normal growth and development ○ Special care for infant	Often new parenting roles must be acquired as there may be no suitable role modeling in parent's own childhood.
• When parents must be absent, maintain communication that is consistent with hopefully the same few individuals to maintain long-term relationship.	Trust and sincerity will foster parents in this demanding role.
• Involve appropriate support services as indicated in a timely manner (e.g., Ronald McDonald House for lodging and local social services agencies).	Support during time of need will enable parents to be near infant as much as possible.
• Ensure appropriate counseling and follow-up for all members as may be deemed essential.	Long-term goals are best established during acute phase of crisis.

Women's Health

ACTIONS/INTERVENTIONS	RATIONALES
PREGNANCY[29] • Encourage the expectant parents to discuss their perceptions and expectations of the pregnancy.	Allows expectant parents to progress through pregnancy in a satisfactory and satisfying manner. Provides knowledge base and helps parents know that what they are experiencing is normal.
• Provide a nonthreatening atmosphere to encourage the parents to discuss their fears and concerns. • Assist parents to dispel myths about birth, postpartum, and early parenthood. • Assist parents to plan for changes in financial requirements of pregnancy, birth, and early parenthood. • Encourage parents to talk to the fetus, spend time together feeling the fetus move, etc. • Encourage attendance in various classes that can assist in the transition to parenthood. • Assist parents in identifying community resources available to expectant and new parents.	

Continued

ACTIONS/INTERVENTIONS	RATIONALES
PARENTHOOD[30,31] • Encourage the new parents to touch, talk to, and observe the newborn as soon as possible (immediately is best). • Encourage comparison of newborn characteristics to fantasized newborn.	Allows expectant parents to progress through pregnancy in a satisfactory and satisfying manner. Provides knowledge base and helps parents know that what they are experiencing is normal.

Psychiatric Health

This diagnosis is more appropriate under Child Health.

Gerontic Health

This diagnosis is not appropriate to use with gerontic clients.

Home Health

ACTIONS/INTERVENTIONS	RATIONALES

• Involve client and family in planning and implementing strategies to decrease or prevent alterations in attachment:
  ○ Identify family strengths and weaknesses.
  ○ Design strategies to support strengths and correct weaknesses.
  ○ Provide safe environment.
	Family involvement enhances effectiveness of intervention.

• Teach parenting strategies and techniques to enhance parent-child interactions.
  ○ Appropriate stimulation for child
  ○ Consistent approach to parenting
	Parenting is learned behavior.

• Consult with or refer parents to community resources as required.	Provides efficient use of existing resources.

Parent, Infant, Child Attachment, Risk for Altered

FLOWCHART EVALUATION: EXPECTED OUTCOME 1

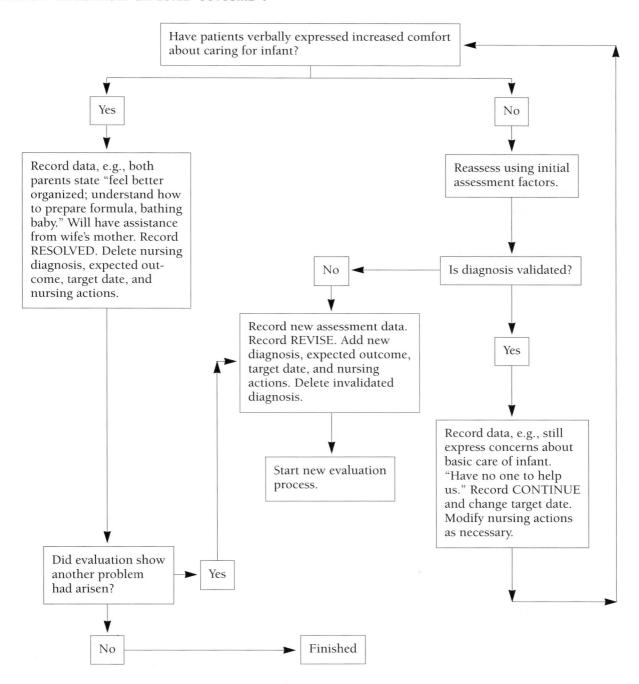

Parent, Infant, Child Attachment, Risk for Altered

FLOWCHART EVALUATION: EXPECTED OUTCOME 2

Have parents shown the stated decrease in risk factors?

Yes

Record data, e.g., state "have arranged better schedule for work and infant care," "Now know how to care for baby." Risks factors now reduced to one—lack of privacy (live with husband's parents). Record RESOLVED. Delete nursing diagnosis, expected outcome, target date, and nursing actions.

Did evaluation show another problem had arisen?

Yes

No → Finished

No → Record new assessment data. Record REVISE. Add new diagnosis, expected outcome, target date, and nursing actions. Delete invalidated diagnosis.

Start new evaluation process.

No

Reassess using initial assessment factors.

Is diagnosis validated?

Yes

Record data, e.g., still expressing concerns about personal needs, lack of experience in caring for a baby. "Scared about baby being too early." Record CONTINUE and change target date. Modify nursing actions as necessary.

Parenting, Altered: Risk for, Actual, and Parental Role Conflict

DEFINITIONS[8]

RISK FOR ALTERED PARENTING The state in which a nurturing figure(s) is at risk to experience an inability to create an environment that promotes the optimum growth and development of another human being.*

ALTERED PARENTING The state in which a nurturing figure(s) experiences an inability to create an environment that promotes the optimum growth and development of another human being.*

PARENTAL ROLE CONFLICT The state in which a parent experiences role confusion and conflict in response to crisis.

NANDA TAXONOMY: RELATING 3.2.1.1.2, 3.2.1.1.1, AND 3.2.3.1

DEFINING CHARACTERISTICS[8]

1. Risk factors for Risk for Altered Parenting
   a. Lack of parental attachment behaviors
   b. Inappropriate visual, tactile, or auditory stimulation
   c. Negative identification of infant or child's characteristics
   d. Negative attachment of meanings to infant or child's characteristics
   e. Constant verbalization of disappointment in gender or physical characteristics of the infant or child
   f. Verbalization of resentment toward the infant or child
   g. Verbalization of role inadequacy
   h. Inattentive to infant or child's needs (*critical*)
   i. Verbal disgust at body functions of infant or child
   j. Noncompliance with health appointments for self and/or infant or child
   k. Inappropriate caretaking behaviors (toilet training, sleep-rest, or feeding) (*critical*)
   l. Inappropriate or inconsistent discipline practices
   m. Frequent accidents
   n. Frequent illness
   o. Growth and development lag in the child
   p. History of child abuse or abandonment by primary caretaker (*critical*)
   q. Verbalizes desire to have child call himself or herself by first name versus traditional cultural tendencies
   r. Child receiving care from multiple caretakers without consideration for the needs of the infant or child
   s. Compulsively seeking role approval from others
2. Altered Parenting
   a. Major defining characteristics
      (1) Abandonment
      (2) Runaway
      (3) Verbalization that cannot control child
      (4) Incidence of physical and psychological trauma
      (5) Lack of parental attachment behaviors
      (6) Inappropriate visual, tactile, or auditory stimulation

   (7) Negative identification of infant or child's characteristics
   (8) Negative attachment of meanings to infant or child's characteristics
   (9) Constant verbalization of disappointment in gender or physical characteristics of the infant or child
   (10) Verbalization of resentment toward the infant or child
   (11) Verbalization of role inadequacy
   (12) Inattentive to infant or child's needs (*critical*)
   (13) Verbal disgust at body functions of infant or child
   (14) Noncompliance with health appointments for self and/or infant or child
   (15) Inappropriate caretaking behaviors (toilet training, sleep-rest, or feeding) (*critical*)
   (16) Inappropriate or inconsistent discipline practices
   (17) Frequent accidents
   (18) Frequent illness
   (19) Growth and development lag in the child
   (20) History of child abuse or abandonment by primary caretaker (*critical*)
   (21) Verbalizes desire to have child call himself or herself by first name versus traditional cultural tendencies
   (22) Child receives care from multiple caretakers without consideration for the needs of the infant or child
   (23) Compulsively seeking role approval from others
   b. Minor defining characteristics
      None given
3. Parental Role Conflict
   a. Major defining characteristics
      (1) Parent(s) expressing concerns or feelings of inadequacy to provide for child's physical and emotional needs during hospitalization or in the home
      (2) Demonstrated disruption in caretaking routines
      (3) Parent(s) expressing concerns about changes in parental role, family functioning, family communication, or family health
   b. Minor defining characteristics
      (1) Expresses concern about perceived loss of control over decisions relating to his or her child
      (2) Reluctant to participate in usual caretaking activities even with encouragement and support
      (3) Verbalizes and/or demonstrates feelings of guilt, anger, fear, anxiety, and/or frustration about effect of child's illness on family process

RELATED FACTORS[8]

1. Risk for and Altered Parenting
   a. Lack of available role model
   b. Ineffective role model
   c. Physical and psychosocial abuse of nurturing figure
   d. Lack of support between or from significant other(s)
   e. Unmet social or emotional maturation needs of parenting figures

*It is important to state as a preface to this diagnosis that adjustment to parenting in general is a normal maturational process that elicits nursing behaviors of prevention of potential problems and health promotion.

f. Interruption in bonding process, that is, maternal, paternal, or other
g. Unrealistic expectation for self, infant, or partner
h. Perceived threat to own survival, physical and emotional
i. Mental and/or physical illness
j. Presence of stress (financial, legal, recent crisis, or cultural move)
k. Lack of knowledge
l. Limited cognitive functioning
m. Lack of role identity
n. Lack of or inappropriate response of child to relationship
o. Multiple pregnancies
2. Parental Role Conflict
a. Separation from child due to chronic illness
b. Intimidation with invasive or restrictive modalities (e.g., isolation or intubation)
c. Specialized care center's policies
d. Home care of a child with special needs (e.g., apnea monitoring, postural drainage, or hyperalimentation)
e. Change in marital status
f. Interruptions of family life due to home care regimen (treatments, caregivers, or lack of respite)

RELATED CLINICAL CONCERNS

1. Birth defect
2. Multiple birth
3. Chronically ill child
4. Substance abuse
5. Parental chronic illness
6. Major depressive episode
7. Manic episode
8. Phobic disorders
9. Dissociative disorders
10. Organic mental disorders
11. Schizophrenic disorders

HAVE YOU SELECTED THE CORRECT DIAGNOSIS?

Family Process, Altered This diagnosis indicates dysfunctioning on part of the entire family, not just the parents. If the entire family is indicating difficulties dealing with current problems or crises, then Altered Family Process is a more correct diagnosis than one of the parenting diagnoses that relate to the parents only.

Family Coping, Ineffective This diagnosis usually arises from the client's perspective that his or her primary support is no longer fulfilling this role. If the problem relates to parents and their child(ren), then one of the parenting diagnoses is the most appropriate diagnosis.

EXPECTED OUTCOMES

1. Will demonstrate appropriate parental role of (specify exactly what, e.g., feeding or medication administration) behavior by (date) and/or
2. Will verbalize realistic expectations of self as parent and for child by (date)

TARGET DATES

The diagnosis will require a lengthy amount of time to be totally resolved. However, progress toward resolutions could be evaluated within 7 days.

NURSING ACTIONS/INTERVENTIONS WITH RATIONALES
Adult Health

ACTIONS/INTERVENTIONS	RATIONALES
• Provide information relative to normal growth and development of self and child by sitting and talking with patient for 30 min twice a day at (times).	Provides knowledge base and assists patient to know that some of the things he or she is experiencing are normal.
• During conference time, assist parent to recognize when stress is becoming distress; e.g., irritability turns to rage and/or verbal or physical abuse, sleeplessness, altered thought process, or tunnel perception of situation.	Prevents a crisis situation. Promotes self-knowledge.
• Teach stress management and parenting techniques, e.g., relaxation, deep breathing, Mother's Day Out, safety precautions, or toileting process.	Provides alternative strategies for coping and provides database needed for dealing with growth and development of child.

- Provide opportunities for parent to participate in child's care.
- Discuss disciplinary methods other than physical, e.g., grounding, taking away privileges, positive reinforcement, and verbal praise for "good" behavior.
- Encourage patient to allow time for own needs.

- Encourage use of support groups. Initiate referrals as needed.

Gives opportunity to practice parenting skills and obtain feedback in supportive environment.
Physical discipline can lead to abuse; sends wrong message to child.

Own needs must be met to decrease stress and facilitate meeting needs of others.

Provides an outlet for parents with other parents in similar situations. Provides long-term support and assistance.

Child Health

ACTIONS/INTERVENTIONS	RATIONALES

• Review current level of knowledge regarding parenting of infant or child to include:
  ◦ Parental perception of infant or child
  ◦ Parental views of expected development of infant or child
  ◦ Health status of infant or child
  ◦ Current needs of infant or child
  ◦ Infant or child communication (remember, behaviors reveal much about feelings)
  ◦ Infant or child usual responsiveness
  ◦ Family dynamics, e.g., who offers support for emotional needs or child's view of mother and father
	Provides database needed to more accurately plan care.

• Determine needs for specific health or developmental intervention from other health care providers as needed.	Needs may be identified with assistance from experts in multidisciplinary domains. Collaboration is essential to avoid fragmentation of care.

• Observe parental readiness and encourage caretaking in a supportive atmosphere in the following ways as applicable:
  ◦ Feeding
  ◦ Bathing
  ◦ Anticipatory safety measures
  ◦ Clarification of medical or health maintenance regimen
  ◦ Play and developmental stimulations for age and capacity
  ◦ Handling and carriage of infant or child
  ◦ Diapering and dressing of infant or child
  ◦ Social interaction appropriate for age and capacity
  ◦ Other specific measures according to patient's status and needs
	Provides data needed to plan teaching and to provide individualization of the plan of care.

• Schedule a daily conference of at least 1 h with parents, and encourage parents to verbalize perceived parenting role, both current and desired.	Provides teaching opportunity. Verbalization reveals thoughts and data needed to more accurately plan care.
• Allow parents to gradually assume total care of infant within hospital setting at least 48 h before dismissal. If more time is required to validate appropriate parenting success, collaborate with pediatrician regarding extending child's stay for 24 h.	Provides opportunity for practice of needed skills or roles; fosters growth and confidence in parenting.
• During conference, assist parents to identify ways of coping with infant and parental demands to include family, community, and health care professional support.	Provides growth opportunities for parents and long-term support.

Women's Health

ACTIONS/INTERVENTIONS	RATIONALES

• Assist patient, through monthly conferences, in completing the tasks of pregnancy by encouraging verbalization of:
   ◦ Fears
   ◦ Mother's perception of marriage
   ◦ Mother's perception of "child within" her
   ◦ Mother's perception of the changes in her life as a result of this birth:
     (1) Relationship with partner
     (2) Relationship with other children
     (3) Effects on career
     (4) Effects on family
• Allow mother to question pregnancy: "Now" and "Who, me?"[32]
	Acceptance of pregnancy and working through the tasks of pregnancy provide a strong basis for positive parenthood and appropriate attachment and bonding.

• Assist mother in realizing existence of child by encouraging mother to:
   ◦ Note when infant moves.
   ◦ Listen to fetal heart tones during visit to clinic.
   ◦ Discuss body changes and their relationship to infant.
   ◦ Verbalize any questions she may have.
• Assist in preparation for birth by:
   ◦ Encouraging attendance at childbirth education classes
   ◦ Providing factual information regarding the birthing experience
   ◦ Involving significant others in preparation for birthing process
• Assist patient in preparing for role transition to parenthood by encouraging:
   ◦ Economic planning, e.g., physician, hospital, or prenatal testing fees
   ◦ Social planning, e.g., changes in lifestyle
	Provides basis for appropriate attachment behaviors and coping skills for transition to maternal role.

• Assist patient in identifying needs related to family's acceptance of the newborn:
   ◦ Mother's perceived level of support from family members
   ◦ Stressors present in family, e.g., economics, housing, or level of knowledge regarding parenting
• Monitor for following behaviors:
   ◦ Refuses to plan for infant
   ◦ No interest in pregnancy or fetal progress
   ◦ Overly concerned with own weight and appearance
   ◦ Refuses to gain weight (diets during pregnancy)
   ◦ Negative comments such as "What this baby is doing to me!"
	Assists in identifying patients at high risk for the development of this diagnosis.

POSTPARTUM

ACTIONS/INTERVENTIONS	RATIONALES

• Assist patient and significant others in establishing realistic goals for integration of baby into family.
• Provide positive reinforcement for parenting tasks:
   ◦ Encourage use of birthing room: Labor, delivery, and recovery (LDR) room and labor, delivery, recovery, and postpartum (LDRP) rooms—for birth to allow active participation in birth process by both parents.
   ◦ Allow mother and partner time with infant (do not remove infant to nursery if stable) following delivery.
   ◦ Provide mother-baby care to allow maximum continuity of mother-infant contact and nursing care.
	Promotes realistic planning for new baby as well as bonding and attachment.

- Assist parents in identifying different kinds of infant behavior and understanding how they allow the infant to communicate with them:
  - Perform gestational age assessment with parents, and explain significance of findings.
  - Perform Brazelton neonatal assessment with parents, and explain significance of findings.
  - Demonstrate how to hold infant for maximum communication.
  - Explain infant reflexes—e.g., rooting or Moro—and the importance of understanding them.
- Assist parents in identifying support systems:
  - Friends from childbirth classes
  - Parents and parents-in-law
  - Siblings
  - Nurse specialists
- Encourage parents to reminisce about birthing experience.
- Assist patient in identifying needs related to family functioning.
- Identify negative maternal behavior:
  - No interest in new baby
  - Talks *excessively* to friends on phone
  - Is more interested in TV than in feeding infant
  - Refuses to listen to infant teaching
  - Asks no questions
  - *Extraordinary* interest in self-appearance:
    (1) *Severe* dieting to gain prepregnancy figure
    (2) *Overutilization* of exercise to gain prepregnancy figure
  - Crying or moodiness
  - Lack of interest in family and other children
  - Failure to perform physical care for infant
  - Noncompliance: Breaks appointments with health care providers for self and infant
- Identify negative paternal behavior:
  - Refusal to support wife by:
    (1) Not assisting in child care
    (2) Not sharing household tasks
    (3) Keeping "his" social contacts and going out while wife remains at home with child
  - Not providing financial support
  - Abandonment
- Assist patient in identifying methods of coping with stress of newborn in family:
  - Seek professional help from nurse specialist, physician (obstetrician or pediatrician), or psychiatrist
  - Identify support system in family or among friends
  - Refer to appropriate community or private agencies

Provides the parents with essential information they need to care for infant.

Provides database need for planning to offset factors that would result in ineffective parenting.

Provides long-term support.

Psychiatric Health

ACTIONS/INTERVENTIONS	RATIONALES
• Monitor the degree to which drugs and alcohol interfere with the parenting process. If this is a factor, discuss a treatment program with the client.	Early intervention and treatment increase the likelihood of a positive outcome.
• Ask client who is caring for children while he or she is hospitalized and assess his or her level of comfort with this arrangement. If a satisfactory arrangement is not present, refer patient to social services so arrangements can be made.	Early intervention and treatment increases the likelihood of a positive outcome.
• Discuss with the client expectations and problem perception.	Promotes the client's sense of control.
• Have client identify support systems and gain permission to include these persons in the treatment plan as necessary. This could include spouse, parents, close friends, etc.	Support system understanding facilitates the maintenance of behaviors after discharge.
• If client desires to maintain parenting role, arrange to have children visit during hospitalization. Assign a staff member to remain with the client during these visits. The staff person can serve as a role model for the client and facilitate communication between the child and the client. Note schedule for these visits here and the staff person responsible for the supervision of these interactions.	A continuous relationship between parent and child is necessary for the normal development of the child.[33]
• Answer client's questions in a clear, direct manner.	Promotes the development of a trusting relationship.
• Spend 15 min twice a day at (times) with the client discussing his or her perception of the parenting role and his or her expectations for self and children.	Promotes the development of a trusting relationship and provides information about the client's worldview that can be utilized in constructing interventions.
• Arrange 30 min a day for interaction between the client and one member of the support system. A staff member is to be present during these interactions to facilitate communication and focus the discussion on parenting issues.	Supports the maintenance of these relationships and provides opportunities for the nurse to do positive role modeling.
• Provide client with information on normal growth and development and normal feelings of parents.	Provides information that will assist the client in making appropriate parenting decisions, enhancing self-esteem.
• Assist client in developing a plan for disciplining children. This plan should be based on behavioral interventions, and the primary focus should be on positive social rewards.[34]	Facilitates the development of positive coping behaviors and promotes a positive expectational set.
• Teach client ways of interacting with child that reduce levels of conflict, e.g., providing child with limited choices, spending scheduled time with the child, or listening carefully to child.	Promotes positive orientation and enhances self-esteem.
• Encourage client to maintain telephone contact with children by providing a telephone and establishing a regular time for the client to call home or have the children call the hospital.	Assists in maintaining these important relationships to make the transition to home easier.
• Encourage support system to continue to include client in decisions related to the children by having them bring up these issues in daily visits and by assisting client and support system to engage in collaborative decision making regarding these issues.	Assists in maintaining client's role functioning, thus enhancing self-esteem.
• Have client identify parenting models, and discuss the effect these persons had on their current parenting style.	Children can be triangled into parental conflicts in an unconscious effort to preserve the marital relationship.[35]
• Observe interaction between parents to assess for problems in the husband-wife relationship that may be expressed in the parenting relationship. If this appears to be happening, refer patient to family therapy.	

• Have client develop a list of problem behavior patterns, and then assist him or her in developing a list of alternative behavior patterns. For example, Current: When I get frustrated with my child, I spank him with a belt. New: When I get frustrated with my child, I arrange to send him to the neighbors for 30 min while I take a walk around the block to calm down.	Promotes client's sense of control and begins the development of alternative, more adaptive coping behaviors.
• Role-play with client those situations that are identified as being most difficult, and provide opportunities to practice more appropriate behavior. This should be done daily in 30-min time periods. Note schedule for this activity here, list time periods, and list those situations that are to be practiced. It would be useful to include spouse.	Behavioral rehearsal provides opportunities for feedback and modeling of new behaviors by the nurse.
• Have client attend group sessions where feelings and thoughts can be expressed to peers and the thoughts and feelings of peers can be heard. Note here the schedule for the group.	Assists client to experience personal importance to others while enhancing interpersonal relationship skills. Increasing these competencies can enhance self-esteem and promote positive orientation.
• Assist client in identifying personal needs and in developing a plan for meeting these needs at home; e.g., parents will exchange babysitting time with neighbors so they can have an evening out once a month. Note this plan here.	Assists parents to develop strategies for coping with role strain.
• Monitor staff attitudes toward client and allow them to express feelings, especially if child abuse is an issue with this client.	Negative attitudes of staff can be communicated to the client, decreasing the client's self-esteem and increasing the client's defensiveness.
• Assist client with grieving separation from child and refer to Anticipatory Grieving for detailed nursing actions.	
• Provide client with positive verbal support for positive parenting behavior and for progress on behavior change goal—e.g., "You demonstrate a great deal of concern for your child's welfare," or "You have taught your child to be very sensitive." Make sure these comments are honest and fit the client's awareness of the situation.	Positive reinforcement encourages behavior and enhances self-esteem.
• Assist client in developing stress reduction skills by: 　○ Teaching deep muscle relaxation and practicing this with client 30 min a day at (time) 　○ Discussing with client the role physical exercise plays in stress reduction and developing a plan for exercise (note plan and type of exercise here). Have staff member remain with the client during these exercise periods. Note time for these periods here.	
• When client's level of tension or anxiety is rising on the unit, remind him or her of the exercise or relaxation technique, and work through one of these with him or her.	
• Assist client in identifying the symptoms he or she has of rising tension so he or she can implement the stress reduction activity when client notices this alteration in his or her feelings and behavior.	Provides parents with positive coping strategies for dealing with role strain.

Gerontic Health

This would be an unusual diagnosis for the gerontic patient, but it might develop if the grandparents had to take grandchildren into their home due to a family crisis. In that instance, the nursing actions would be the same as those given in Adult Health and Child Health.

Home Health

ACTIONS/INTERVENTIONS	RATIONALES
• Act as role model through use of positive attitude when interacting with the child and parents.	Role modeling provides example for parenting skills.
• Report child abuse and neglect to the appropriate authorities.	Meets legal requirements and provides for intervention.

• Teach client and family appropriate information regarding the care and discipline of children:
  ○ Cultural norms
  ○ Normal growth and development
  ○ Anticipatory guidance regarding psychosocial, cognitive, and physical needs for children and parents
  ○ Expected family life cycles
  ○ Development and use of support networks
  ○ Safe environment for family members
  ○ Nurturing environment for family members
  ○ Special needs of child requiring invasive or restrictive treatments
	Knowledge is necessary to provide appropriate child care.

• Involve client and family in planning and implementing strategies to decrease or prevent alterations (risk for or actual) in parenting:
  ○ Family conference: Identify each member's perspective of the situation.
  ○ Mutual goal setting: Develop short-term, realistic goals with evaluation criteria.
  ○ Communication: Use open, honest communication with positive feedback.
  ○ Distribution of family tasks: Tasks are performed by all family members as developmentally and physically appropriate.
  ○ Promoting parent's self-esteem: Provide positive support of existence and positive parenting skills.
	Involvement of family in planning enhances the effectiveness of the interventions.

• Assist client and family in lifestyle adjustments that may be required:
  ○ Development of parenting skills
  ○ Use of support network
  ○ Establishment of realistic expectations of children and spouse
	Long-term behavioral changes require support.

• Refer patient to appropriate assistive resources.	Support groups, family therapist, school nurse, and teachers can enhance the treatment plan.

Parenting, Altered: Risk for, Actual, and Parental Role Conflict

FLOWCHART EVALUATION: EXPECTED OUTCOME 1

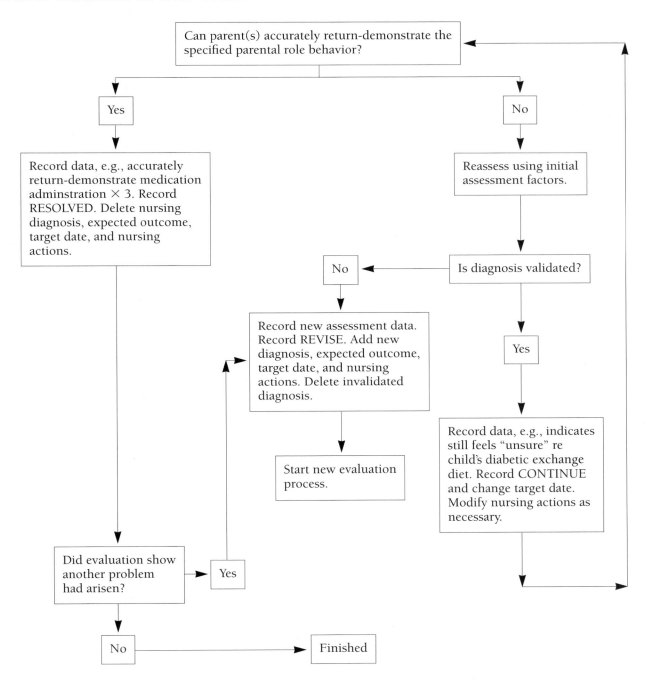

Parenting, Altered: Risk for, Actual, and Parental Role Conflict

FLOWCHART EVALUATION: EXPECTED OUTCOME 2

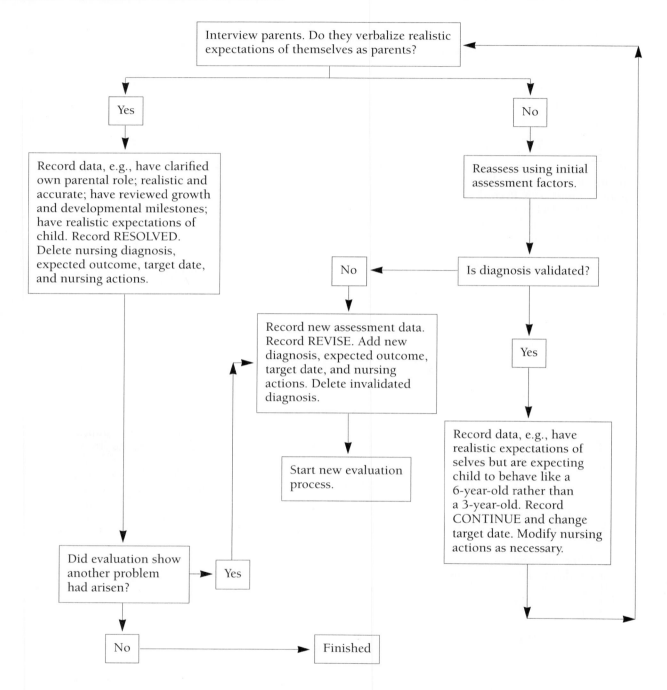

Relocation Stress Syndrome

DEFINITION[8]

Physiological and/or psychosocial disturbances as a result of transfer from one environment to another.

NANDA TAXONOMY: MOVING 6.7

DEFINING CHARACTERISTICS[8]

1. Major defining characteristics
   a. Change in environment or location
   b. Anxiety
   c. Apprehension
   d. Increased confusion (elderly population)
   e. Depression
   f. Loneliness
2. Minor defining characteristics
   a. Verbalization of unwillingness to relocate
   b. Sleep disturbance
   c. Change in eating habits
   d. Dependency
   e. Gastrointestinal disturbances
   f. Increased verbalization of needs
   g. Insecurity
   h. Lack of trust
   i. Restlessness
   j. Sad affect
   k. Unfavorable comparison of post- or pretransfer staff
   l. Verbalization of being concerned or upset about transfer
   m. Vigilance
   n. Weight change
   o. Withdrawal

RELATED FACTORS[8]

1. Past, concurrent, and recent losses
2. Losses involved with decision to move
3. Feeling of powerlessness
4. Lack of adequate support system
5. Little or no preparation for the impending move
6. Moderate to high degree of environmental change
7. History and types of previous transfers
8. Impaired psychosocial health status
9. Decreased physical health status

RELATED CLINICAL CONCERNS

1. Any diagnosis that would require transfer of the patient to a long-term care facility.
2. A chronic disease that would require the older adult to move in with his or her children.

HAVE YOU SELECTED THE CORRECT DIAGNOSIS?

Ineffective Individual Coping This diagnosis and Relocation Stress Syndrome do sound similar; however, the differentiating factor is whether or not the individual is being or recently has been involved in a transfer from one care setting to another. If such a transfer is being considered or has occurred, initial interventions should be directed toward resolving the problems associated with relocation of the patient.

Impaired Adjustment Certainly any move, whether ill or healthy, would require some adjustment. However, this diagnosis relates to an individual's adjusting to his or her own illness or health problem, not adjusting to a change in the health care setting.

EXPECTED OUTCOMES

1. The patient will verbalize increased satisfaction with new environment by (date) and/or
2. The patient will demonstrate a decrease in the major defining characteristics for Relocation Stress Syndrome by (date)

TARGET DATES

An initial target date of 7 days would be reasonable to assess for progress toward meeting the expected outcome.

NURSING ACTIONS/INTERVENTIONS WITH RATIONALES

Adult Health

ACTIONS/INTERVENTIONS	RATIONALES
• Encourage verbalization of feelings, both positive and negative, by actively listening, using reflection, asking open-ended questions, etc., about relocation. Schedule 30 min twice a day at (times) to focus on this topic.	Brings feelings out into the open and clarifies emotions and makes them easier to cope with.
• Determine any previous experience with relocation and the strategies used to cope with the experience during discussions with the patient.	Provides understanding of problem and information to further develop interventions. Determines previously used coping strategies, which ones were successful or unsuccessful, and what alternative strategies may be tried. Increases self-confidence and decreases feeling of powerlessness.
• Allow patient to control, to the extent possible, his or her environment.	
• Provide consistency in daily care such as same primary nurse, same daily routines, and same environment.	Provides security, thus facilitating adjustment.
• Explain all procedures prior to implementation.	Decreases anxiety.
• Teach stress management techniques such as relaxation, meditation, deep breathing, exercise, diversional activities. Have patient return-demonstrate technique for 15 min twice a day at (times).	Decreases anxiety so that energy can be used to implement effective coping strategies.
• Consult with other health care professionals as necessary.	Collaboration promotes care that incorporates physiologic and psychosocial interventions that may be needed as a result of relocation stress.
• Help patient maintain former relationships by providing letter-writing materials or a telephone.	Decreases feelings of isolation and depression.
• Provide patient with a list of organizations and community services available for newcomers, e.g., Welcome Wagon, senior citizens' groups, churches, or singles' groups.	Assists patient to develop new relationship and may hasten adjustment.

Child Health

ACTIONS/INTERVENTIONS	RATIONALES
• Assess, to the degree possible, the emotional stability of the patient and family (can use Chess-Thomas Temperament Scale[36]).	Adaptability to change is determined to a large degree by temperament and previous coping.

• Schedule a family conference of at least 1 h daily and focus on:
  ○ Feelings of patient or family regarding move
  ○ Aspects of relocation that are problematic, e.g., school or friends
  ○ Identification of potential benefits and growth the relocation might offer
	Provides support to cope with changes caused by relocation.

• Encourage plans for maintaining desired past relationships despite physical move, e.g., letters, telephone calls, or visits.	

Women's Health

The nursing actions for a woman with this nursing diagnosis are the same as those found in Adult Health and Gerontic Health.

Psychiatric Health

The nursing actions for the mental health client with this diagnosis are the same as those found in Adult Health and Gerontic Health.

Gerontic Health

> NOTE: These actions apply to patient entering an acute care facility.

ACTIONS/INTERVENTIONS	RATIONALES
• Identify if the patient is at risk for relocation syndrome. In older adults this may include those with no confidant (social support), those who perceive themselves as worriers, those in poor health, and those with low self-esteem.[37]	Early identification of patients at risk can mean earlier intervention and a possible decrease in the negative consequences of relocation.
• Assist patient in realistic perception of event: What has occurred, reasons for transfer based on physical needs, changed health status.	May assist in accepting need for relocation.
• Provide supportive care as the situation requires such as answering questions regarding the routines in the hospital or expected course of treatment.	Allows responses that are tailored to the individual's expressed needs.
• Discuss possible occurrence of syndrome with significant others.	Provides anticipatory information that avoids undue stress on family.
• Discuss with the patient and significant others the patient's usual coping skills.	Provides database to build on prior to discharge from acute care facility.
• Discuss transfer with patient and family.	Provides time to question and promote positive adjustment to the change in location.
• If not returning to prehospitalization location, discuss with the patient his or her proposed plans, reasons for transfer, and patient's response to proposal.	Allows time for ventilation of feelings related to the relocation.

Home Health

> NOTE: See Psychiatric Health for additional interventions.

ACTIONS/INTERVENTIONS	RATIONALES
• Monitor for signs of relocation stress syndrome.	Provides database for early recognition and intervention. Family involvement enhances effectiveness of interventions. If client is moving into a family member's residence, entire family will experience change.
• Involve client and family in planning, implementing, and promoting reduction or elimination of relocation stress:	
○ Family conference: Discuss each member's perspective of the situation. Clarify potential responses to move.	
○ Mutual goal setting: Identify goals and evaluation criteria. Specify tasks and roles for each member.	
○ Communication: Use open, direct communication, and give positive feedback.	
• Assist client and family in lifestyle adjustments that may be required:	
○ Adjustment to changing role functions and relationships	
○ Requirements for redistribution of family tasks	

ACTIONS/INTERVENTIONS	RATIONALES
○ Redistribution of space in the household ○ Preparation for the move ○ Orientation to new surroundings ○ Provision of selected items that are meaningful to the client ○ Preparation for the potential responses, e.g., sleep and eating ○ Provision of any special treatments or equipment ○ Changes in financial situation • Consult with or refer patient to assistive resources as indicated.	Social services, support groups, and a psychiatric nurse clinician can enhance the treatment plan.

Relocation Stress Syndrome

FLOWCHART EVALUATION: EXPECTED OUTCOME 1

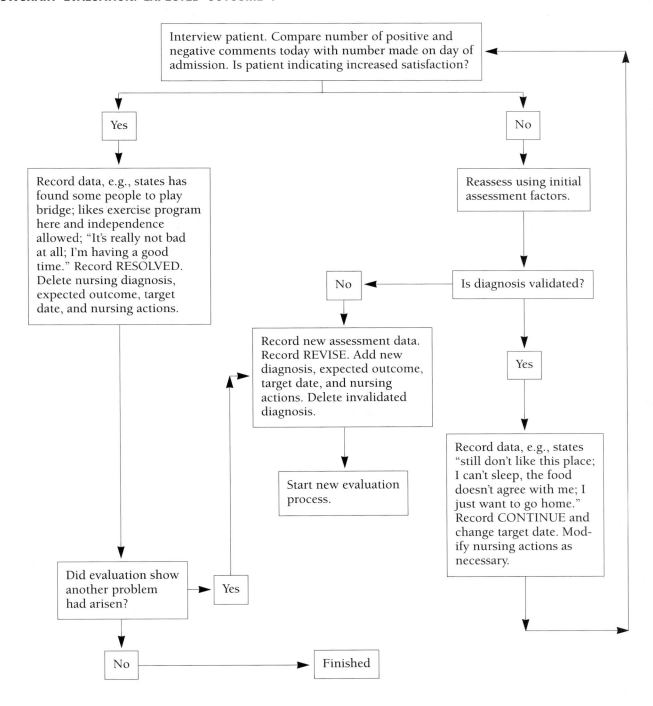

Relocation Stress Syndrome

FLOWCHART EVALUATION: EXPECTED OUTCOME 2

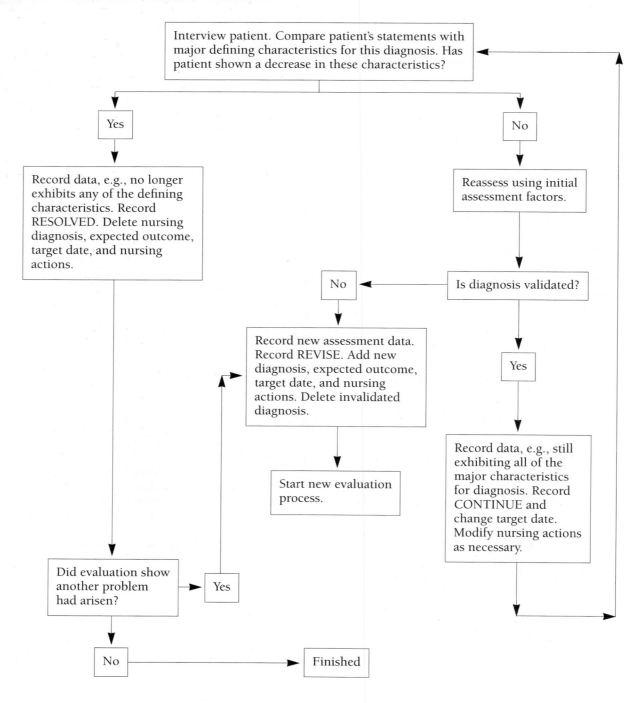

Role Performance, Altered

DEFINITION[8]

Disruption in the way one perceives one's role performance.

NANDA TAXONOMY: RELATING 3.2.1

DEFINING CHARACTERISTICS[8]

1. Major defining characteristics
   a. Change in self-perception of role
   b. Denial of role
   c. Change in others' perception of role
   d. Conflict in roles
   e. Change in physical capacity to resume role
   f. Lack of knowledge of role
   g. Change in usual patterns of responsibility
2. Minor defining characteristics
   None given

RELATED FACTORS[8]

To be developed

RELATED CLINICAL CONCERNS

1. Any major surgery
2. Any chronic disease
3. Any condition resulting in hemiplegia, paraplegia, or quadriplegia
4. Chemical abuse
5. Cancer

HAVE YOU SELECTED THE CORRECT DIAGNOSIS?

Social Isolation   This diagnosis relates to the patient who, because of physical, communicative, or social problems, chooses to be alone or perceives that he or she is alone and therefore isolated from society. This diagnosis deals mainly with the individual who cannot or will not perform any role.

Altered Family Process   This diagnosis refers to an entire family that must in one way or another alter the processes that go on within the family. Many times this will involve altered role performances of the individual family members; however, the overall focus is on the alteration within the family and not with the individual members of the family.

EXPECTED OUTCOMES

1. Will list at least (number) factors contributing to disturbance in role performance by (date) and/or
2. Will implement plan to offset factors contributing to disturbance in role performance by (date)

TARGET DATES

Target dates for this diagnosis will have to be highly individualized according to each situation. A minimum target date would be 5 days to allow time to identify impinging factors and methods to cope with those factors.

NURSING ACTIONS/INTERACTIONS WITH RATIONALES

Adult Health

ACTIONS/INTERVENTIONS	RATIONALES
• Encourage patient to express his or her perception of role responsibilities by active listening, using reflection, asking open-ended questions, accepting patient's feelings, and maintaining a nonjudgmental attitude.	Relieves stress and helps patient to clarify feelings in a safe environment.
• Help patient and significant others realistically negotiate role responsibilities by assisting in the problem-solving process—What is the role? What are its responsibilities? How can responsibilities be shared? What outcomes are expected of the role? Have patient and significant other(s) meet together for 1 h every other day.	Facilitates problem solving. Promotes cooperation among involved persons.
• Teach patient about his or her role, e.g., parent, caregiver, or breadwinner. Allow time for discussion, return-demonstrations, and questioning prior to discharge.	Clarifies misconceptions and provides realistic role expectations.
• Help patient identify community resources to assist in role responsibilities prior to discharge.	Provides support for short-term and long-term problem solving.
• Refer to psychiatric nurse clinician as needed (see Psychiatric Health nursing actions for more detailed interventions).	Collaboration promotes holistic plan of care, and problem may need specialized interventions.

Child Health

ACTIONS/INTERVENTIONS	RATIONALES
• Determine how child and parent perceive the expected role for the child.	Provides essential database necessary to plan care.
• Identify confusion or diffusion of role according to child's and parent's expectations versus actual role.	Problem identification serves to establish common areas to be further explored in role performance.
• Determine value the child has in the family.	The value a child has for each family is critical to expectations for all involved.
• Determine child's self-perception.	One's self-perception provides insight into how one evaluates his or her own performance.
• Identify ways to alleviate role performance alteration according to actual cause. If child is temporarily unable to participate in certain physical activities, explore other nonphysical ways the child can participate.	Alleviation of one or more role performance alterations may prevent further deterioration in role functioning with a greater appreciation for the value of all roles.
• Allow for ventilation of feelings by child via puppetry, art, or other age-appropriate methods. Schedule at least 30 min during each 8-h shift, while awake, for this activity. Note times here.	Feelings are most critical in exploring one's role performance. Appropriate aids in communication serve to foster focused play or behaviors to reveal thoughts of the child who is unable to express himself or herself.
• Provide patient and parents with options to best facilitate needs for future implications of compromised role performance—for example, shared experiences with peers who have temporarily had to forsake physical activities due to illness. How did they keep up with the team?	Vicarious involvement allows for shared activities and the sense of maintaining closeness with the desired groups or person.
• Allow for family time and support for choices to uphold role needs, e.g., visitation by peers.	Shared time of family and friends is important especially in times of role stress to maintain value of self.
• Provide for safety needs of child and family.	Standard care includes safety. The tendency is to relax concerns in times of less stressful activity.
• Assist in follow-up plans with appropriate appointments for psychiatric or pediatric care.	Arrangements for follow-up promote valuing of follow-up and increase the likelihood for compliance.
• Provide support in identification of risk to normal actualization of potential of child.	Early identification of primary or secondary risks may prevent or minimize tertiary risks for the child and family.

Women's Health

ACTIONS/INTERVENTIONS	RATIONALES
• Allow patient to describe her perception of her role as a mother, wife, and working woman.	Provides database to initiate care planning.
• Identify sources of role stress and strain that contribute to role conflict and fatigue.	
• Assist in developing a schedule that manages time well, both at home and at work.	

• Involve significant others in planning methods of reducing role stress and strain at home by:
  ○ Assisting with child care
  ○ Assisting with household duties
  ○ Sharing carpooling and children's activities
	Encourages patient to identify various roles she is currently fulfilling and provides support that allows planning of coping strategies and techniques.

• Encourage patient to use time at work for "work activities" and time at home for "home activities"—i.e., do not take work home.	
• Look at possibility of job sharing or part-time employment while children are at home.	
• Plan home activities in advance, such as shopping and cooking meals in advance and freezing them for later use.	
• Encourage division of workload by exchanging child care activities with friends or other families in the neighborhood.	

Psychiatric Health

ACTIONS/INTERVENTIONS	RATIONALES

• Sit with client (number) minutes (number) times per day to discuss client's feelings about self and role performance.
• Answer questions honestly.
• Provide feedback to client about nurse's perceptions of client's abilities and appearance by:
  ◦ Using I statements
  ◦ Using references related to the nurse's relationship to the client
  ◦ Describing the nurse's feelings in the relationship
	Provides information about client's perceptions and expectations that can be utilized in developing specific interventions.
	Promotes the development of a trusting relationship.
	Assists the client in realistically evaluating his or her perceptions.

• Provide positive reinforcement. List here those things, including social rewards, that are reinforcing for the client and when they are to be used. Also list those things that have been identified as nonreinforcers for this client.	Reinforcement encourages positive behavior and enhances self-esteem.
• Provide group interaction with (number) persons (number) minutes 3 times a day at (times). This activity should be gradual within client's ability—e.g., on admission client may tolerate 1 person for 5 min. If the interactions are brief, the frequency should be high—e.g., 5-min interactions should occur at 30-min intervals.	Assists client to experience personal importance to others while enhancing interpersonal relationship skills. Increasing these role competences can enhance self-esteem and promote a positive orientation.
• Reflect back to client negative self-statements made by the client. This should be done with a supportive attitude in a manner that will increase client's awareness of these negative evaluations of self.	This will increase the client's awareness of these statements and facilitate the development of alternative cognitive patterns. Achievement of goals provides reinforcement, which encourages the positive behavior and enhances self-esteem.
• Set achievable goals for the client. • Provide activities that the client can accomplish and that the client values. Care should be taken not to provide tasks that the client finds demeaning, which could actually reinforce client's negative self-evaluation.	Accomplishment of valued tasks provides reinforcement, which encourages positive behavior and enhances self-esteem.
• Provide verbal reinforcement for the achievement of steps toward a goal. • Have client develop a list of his or her strengths and potentials.	Promotes a positive orientation.
• Define the client's lack of goal achievement or failures as simple mistakes that are bound to occur when one attempts something new—e.g., learning comes with mistakes; if one does not make mistakes, one does not learn. • Define past failures as the client's best attempts to solve a problem—e.g., if the client had known of a better solution, he or she would have used it; one does not set out to fail.	Promotes a positive orientation.
• Make necessary items available for the client to groom self. • Spend (number) minutes at (time) assisting the client with grooming, providing necessary assistance and positive reinforcement for accomplishments. • Focus client's attention on the here and now.	Appropriate grooming improves the client's self-evaluation. The nurse's presence can provide positive reinforcement, and reinforcement encourages positive behavior. Past happenings are difficult for the nurse to provide feedback on.
• Present the client with opportunities to make decisions about care, and record these decisions on the chart. • Develop with the client alternative coping strategies.	Promotes client's sense of control and enhances self-esteem. Promotes the development of more adaptive coping behaviors and increases the client's role competence.

Continued

ACTIONS/INTERVENTIONS	RATIONALES
• Practice new coping behavior with client (number) minutes at (time).	Repeated practice of a behavior internalizes and personalizes the behavior.
• Discuss with the client ideal versus current perceptions of role performance.	Assists client in a cognitive appraisal of perceptions to eliminate unrealistic or irrational beliefs.
• Discuss with the client those factors that are perceived to be interfering with role performance.	Assists client in cognitive evaluation of perception of role performance.
• Have the client develop a list of alternatives for resolving interfering factors. This list should be noted here.	Facilitates the development of alternative coping behaviors.
• Establish an appointment with significant others to discuss their perceptions of the client's role performance and their perceptions of the various roles involved in the identified situations. Date and time of this meeting should be written here.	Assists in establishing agreement on the performance of role pairs to decrease role conflict and strain. This is of primary importance since roles occur in interactions.
• Discuss with the client and significant others alterations in role that will facilitate successful performance. Date and time of this meeting should be written here.	
• Develop a specific list of necessary changes, and provide the client system with a written copy.	
• Role-play altered role situations with the client system for 1 h once a day at (time). This would include opportunities for clients to practice those areas of role performance that may be new or unique.	Repeated practice of a behavior internalizes and personalizes the behavior.

• If client and client system cannot achieve agreement on the problematic role refer client to:
  ○ Psychiatric mental health clinical nurse specialist
  ○ Family therapist
  ○ Social worker
	Interactions with the health care system involve role pairs with the role expectations that are present in any social situation. As in any interaction, there can be differing expectations about role performance, which can lead to role conflict and strain.

• If problematic roles involve interactions between client and members of the health care team (nurses, physicians, etc.), request consultation with psychiatric mental health clinical nurse specialist or mental health specialist with experience in the area of resolving system problems, i.e., family therapists or social workers.	

Gerontic Health

ACTIONS/INTERVENTIONS	RATIONALES
• Discuss, with the patient, how he or she perceives that his or her role performance has altered.	Provides opportunity to gain patient's exact perspective on situation. Provides database needed for most effective planning.
• Discuss, with patient, potential role modifications or substitutions, such as foster grandparenting, friendly visitor at a long-term-care facility, participant in intergenerational programs, or telephone reassurance visitor or caller.	Depending on the patient's interests and abilities, these measures would provide an alternate method to achieve role satisfaction.

Home Health

ACTIONS/INTERVENTIONS	RATIONALES
• Monitor for factors contributing to disturbed role performance.	Provides database for early recognition and intervention.
• Involve client and family in planning, implementing, and promoting reduction or elimination of disturbance in role function:	Family involvement in planning increases the likelihood of effective intervention.
∘ Family conference: Clarify expected role performance of all family members.	
∘ Mutual goal setting: Set realistic goals and evaluation criteria. Identify tasks for each family member.	
∘ Communication: Use open, direct communication, and provide positive feedback.	
• Assist client and family in lifestyle adjustments that may be required:	Long-term behavioral changes require support.
∘ Treatment of physical or emotional disability	
∘ Stress management	
∘ Adjustment to changing role functions and relationships	
∘ Development and use of support networks	
∘ Requirements for redistribution of family tasks	
• Consult with assistive resources as indicated.	Utilization of existing services is efficient use of resources. Psychiatric nurse clinician, occupational and physical therapists, and support groups can enhance the treatment plan.

Role Performance, Altered

FLOWCHART EVALUATION: EXPECTED OUTCOME 1

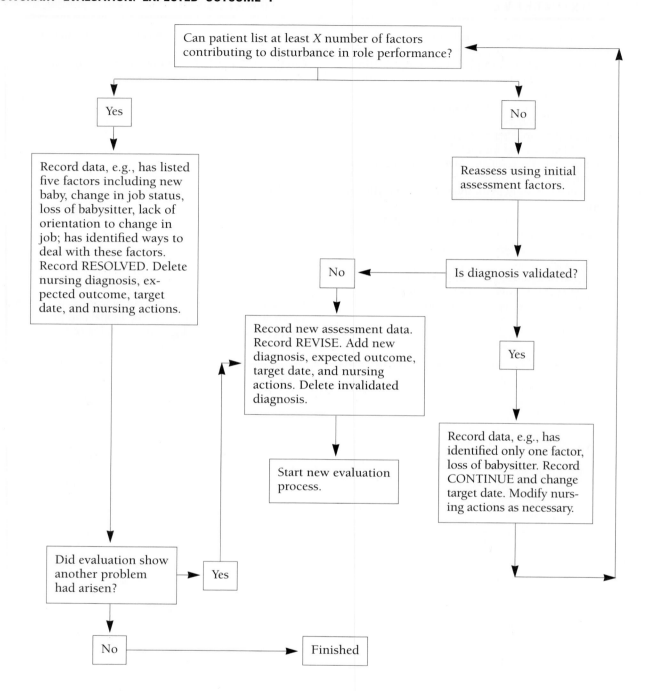

Role Performance, Altered

FLOWCHART EVALUATION: EXPECTED OUTCOME 2

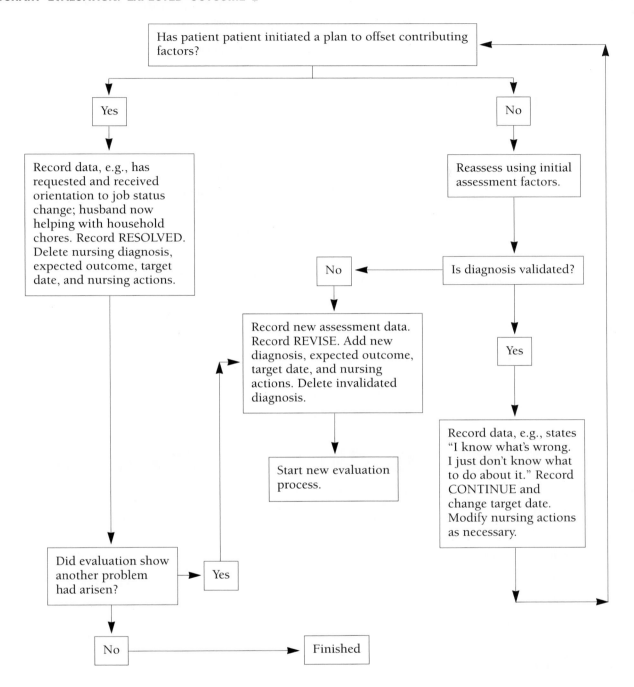

Social Interaction, Impaired

DEFINITION[8]

The state in which an individual participates in an insufficient or excessive quantity or ineffective quality of social exchange.

NANDA TAXONOMY: RELATING 3.1.1

DEFINING CHARACTERISTICS[8]

1. Major defining characteristics
   a. Verbalized or observed discomfort in social situations
   b. Verbalized or observed inability to receive or communicate a satisfying sense of belonging, caring, interest, or shared history
   c. Observed use of unsuccessful social interaction behaviors
   d. Dysfunctional interaction with peers, family, and/or others
2. Minor defining characteristics
   a. Family report of change of style or pattern of interaction

RELATED FACTORS[8]

1. Knowledge or skill deficit about ways to enhance mutuality

2. Communication barriers
3. Self-concept disturbance
4. Absence of available significant others or peers
5. Limited physical mobility
6. Therapeutic isolation
7. Sociocultural dissonance
8. Environmental barriers
9. Altered thought process

RELATED CLINICAL CONCERNS

1. Any condition causing paraplegia, hemiplegia, or quadriplegia
2. AIDS
3. Alzheimer's disease
4. Cancer of the larynx
5. Mental retardation
6. Substance abuse
7. Communicable disease
8. Altered physical appearance secondary to disease or trauma
9. Psychiatric disorders, for example, major depression, borderline personality disorder, or schizoid personality disorder

HAVE YOU SELECTED THE CORRECT DIAGNOSIS?

Knowledge Deficit   This diagnosis, particularly as related to mutuality, would be the most appropriate alternate diagnosis if the individual verbalized or demonstrated an inability to attend to significant others' social actions in the context of independent and dependent aspects of their role.

Impaired Verbal Communication   This would be the most appropriate diagnosis if the individual is unable to receive or send communication. Certainly Impaired Verbal Communication could relate to Impaired Social Interaction and would be the primary problem that has to be resolved.

Social Isolation   This would be the more appropriate diagnosis when the individual is placed in or chooses isolation due to physiologic, sociologic, or emotional concerns. Further assessment is required to completely delineate the exact problem when self-isolation is chosen as the diagnosis.

EXPECTED OUTCOMES

1. Will verbalize satisfaction with quantity and quality of social interactions by (date) and/or
2. Will demonstrate (increased) (decreased) involvement in social interactions by (date)

TARGET DATES

Assisting the patient to modify social interactions will require a significant amount of time. A target date ranging between 7 and 10 days would be appropriate for evaluating progress.

NURSING ACTIONS/INTERVENTIONS WITH RATIONALES
Adult Health

ACTIONS/INTERVENTIONS	RATIONALES
• Encourage patient to express how he or she feels or what he or she fears in a social situation by scheduling at least 10 min twice a day at (times) to focus on this topic.	Assists patient to examine social experience and verbalize feelings. Encourages therapeutic relationship.
• Evaluate patient's communication skills, and help him or her to find alternative ones during interactions with patient.	Improves communication skills.
• Help patient obtain a realistic perception of self by focusing on and enhancing strengths during conferences with patient.	Helps patient to see that no one is perfect, and improves self-concept.
• Role-play social interactions with patient. Allow patient to choose which social interactions he or she wishes to role-play for 10 min twice a day at (times).	Promotes self-confidence in social situations by allowing practice in a safe environment.
• Help patient participate in group interactions; use crutches, wheelchair, or stretcher to get patient out of his or her room at least 2 times per shift, while awake, at (times).	Increases social skills by providing social contact.
• Involve patient in daily care. Help the patient to make decisions about own care.	Improves self-concepts. Increases motivation. Decreases feeling of powerlessness.
• If patient is in isolation, spend at least 10 min every hour with the patient.	Avoids feeling of total isolation for patient.
• Consult with patient's minister, priest, or rabbi as patient desires.	Provides reinforcement for worth of self.
• Initiate referrals to support groups prior to discharge.	Puts patient in contact with community groups to interact with patient to decrease social isolation.

Child Health

ACTIONS/INTERVENTIONS	RATIONALES
• Monitor for contributory factors to altered social interaction pattern, e.g., role-play with puppets.	Provides database needed to plan appropriate care.
• Determine the effect the altered social interaction has on the child, parent, family, and school.	Provides database needed to accurately plan intervention.
• Develop a plan of care to best meet child's potential for succeeding with appropriate social interaction—this will be highly qualified by social class and values.	Individual family values will dictate the way in which social interaction is dealt with.
• Determine if conflict exists between parent's and child's desired social interaction.	Conflict may prevent appropriate attention to actual social interaction but must be dealt with as it will remain a critical component. This may be true particularly at times of authority issues, e.g., adolescence.
• If conflict exists regarding social interaction, deal with this as needed in values or beliefs pattern.	Values and beliefs may be in conflict, and some resolution of the problem is essential to prevent further long-term effects.
• Assist child, parents, and family in ventilation of feelings regarding social interaction impairment, including actual consequences of the impairment.	Ventilation of feelings and the opportunity to do so serve to value the importance for the patient to help reduce anxiety and initiate problem resolution.
• Make referrals as appropriate to professionals best able to assist in dealing with problem, e.g., psychiatric nurse clinical specialist, play therapist, or family therapist.	Referral serves to best deal with problems according to a match of needs and resources.

Continued

ACTIONS/INTERVENTIONS	RATIONALES
• Identify local support groups to appropriately match needs, e.g., parent-child support groups for the handicapped, United Cerebral Palsy Association, or Spina Bifida Association.	Resource groups provide vital support through provision of a common shared sense of concern, coping, and empowerment.
• If impaired social interaction also relates to school, include teacher and essential school personnel in plans for resolving the impairment and for best follow-up.	Valuing the importance of school and the need to provide the best for the child and family in the development of positive social interaction is showing respect for the patient and family.
• Identify follow-up appointment needs and ways to monitor progress for child and family—e.g., stickers as incentives to reinforce desired behavior.	Provides reinforcement and attaches value to follow-up.
• Anticipate discrepant or unrealistic expectations by parents of children. Monitor for potential abuse of child according to pattern for this.	Unrealistic demands or expectations are risk indicators for abuse.

Women's Health

This nursing diagnosis will pertain to women the same as to any other adult. The reader is referred to the other sections—Adult Health, Child Health, Psychiatric Health, Gerontic Health, and Home Health—for specific nursing actions.

Psychiatric Health

ACTIONS/INTERVENTIONS	RATIONALES
• If delusions or hallucinations are present, refer to Sensory-Perceptual Alteration for detailed interventions.	Promotes the development of a trusting relationship.
• Assign primary care nurse to client.	
• Primary nurse will spend (number) minutes twice a day at (times) with client. The focus of this interaction will change as a relationship is developed. Initially the nurse should model for the client how to develop a relationship through his or her behavior in developing this relationship with the client. This modeling should include demonstrating respect for the client, consistency in interaction, congruence between thoughts, feelings, and actions, and empathy.	Promotes the development of a trusting relationship and provides opportunities for the client to observe the nurse in appropriate interpersonal interactions.
• Have client identify those persons in the environment who are considered family, friends, and acquaintances. Then have client note how many interactions per week occur with each person. Have client identify his or her thoughts, feelings, and behavior about these interactions.	Assists the client in reality testing of the belief that he or she is having difficulty with interpersonal relationships.
• Provide appropriate confrontation with client about his or her behavior patterns that inhibit interaction in relationships with the nurse.[13]	Assists client in developing alternative coping behaviors that are adaptive.
• Observe client in interactions with others on the unit, and identify patterns of behavior that inhibit social interaction.	Facilitates the provision of feedback to the client on methods he or she could use to improve interpersonal effectiveness.
• Develop a list of those things the client finds rewarding, and provide these rewards as client successfully completes progressive steps in treatment plan.	Positive reinforcement encourages behavior.
• When client is demonstrating socially inappropriate behavior, keep interactions to a minimum and escort client to a place away from activities.	Continuing the interaction could provide positive reinforcement and encourage inappropriate behavior.

- When inappropriate behavior stops, discuss the behavior with the client and develop a list of alternative kinds of behavior for the client to use in situations where the inappropriate behavior is elicited. Note here those kinds of behavior that are identified as problematic with the action to be taken if they are demonstrated—e.g., client will spend time out in seclusion and away from group activity.

Promotes the client's sense of control and begins the development of alternative, more adaptive coping behaviors. Social isolation assists in decreasing behaviors.

- Develop a schedule for gradually increasing time that the client spends in group activities. For example, client will spend (number) minutes in the group dining hall during mealtimes or will spend (number) minutes in a group game. Note client's specific activities here.

Social interaction can provide positive reinforcement and opportunities for the client to practice new behaviors in a supportive environment.

- Primary nurse will spend 30 min a day with client exploring thoughts and feelings about social interactions and in assisting with reality testing of social interaction—e.g., what others might mean by silence and other nonverbal responses.

- Identify with client areas of social skill deficit, and develop a plan for improving these areas. This could include:
  - Assertiveness training
  - Role-playing difficult situations
  - Teaching client relaxation techniques to reduce anxiety in social situations. (Note here the plan and schedule for implementation. This should be a progressive plan with rewards for accomplishment of each step.)

Promotes the client's sense of control and begins the development of alternative, more adaptive coping behaviors by increasing role competence.

- Consult with occupational therapist if client needs to learn specific skills to facilitate social interactions— e.g., cooking skills so friends can be invited to dinner or craft skills so client can join others in social interactions around these activities.

Increasing behavioral repertoire increases role competence, which enhances self-esteem.[1]

- Include client in group activities on the unit, and assign client activities that can be easily accomplished and that will provide positive social reinforcement from other persons involved in the activities.

Reinforcement encourages positive behavior and enhances self-esteem.

- When client demonstrates tolerance for group interactions, schedule time for the client to participate in a group therapy that provides opportunities for feedback about relationship behavior from peers and for listening to the thoughts and feelings of peers.

Disconfirms the client's sense of aloneness and assists client to experience personal importance to others while enhancing interpersonal relationship skills. Increasing these competencies can enhance self-esteem and promote positive orientation.

- Discuss with support system ways in which they can facilitate client interaction.

Support system understanding facilitates the maintenance of new behaviors after discharge.

- Have client identify those activities in the community that are of interest and would provide opportunities for interaction. List those activities here and develop a plan for client to develop necessary skills to ensure opportunities for interactional success during these activities, e.g., practice a card game or tennis while in the hospital.

Increases the client's ability to successfully perform these roles, which provides positive reinforcement encouraging the behavior and enhancing self-esteem.

- When client reports problems in an interaction, review his or her perceptions of the interaction and evaluation of when the problems began.

Assists the client with reality testing of their perceptions.

- Limit amount of time client can spend alone in room. This should be a gradual alteration and done in steps that can easily be accomplished by the client. Note specific schedule for client here. Have staff person remain with client during these times until client demonstrates an ability to interact with others.

Successful accomplishment of a task provides positive reinforcement and promotes a positive orientation.

- Have referral source make contact with client before discharge and schedule a postdischarge meeting.

Promotes the development of a trusting relationship while the client is in a safe environment.

Gerontic Health

The nursing actions for the gerontic patient with this diagnosis are the same as those given in Adult Health and Psychiatric Health.

Home Health

ACTIONS/INTERVENTIONS	RATIONALES
• Monitor for factors contributing to the impaired social interaction, e.g., psychologic, physical, economic, or spiritual.	Provides database for early recognition and intervention.

• Involve client and family in planning, implementing, and promoting reduction or elimination of impaired social interaction:
  ◦ Family conference: Identify perspective of each member. Establish consistent rules for behaviors.
  ◦ Mutual goal setting: Set consistent rules for behavior and provide support for care providers. Identify tasks for each member.
	Family involvement enhances the effectiveness of the interventions.

• Assist patient and family in lifestyle adjustments that may be required:
  ◦ Providing safe environment
  ◦ Development and use of support networks
  ◦ Change in role functions
  ◦ Prescribed treatments, e.g., medications or behavioral interventions
  ◦ Assistance with self-care activities
  ◦ Possible hospitalization or placement in halfway house
  ◦ Treatment of drug or alcohol abuse
  ◦ Development and practice of social skills
  ◦ Independent living skills
  ◦ Finances
  ◦ Stress management
  ◦ Suicide prevention
	Permanent changes in behavior and family roles require support.

• Assist client and family to develop criteria to determine when crisis exists and professional intervention is necessary:
  ◦ Violence
  ◦ Sudden change in ability to care for self
  ◦ Hallucinations or delusions
	Provides database for early recognition and intervention.

• Consult with or refer patient to assistive resources as indicated.	Utilization of existing services is efficient use of resources. Respite care and support groups can enhance the treatment plan.

Social Interaction, Impaired

FLOWCHART EVALUATION: EXPECTED OUTCOME 1

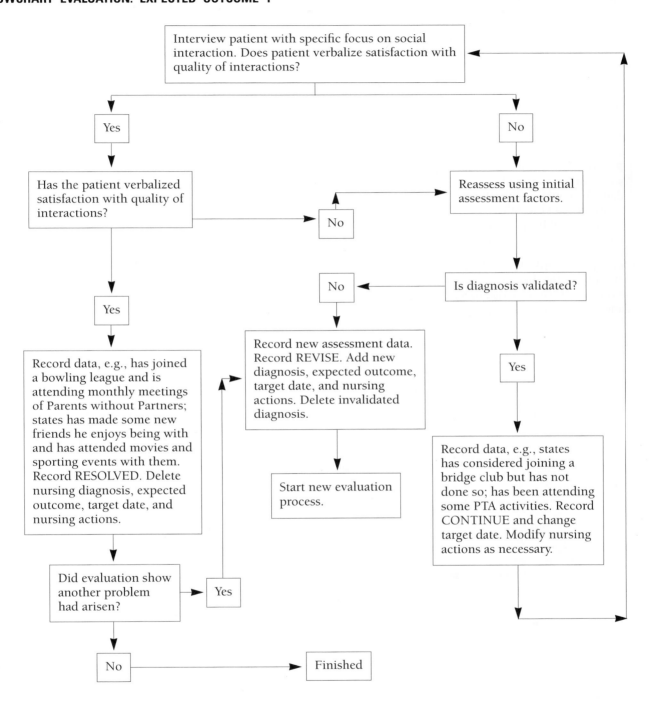

Social Interaction, Impaired

FLOWCHART EVALUATION: EXPECTED OUTCOME 2

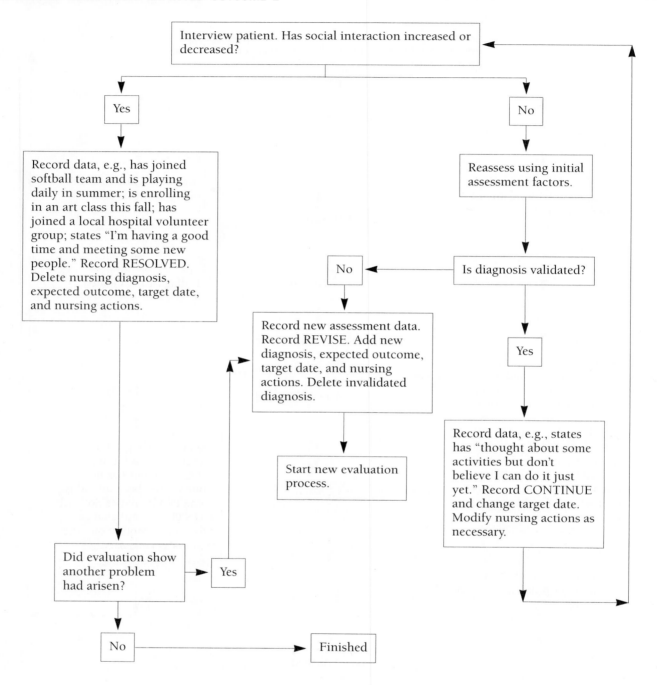

Social Isolation

DEFINITION[8]

Aloneness experienced by the individual and perceived as imposed by others and as a negative or threatened state.

NANDA TAXONOMY: RELATING 3.1.2

DEFINING CHARACTERISTICS[8]

1. Objective
   a. Absence of supportive significant other(s) (family, friends, or group) (*critical*)
   b. Sad, dull affect
   c. Inappropriate or immature interests or activities for development age or stage
   d. Uncommunicative
   e. Withdrawn
   f. No eye contact
   g. Preoccupation with own thoughts
   h. Repetitive meaningless actions
   i. Projects hostility in voice or behavior
   j. Seeks to be alone, or exists in a subculture
   k. Evidence of physical or mental handicap or altered state of wellness
   l. Shows behavior unaccepted by dominant cultural group
2. Subjective
   a. Expresses feelings of aloneness imposed by others (*critical*)
   b. Expresses feelings of rejection (*critical*)
   c. Experiences feelings of difference from others
   d. Inadequacy in or absence of significant purpose in life
   e. Inability to meet expectations of others
   f. Insecurity in public
   g. Expresses values acceptable to the subculture but unacceptable to the dominant cultural group
   h. Expresses interests inappropriate to the developmental age or state

RELATED FACTORS[8]

Factors contributing to the absence of satisfying personal relationships such as:

1. Delay in accomplishing developmental tasks
2. Immature interests
3. Alterations in physical appearance
4. Alterations in mental status
5. Unaccepted social behavior
6. Unaccepted social values
7. Altered state of wellness
8. Inadequate personal resources
9. Inability to engage in satisfying personal relationships

RELATED CLINICAL CONCERNS

1. Any condition that has resulted in scarring
2. Alzheimer's disease
3. AIDS
4. Tuberculosis
5. Any condition causing impaired mobility
6. Psychiatric disorders such as major depression, schizophrenic disorders, paranoid disorders, or conduct disorders

HAVE YOU SELECTED THE CORRECT DIAGNOSIS?

Knowledge Deficit   This diagnosis, particularly as related to mutuality, would be the most appropriate alternate diagnosis if the individual verbalized or demonstrated an inability to attend to significant others' social actions in the context of independent and dependent aspects of his or her role.

Impaired Verbal Communication   This would be the most appropriate diagnosis if the individual is unable to receive or send communication. Certainly Impaired Verbal Communication could relate to Impaired Social Interaction and would be the primary problem that has to be resolved.

Impaired Social Interaction   Impaired social interaction can be either too much or too little in terms of social activity and is more focused on the individual's choice. In Social Isolation the patient sees this problem as being caused by others.

EXPECTED OUTCOMES

1. Will identify at least (number) ways to increase social interaction by (date) and/or
2. Will participate in social activities at least weekly by (date)

TARGET DATES

A target date range of 2 to 7 days would be acceptable depending on the exact social interaction chosen.

NURSING ACTIONS/INTERVENTIONS WITH RATIONALES
Adult Health

ACTIONS/INTERVENTIONS	RATIONALES
• Encourage patient to verbalize feelings of isolation and aloneness by visiting patient every hour and scheduling a discussion for at least 10 min each shift while awake.	Promotes a therapeutic relationship where patient can verbalize in a nonthreatening environment.
• Provide positive feedback and support for social interactional skills as appropriate.	Increases self-confidence. Decreases anxiety in social situations.
• Encourage patient to use assistive or corrective devices such as artificial vocal cord; limb, eye, or breast prosthesis; or special makeup. Have patient return-demonstrate self-care management activities at least daily.	Increases self-esteem and self-confidence.
• Encourage visits from family and significant others daily.	Increases social contacts and interactional skills.
• Encourage patient to participate in diversional activities, especially those involving groups, daily.	Increases social contacts and interactional skills.
• Encourage patient to identify and use community support systems and groups prior to discharge.	Increases social contacts. Promotes assistance with short-term and long-term goals.

Child Health

ACTIONS/INTERVENTIONS	RATIONALES
• Provide opportunities for expression of feelings about desired social activity by spending 15–20 min per shift, during waking hours, at (times) with patient and family.	Ventilation allows for insight into patient's thinking and assists in reducing anxiety.
• Determine what obstacles are perceived by patient and family in pursuit of desired social activities by asking both direct and open-ended questions—e.g., "What do you think prevents you from doing what you want to?"	Directed inquiry into obstacles that prevent the patient from engaging in desired social interaction increases the likelihood of a more complete database that will allow more individualized planning.
• Identify what realistic patterns for socialization are applicable for patient and family in collaboration with the patient and family.	Realistic goals are more likely to bring about the desired changes for more effective social interaction.
• Collaborate with other health care professionals to meet realistic goals for patient and family socialization.	Appropriate use of resource personnel ensures optimal likelihood for goal attainment.
• Monitor for contributory related factors to best consider social activity pattern.	All factors must be considered to provide a holistic plan of care.
• Identify support groups to assist in realization of desired social activities.	Support groups provide a sense of sharing and empowerment.
• Monitor patient's and family's perceptions of the effect desired social activities might have on current role-relationship pattern.	Roles are closely impacted by patterns of social interaction.
• Provide appropriate opportunities for assessment of young child's perceptions of situational needs and how he or she views self.	The child's view of self in relationship to social patterns is vital to planning the most effective interventions.
• Assist patient to develop schedule for consideration of desired social activities at least 2 days before dismissal from hospital.	Appropriate planning serves to increase success with desired activities.
• Provide for appropriate follow-up appointment as needed previous to dismissal from hospital.	Follow-up plans attach value to long-term care for the patient.

Women's Health

The following nursing actions apply to the social isolation experienced by the patient who has sexually transmitted diseases such as herpes genitalis, syphilis, chlamydia, gonorrhea, and AIDS.

ACTIONS/INTERVENTIONS	RATIONALES

• Assure patient of confidentiality.
• Refer for counseling and/or treatment to:
  ○ Support groups
  ○ Professionals, e.g., public health clinic, nurse specialists, or physician
	Promotes sharing of information by patient.
	Provides long-term support and care for patient.

• Provide a nonjudgmental atmosphere to[38] encourage verbalization of concerns:
  ○ Recurrent nature of disease, especially herpes and chlamydia
  ○ Lack of cure for disease (AIDS)
  ○ Economics in treating disease
  ○ Social stigma associated with disease
  ○ Opportunity for entrance into health care system
• Encourage honesty in answers to such questions as:
  ○ Multiple sexual partners (identify contacts)
  ○ Describing sexual behavior
	Provides database needed to provide appropriate care and teaching.

• Encourage honest communication with sexual partners.	Sexual partners will need to seek health care also.

Psychiatric Health

ACTIONS/INTERVENTIONS	RATIONALES
• If delusions and/or hallucinations are present, refer to Sensory-Perceptual Alteration for detailed interventions.	Assists in understanding the client's worldview, which facilitates the development of specific interventions.
• If social isolation is related to client's feelings of powerlessness, refer to Powerlessness (Chap. 8) for detailed interventions. • Discuss with client his or her perception of the source of the social isolation and have him or her list those things he or she has tried to resolve the situation.	
• Have client list those persons in the environment that are considered family, friends, and acquaintances. Then have client note how many interactions per week occur with each person. Have client identify what interferes with feeling connected with these persons. This activity should be implemented by the primary nurse. Note schedule for this interaction here.	Facilitates the client's reality testing of his or her perception of being socially isolated.

• When contributing factors have been identified, develop a plan to alter these factors. This could include:
  ○ Assertiveness training
  ○ Role-playing difficult situations
  ○ Teaching client relaxation techniques to reduce anxiety in social situations. (Note plan and schedule for implementation here.)
	Facilitates the development of alternative coping behaviors that enhance role performance.

• Develop a list of those things the client finds rewarding and provide these rewards as client successfully completes progressive steps in treatment plan. This schedule should be developed with the client. Note here the schedule for rewards and the kinds of behavior to be rewarded.	Reinforcement encourages positive behavior and enhances self-esteem.

Continued

ACTIONS/INTERVENTIONS	RATIONALES
• Consult with occupational therapist if client needs to learn specific skills to facilitate social interactions— e.g., cooking skills so friends can be invited to dinner, craft skills so client can join others in social interactions around these activities, or dancing.	Increases the client's competencies, which enhances role performance and self-esteem.
• Provide client with those prostheses necessary to facilitate social interactions, e.g., hearing aids or eyeglasses. Note here the assistance needed from nursing staff in providing these to client. Also note where they are to be stored while not in use.	
• Include client in group activities on the unit. Assign client activities that can be easily accomplished and that will provide positive social reinforcement from another person involved in the activities. This could include things like having client assume responsibility for preparing a part of a group meal or for serving a portion of a meal, etc.	Successful accomplishment of a valued task can provide positive reinforcement that encourages behavior.
• Role-play with client those social interactions identified as most difficult. This will be done by primary nurse. Note schedule for this activity here.	Repeated practice of a behavior internalizes and personalizes the behavior.
• Discuss with client those times it would be appropriate to be alone, and develop a plan for coping with these times in a positive manner—e.g., client will develop a list of books to read, music to listen to, or community activities to attend.	Promotes the client's sense of control while facilitating the development of alternative coping behaviors.
• When client is demonstrating socially inappropriate behavior, keep interactions to a minimum, and escort him or her to a place away from group activities.	Lack of positive reinforcement decreases a behavior.
• When inappropriate behavior stops, discuss the behavior with the client, and develop a list of alternative kinds of behavior for the client to use in situations in which the inappropriate behavior is elicited. Note here those kinds of behavior that are identified as problematic with the action to be taken if they are demonstrated—e.g., client will spend a time-out in seclusion or sleeping area.	Promotes client's sense of control while facilitating the development of alternative coping behaviors.
• Develop a schedule of gradually increasing time for client in group activities—e.g., client will spend (number) minutes in the group dining hall during meal times or will spend (number) minutes in a group game twice a day. Note specific goals for client here.	Provides client with opportunities to practice new behaviors in a safe, supportive environment.
• Primary nurse will spend 30 min once a day with client at (time) discussing client's reactions to social interactions and in assisting client with reality testing social interactions—e.g., what others might mean by silence or various nonverbal and verbal expressions. This time can also be used to discuss relationship roles and client's specific concerns about relationships.	
• Assign client a room near areas with high activity.	Facilitates client's participation in unit activities. Decreases the client's opportunities for socially isolating self.
• Assign one staff person to the client each shift, and have this person interact with client every 30 min while awake.	
• Be open and direct with client in interactions, and avoid verbal and nonverbal behavior that requires interpretation from client.	Promotes a trusting relationship.
• Have client tell staff his or her interpretation of interactions.	Assists client in reality testing his or her perceptions that might inhibit social interactions.
• Have client identify those activities in the community that are of interest and would provide opportunities for interactions with others. List client's interests here.	Promotes the client's sense of control.

- Develop, with the client, a plan for making contact with the identified community activities groups before discharge.
- When client demonstrates tolerance for group interactions, schedule time for the client to participate in a therapy group that provides opportunities for feedback about relationship behavior from peers and for listening to the thoughts and feelings of peers.
- Arrange at least 1 h a week for client to interact with support system in the presence of the primary nurse. This will allow the nurse to assess and facilitate these interactions.
- Discuss with support system ways in which they can facilitate client interaction.
- Model for support system and for client those kinds of behaviors that facilitate communication.[39]
- Limit the amount of time client can spend alone in room. This should be a gradual alteration and should be done in steps that can be easily accomplished by client. Note specific schedule for client here—e.g., client will spend 5 min per hour out in day area. Have staff person remain with client during these times until client demonstrates an ability to interact with others.
- Refer client to appropriate community agencies.

Promotes the client's sense of control and begins the development of adaptive coping behaviors.

Disconfirms the client's sense of aloneness and assists client to experience personal importance to others while enhancing interpersonal relationship skills. Increasing these competencies can enhance self-esteem and promote positive orientation.
Support system understanding facilitates the maintenance of new behaviors after discharge.

Provides opportunities for client to practice new role behaviors in a safe, supportive environment.

Gerontic Health

ACTIONS/INTERVENTIONS	RATIONALES
• Discuss with patient what efforts he or she has made to increase social contacts and what results have been obtained.	Assists in determining what interventions may result in positive outcomes.
• Ask patient to identify hobbies and activities that have been a part of his or her adult life.	Provides information on preferred activities and guides the nurse in seeking resources that match the patient's interests.
• Ask patient to identify barriers to continuing with the hobbies and activities he or she enjoyed.	Barriers may be indicators of need for use of specific resources such as adaptive equipment or transportation.
• Assist patient in identifying and contacting community support services.	In many areas, initial contact with support services can entail numerous telephone calls to reach the appropriate resource.

Home Health

NOTE: See Psychiatric Health nursing actions for detailed interventions.

ACTIONS/INTERVENTIONS	RATIONALES

• Involve client and family in planning and implementing strategies to reduce social isolation:
  ○ Family conference: Discuss perceptions of source of social isolation and list possible solutions.
  ○ Mutual goal setting: Set realistic goals with evaluation criteria. List specific tasks for each family member.
	Family involvement in planning enhances the effectiveness of interventions.

Continued

ACTIONS/INTERVENTIONS	RATIONALES

○ Communication: Provide positive feedback.
• Assist family and patient with lifestyle adjustments that may be required:
  ○ Promote social interaction.
  ○ Provide transportation.
  ○ Provide activities to keep busy during lonely times.
  ○ Provide communication alternatives for those with sensory deficits.
  ○ Assist with disfiguring illness—e.g., refer patient to enterostomal therapist or prosthesis manufacturer.
  ○ Control incontinence or provide absorbent undergarments when socializing.
  ○ Promote self-worth.
  ○ Promote self-care.
  ○ Develop and utilize support groups.
  ○ Use pets.
  ○ Establish regular telephone contact.
  ○ Inform patient of volunteer programs in the community that he or she could work for.
• Consult with or refer patient to assistive resources as indicated.
	Permanent changes in behavior and family roles require support.
	
	Utilization of existing services is efficient use of resources. Self-help groups, occupational therapists, or home-bound programs can enhance the treatment plan.

Social Isolation

FLOWCHART EVALUATION: EXPECTED OUTCOME 1

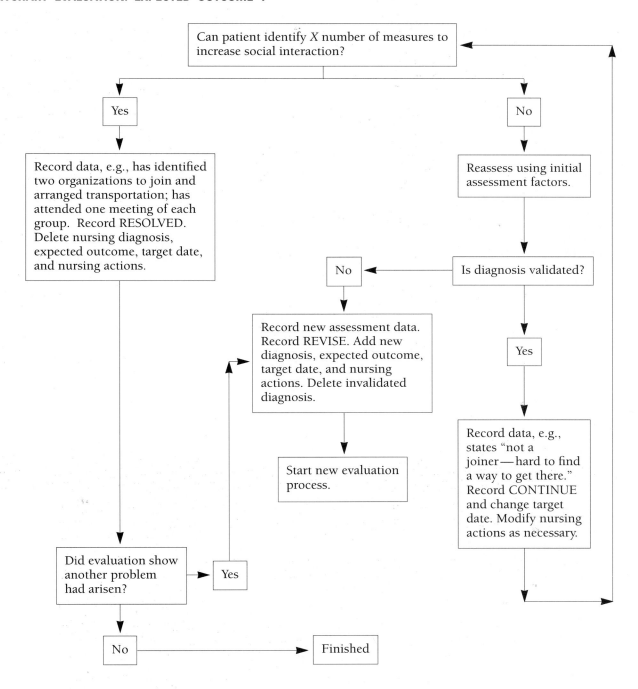

Social Isolation

FLOWCHART EVALUATION: EXPECTED OUTCOME 2

Verbal Communication, Impaired

DEFINITION[8]

The state in which an individual experiences a decreased or absent ability to use or understand language in human interaction.

NANDA TAXONOMY: COMMUNICATING 2.1.1.1

DEFINING CHARACTERISTICS[8]

1. Major defining characteristics
   a. Is unable to speak dominant language (*critical*)
   b. Speaks or verbalizes with difficulty (*critical*)
   c. Does not or cannot speak (*critical*)
   d. Stutters
   e. Slurs speech
   f. Has difficulty forming words or sentences
   g. Has difficulty expressing thought verbally
   h. Uses inappropriate verbalization
   i. Experiences dyspnea
   j. Experiences disorientation
2. Minor defining characteristics
   None given

RELATED FACTORS[8]

1. Decrease in circulation to brain
2. Brain tumor
3. Physical barrier (tracheostomy or intubation)
4. Anatomical defect such as cleft palate
5. Psychological barriers (psychosis or lack of stimuli)
6. Cultural difference
7. Developmental or age-related impairments

RELATED CLINICAL CONCERNS

1. Laryngeal cancer
2. Cleft lip or cleft plate
3. Cerebrovascular accident
4. Facial trauma
5. Respiratory distress
6. Late-stage Alzheimer's disease
7. Tourette's disorder
8. Psychiatric disorders such as schizophrenic disorders, delusional disorders, psychotic disorders, or delirium
9. Autism

HAVE YOU SELECTED THE CORRECT DIAGNOSIS?

Social Isolation   Social Isolation can occur because of the reduced ability or inability of an individual to use language as a means of communication. The primary diagnosis would be Impaired Verbal Communication since resolution of the problem would assist in alleviating Social Isolation.

Sensory-Perceptual Alteration (Auditory)   If the individual has difficulty in hearing, then he or she would also reflect Impaired Verbal Communication. The primary problem would be the Auditory difficulty since correcting of this deficit would help improve communication.

EXPECTED OUTCOMES

1. Will verbalize satisfaction with communication process by (date) and/or
2. Will communicate in a clear manner via (state specific method, e.g., orally, esophageal speech, or computer) by (date)

TARGET DATES

The target date for resolution of this diagnosis will be long-range. However, 7 days would be appropriate for an initial evaluation.

NURSING ACTIONS/INTERVENTIONS WITH RATIONALES
Adult Health

ACTIONS/INTERVENTIONS	RATIONALES

• Maintain a patient, calm approach by:
  ○ Allowing adequate time for communication
  ○ Not interrupting the patient or attempting to finish sentences for him or her
	Avoids interfering with patient's communication attempts.

Continued

ACTIONS/INTERVENTIONS	RATIONALES
○ Asking questions that require short answers or a nod of the head ○ Anticipating needs • Provide materials that can be used to assist in communication—e.g., magic slate, flash cards, pad and pencil, "Speak and Spell" computer toy, pictures, or letter board.	Provides alternative methods of communication. Decreases anxiety and feelings of powerlessness and isolation.
• Inform family, significant others, and other health care personnel of the effective ways patient communicates.	Promotes effective communication. Prevents frustration in patient.
• Answer call bell promptly rather than using the intercom system.	Decreases stress for patient by not straining communication resources.
• Assure patient that parenteral therapy does not interfere with patient's ability to write.	Decreases anxiety.
• Initiate referral to speech therapist if appropriate.	Initial teaching regarding speech may need interventions by specialist.
• Initiate referrals to support agencies such as Lost Chord Club or New Voice Club as appropriate.	Groups that experienced the same problems can assist in rehabilitation and decrease social isolation. Promotes patient's comfort.
• Discuss use of electronic voice box and esophageal speech prior to discharge. Have patient practice using device.	Reduces anxiety and increases self-confidence.
• Encourage patient to have recordings made for reaching police, fire department, doctor, or emergency medical service if impaired verbal communication is a long-term condition.	Promotes safety, increases comfort, and decreases anxiety.

Child Health

ACTIONS/INTERVENTIONS	RATIONALES
• Monitor patient's potential for speech according to subjective and objective components to include: ○ Reported or documented previous speech capacity or potential ○ Health history for evidence of cognitive, sensory, perceptual, or neurologic dysfunction ○ Actual auditory documentation of speech potential ○ Assessment done by speech specialist ○ Patterns of speech of parents and significant others ○ Cultural meaning attached to speech or silence of children ○ Any related trauma or pathophysiology ○ Parental perception of child's status, especially in instances of congenital anomaly such as cleft lip or palate ○ Identification of dominant language and secondary languages heard or spoken in family	Provides database needed to plan more complete and accurate interventions.
• Assist the patient and parents to understand needed explanations for procedures, treatments, and equipment to be used in nursing care.	Provides teaching opportunity. Decreases anxiety, which can interfere with communication.
• Encourage feelings to be expressed by taking time to understand possible attempts at speech. Use pictures if necessary for young children.	Alternate methods of communication and sensitivity to attempts at communication attach value to the patient and serve to reinforce future attempts at communication.
• Encourage family participation in care of patient as situation allows.	Family input provides an opportunity for communication and fosters parent-child relationship.
• Assist family to identify community support groups.	Provides long-term support for coping.

- Assist patient and family in determining the impact Altered Verbal Communication may have for family functioning.
- Provide information for long-term medical follow-up as indicated, especially for congenital anomalies.
- Assist in identification of appropriate financial support if child is able to qualify for help according to state and federal legislation.
- Monitor for potential for related alterations in role-relationship patterns as a result of Altered Verbal Communication.
- Monitor potential for related alterations in self-concept or coping patterns as a result of Altered Verbal Communication.
- Provide appropriate patient and family teaching for care of patient if permanent tracheostomy or related prosthetic is to be used to include:
  - Appropriate number or size of tracheostomy tube
  - Appropriate duplication of size of tracheostomy tube in place in event of accidental dislodging or loss
  - Appropriate administration of oxygen via trach adapter
  - Appropriate suctioning technique, sterile and nonsterile
  - Appropriate list of supplies and how to procure them
  - Resources for actual care in emergency, with list of numbers including ambulance and nearest hospital
  - Appropriate indications for notification of physician (*Note*: These may vary slightly according to physician's plan or actual patient status.)
    (1) Bleeding from tracheostomy
    (2) Coughing out or dislodging of tracheostomy
    (3) Difficulty in passing catheter to suction tracheostomy
    (4) Fever above 101°F
    (5) Appropriate daily hygiene of tracheostomy
    (6) Caution regarding use of regular gauze or other substances that might be inhaled or ingested through tracheostomy
    (7) Need for humidification of tracheostomy

Provides long-term support for coping.
Family functioning relies heavily on communication.

Knowledge helps to prepare family for long-term needs and helps reduce anxiety about unknowns.
Funding by third-party payment may be available depending on patient's medical status.

Alterations in communication can affect the role-relationship pattern.

Alterations in communication may impact self-esteem and should be considered as a risk factor.

Basic standards of care for the patient with a tracheostomy.

Women's Health

This nursing diagnosis will pertain to women the same as to any other adult. The reader is referred to the other sections—Adult Health, Psychiatric Health, and Home Health.

Psychiatric Health

If impaired communication is related to alterations in physiology or surgical alterations, refer to Adult Health nursing actions.

ACTIONS/INTERVENTIONS	RATIONALES
- Establish a calm, reassuring environment.	Inappropriate levels of sensory stimuli can increase confusion and disorganization.
- Provide client with a private environment if experiencing high levels of anxiety to assist him or her in focusing on relevant stimuli.	High levels of anxiety decrease the client's ability to process information.

Continued

ACTIONS/INTERVENTIONS	RATIONALES

• Communicate with client in clear, concise language:
  ○ Speak slowly to client.
  ○ Do not shout.
  ○ Face client when talking to him or her.
  ○ Role-model agreement between verbal and nonverbal behavior.
	Inappropriate levels of sensory stimuli can increase confusion and disorganization. When verbal and nonverbal behavior are not in agreement, a double-bind or incongruent message may be sent. These incongruent messages place the receiver in a "darned if you do, darned if you don't" situation and promote interpersonal ineffectiveness.

• Spend 30 min twice a day at (times) with client discussing communication patterns. This time could also include, as the client progresses:
  ○ Constructive confrontation about the effects of the dysfunctional communication pattern on relationships
  ○ Role-playing appropriate communication patterns
  ○ Pointing out to client the lack of agreement between verbal and nonverbal behavior and context
  ○ Helping client to understand purpose of dysfunctional communication patterns
  ○ Developing alternative ways for client to have needs met
	Promotes the development of a trusting relationship while providing the client a safe environment in which to practice new behaviors. Behavioral rehearsal helps to facilitate the client's learning new skills through the use of feedback and modeling by the nurse.

• Develop, with the client's assistance, a reward program for appropriate communication patterns and for progress on goals. Note here the kinds of behavior to be rewarded and schedule for reward.	Reinforcement encourages positive behavior while enhancing self-esteem.
• Instruct client in assertive communication techniques, and practice these in daily interactions with the client. Note here those assertive skills client is to practice and how these are to be practiced—e.g., each medication is to be requested by the client in an assertive manner.	Assertiveness improves the individual's ability to act appropriately and effectively in a manner that maximizes coping resources.[35]
• Provide the client with positive verbal rewards for appropriate communication.	Reinforcement encourages positive behavior.
• Sit with client while another client is asked for feedback about an interaction.	The nurse's presence provides support while the client can receive feedback on interpersonal skills from a peer.
• Keep interactions brief and goal directed when client is communicating in dysfunctional manner.	Inappropriate levels of sensory stimuli can increase confusion and disorganization.
• Spend an extra 5 min in interactions in which client is communicating clearly, and inform client of this reward of time.	Time with the nurse can provide positive reinforcement.
• Reward improvement in client's listening behavior. This can be evaluated by having the client repeat what has just been heard. Provide clarification for the differences between what was heard and what was said.	Improved attending skills improve the client's ability to understand communication from others and to clarify unclear portions of communication.
• Have support system participate in one interaction per week with the client in the presence of a staff member. The staff member will facilitate communication between the client and the support system. Note time for these interactions here with the name of the staff person responsible for this process.	Behavioral rehearsal provides opportunities for feedback and modeling from the nurse. Support system understanding facilitates the maintenance of new behaviors after discharge.
• Arrange for client to participate in a therapeutic group. Note schedule for these groups here.	Provides an opportunity for the client to receive feedback on communication from peers and to observe the interactions of peers so that they may increase their requisite variety of responses in social situation. Models appropriate communication skills for the client.
• Request that client clarify unclear statements or communications in private language.	
• Teach client to request clarification on confusing communications. This may be practiced with role-play.	Repeated practice of a behavior internalizes and personalizes the behavior.
• Include client in unit activities and assign appropriate tasks to client. These should require a level of communication the client can easily achieve so that a positive learning experience can occur. Note level of activity appropriate for client here.	Provides opportunities for the client to practice new behaviors in a supportive environment.

- If communication problems evolve from a language difference, have someone who understands the language orient the client to the unit as soon as possible and answer any questions the client might have.
- Use nonverbal communication to interact with client when there is no one available to translate.
- Obtain information about nonverbal communication in the client's culture and about appropriate psychosocial behavior. Alter interactions and expectations to fit these beliefs as they fit the client. Note here that information that is important in providing daily care for this client.
- Determine if the client understands any English and if so how it is best understood—i.e., written or spoken.
- If client does not understand English, determine if a language other than the one from the culture of origin is spoken. Perhaps a common language for staff and client can be found—e.g., few people other than Navajos speak Navajo, but some older Navajos also speak Spanish.
- Do not shout when talking with someone who speaks another language. Speak slowly and concisely.
- Use pictures to enhance nonverbal communication.

- If a staff member does not speak the client's language, arrange for a translator to visit with the client at least once a day to answer questions and provide information. Have a schedule for the next day available so that it can be reviewed with the client and information can be provided about complex procedures. Have a staff member remain with the client during these interactions to serve as a resource person for the translator. Allow time for the client to ask questions and express feelings. Note schedule for these visits here with the name of the translator.

Decreases the client's sense of isolation and anxiety.

Decreases the client's sense of social isolation and promotes the development of a trusting relationship. Decreases the possibilities for misunderstandings to develop.

Promotes the development of a trusting relationship.

Communication facilitates social interaction and increases the client's sense of control.

Inappropriate levels of sensory stimulation can increase confusion and disorganization.
Pictures facilitate communication when the caregiver and client do not share the same language.
Promotes the client's sense of control and decreases social isolation.

Gerontic Health

The nursing actions for a gerontic patient with this diagnosis are the same as those given in Adult Health and Psychiatric Health.

Home Health

ACTIONS/INTERVENTIONS	RATIONALES
• Involve client and family in planning and implementing strategies to decrease, prevent, or cope with impaired verbal communication: ○ Family conference: Discuss each member's perspective of the situation.	Family involvement enhances effectiveness of interventions.

Continued

ACTIONS/INTERVENTIONS	RATIONALES
○ Mutual goal setting: Set short-term accomplishable goals with evaluation criteria; specify tasks for each member.	
○ Communication: Identify ways to communicate with client.	
• Teach client and family appropriate information regarding the care of a person with impaired verbal communication:	Knowledge bases required to interact with family member who is verbally impaired.
○ Use of pencil and paper, alphabet letters, head signals, sign language, pictures, flash cards, or computer	
○ Use of repetition	
○ Facing the person when communicating	
○ Use of simple, one-step commands	
○ Allowing time for person to respond	
○ Use of drawing, painting, coloring, singing, or exercising	
○ Identifying tasks the person with impaired verbal communication can do well	
○ Decreasing external noise	
• Assist patient and family in lifestyle adjustments that may be required:	Lifestyle changes require long-term behavioral changes. Support enhances permanent changes in behavior.
○ Stress management	
○ Changing role functions and relationships	
○ Learning a foreign language	
○ Acknowledging and coping with frustration with communication efforts	
○ Obtaining necessary supportive equipment, e.g., hearing aid, special telephone, or artificial larynx	
• Consult with or refer patient to appropriate assistive resources as required.	Self-help groups and rehabilitation services can enhance the treatment plans.

Verbal Communication, Impaired

FLOWCHART EVALUATION: EXPECTED OUTCOME 1

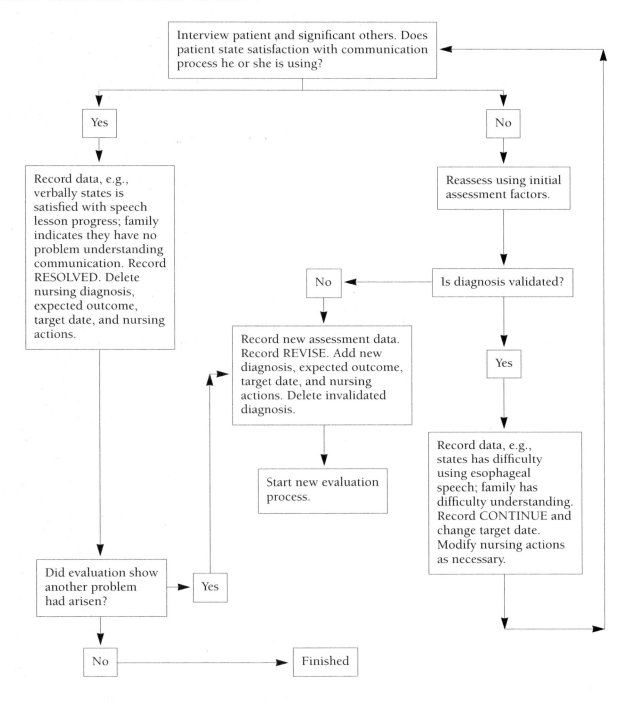

Verbal Communication, Impaired

FLOWCHART EVALUATION: EXPECTED OUTCOME 2

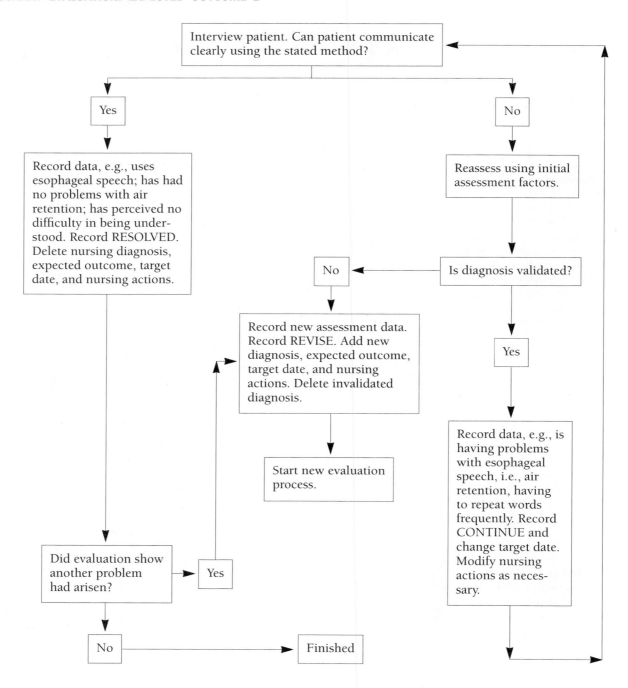

Violence, Risk for: Self-Directed or Directed at Others

DEFINITION[8]

RISK FOR VIOLENCE: DIRECTED AT OTHERS Behaviors in which an individual demonstrates that he or she can be physically, emotionally, and/or sexually harmful to others.

RISK FOR VIOLENCE: SELF-DIRECTED Behaviors in which an individual demonstrates that he or she can be physically, emotionally, and/or sexually harmful to self.

NANDA TAXONOMY: FEELING 9.2.2

DEFINING CHARACTERISTICS[8]

1. Risk factors—Risk for Violence: Directed at others
   a. History of violence:
      (1) *Against others*: Hitting someone, kicking someone, spitting at someone, scratching someone, throwing objects at someone, biting someone, attempted rape, rape, sexual molestation, or urinating or defecating on a person
      (2) *Threats*: Verbal threats against property, verbal threats against person, social threats, cursing, threatening notes or letters, threatening gestures, or sexual threats
      (3) *Against self*: Suicidal threats or attempts, hitting or injuring self, or banging head against wall
      (4) *Social*: Stealing, insistent borrowing, insistent demands for privileges, insistent interruption of meetings, refusal to eat, refusal to take medication, or ignoring instructions
      (5) *Indirect*: Tearing off clothes, ripping objects off walls, writing on wall, urinating on floor, defecating on floor, stamping feet, temper tantrums, running in corridors, yelling, throwing objects, breaking a window, slamming doors, or sexual advances
   b. Neurological impairment: Positive EEG, CAT, or MRI; head trauma; positive neurological findings; or seizure disorders
   c. Cognitive impairment: Learning disabilities, attention deficit disorder, or decreased intellectual functioning
   d. History of childhood abuse
   e. History of witnessing family violence
   f. Cruelty to animals
   g. Firesetting
   h. Prenatal and perinatal complications or abnormalities
   i. History of drug or alcohol abuse
   j. Pathological intoxication
   k. *Psychotic symptomatology*: Auditory, visual, or command hallucinations; paranoid delusions; or loose, rambling, or illogical thought processes
   l. *Motor vehicle offenses*: Frequent traffic violations, or use of motor vehicle to release anger
   m. Suicidal behavior
   n. Impulsivity
   o. Availability and/or possession of weapon(s)
   p. *Body language*: Rigid posture, clenching of fists and jaw, hyperactivity, pacing, breathlessness, and threatening stances

2. Risk factors—Risk for Violence: Self-directed
   a. Age 15 to 19 or over 45
   b. *Marital status*: Single, widowed, or divorced
   c. *Employment*: Unemployed; or recent job loss or failure
   d. *Occupation*: Executive, administrator, owner of business, professional, or semiskilled worker
   e. *Interpersonal relationships*: Conflictual
   f. *Family background*: Chaotic or conflictual or history of suicide
   g. *Sexual orientation*: Active bisexual or inactive homosexual
   h. *Physical health*: Hypochondriac or chronic or terminal illness
   i. *Mental health*: Severe depression, psychosis, severe personality disorder, or alcohol or drug abuse
   j. *Emotional status*: Hopelessness, despair, increased anxiety, panic, anger, or hostility
   k. History of multiple attempts
   l. *Suicidal ideation*: Frequent, intense, or prolonged
   m. *Suicidal plan*: Clear and specific
   n. *Lethality*: Method and availability of destructive means
   o. *Personal resources*: Poor achievement, poor insight, or affect unavailable and poorly controlled
   p. *Social resources*: Poor rapport, socially isolated, or unresponsive family
   q. *Verbal clues*: Talking about death, "better off without me," or asking questions about lethal dosages of drugs
   r. *Behavioral clues*: Writing forlorn love notes, directing angry messages at a significant other who has rejected the person, giving away personal items, or taking out a large life insurance policy
   s. Persons who engage in autoerotic sexual acts

RELATED FACTORS[8]

1. Antisocial character
2. Battered women
3. Catatonic excitement
4. Child abuse
5. Manic excitement
6. Organic brain syndrome
7. Panic states
8. Rage reactions
9. Suicidal behavior
10. Temporal lobe epilepsy
11. Toxic reactions to medication

RELATED CLINICAL CONCERNS

1. Physical abuse
2. Organic brain syndrome; Alzheimer's disease
3. Attempted suicide
4. Epilepsy, temporal lobe
5. Panic episode

STOP

HAVE YOU SELECTED THE CORRECT DIAGNOSIS?

Ineffective Family Coping, Disabled or Compromised This diagnosis relates to the inability of the primary caregiver or caretaker to meet the needs of the patient. No violence is included in this diagnosis. If abuse has been assessed, then the diagnosis should be changed.

Altered Parenting This diagnosis relates to the relationship between the nurturing figure and the child. Child abuse is included within this diagnosis, but as an actual fact, not as a risk for. If a risk for abuse exists, then Risk for Violence is the most appropriate diagnosis.

EXPECTED OUTCOMES

1. Will demonstrate at least (number) alternative methods for releasing anger by (date) and/or
2. Will identify factors that contribute to risk for violence by (date)

TARGET DATES

For the sake of all concerned, the patient should begin to demonstrate progress within 3 to 5 days. However, the patient must be monitored on a daily basis. To totally control violent behavior may take months.

NURSING ACTIONS/INTERVENTIONS WITH RATIONALES

Adult Health

ACTIONS/INTERVENTIONS	RATIONALES
• Refer patient to psychiatric nurse clinician (see Psychiatric Health nursing actions).	Violence or risk for violence requires specific interventions by a specialist in the area of mental health. Monitors for deterioration of condition and promotes early intervention.
• Monitor for signs of anger or distress such as restlessness, pacing, wringing of hands, or verbally abusive behavior.	
• Accept anger of patient, but do not participate in it when interacting with patient.	Anger is an acceptable emotion if appropriately handled but escalation of anger is to be avoided.
• Remain calm. Set limits on patient's behavior, and reduce environmental stimuli.	Decreases sensory stimuli. Decreases anxiety- and violence-provoking situations.
• Encourage patient to verbalize angry feelings rather than physically demonstrating them or to physically demonstrate them in a constructive way—e.g., working out on a punching bag, banging a trash can, or taking a walk. Schedule 30 min twice a day at (times) to confer with patient regarding this topic.	Promotes an acceptable alternative strategy for dealing with anger.
• Let the patient know that he or she has control of and is responsible for own actions. Help patient identify situations that interfere with his or her control during conferences with patient.	Reinforces reality and maintains limits on behavior.
• Provide a safe environment by removing clutter, breakables, or potential weapons. Restrain or seclude patient as needed.	Promotes safety and reduces risk of harm to patients or others.
• Observe, at least once an hour, for indications of suicidal behavior, e.g., withdrawal, depression, or ~ning and organizing for attempt.	Prevents self-inflicted violence.
~ lications as ordered (tranquilizer, sedative, ~itor effects of medication.	Determines effectiveness of medication as well as monitoring for unwanted side effects.

Child Health

ACTIONS/INTERVENTIONS	RATIONALES
• Assist patient and family to describe usual patterns of role-relationship activities.	Insight into role-relationships is basic in determining the risk for violence.
• Monitor for precipitating or triggering events that seem to recur as the pattern for violence is explored.	Risk indicators can be identified as assessment for repeated violence is made.
• Assist the patient and family to describe own perception of the actual or potential violence pattern.	Insight of patient or parents reveals basic data about the violence pattern that assists in accurate intervention.
• Provide opportunities for expression of emotions related to the violence appropriate for age and developmental capacity—e.g., a toddler could use dolls, puppets, or other noninvasive methods.	Expression of thoughts and feelings in a directed age-appropriate manner helps the child understand the impact of the violence and assists in reducing his or her anxiety.
• Provide appropriate collaboration for long-term follow-up regarding appropriate intervention.	Valuing long-term follow-up fosters compliance and shows sensitivity to the patient's needs for long-term support. Safety is also at risk. In many instances, legal mandates will dictate exact protocols to be enforced.
• Provide for role-taking by parents in a supportive manner when possible.	Supportive role-modeling provides a safe and nonjudgmental milieu for parents to practice parenting and appropriate behaviors with child. It also allows for observation of behaviors to follow reciprocity of parental-infant dyad or triad.
• Provide consistency in caregivers to best develop a trust for nursing staff during hospitalization.	Consistency increases trust in caregivers.
• Provide for confidentiality and privacy.	Standards that are too often overlooked.
• Ensure that discussions regarding child and family are carried out with objectivity.	Objective dialogues are less threatening for all involved.
• Address appropriate authorities as needed for protection of child and family members to include security or police members according to institutional policy.	Appropriate child protective measures must be taken.
• Provide support in determining usual coping patterns and how these may be enhanced to deal with altered role-relationship pattern of violence.	Support in coping and dealing with violence will help reduce likelihood of increasing violence and assist in reducing anxiety.
• Assist in plans for placement, transitional placement, or dismissal to return home for family.	Appropriate planning for changes in care and the environment lessens the emotional trauma of these changes.
• Assist in identification of specific resources for long-term planning as appropriate.	Follow-up ensures attention to long-term needs and attaches value to follow-up care.
• Maintain objectivity in documentation of parent-child interactions.	

Women's Health

NOTE: These actions relate specifically to the abused, battered woman.[38,40-43]

ACTIONS/INTERVENTIONS	RATIONALES
• Be alert for cues that might indicate battering such as: ○ Hesitancy in providing detailed information about injury and how it occurred ○ Inappropriate affect for the situation ○ Delayed reporting of symptoms ○ Types and sites of injuries such as bruises to head, throat, chest, breast, or genitals ○ Inappropriate explanations ○ Increased anxiety in presence of the batterer	Provides database necessary to accurately assess the true causative factor.

Continued

ACTIONS/INTERVENTIONS	RATIONALES
• Provide a quiet, secure atmosphere to facilitate verbalization of fears, anger, rage, guilt, and shame.	Provides emotional support to patient. Fosters security for patient so that she will realize that she is not alone or the only person to have had this experience.
• Provide information on options available to patient, e.g., women's shelters and legal aid societies.	Provides basic information needed by the patient for future planning.

• Assist the patient in raising her self-esteem by:
  ○ Asking permission to do nursing tasks
  ○ Involving patient in decision making
  ○ Providing patient with choices
  ○ Encouraging patient to ask questions
  ○ Assuring patient of confidentiality	

• Assist patient in reviewing and understanding family dynamics.	
• Encourage and assist patient in planning for economic and financial needs such as housing, job, childcare, food, clothing, school for the children, and legal assistance.	Provides the information, long-range support, and essentials for resolving the problem.
• Refer patient to social services for immediate financial assistance for shelter, food, clothing, and childcare.	
• Assist patient in identifying lifestyle adjustments that each decision could entail.	
• Encourage development of community and social network systems.	

Psychiatric Health

ACTIONS/INTERVENTIONS	RATIONALES
• Introduce self to client, and call client by name.	Conditions that make people feel anonymous facilitate aggressive behavior.[44]
• If aggressive behavior is resulting from toxic substances, consult with physician for medication and detoxification procedure.	Staff and client safety is of primary concern.
• Observe client every 15 min during detoxification, assessing vital signs and mental status until condition is stable.	Client safety is of primary concern.
• Place client in quiet environment for detoxification.	Inappropriate levels of sensory stimuli can increase confusion and disorganization.
• Eliminate environmental stimuli that affect client in a negative manner. This could include staff, family, and other clients. Establish balance between being in control and being controlling.	Inappropriate levels of sensory stimuli can increase confusion and disorganization, increasing the risk for violent behavior.
• Provide a calm, reassuring environment. Respect client's requests for quiet, alone time.	

• Protect client from harm by:
  ○ Removing sharp objects from environment
  ○ Removing belts and strings from environment
  ○ Providing a one-to-one constant interaction if risk for self-harm is high
  ○ Checking on client's whereabouts every 15 min
  ○ Removing glass objects from environment
  ○ Removing locks from room and bathroom doors
  ○ Providing a shower curtain that will not support weight
  ○ Checking to see if client swallows medication
	Provides basic client safety.

• Observe client's use of physical space, and do not invade client's personal space.	Encroachment of the client's personal space may be perceived as a threat.[45]

- If it is necessary to have physical contact with the client, explain this need to the client in brief, simple terms before approaching.
- Remove unnecessary clutter and excess stimuli from the environment.
- Talk with client in calm, reassuring voice.
- Do not make sudden moves.
- Remove persons who irritate the client from the environment. Remember the best intervention for violent behavior is prevention. Observe client carefully for signs of increasing anxiety and tension.
- Do not assume physical postures that are perceived as threatening to the client.
- If increase in tension is noted, talk with client about feelings.
- Help client attach feelings to appropriate persons and situations — e.g., "Your boss really made you angry this time."
- Suggest to client alternative behavior for releasing tension — e.g., "You really seem tense right now. Let's go to the gym so you can use the punching bag." Or, "Let's go for a walk."
- Provide medication as ordered, and observe client for signs of side effects, especially orthostatic hypotension.
- Answer questions in an open, direct manner.

- Orient client to reality in interactions. Use methods of indirect confrontation that do not pose a personal threat to client. Do not agree with delusions — e.g., "I do not hear voices other than yours or mine" or "This is the mental health unit at (name) Hospital."
- Refer to Altered Thought Process (Chap. 7) for detailed interventions for delusions and hallucinations.

- Assign one staff member to be primary caregiver to client to facilitate the development of a therapeutic relationship.
- Inform client before any attempts to make physical contact are made in the process of normal provision of care — e.g., explain to client that you would like to assist him or her with dressing, would this be all right?
- Assist client in identifying potential problem behavior with feedback about his or her behavior.
- Have client talk about angry feelings toward self and others.
- Contract with client to talk with staff member when he or she feels an increase in internal tension or anger.

- Set limits on inappropriate behavior, and discuss these limits with the client. Note these limits here as well as the consequences for these kinds of behaviors. This information should be very specific so the intervention is consistent from shift to shift. Present these limits as choices.
- If conflict occurs between client and someone else, sit with them as they resolve the conflict in an appropriate manner. The nurse will serve as a facilitator during this interaction.
- Discuss tension reduction techniques with client, and develop a plan for client to learn these techniques and apply them in difficult situations. Note the plan here.

Clarifies role of staff to client so that the intent of these interactions can be framed in a positive manner.

Inappropriate levels of sensory stimuli can increase the client's confusion and disorganization, thus increasing the risk for violent behavior.

Assists client in developing coping behaviors.

Assists client in developing coping behaviors that are appropriate to the situation. Promotes the client's sense of control.[45]
Assists client in releasing physical tension associated with high levels of anger.

Provides the least restrictive way of assisting client to control behavior.
Promotes the development of a trusting relationship and promotes consistency in interventions.[45]
Direct confrontations could be perceived as a threat to the client and precipitate violent behavior.[46]

Promotes the development of a trusting relationship. In crisis, clients are more likely to respond positively to someone with whom they have a trusting relationship. Increases consistency in interventions.[45]

Clients who are prone to violence need increased personal space. Intrusions could provoke violent behavior.[45]

Promotes client's sense of control, which decreases risk for violent behavior.[45]
Assists client to understand the reasons for the anger, which can defuse the situation.[45]
Promotes client's sense of control by assuring the client that if he or she can no longer maintain control, the staff has a specific plan to assist him or her.[45]

Staff presence can reinforce using appropriate problem-solving skills as the client practices these new behaviors.

Promotes the client's sense of control. Repeated practice of a behavior internalizes and personalizes the behavior.

Continued

ACTIONS/INTERVENTIONS	RATIONALES
• Develop with the client a reward system for appropriate behavior. Note reward system here.	Positive reinforcement encourages behavior.
• Talk with client about the differences between feelings and behavior. Role-play with client, attaching different kinds of behavior to feelings of anger.	Promotes the client's sense of control by establishing limits around feelings in the cognitive realm. Repeated practice of a behavior internalizes and personalizes the behavior.
• Help client in determining if the feeling being experienced is really anger. Explain that at times of high stress we can misinterpret feelings and must be very careful not to express the wrong feeling. What we are expressing as anger may actually be, for example, anxiety or frustration.	Placing other names on the feeling may open new behavior possibilities to the client while promoting a positive orientation—e.g., if this were anger, lashing out would be appropriate, but since it is anxiety, it is more appropriate to relax.
• When client is capable, assign him or her to group in which feelings can be expressed and feedback can be obtained from peers. Note schedule for group activity here.	Promotes the client's sense of control by providing role models for alternative ways of coping with feelings.
• Review with client the consequences of inappropriate behavior, and assess the gains of this behavior over the costs.	Assesses the possibility for secondary gain from inappropriate behavior.
• Accept all threats of aggressive behavior as serious.	Client and staff safety is of primary importance.
• Remind staff to not take aggressive acts personally even if they appear to be directed at one staff member.	As the nurse's level of arousal increases, judgment decreases, making the nurse less effective when working with the client experiencing difficulty.[45]
• Provide client with positive verbal feedback about positive behavior changes..	Positive feedback encourages behavior.
• Do not place client in frustrating experiences without a staff member to support client during the experience.	Frustration can increase the risk for aggression.[44]
• If client is suicidal, place him or her in a room with another client.	Decreases the amount of time the client is alone.
• Provide client with opportunities to regain self-control without aggressive interventions by giving client choices that will facilitate control—e.g., "Would you like to take some medication now or spend some time with a staff member in your room?" Or, "We can help you into seclusion, or you can walk there on your own."	Promotes the client's perception of control while supporting self-esteem.
• Provide client with opportunities to maintain dignity.	
• Assure client that you will not allow him or her to harm self or someone else.	
• Reinforce this by having more staff present than necessary to physically control client if necessary. Persons from other areas of the institution may be needed in these situations. If others are used, they should be trained in proper procedures.	Client and staff safety are of primary concern.
• If potential for physical aggression is high[45,46]: ◦ Place one staff member in charge of the situation.	Promotes consistency in intervention and decreases inappropriate levels of sensory stimulation.
◦ As primary person attempts to talk client down, other staff member should remove other clients and visitors from the situation.	Client and staff safety are of primary concern.
◦ Other staff members should remove potential weapons from the environment in an unobtrusive manner. This could include pool cues and balls, chairs, flower vases, or books.	Assists in reducing levels of emotion.
◦ Avoid sudden movements.	
◦ Never turn back on client.	
◦ Maintain eye contact (this should not be direct, for this can be perceived as threatening to the client), and watch client's eyes for cues about potential targets of attack.	Assists in assessing the client's intentions without appearing threatening.

- Do not attempt to subdue client without adequate assistance.
- Put increased distance between client and self.

- Tell client of the concern in brief, concise terms.
- Suggest alternative behavior.
- Help client focus aggression away from staff.
- Encourage client to discuss concerns.

- If talking does not resolve the situation:
  - Have additional assistance prepared for action (at least 4 persons should be present).
  - Have those who are going to be involved in the intervention remove any personal items that could harm client or self, e.g., glasses, guns, long earrings, necklaces, or bracelets.
  - Have seclusion area ready for client, remove glass objects and sharp objects, and open doors for easy entry.
  - Briefly explain to client what is going to happen and why.
  - Use method practiced by intervention team to place client in seclusion or restraints.
  - Protect self with blankets with arms bent in front of body to protect head and neck.
  - Be prepared to leave the situation, and be aware of location of exits.
- See Impaired Physical Mobility (Chap. 5) for care of client in seclusion or restraints.
- Discuss the violent episode with the client when control has been regained. Answer questions client has about the situation and provide client with opportunities to express thoughts and feelings about the episode.
- Inform client of the behavior that is necessary to be released from seclusion or restraints.
- Process situation with client after incident.
- Assess milieu for "organizational provocation."

Client and staff safety are of primary concern.

Clients who have a potential for violent behavior need more personal space.
Maintains appropriate levels of sensory stimuli.
Promotes the client's sense of control.
May prevent the need for more restrictive interventions.
Assists in reducing levels of emotion and deescalation of behavior.

Client and staff safety are of primary concern.

Prevents sensory overload while providing reassurance to the client.

Client and staff safety and coordination are of primary concern.
Contains the client's body and blocks the client's vision if it is necessary to disarm the client.[46]
Client and staff safety are of primary concern.

Debriefing diminishes the emotional impact of the intervention and provides an opportunity to clarify the circumstances for the intervention, offer mutual feedback, and promote the client's self-esteem.[47]
Promotes the client's sense of control and enhances self-esteem.

Gerontic Health

ACTIONS/INTERVENTIONS	RATIONALES
- In cases of dementia, discuss with the caregiver if there is a usual pattern of violence, e.g., does startling or speaking in loud tones or having several people speaking at once usually result in a violent outburst by the patient?	Awareness of violence triggers provides guidelines for adjusting environment and staff behaviors.

Home Health

ACTIONS/INTERVENTIONS	RATIONALES

• Teach client and family appropriate monitoring of signs and symptoms of the risk for violence:
  ○ **Substance abuse**
  ○ Increased stress
  ○ Social isolation
  ○ Hostility
  ○ Increased motor activity
  ○ Disorientation to person, place, and time
  ○ Disconnected thoughts
  ○ Clenched fists
  ○ Throwing objects
  ○ Verbalizations of threats to self or others
	Provides database for early recognition and intervention.

• Assist client and family in lifestyle adjustments that may be required:
  ○ Recognition of feelings of anger or hostility
  ○ Developing coping strategies to express anger and hostility in acceptable manner—exercise, sports, art, music, etc.
  ○ Prevention of harm to self and others
  ○ Treatment of substance abuse
  ○ Management of debilitating disease
  ○ Coping with loss
  ○ Stress management
  ○ Decreasing sensory stimulation
  ○ Provision of safe environment
  ○ Removal of weapons, toxic drugs, etc.
  ○ Development and use of support network
  ○ Restriction of access to weapons, especially handguns[48,49]
	Permanent changes in behavior require support.

• Discuss workplace issues related to violence.[50]	Homicide is a leading cause of occupational death. Prevention is needed.
• Develop anticipatory guidance materials for violence prevention.[50,51]	Age-appropriate prevention strategies provide support for change.

• Involve patient and family in planning and implementing strategies to reduce the risk for violence:
  ○ Family conference
  ○ Mutual goal setting
  ○ Communication
	Provides for early intervention.

• Assist client and family to set criteria to help them to determine when intervention of law enforcement officials or health professionals is required—e.g., if patient becomes a threat to self or others.	
• Consult with or refer patient to assistive resources as appropriate.	Utilization of existing services is efficient use of resources. Psychiatric nurse clinician and support groups can enhance the treatment plan.

Violence, Risk for: Self-Directed or Directed at Others

FLOWCHART EVALUATION: EXPECTED OUTCOME 1

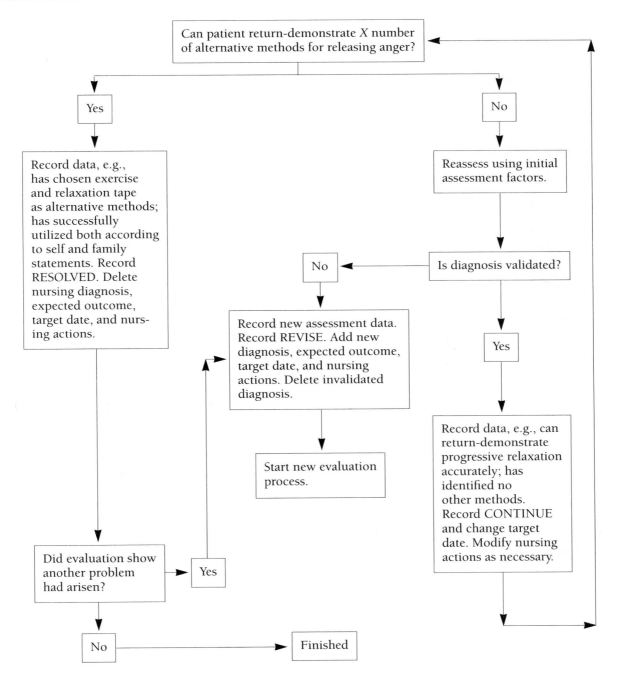

Violence, Risk for: Self-Directed or Directed at Others

FLOWCHART EVALUATION: EXPECTED OUTCOME 2

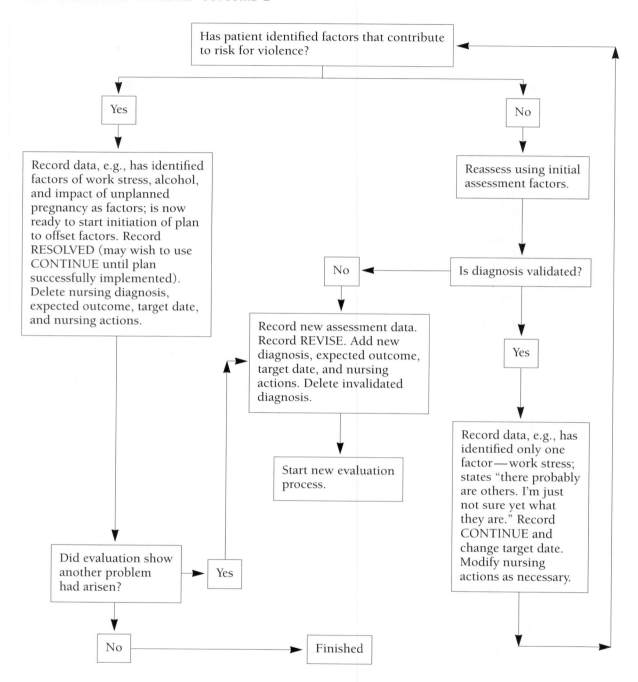

Sexuality-Reproductive Pattern

Pattern Description

This pattern focuses on the sexual-reproductive aspects of individuals over the entire lifespan. Sexuality patterns involve sex role behavior, gender identification, and physiologic and biologic functioning, as well as the cultural and societal expectations of sexual behavior. An individual's anatomic structure identifies sexual status, which determines the social and cultural responses of others toward the individual and, in turn, the individual's responsive behavior toward others.

Reproductive patterns involve the capability to procreate, actual procreation, and the ability to express sexual feelings. The success or failure of psychologically and physically expressing sexual feelings and procreating can affect an individual's lifestyle, health, and self-concept.

The nurse may care for clients who, because of illness, violence, or lifestyle, experience alterations or disturbances in their sexual health that affect their sexuality and reproductive patterns.

Pattern Assessment

1. Following a rape, is the patient experiencing multiple physical symptoms?
   a. Yes (Rape-Trauma Syndrome, Compound Reaction)
   b. No
2. Following a rape, is the patient indicating severe emotional reactions?
   a. Yes (Rape-Trauma Syndrome, Compound Reaction)
   b. No
3. Is the client using alcohol or drugs to cope following a rape?
   a. Yes (Compound Reaction)
   b. No
4. Has the client changed her relationship with males?
   a. Yes (Silent Reaction)
   b. No
5. Does the client indicate increased anxiety in follow-up counseling?
   a. Yes (Silent Reaction)
   b. No
6. Does the client verbalize any problems related to sexual functioning?
   a. Yes (Sexual Dysfunction)
   b. No
7. Does the client exhibit any indications of physical or psychosocial abuse?
   a. Yes (Sexual Dysfunction)
   b. No
8. Does the client relate any changes in sexual behavior?
   a. Yes (Altered Sexuality Pattern)
   b. No
9. Does the client report any difficulties or limitations in sexual behavior?
   a. Yes (Altered Sexuality Pattern)
   b. No

Conceptual Information

Gender development and sexuality are closely entwined with biologic, psychologic, sociologic, spiritual, and cultural aspects of human life. The biologic sex of an individual is decided at the time of conception, but sexual patterning is influenced from the moment of birth by the actions of those surrounding the individual. From this moment, males and females receive messages about who they are and what it means to be masculine or feminine.[1]

The sexuality of an individual is composed of biologic sex, gender identity, and gender role. The biologic and psychologic perspectives of culture and society determine how an individual develops sexually, particularly in the sense that one has of being male or female (gender identity). Biologic identity begins at the moment of fertilization when chromosomal sex is determined and becomes even more defined at 5 to 6 weeks of fetal life. At this time the undifferentiated fetal gonads become ovaries (XX, female chromosomal sex) or testes (XY, male chromosomal sex), and hormones finalize the genital appearance between the seventh and twelfth weeks. Fetal androgens (testicular hormones) must be present for male reproductive structures to develop from the wolffian ducts. If fetal androgens are not present, the fetus will develop female reproductive structures. By the twelfth week of fetal life, biologic sex is well established.[1,2]

Reactions by others begin the moment the biologic sex of the fetus or infant is known. Whether the sex of the infant is known before birth or not until the time of birth, the parents and those about them prepare for either a boy or a girl by buying clothes and toys for a boy (color blue, pants, shirts, football) or a girl (color pink, frilly dresses, dolls), as well as speaking to the infant differently according to sex. Girls are usually spoken to in a high, singsong voice: "Oh, isn't she cute!"; while boys are spoken to in a low-pitched, matter-of-fact voice: "Look at that big boy. He will really make a good football player one of these days!" These actions contribute to the infant's gender identity and perception of self. Behavioral responses from the infant are elicited by the parents based on their views of what roles a boy or girl should fulfill.

Gender role is determined by the kinds of sex behavior that are performed by individuals to symbolize to themselves and others that they are masculine or feminine.[3] Early civilizations assigned roles according to who performed what tasks for survival. Women were relegated to specific roles because of the biologic nature of bearing children, rearing children, and gathering food. The men were the hunters and soldiers. Advanced technologies, changing mores, birth control, and alternative methods of securing food and rearing children have led to changes in roles based on gender in Western society. Gender roles are influenced by cultural, religious, and social pressures. "Gender role stereotypes are culturally assigned clusters of behaviors or attributes covering everything from play activities and personal traits to physical appearance, dress and vocational activities."[4]

As in gender identity, researchers have noticed gender role-play in children as young as 13 months. Schoolchildren are particularly exposed and pressured into gender role stereotyping by parents, teachers, and peers, who demand expected, rigid behavior patterns according to the sex of the child. Molding into gender roles is often accomplished by handling girls and boys differently; little girls are usually handled gently as infants, and adults fuss with their baby's hair and telling them how pretty they are; little boys are usually roughhoused and are told, "What a big boy you are." Sex directional training is also accomplished by such verbalizations as "Where's Daddy's girl?" and "Big boys don't cry, be a man."[5]

Western North American society is moving toward a blending of male and female roles; however, stereotyping still exists. According to Schuster and Ashburn,[4] stereotyping is not all bad, as it can help "reduce anxiety arising from gender differences and may aid in the process of psychic separation from one's parents." Therefore, they conclude that stereotypes can provide structure and facilitate development as well as restrict development and become too rigid, thus interfering with a child's potential.

One's sexuality is a continuing lifetime evolution, changing as one matures and progresses through the life cycle. It is impossible to separate an individual's sexuality from his or her development, as sexuality combines the interaction of the biophysical and psychosocial elements of the individual.

According to a recent national research study,[6] "Rape in America," rape occurs far more often than previously recognized. This study found that 683,000 American women were raped in 1990, which is far higher than had been estimated. Almost 62 percent of these women stated that they were minors when they were raped, and about 29 percent stated they were younger than 11 when the rape occurred. This research indicates that rape is most definitely a traumatic event for our young in America. Of the rapists, 75 percent were known by the victim and included such persons as neighbors, friends, relatives, boyfriends, ex-boyfriends, husbands, or ex-husbands. Only 22 percent of the rapists were strangers to the victim. In 28 percent of the cases, injuries to the victim, beyond the rape itself, occurred. Sadly, only 16 percent of the victims tell police about the attack with the victims' being concerned about the family finding out, being blamed by others for the attack, and others' knowing about the attack. These concerns have decreased in victims raped in the past 5 years; however, in this group, there were increased concerns about having their names become public, getting AIDS and other sexually transmitted diseases, and becoming pregnant. Confidentiality of name is a high priority for these victims.

Developmental Considerations

INFANT

Erickson[4] defines the major task of infancy as the development of trust versus mistrust. The act of the parents' nurturing and providing caretaking activities allows the infant to begin experiencing various pleasures and physical sensations such as warmth, pleasure, security, and trust,[1] and it is through these acts of nurturing that the infant begins to develop a sense of masculinity or femininity (gender identity). The infant is further molded by the parents' perceptions of sex-appropriate behavior through reward and punishment. Female infants tend to be less aggressive and develop more sensitivity because girls are usually rewarded for "being good," and male infants develop more aggressively and learn

to be independent because boys are told that "big boys don't cry" and he learns to comfort himself. By the age of 13 months, sexual behavior patterns and differences are in place,[1,4] and core gender identity is theorized to be formed by 18 months.[7] "These early behaviors are so critical to one's core gender-identity that children who experience gender reassignment after the age of 2 years are high-risk candidates for psychotic disorders"[4] (p. 321).

The infant who is sexually abused is usually physically traumatized and many times dies. Developmental delays can be recognized in these children by failure to thrive, low weight or no weight gain, lethargy, and flat affect.

TODDLER AND PRESCHOOLER

Neuromuscular control allows toddlers to explore their environment, interact with their peers,[1,4] and develop autonomy and independence.[7] Genital organs continue to increase in size but not in function. The toddler's vocabulary increases, he or she distinguishes between male and female by recognizing clothing and body parts, and he or she develops pride in his or her own body, especially the genital area, as he or she becomes aware of elimination or excretory functions. They need guidance and require parents to set limits as they learn to "hold on" or "let go" in order to achieve a sense of autonomy.[4] By the age of 3, they have perfected verbal terms for the sexes, understand the meaning of gender terms and understand the roles associated with those terms (for example, girl is sister or mother, and boy is brother or father),[1] and receive pleasure from kissing and hugging.[7]

The preschooler is busy developing a sense of socialization and purpose. Learning suitable behavior for girls and boys or sex role behavior is the major task during the preschool years. Preschoolers will often identify with the parent of the same sex while forming an attachment to the parent of the opposite sex. They are inquisitive about sex and are often occupied in exploration of their own bodies and friends' bodies. This will often be exhibited in group games such as "doctor-nurse," urinating "outside," or masturbating.[7] The toddlers' concept of their bodies, not as a whole but as individual parts, changes when as preschoolers they begin to develop "an awareness of themselves as individuals, and become more concerned about body integrity and intactness."[4]

It is important to note that 6-year-olds are the age group most subjected to sexual abuse.[8] How a child handles this experience and his or her future developmental and psychological growth depend largely on the reactions and actions of the significant adult in the child's life.[7] Rape that occurs during early childhood may simply be acknowledged by the child as part of the experience of growing up and may have no long-term effects if not repeated. Usually counseling during this developmental age has great effect. All claims of abuse by a child should be investigated and should be handled by someone who has the experience and knowledge to deal with the child and his or her parents in a professional and understanding manner.

SCHOOL-AGE CHILD

Play is the most important work of children—it allows them to be curious and investigate social, sexual, and adult behavior. "Through play children learn how to get their needs met and how to meet the needs of others."[4] Different socialization of boys and girls tends to become apparent in play during the school years, with boys engaging in aggressive team play and girls in milder play and forming individual friendships. These activities can lead to stereotyping and exaggeration of gender difference.

Going to school allows children to begin to be more independent and form peer groups of the same sex. Although the peer group becomes very important to them, they need adult direction in learning socially acceptable forms of sexual behavior and when they may engage in them. If they do not receive the information they are seeking, negative feelings and apprehension about sexuality may develop.[1]

Great trauma can occur when rape occurs during these years. It is very damaging to the value systems that are being formed. Sexual identity can be disturbed, and sexual confusion can occur.

ADOLESCENT

Puberty, "the period of maturation of the reproductive system,"[4] causes profound changes in the individual's sexual anatomy and physiology and is a major developmental crisis for the adolescent. Secondary sex characteristics appear— breasts, pubic hair, and menstruation in girls, and testicular enlargement, penile enlargement, pubic hair, ejaculation, and growth of muscle mass in boys. The configuration, contour, and function of the body change rapidly and dramatically point out sexual differences and the onset of adulthood. These changes bring new feelings that create role confusion and increase awareness of sexual feelings. "The major task of adolescence is the establishment of identity in the fact of role confusion."[1]

Peer groups have an important influence on the young adolescent (12 to 15 years), but during late adolescence (16 to 19 years) the peer group influence lessens and more intimate relationships with the opposite sex develop.[7] These relationships can involve a wide range of sexual behavior from exploring behavior to intercourse, sometimes with the result of teenage pregnancy. Exploring behavior can be either with the opposite sex (foreplay and intercourse), the same sex (homosexuality), or self (masturbation). How the teenager views himself or herself sexually will depend on the reassurance and guidance he or she receives from a significant adult in his or her life. The greatest misunderstandings of teenagers involve homosexuality, masturbation, and conception and contraception. How these subjects are approached, taught, and supported can influence their adult sexuality.[1,7]

It is during adolescence, when new experiences of sexual maturity begin, that questions about maleness or femaleness are asked by the individual and concerns arise about "who one is within the peer group."[1] Adolescents must evaluate their masculinity and femininity, question and then decide on their gender identity, gender orientation, and gender preference. The adolescent deals not only with physical changes but integrates past experiences and role models with new experiences and new role models into his or her own gender identity.

Violent sexual occurrences during this period of life can devastate a person for the rest of his or her life. Adolescents are dealing with sexual confusion and identification; rape can

stop or slow or change this process. Fear and loss of self-esteem can dictate actions and influence sexual identity and gender expression.

YOUNG ADULT

This period of an individual's life (usually 20s and early 30s) is concerned with selecting a vocation, obtaining an education, military service, choosing a partner, building a career, and establishing an intimate relationship. This is a period of maximal sexual self-consciousness, commitment to a relationship, and social legitimization of sexual experiences.[1,4,7] There is a concern with parenting and establishment of the marital relationship.

Rape can slow or stop normal sexual relationships during the adult years. Fear can become the greater part of life for the victim. These years are ones for forming lasting relationships with the opposite sex, marrying, and beginning families. Rape can cause withdrawal from any interaction with the opposite sex; relationships can break up not only because of the reaction of the victims of rape but also because of the reactions of the families and spouses of the victim.

ADULT

Demands placed on adults by their careers and rearing children may interfere with their sexual interest and activity.[1] The major task of this period of life is to accept one's own lifestyle and decisions rather than feeling frustrated and disappointed. "Social pressures and expectations, feedback from significant others and finally self-perception all influence how one evaluates the success of one's life."[1]

Although the adult is at the peak of his or her career or profession, physiologic changes begin to influence the adult's lifestyle. The aging process, illnesses, and menopause (male and female) cause changes in lifestyles and everyday activities. Sexual activities can undergo changes because of these physical and physiologic changes; however, the adult who lives a healthy lifestyle, has good nutrition, exercises, and has an optimistic outlook usually feels good and functions well sexually. Often middle-aged adults, just as they have finished rearing their children, are faced with the task of caring for their elderly parents.

OLDER ADULTS

As in adolescence, dramatic body changes begin in late adulthood and continue into old age. There is no reason that healthy men and women cannot continue to enjoy their sexuality into old age. Women must deal with menopause and postmenopause, and men must often deal with impotence; however, with an interested sexual partner, good healthy sexuality can continue.

Older women are viewed by rapists as easy victims. Slowing of physical reactions and disabilities of old age (seeing, hearing, or slow gait) keep them from being alert to danger and from reacting quickly. More important, the older woman often views herself as inferior, and this contributes to her own victimization.[9] Because most women outlive men and face changes in lifestyles and economic status, they are reluctant, and often cannot afford, to leave familiar older parts of cities that often change and deteriorate. This may expose them to the accompanying increase in crime rate.[9]

APPLICABLE NURSING DIAGNOSES

Rape-Trauma Syndrome

DEFINITION

Forced, violent sexual penetration against the victim's will and consent. The trauma syndrome that develops from this attack or attempted attack includes an acute phase of disorganization of the victim's lifestyle and a long-term process of reorganization of lifestyle. This syndrome includes the following three subcomponents: Rape-Trauma, Compound Reaction, and Silent Reaction.[10]

NANDA TAXONOMY: FEELING 9.2.3.1, 9.2.3.1.1, AND 9.2.3.1.2

DEFINING CHARACTERISTICS[10]

1. Rape-Trauma Syndrome
   a. Acute phase:
      (1) Emotional reactions (anger, embarrassment, fear of physical violence and death, humiliation, revenge, or self-blame)
      (2) Multiple physical symptoms (gastrointestinal irritability, genitourinary discomfort, muscle tension, or sleep pattern disturbance)
   b. Long-term phase:
      (1) Changes in lifestyle (change in residence, dealing with repetitive nightmares and phobias, seeking family support, or seeking social network support)
2. Compound Reaction
   Same as Rape-Trauma Syndrome.
3. Silent Reaction
   a. Major defining characteristics
      (1) Abrupt changes in relationships with men
      (2) Increase in nightmares
      (3) Increased anxiety during interview, that is, blocking of associations, long periods of silence, minor stuttering, or physical distress
      (4) Pronounced changes in sexual behavior
      (5) No verbalization of the occurrence of rape
      (6) Sudden onset of phobic reactions
   b. Minor defining characteristics
      None given.

RELATED FACTORS[10]

Included in definition of diagnosis.

RELATED CLINICAL CONCERNS

Not applicable.

HAVE YOU SELECTED THE CORRECT DIAGNOSIS?

Sexual Dysfunction   Rape can be the cause of Sexual Dysfunction in a patient who cannot learn to put into perspective or deal with the rape experience. Rape-Trauma is always the result of a violent act and must be dealt with according to the individual situation. Although Sexual Dysfunction can occur as the result of rape, the nurse must assist the patient to deal with the trauma of the rape in order to assist with the sexual dysfunction.

EXPECTED OUTCOMES

1. Will identify and use at least (number) support systems by (date) and/or
2. Will verbalize (number) positive self-statements related to personal response to the incident by (date)

TARGET DATES

Due to the varied physical and emotional impact of rape, a target date of 3 days would not be too soon to evaluate for progress.

NURSING ACTIONS/INTERVENTIONS WITH RATIONALES

Adult Health

ACTIONS/INTERVENTIONS	RATIONALES
• Explore your own feelings about rape prior to initiating patient care. Maintain nonjudgmental attitude. Actively listen when survivor wants to talk about event. Encourage verbalization of thoughts, feelings, and perceptions of the event. Explore basis for and reality of thoughts, feelings, and perceptions.	The nurse's feelings can be sensed by the survivor and can influence the survivor's coping and sense of self.

Continued

ACTIONS/INTERVENTIONS	RATIONALES
• Attend to physical and health priorities such as lacerations or infection with appropriate explanations and preparation.	Prompt attention to physical needs provides comfort and facilitates a trusting relationship.
• Promote trusting, therapeutic relationship by spending at least 30 min every 4 h (while awake) at (times) with survivor.	Promotes expression of feelings and validates reality.
• Use calm, consistent approach when interacting with survivor. Respect survivor's rights.	Assists in reducing anxiety.
• Be supportive of survivor's values and beliefs.	Survivor's sexuality is intimately linked to her value-belief system.
• Explain need for medicolegal procedures, procedures to assess for sexually transmitted diseases, prophylactic medications, and medications to avoid postcoital contraception before performing procedures. Refer to women's health nursing actions for specifics about procedures.	Enlists survivor's cooperation and prepares her for events in case charges are filed against the alleged rapist.
• Provide for appropriate privacy and health teaching as care is administered. Allow survivor to see own anatomy if this seems appropriate as part of health teaching.	Avoids perpetuating survivor's fear due to necessity of examination and treatment in the same body area involved in the rape. Could promote a sensation of rape recurrence.
• Assist survivor in activities of daily living after examination.	Promotes a slight sense of return to normalcy. Emotional shock may render survivor temporarily unable to perform basic ADLs.

• Determine to what degree or extent symptoms of physical reactions exist such as:
  ◦ Pain or body soreness
  ◦ Disturbances in sleep
  ◦ Altered eating patterns
  ◦ Anger
  ◦ Self-blame
  ◦ Mood swings
  ◦ Feelings of helplessness
	Basic database needed to plan for long-term effects of rape.

• Administer medications as ordered to alleviate pain, anxiety, or inability to sleep, and teach survivor how to safely take such medications.	Allows time for survivor to process event in a way that maintains self-integrity and self-esteem.
• When interacting with the survivor, recognize that she will proceed at her own rate in resolving rape trauma. Do not rush or force survivor.	
• Identify available support systems, e.g., rape crisis center, and involve significant other as appropriate.	Support systems that know signs and symptoms of rape-trauma syndrome can provide help for both short-term and long-term interventions. Promotes effective coping for the survivor.
• Monitor coping in survivor and significant other until discharged from hospital.	Monitors for adaptive and maladaptive coping strategies. Provides opportunity to assist survivor and significant other to practice alternative coping strategies.
• Assist survivor to identify own strengths in dealing with the rape.	Helps to build survivor's self-esteem and overcome self-blame.
• Provide anticipatory guidance about the long-term effects of rape. Promote self-confidence and self-esteem through positive feedback regarding strengths, plans, and reality.	Helps to prepare for expected and unexpected reactions in self, friends, and significant others.
• Provide for appropriate epidemiologic follow-up in cases of venereal disease.	Required by law.
• Collaborate with other health care professionals as needed.	Promotes holistic approach and more complete plan of care.
• Arrange for appropriate long-term follow-up before dismissal from hospital, e.g., counseling.	Provides for long-term support.

MALE RAPE VICTIM

- Provide same considerations as with female survivor. (Usually these are the result of homosexual relationships. Most reported cases are children and early adolescents.)
- Refer patient to trained male counselor (rape crisis center).

The act of rape is an act of violence regardless of the gender of the patient and requires the same type of care and concern.

Child Health

ACTIONS/INTERVENTIONS	RATIONALES
• Encourage collaboration among health professionals to best address patient's needs.	Specialist will be required to deal with the unique needs of the young child enduring rape. The likelihood exists for incest or a closely related individual's being identified as the one who committed the act.
• Try to establish trust as dictated by age and circumstances related to rape trauma (with nurse being same sex as patient). **Do not** leave alone. Be gentle and patient.	
○ Infants and toddlers: Ensure continuity of caregivers. Explain procedures with dolls and puppets.	
○ Preschoolers: Ensure continuity of caregivers. Allow patient to perform self-care behavior as ability presents. Use art and methods that deal with general view of what happened, singling out child as not being the "cause" of this incident.	
○ School-agers: Maintain continuity of caregivers. Assist patient to express concerns related to incident. Use appropriate techniques in interviewing to determine extent of sexual dysfunction or potential threat to future functioning.	
○ Adolescents: Maintain continuity of caregivers. Encourage patient to express how this experience affects own self-identity and future sexual activities. Encourage psychiatric assistance in resolving this crisis for any patients of this age group. Look for signs of growth of secondary sex characteristics.	
• Follow up with appropriate documentation and coordination of child protective service needs. Assist parents or guardians in signing proper release forms. Determine if situation involves incest.	Appropriate protocols for documentation and reporting of rape or incest must be followed according to state and federal guidelines.
• Assist patient to deal with residual feelings such as guilt for revealing or identifying assailant (in young children this often must be dealt with within family or extended-family situations) by allowing at least 30 min per shift (while awake) at (times). Use simple language when dealing with child.	Resolution of unresolved guilt or feelings about the event must be dealt with as soon as client's condition permits.
• Encourage family members to assist in care and follow-up of patient's reorganization plans:	Risk behaviors serve as cues to alert the family or caregiver to monitor the child's progress in resolving the crisis.
○ Be alert for signs of distress such as refusing to go to school, dreams, nightmares, or verbalized concerns.	

Continued

ACTIONS/INTERVENTIONS	RATIONALES
○ Identify ways to gradually resume normal daily schedule. ○ Assist family to identify how best to resolve and express feelings about the incident. • Carry out appropriate health teaching regarding normal sexual physiology and functioning according to age and developmental capacity.	Normalcy is afforded as attempts are realistically made to resolve any aspects of rape trauma.
INCEST • Monitor for inappropriate sexual behavior among family members. • Monitor for children who know more about the actual mechanics of sexual intercourse than their developmental age indicates they would. • Monitor for girls who seem to have taken over the mother's role in the home. • Monitor for mothers who have withdrawn from the home, either emotionally or physically.	Provides database needed to accurately assess for incest.

Women's Health

ACTIONS/INTERVENTIONS	RATIONALES
• Assist the survivor through the procedures for provision of necessary health care treatment. Explain each phase of examination to survivor. Remain with the survivor at all times. • History: ○ List of previous venereal diseases ○ List of previous pelvic infections ○ Any injuries that were present before attack ○ Obstetric/menstrual history • Assist in gathering information to provide proper health and legal care. • Secure survivor's description of any objects used in the attack and how these objects were used in the attack. • Maintain sequencing and collection of evidence (chain of evidence): ○ Label each specimen with: (1) Survivor's name and hospital number (2) Date and time of collection (3) Area from which specimen was collected (4) Collector's name ○ Ensure proper storage and packaging of specimens: (1) Clothing and items that are wet, e.g., with blood or semen, should be put in paper bags, not plastic. (2) Specimens obtained on microscopic slides or swabs need to be air dried before packaging. ○ Comb pubic hair for traces of attacker's pubic hair or other evidence: (1) Submit paper towel placed under victim to catch combings, as well as the comb used, along with pubic hair. (2) Pluck (do not cut) 2–3 pubic hairs from the patient, and label properly. These are used for comparison.	Provides database necessary for intervention. Secures chain-of-evidence procedure and assists in reducing anxiety for client. Plastic bags will cause molding of wet items.

○ When custody of evidence is transferred to police, be certain written evidence of transfer is properly recorded:
  (1) Signatures of individuals involved in transfer
  (2) Name of person to whom the evidence is being transferred
  (3) Date and time
○ Take photographs of injuries or torn clothing.
○ Have survivor sign forms for release of information to authorities.
○ Provide medical treatment and follow-up for:
  (1) Injuries
  (2) Sexually transmitted disease: AIDS, gonorrhea, or syphilis
  (3) Pregnancy

ACTIONS/INTERVENTIONS	RATIONALES
• Report to proper authorities any suspicion of family violence.	Initiates long-range support for patient.
• Evaluate for increased rate of changing residences, repeated nightmares, and sleep pattern disturbance.	Provides database that allows accurate interpretation of long-range impact. Provides information needed to plan long-term care.
• Encourage patient to discuss phobias, frustrations, and fears.	
• Be available and allow patient to express difficulties in establishing normal activities of daily living and redescribe attack as needed.	Provides long-term essential support.
• Assist patient in developing a plan of reorganization of activities of daily living.	Promotes realistic planning for problem while avoiding continued denial of problem.

Psychiatric Health

ACTIONS/INTERVENTIONS	RATIONALES
• Assign a primary care nurse to client. This nurse should be of the sex the client demonstrates most comfort with at the current time.	Promotes the development of a trusting relationship.
• Primary care nurse will remain with the client during the orientation to the unit.	Promotes the development of a trusting relationship.
• Limit visitors as client feels necessary.	Promotes the client's sense of control while meeting security needs.
• Answer client's questions openly and honestly.	Promotes the development of a trusting relationship.
• Primary care nurse will be present to provide support for client during medical or legal examinations if the client has not identified another person.	Promotes the development of a trusting relationship while meeting the client's security needs.
• Assist client in identifying a support person, and arrange for this person to remain with the client as much as necessary. Note the name of this person here.	Promotes the client's sense of control while meeting security needs.
• Provide information to the client's support system as the client indicates is needed.	Support system understanding enhances their ability to support the client in a constructive manner.
• Allow client to talk about the incident as much as is desired. Sit with client during these times, and encourage expression of feelings.	Facilitates the confrontation of the memories of the event and attachment of meaning to the situation, which will promote a sense of control.[11]
• Communicate to client that his or her response is normal. This could include expressions of anger, fear, discomfort with persons of the opposite sex, discomfort with sexuality, or personal blame.	Normalization of the client's feelings without diminishing his or her experience enhances self-esteem and helps him or her to move from a position of victim to that of a survivor.[12]
• Inform client that rape is a physical assault rather than a sexual act and that rapists choose victims without regard for age, physical appearance, or manner of dress.	Promotes the client's resolution of guilt and feelings of responsibility.

Continued

ACTIONS/INTERVENTIONS	RATIONALES
• Assist client in developing a plan to return to activities of daily living. The plan should begin with steps that are easily accomplished so that the client can regain a sense of personal control and power. Note the steps of the plan here.	Promotes the client's sense of control and inhibits the tendency toward social isolation.[12]
• Provide positive social rewards for the client's accomplishment of established goals. Note here the kinds of behavior that are to be rewarded and the rewards to be used.	Positive reinforcement encourages behavior while enhancing self-esteem.
• Provide the client with opportunities to express anger at the assailant in a constructive manner, e.g., talking about fantasies of revenge, use of punching bag or pillow, or physical activity.	Assists client in moving from the powerless position of victim to a position of survivor.
• When client can interact with small groups, arrange for client's involvement in a therapeutic group that provides interaction with peers. Note time of group meetings here.	Provides the client opportunities to resolve his or her feelings of being different while decreasing social isolation. Promotes consensual validation of experience with others from similar situations, which enhances self-esteem and emotional resources available for coping.[12]
• Involve client in unit activities. Assign client activities that can be easily accomplished. Note client's level of functioning here along with those tasks that are to be assigned to the client.	Prevents social isolation. Accomplished tasks enhance self-esteem with positive reinforcement. Also provides opportunities to reality test self-perceptions against those of peers on the unit.
• Primary nurse will spend (number) minutes with client twice a day at (times) to focus on expression of feelings related to the rape. Encourage client not to close these feelings off too quickly. Assist client in reducing stress in other life situations while healing emotionally from the rape experience. Begin to facilitate client's use of cognitive coping resources by logically assessing various aspects of the situation.	Promotes reality testing of feelings related to the rape and inhibits the development of self-blame and guilt, which often occur in survivors.
• Assist client in developing a plan to reduce life stressors so emotional healing can continue. Note this plan here with the support needed from the nursing staff in implementing this plan.	Promotes the client's sense of control and provides a positive orientation.
• Primary nurse will meet with client and primary support person once per day to facilitate their discussion of the rape. If the client is involved in an ongoing relationship, such as a marriage, this interaction is very important. The support person should be encouraged to express his or her thoughts and feelings in a constructive manner. If it is assessed that the rape has resulted in potential long-term relationship difficulties such as rejection or sexual problems, refer to couple therapy.	Support system understanding and acceptance facilitate the client's coping and the maintenance of these relationships.
• Refer client to appropriate community support groups, and assist him or her with contacting these groups before discharge.	Promotes the client's reintegration into the community and inhibits the isolating behavior often exhibited by these clients.[12]

Gerontic Health

ACTIONS/INTERVENTIONS	RATIONALES
• In the event of the rape being secondary to elder abuse, refer the patient to adult protective services.	Provides a resource for the older adult to explore options and prevent recurrence of problem.

Home Health

ACTIONS/INTERVENTIONS	RATIONALES
• During the acute phase, be sure that appropriate assessment, law enforcement involvement, and treatment of physical injuries or sexually transmitted diseases are provided.	Early and accurate intervention decreases sequelae and provides documentation for any legal action.
• Assist client and family in lifestyle changes that may be needed:	Provides support and enhances recovery.
○ Treatment for physical injuries or sexually transmitted diseases	
○ Testimony in court	
○ Protection	
○ Coping with terror, nightmares, or fear	
○ Coping with alterations in sexual response to significant others	
○ Development and use of support networks	
○ Stress management	
○ Changing phone number or moving	
○ Traveling with companion	
○ Strategies for prevention of rape	
• Assist client and family in planning and implementing strategies for resolution of rape-trauma syndrome:	Crimes of violence upset the family equilibrium and require support to correct.
○ Communication, e.g., discussion of feelings among family members	
○ Mutual sharing and trust	Involvement of client and significant others is important to ensure successful resolution.
○ Problem solving, e.g., providing support for family members and client; strategies to reduce possibility of future attacks	
• Consult with or refer patient to assistive resources as appropriate.	Use of existing resources and expertise provides high-quality care and is effective use of already available resources.

Rape-Trauma Syndrome, Compound Reaction and Silent Reaction

FLOWCHART EVALUATION: EXPECTED OUTCOME 1

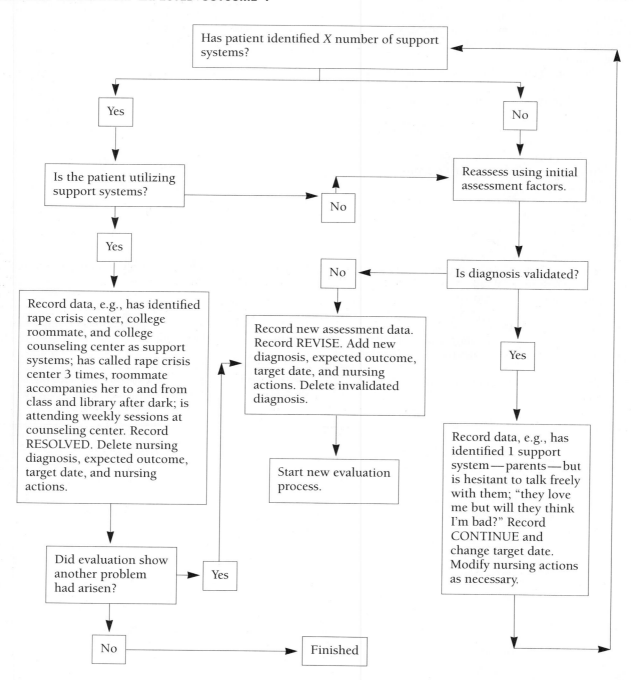

Has patient identified *X* number of support systems?

Yes

No

Is the patient utilizing support systems?

No

Reassess using initial assessment factors.

Yes

No

Is diagnosis validated?

Record data, e.g., has identified rape crisis center, college roommate, and college counseling center as support systems; has called rape crisis center 3 times, roommate accompanies her to and from class and library after dark; is attending weekly sessions at counseling center. Record RESOLVED. Delete nursing diagnosis, expected outcome, target date, and nursing actions.

Record new assessment data. Record REVISE. Add new diagnosis, expected outcome, target date, and nursing actions. Delete invalidated diagnosis.

Yes

Start new evaluation process.

Record data, e.g., has identified 1 support system—parents—but is hesitant to talk freely with them; "they love me but will they think I'm bad?" Record CONTINUE and change target date. Modify nursing actions as necessary.

Did evaluation show another problem had arisen?

Yes

No

Finished

Rape-Trauma Syndrome, Compound Reaction and Silent Reaction

FLOWCHART EVALUATION: EXPECTED OUTCOME 2

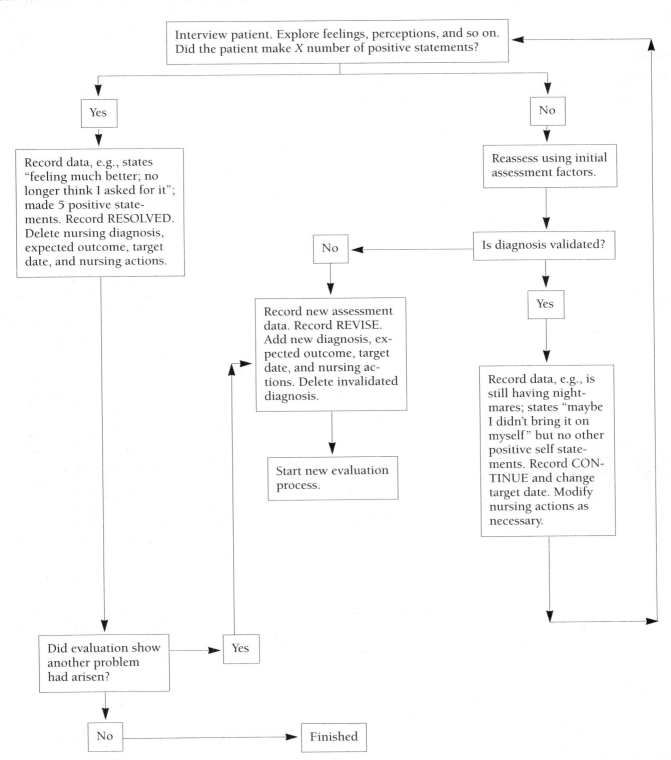

Sexual Dysfunction

DEFINITION

The state in which an individual experiences a change in sexual function that is viewed as unsatisfying, unrewarding, or inadequate.[10]

NANDA TAXONOMY: RELATING 3.2.1.2.1

DEFINING CHARACTERISTICS[10]

1. Major defining characteristics
   a. Verbalization of problem
   b. Alterations in achieving perceived sex role
   c. Actual or perceived limitation imposed by disease and/or therapy
   d. Conflicts involving values
   e. Alteration in achieving sexual satisfaction
   f. Inability to achieve desired satisfaction
   g. Seeking confirmation of desirability
   h. Alteration in relationship with significant other
   i. Change of interest in self and others
2. Minor defining characteristics
   None given

RELATED FACTORS[10]

1. Biopsychosocial alteration of sexuality
2. Ineffectual or absent role models

3. Physical abuse
4. Psychosocial abuse, for example, harmful relationships
5. Vulnerability
6. Values conflict
7. Lack of privacy
8. Lack of significant others
9. Altered body structure or function (pregnancy, recent childbirth, drugs, surgery, anomalies, disease process, trauma, or radiation)
10. Misinformation or lack of knowledge

RELATED CLINICAL CONCERNS

1. Endocrine, urological, neuromuscular, and skeletal disorders
2. Genital trauma
3. Agoraphobia
4. Pelvic surgery
5. Malignancies of the reproductive tract
6. Female circumcision[13]
7. Psychiatric disorders such as mania, major depression, dementia, borderline personality disorder, substance abuse or use, anxiety disorder, and schizophrenia.

HAVE YOU SELECTED THE CORRECT DIAGNOSIS?

Altered Sexuality Pattern   In this diagnosis, the individual is expressing concern about his or her sexuality. This diagnosis could be a result of Sexual Dysfunction but it is not necessarily a problem to the patient. Altered Sexuality Patterns can be compatible with the patient's lifestyle for whatever reason and create no overwhelming problems for the patient.

Rape-Trauma Syndrome   This diagnosis could result in Sexual Dysfunction because of the patient's inability to deal with the violence, trauma, and lifestyle changes as a result of rape. It is absolutely essential for the nurse to ascertain the cause of the Sexual Dysfunction and to determine if it is the result of the patient's perception of sexuality in general, pathophysiology, or trauma.

EXPECTED OUTCOMES

1. Will have decreased complaints of sexual dysfunction by (date) and/or
2. Will report return, as near as possible, to previous levels of sexual functioning by (date)

TARGET DATES

Depending on the patient's perception of the sexual dysfunction, target dates may range from 1 week to several months.

NURSING ACTIONS/INTERVENTIONS WITH RATIONALES
Adult Health

ACTIONS/INTERVENTIONS	RATIONALES
• Facilitate communication between patient and partner by providing at least (number) minutes per day for privacy to communicate.	Promotes identification of issues involved in sexual dysfunction.
• Encourage patient and partner to talk about concerns and problems during conference.	Sexual behavior includes verbal, nonverbal, genital, and nongenital activities.
• Talk with patient and partner about alternate ways to attain sexual satisfaction and express sexuality, e.g., hugging, touching, kissing, masturbation, hand holding, or sexual aids. Provide factual informational material.	
• Clarify misconceptions as needed—e.g., sexual activity is dangerous after a heart attack, older people don't engage in sexual activity, or a hysterectomy decreases sexual drive.	Misinformation and myths contribute to sexual dysfunction.
• Be nonjudgmental in your attitudes.	Sexuality is a highly personal experience. Nonjudgmental attitudes reduce anxiety and open the way for therapeutic communication.
• Respect patient's values and attitudes about sexuality and sexual functioning.	Sexual behavior is intimately linked to the value-belief system. Demeaning these values and beliefs will cause anxiety in patient.
• Provide accurate information on effects of medical diagnosis or treatment on sexual functioning.	Clarifies misconceptions. Provides information on changes or modifications in sexual activities that may need to occur due to disease process.
• Implement measures to improve self-concept, e.g., positive self-talk, assertiveness, new hairdo, new clothes, or new social surroundings.	How one feels about self is important in self-perception of sexuality.
• Provide privacy for expressing sexuality, e.g., masturbation, sexual intercourse, particularly when patient has been hospitalized for a significant length of time or has been separated from significant other for a significant length of time.	Sexuality expression may be inhibited by hospitalization, but need exists.
• Teach patient importance of adequate rest before and after sexual activity.	Sexual activity increases basal metabolic rate and initiates the sympathetic nervous system, creating a high level of stress.

• If dyspareunia is a problem, teach patient and significant other to:
  ○ Use adequate amounts of water-soluble lubricant.
  ○ Use vaginal steroid cream.
  ○ Take sitz baths.
	Increases comfort and reduces trauma. Eases dryness and avoids irritation.

• If impotence is a problem, advise patient to:
  ○ Consult with a physician regarding a complete physical examination.
  ○ Consult with sex therapist.
  ○ Consider penile prosthesis.
	Discovers underlying causes of impotence. Provides an alternative method of penile erection to find satisfaction in intercourse.

Child Health

This diagnosis is not appropriate for a child.

Women's Health

NOTE: Very little information is found in the literature on Sexual Dysfunction of lesbian women, as they often conceal their sexual orientation when they receive health care and some choose not to receive health care if there is a danger of exposure.[14] The following actions refer to those who have a heterosexual relationship.

ACTIONS/INTERVENTIONS	RATIONALES

• Obtain detailed sexual history.
• Determine who the patient is:
  ◦ Female
  ◦ Male
  ◦ Couple or partners
  ◦ Review communication skills between partners.
• Ascertain couple's knowledge of:
  ◦ Sexual performance
  ◦ Female and male anatomy and physiology
  ◦ Female and male orgasm
  ◦ Anticipatory performance anxiety
  ◦ Unrealistic romantic ideas
  ◦ Rigid religious conformity
  ◦ Negative conditioning in formative years
  ◦ Erection and ejaculation
  ◦ Stimulation
  ◦ Arousal
  ◦ Sexual anxiety
  ◦ Fear of failure
  ◦ Demand for performance
  ◦ Fear of rejection
	Provides database needed to plan accurate intervention.

• Dispel sexual myths and fallacies or misinformation about sexuality by:
  ◦ Allowing patient to talk about beliefs and practices in a nonthreatening atmosphere
  ◦ Providing correct information
  ◦ Answering questions in an honest manner
  ◦ Referring to the appropriate agencies or health care providers
	Provides basic information and support that can assist patient in long-term care.

• Obtain description of current problem:
  ◦ Psychological
  ◦ Physical
  ◦ Social
	Provides essential database to permit narrowing of focus for intervention.

• Determine type of sexual dysfunction:
  ◦ General
  ◦ Lack of erotic feeling
  ◦ Lack of sexual responses
  ◦ No pleasure in sexual act
  ◦ Consider it an ordeal
  ◦ Avoidance
  ◦ Frustration
  ◦ Disappointment
  ◦ Fear
  ◦ Disgust
  ◦ Orgasmic difficulties
• If client is sexually responsive but cannot complete sexual response cycle, determine if this is:
  ◦ Situational: Client is inhibited, disappointed, or disinterested.
  ◦ Physiologic: Interruption results from lack of lubrication, impotence, or interference with sexual response cycle.
  ◦ Psychologic: Ambivalence, guilt, or fear is present.
• If vaginismus (tight closing of vaginal muscle with any attempt at penetration) is present, determine if this results from:
  ◦ Fear of vaginal penetration
  ◦ Spasm of vaginal muscles
  ◦ Frustration	

- ○ Frustration
- ○ Fear of inadequacy
- ○ Guilt
- ○ Pain
- ○ Prior sexual trauma
- ○ Strict religious code
- ○ Rape
- ○ Dyspareunia
- Discuss consequences of sexual acts and situations in an honest and nonthreatening manner.
- Collaborate with appropriate therapists.

Initiates intervention in a supportive environment.

Provides the long-term care and support that are needed to resolve the basic problem.

Psychiatric Health

NOTE: If sexual dysfunction is related to physiologic limitations, loss of body part, or impotence, refer to Adult Health care plan. If dysfunction is related to ineffective coping or poor social skills, initiate the following actions.

ACTIONS/INTERVENTIONS	RATIONALES
• Set limits on the inappropriate expression of sexual needs. Note the kinds of behavior to be limited and the consequences for inappropriate behavior here—e.g., when client approaches staff member with sexually provocative remarks, the staff member will use constructive confrontation and discontinue the interaction.[15] Inform client of these limits.	Promotes client's sense of control while maintaining the safety of the milieu.
• Assign primary care nurse to client on each shift. The primary care nurse will spend 15 min with the client twice per shift at (times) to develop a relationship and then begin to explore with the client the effects this behavior has on others and the needs that are being met by the behavior.	Promotes the development of a trusting relationship.
• Assist client in identifying environmental stimuli that provoke sexual behavior and in developing alternative responses to these stimuli in inappropriate situations.	
• Develop with the client a list of alternative kinds of behavior to meet the need currently being met by the sexual behavior. Note alternative behavior patterns here with plan for implementing them.	Promotes the client's sense of control.
• Provide client with information about appropriate sexual behavior—e.g., what are "normal" sexual expressions or what are appropriate ways to meet sexual needs (intercourse with appropriate person or masturbation at suitable time in an appropriate place).	Facilitates the development of appropriate coping behaviors.
• Role-play with client those social situations that have been identified as problematic. These could include setting limits on others' inappropriate behavior toward the client or situations in which the client needs to practice appropriate social responses.	Behavioral rehearsal provides opportunities for feedback and modeling of new behaviors by the nurse.
• Assist client in appropriate labeling of feelings and needs—e.g., anxiety may be inappropriately labeled as "sexual tension."	Promotes the client's sense of control and facilitates the development of adaptive coping behaviors.
• Plan a private time and place for client. Inform client that this can be used for appropriate sexual expression. Note this plan here.	Social isolation inhibits inappropriate behavior by removing social rewards.

Continued

ACTIONS/INTERVENTIONS	RATIONALES
• If client begins inappropriate sexual behavior while involved in group activities, remove client from group to a private place and explain to client purpose of this action. Inform client that he or she may return to the group when (the limit set by the care team will be noted here).	
• If sexual behavior results from anxiety, refer to Anxiety for detailed care plan.	Promotes the development of adaptive interpersonal skills in an environment that provides supportive feedback from peers.
• Assign client tasks in unit activities that are appropriate for client's level of comfort with group interaction — e.g., if client is uncomfortable with persons of opposite sex, assign a task that requires involvement with a same-sex group or involvement with an opposite-sex staff member who can begin a relationship.	
• Recognize and support client's feelings — e.g., "You sound confused."	Promotes the development of a trusting relationship. Models for the client appropriate expressions of feelings in a supportive environment. Helps the client to learn to talk about feelings rather than act on them.
• Engage client in a socialization group once a day at (time). This should provide the client with an opportunity to interact with peers in an environment that provides feedback to the client in a supportive manner.	Decreases social isolation and provides the client with an opportunity to practice interpersonal skills in a supportive environment.
• Arrange a consultation with occupational therapist to assist client in developing needed social skills — e.g., cooking skills or skills at games that require socialization.	Increases the client's interpersonal competence and enhances self-esteem.
• Provide an environment that does not stimulate inappropriate sexual behavior — e.g., staff member indirectly encourages client's behavior with dress or verbal comments or other clients interact with client in a sexual manner.	Promotes an environment that increases the opportunities for the client to succeed with new behaviors. This success serves as reinforcement which encourages positive behavior and enhances self-esteem.
• Sit with client (number) minutes once a shift at (time) to discuss nonsexual-related information.	Nurses' interactions can provide social reinforcement for the client's appropriate interactions. Provides opportunity for the client to practice new behaviors in a supportive environment. Success in this situation provides reinforcement, which encourages positive behavior and enhances self-esteem.
• Provide positive social rewards for appropriate behavior (the rewards as well as the kinds of behavior to be rewarded should be noted here).	Reinforcement encourages positive behavior and enhances self-esteem.
• Evaluate the effects of the client's current medication on sexual behavior, and consult with physician as needed for necessary alterations.	Basic monitoring of medication efficiency.
• Develop a structured daily activity schedule for the client, and provide client with this information.	Assists the client in focusing away from issues of sexuality and engaging in socially appropriate activity.
• Schedule time for client to engage in physical activity. This activity should be developed with the client's assistance and could include walking, jogging, basketball, cycling, dancing, "soft" aerobics, etc. A staff member should participate with the client in these activities to provide positive social reinforcement. Note schedule and type of activity here.	Physical activity decreases anxiety and increases the production of endorphins, which increase the client's feelings of well-being.[16] Provides opportunities for the client to learn alternative ways of coping with anxiety in a supportive environment.

Gerontic Health

ACTIONS/INTERVENTIONS	RATIONALES
• Monitor for use of medications that may induce sexual dysfunction. Male impotency may be related to antihypertensive medications.	Identifies correctable source of impotency.
• Determine individual patient's knowledge of facts and myths regarding sexual changes in aging.	Knowledge of expected aging changes may encourage the individual to discuss changes experienced and seek treatment for dysfunction.
• Identify resources for assistance with sexual dysfunction such as Impotents Anonymous groups.[17]	Provides an information source and support for individuals with a common problem. Impotence, regardless of etiology, shows marked increase beyond age 65.
• Provide resources for patients with chronic illnesses, such as COPD or arthritis, that address and assist in problem solving regarding disease-related sexual difficulties.[18]	
• Provide uninterrupted time for couples, particularly in long-term-care settings, where it may be difficult to maintain or attain privacy.	Assists patients in maintaining sexuality as long as possible.

Home Health

ACTIONS/INTERVENTIONS	RATIONALES
• Involve client and significant other in planning and implementing strategies for reducing sexual dysfunction and enhancing sexual relationship: ○ Communication, e.g., discussion of concerns and ideas for intervention ○ Mutual sharing and trust ○ Problem solving—e.g., identification of specific strategies with roles defined, such as second honeymoon or specific sexual arousal exercises	Sexual dysfunction affects and is affected by relationships. Involvement of significant people in strategies is vital to enhance the potential for success.
• Assist patient and significant other with lifestyle adjustments that may be required by: ○ Providing accurate and appropriate information regarding contraception ○ Teaching stress management ○ Providing information regarding sexuality and clarifying myths regarding sexuality ○ Exploring strategies for coping with disabling injury or disease ○ Using massage ○ Using touch ○ Treating substance abuse ○ Exercising regularly ○ Coping with changes in role functions and role relationships ○ Using water-soluble lubricants ○ Obtaining treatment for physical problems, e.g., vaginal infections or penile discharge ○ Teaching changes accompanying pregnancy ○ Teaching side effects of medication	Lifestyle changes require permanent behavior changes. Support and self-evaluation can improve the probability of successful change.
• Consult with or refer patient to assistive resources as indicated.	Use of existing resources provides for high-quality care and effective use of services.

Sexual Dysfunction

FLOWCHART EVALUATION: EXPECTED OUTCOME 1

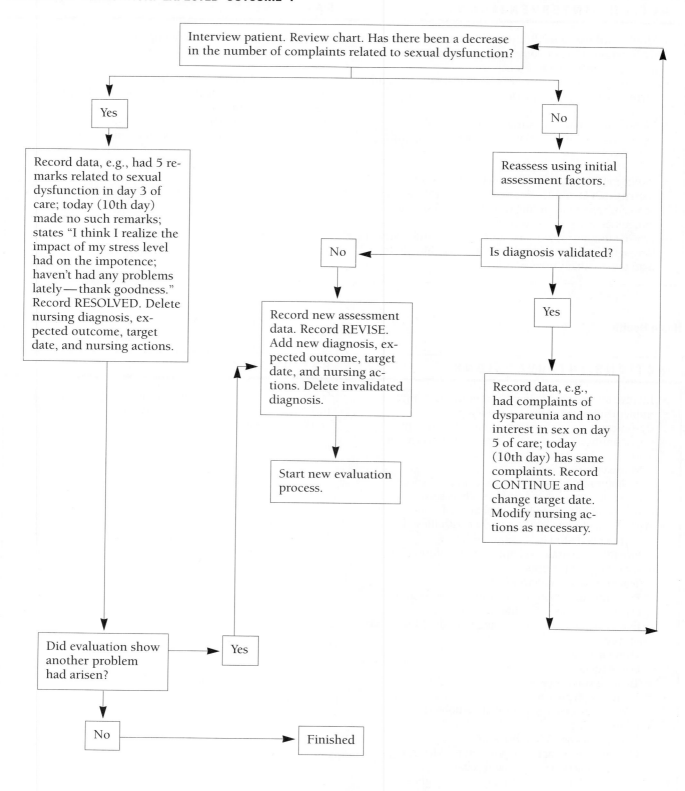

Sexual Dysfunction

FLOWCHART EVALUATION: EXPECTED OUTCOME 2

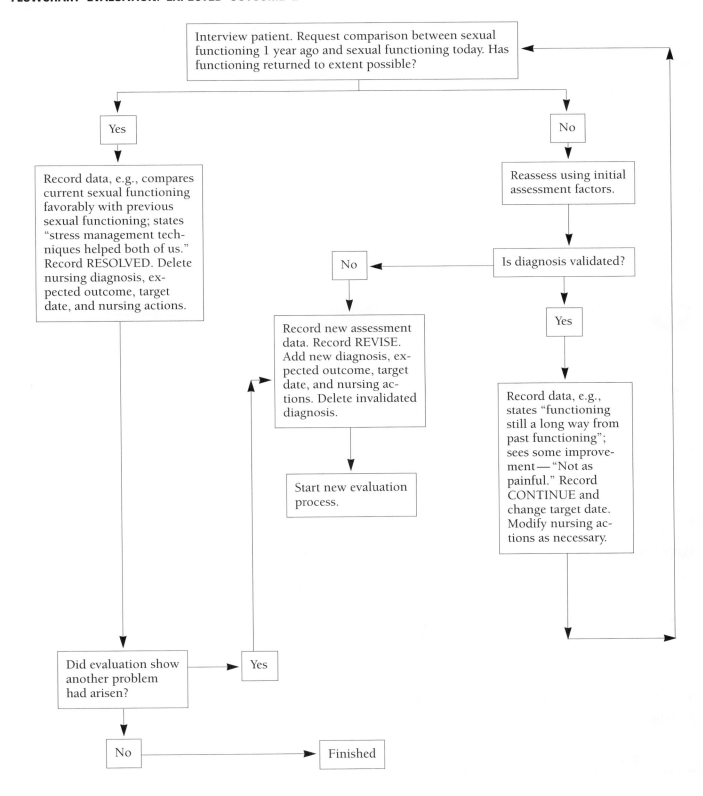

Sexuality Patterns, Altered

DEFINITION

The state in which an individual expresses concern regarding his or her sexuality.[10]

NANDA TAXONOMY: RELATING 3.3

DEFINING CHARACTERISTICS[10]

1. Major defining characteristics
   a. Reported difficulties, limitations, or changes in sexual behaviors or activities
2. Minor defining characteristics
   None given

RELATED FACTORS[10]

1. Knowledge or skills deficit about alternative responses to health-related transitions or altered body function or structure, illness or medical

2. Lack of privacy
3. Lack of significant others
4. Ineffective or absent role models
5. Conflicts with sexual orientation or variant preferences
6. Fear of pregnancy or of acquiring a sexually transmitted disease
7. Impaired relationship with a significant other

RELATED CLINICAL CONCERNS

1. Mastectomy
2. Hysterectomy
3. Cancer of the reproductive tract
4. Any condition resulting in paralysis
5. Sexually transmitted disease, for example, syphilis, gonorrhea, or AIDS

HAVE YOU SELECTED THE CORRECT DIAGNOSIS?

Sexual Dysfunction Sexual Dysfunction indicates that there are problems in sexual functioning. Altered Sexual Patterns refers to concerns about sexuality but does not necessarily mean an overwhelming problem. In some instances this diagnosis may involve a lifestyle different from heterosexual norms.

Rape-Trauma Syndrome Certainly a traumatic event such as a rape could result in an Altered Sexuality Pattern. The nurse would focus, however, in assisting the patient to deal with the rape trauma first. Resolving this problem would assist in resolving the Altered Sexuality Pattern. Many of the other nursing diagnoses can impact sexual feelings and functioning in both men and women. Examples are Body Image Disturbance, Pain, Chronic Pain, Fear, Anxiety, Dysfunctional Grieving, and Altered Role Performance.

EXPECTED OUTCOMES

1. Will identify at least (number) factors contributing to altered sexual pattern by (date) and/or
2. Will verbalize fewer complaints regarding altered sexual pattern by (date)

TARGET DATES

Because of the extremely personal nature of sexuality, the patient may be reluctant to express needs or problems in this area. For this reason, a target date of 5 to 7 days would be acceptable.

NURSING ACTIONS/INTERVENTIONS WITH RATIONALES
Adult Health

ACTIONS/INTERVENTIONS	RATIONALES
• Establish therapeutic and trusting relationship with patient and significant others.	Promotes therapeutics and open communication.
• Address other primary nursing needs, especially physiologically related and self-image related.	Meeting these needs promotes solving of the altered sexuality pattern.

ACTIONS/INTERVENTIONS	RATIONALES
• Actively listen to patient's and significant other's efforts to talk about fears or changes in body image affecting sexuality or altered sexual preferences. Assist patient and family to identify how the desired sexual function may be attained.	Promotes open and therapeutic communications.
• Help patient and significant other to understand that sexuality does not necessarily mean intercourse.	Misinformation and myths may create unrealistic expectations about sexuality and the sexual experience.
• Discuss alternate methods for expressing sexuality, including masturbation.	Sexuality includes verbal, nonverbal, genital, and nongenital sexual activities.
• Do not be judgmental with patient or significant other.	Sexuality is a highly personal behavior. The nurse's attitude can create guilt feelings and stress in the patient.
• Provide privacy and time for patient and significant other to be alone if so desired.	Allows for sexual expressions.
• Administer medications as ordered with monitoring of potential side effects.	
• Monitor for contributory causative components, and provide appropriate education and follow-up.	Permits a more fully developed and accurate plan of care. Provides for long-term support.

Child Health

ACTIONS/INTERVENTIONS	RATIONALES
• Encourage child and family to verbalize perception of altered sexual functioning, e.g., undescended testicle.	Provides the database necessary to accurately plan intervention.
• Assist patient and family to identify how the desired sexual function may be attained.	Specific plans for goals of sexual function desired will assist in how the client will be treated, e.g., surgeries for future procreation.
• Include appropriate collaboration with other health care team members as needed.	Specialist may best meet the unique needs represented with altered sexual functioning.
• Provide attention to developmentally appropriate role-modeling for age and situation.	Opportunities appropriate for age with role models serve as valuable learning modes.
• Encourage peer support during hospitalization as appropriate.	Peer support fosters sense of self, which is also a composite of sexuality.
• Plan for potential long-term nursing follow-up.	The chronic nature of many physiologic components will necessitate serial rechecks and treatment over time as the child grows and matures.

Women's Health

ACTIONS/INTERVENTIONS	RATIONALES
• Assist the patient to describe her sexuality and understanding of sexual functioning as it relates to her lifestyle and lifestyle decisions.	Provides database needed to plan for successful interventions.
• Allow patient time to discuss sexuality and sex-related problems in a nonthreatening atmosphere. Obtain a complete sexual history including current emotional state.	
• Assist patient in listing lifestyle adjustments that need to be made—e.g., different methods of achieving sexual satisfaction in the presence of mutilating surgery.	
• Identify significant others in patient's life and involve them, if so desired by patient, in discussion and problem-solving activities regarding sexual adjustments.	

Continued

ACTIONS/INTERVENTIONS	RATIONALES

• Provide atmosphere that allows patient to discuss freely:
  ○ Partner choice
  ○ Sexual orientation
  ○ Sexual roles
• Assist patient in identifying lifestyle adjustments to each different cycle of reproductive life:
  ○ Puberty
  ○ Pregnancy
  ○ Menopause
  ○ Postmenopause
	Assists patient in planning coping strategies to various life situations and provides information the patient needs to achieve the planning.

• Discuss pregnancy and the changes that will occur during pregnancy and the postpartum period:
  ○ Sexuality
  ○ Mood swings
• Discuss aspects of sexuality and intercourse during pregnancy. Answer questions promptly and factually:
  ○ Positions
  ○ Frequency
  ○ Effects on fetus
  ○ Effects on pregnancy
  ○ Fears about sexual changes
• Discuss postpartum healing process and timing of resumption of intercourse.
• Assist patient facing surgery or body structure changes in identifying lifestyle adjustments that may be needed—e.g., ileostomy, colostomy, mastectomy, or hysterectomy.
• Allow patient to grieve loss of body image.
	Provides essential information needed by patient to offset concerns regarding maintaining sexuality during and after pregnancy.

• Reassure patient that she can still participate in sexual activities.
• Assure confidentiality for patient with sexually transmitted diseases.
• Encourage verbalization of concerns with sexually transmitted diseases:
  ○ Recurrent nature of disease, especially herpes and *Chlamydia*
  ○ Lack of cure for disease (AIDS)
  ○ Economics in treating disease
  ○ Social stigma associated with disease
• Encourage honesty in answering questions about:
  ○ Multiple sex partners
  ○ Describing sexual behavior
	Provides support to patient who is questioning continuance of sexuality.
	Promotes sharing of information necessary to plan care.
	
	Provides the database needed to most accurately plan care.

• Encourage honest communication with sexual partners(s).	Sexual partner will require health care.

Psychiatric Health

NOTE: If alteration is related to altered body function or structure or illness, refer to Adult Health nursing actions.

ACTIONS/INTERVENTIONS	RATIONALES
• Assign primary care nurse who is comfortable discussing sexually related material with client.	Promotes the development of a trusting relationship.
• Primary nurse will spend (number) minutes (number) times a day with client discussing issues related to diagnosis. These discussions will include: ○ Client's thoughts and feelings about alteration ○ Other stressors and concerns in the client's life that could affect sexual patterns ○ Client's perceptions of partner's responses ○ Client's perceptions of self as a sexual person without a partner ○ Client's perceptions of social or cultural expectations ○ Client's thoughts and feelings about sexuality	Expression of feelings and perceptions in a supportive environment facilitates the development of alternative coping behaviors.
• If alteration is related to lack of information, develop a teaching plan and note teaching plan here.	Provides guide to ensure that client gets accurate and consistent information.
• When client identifies *specific* difficulties that contribute to the concern, develop specific action plan to cope with these and note the plan here.	Promotes the client's sense of control and enhances self-esteem.
• If alteration is related to problems with the significant other, arrange a meeting with client and significant other to discuss the perceptions each has about the problem. If these difficulties are related to a lack of information, develop a teaching plan and note it here. If alteration is related to long-term relationship or if alteration is only one of several problems, refer partners to marriage and family therapist or clinical nurse specialist.	Provides opportunity for nurse to facilitate communication between the partners and for the partners to communicate their relationship needs as well as personal needs in a nonthreatening environment.
• Arrange private time for client and partner to discuss relationship issues, including sexuality. Note time and place arranged for this discussion here.	Provides recognition and support for this relationship.
• During interactions with client and significant other, have them express feelings about their relationship. These should be both positive and negative feelings.	Promotes the development of a positive expectational set. Positive feelings enhance self-esteem and enhance personal psychologic resources for coping with the difficult aspects of the relationship.

Gerontic Health

The nursing actions for the older adult with this diagnosis are the same as for the adult health patient.

Home Health

ACTIONS/INTERVENTIONS	RATIONALES
• Monitor for factors contributing to altered sexuality patterns by (date).	Provides database for early identification and intervention.
• Involve appropriate family members—e.g., significant others or parents of child—in planning, implementing, and promoting reduction or elimination of Altered Sexuality Patterns: ○ Communication, e.g., discussion of values and sexual mores	Sexual behavior can affect the entire family. Involvement of family in problem identification and intervention enhances the probability of successful intervention.

Continued

ACTIONS/INTERVENTIONS	RATIONALES

◦ Mutual sharing and trust
◦ Problem solving—e.g., identification of strategies acceptable to all involved with the role of each person identified
◦ Sex education, e.g., clarifying any misconceptions regarding sexual behavior and sexuality
• Assist client and family with lifestyle adjustments that may be required:
  ◦ Providing accurate and appropriate information regarding sexuality and contraception
  ◦ Providing time and privacy for development and improvement of sexual relationship
  ◦ Teaching stress management
  ◦ Coping with loss of sexual partner
  ◦ Providing accurate and appropriate information regarding sexually transmitted diseases
  ◦ Providing accurate and appropriate information regarding sexual orientation, e.g., homosexuality, heterosexuality, or transexuality
  ◦ Coping with physical disability
  ◦ Side effects of medical treatment
• Consult with assistive resources as indicated.
	Provides knowledge and support necessary for permanent behavioral change.
	
	Specialized counseling may be indicated. Use of existing resources provides effective use of resources.

Sexuality Patterns, Altered

FLOWCHART EVALUATION: EXPECTED OUTCOME 1

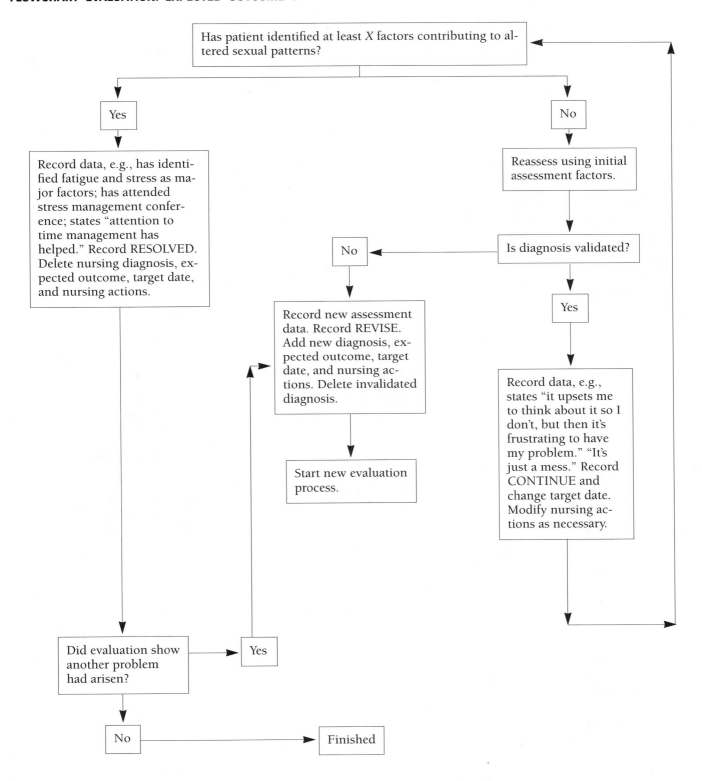

Sexuality Patterns, Altered

FLOWCHART EVALUATION: EXPECTED OUTCOME 2

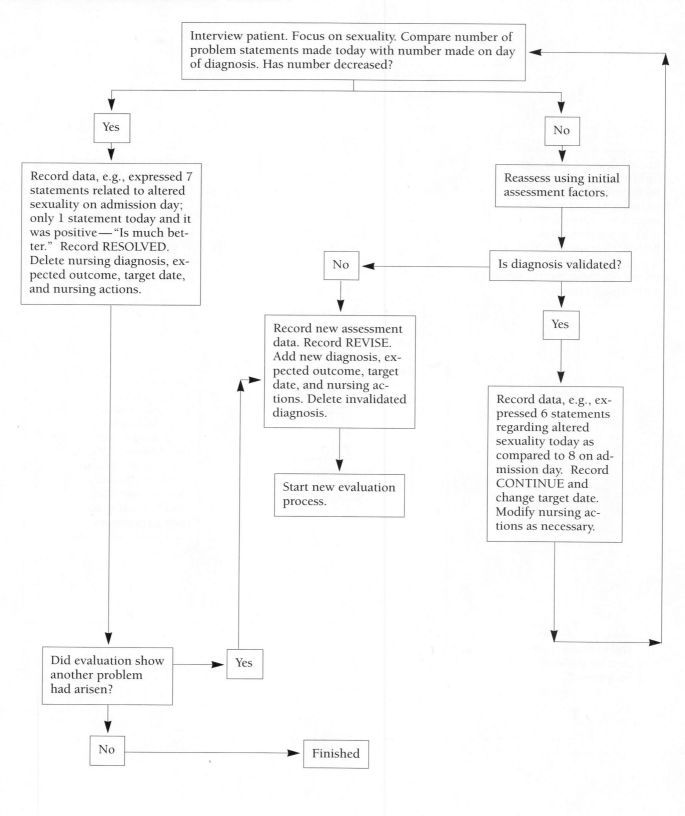

Interview patient. Focus on sexuality. Compare number of problem statements made today with number made on day of diagnosis. Has number decreased?

Yes

No

Record data, e.g., expressed 7 statements related to altered sexuality on admission day; only 1 statement today and it was positive—"Is much better." Record RESOLVED. Delete nursing diagnosis, expected outcome, target date, and nursing actions.

Reassess using initial assessment factors.

Is diagnosis validated?

No

Yes

Record new assessment data. Record REVISE. Add new diagnosis, expected outcome, target date, and nursing actions. Delete invalidated diagnosis.

Record data, e.g., expressed 6 statements regarding altered sexuality today as compared to 8 on admission day. Record CONTINUE and change target date. Modify nursing actions as necessary.

Start new evaluation process.

Did evaluation show another problem had arisen?

Yes

No

Finished

Coping-Stress Tolerance Pattern

Pattern Description

Stress has been defined as the response of the body or the system to any demand made on it[1]. This response can be both physiologic and psychosocial. Since demands are synonymous with living, stress has been defined as "life itself."[1] The system's (individual, family, or community) ability to respond to these demands has an effect on the well-being of the system. *Stress tolerance pattern* refers to the system's usual manner of responding to stress or to the amount of stress previously experienced. This includes the stress response history of the individual, family, or community.[2] *Coping* has been defined as "efforts to master condition of harm, threat, or challenge when a routine or automatic response is not readily available."[3] Thus, the coping pattern is the system's pattern of responding to nonroutine threats. The client's ability to respond to stress is affected by a complex interaction of physical, social, and emotional reactions. Assessment of this pattern focuses on gaining an understanding of the interaction of these factors within the system. Interventions are related to maximizing the system's well-being.[1,3]

Pattern Assessment

1. Does the client verbalize inability to cope?
   a. Yes (Ineffective Individual Coping)
   b. No
2. Does the client demonstrate inability to problem solve?
   a. Yes (Ineffective Individual Coping)
   b. No
3. Does the client deny problems or weaknesses in spite of evidence to the contrary?
   a. Yes (Defensive Coping)
   b. No
4. Is the client projecting blame for current situation on other persons or events?
   a. Yes (Defensive Coping)
   b. No
5. Did the patient delay seeking health care assistance to the detriment of his or her health?
   a. Yes (Ineffective Denial)
   b. No
6. Does the patient downplay condition?
   a. Yes (Ineffective Denial)
   b. No
7. Does the patient verbalize nonacceptance of health status change?
   a. Yes (Impaired Adjustment)
   b. No
8. Is the patient moving toward independence?
   a. Yes
   b. No (Impaired Adjustment)
9. Is the client's primary caregiver denying the severity of the client's problem?
   a. Yes (Ineffective Family Coping, Disabling)
   b. No
10. Does the client demonstrate indications of neglect?
    a. Yes (Ineffective Family Coping, Disabling)
    b. No
11. Does the client state concerns about care being received from primary caregiver?
    a. Yes (Ineffective Family Coping, Compromised)
    b. No
12. Can the primary caregiver verbalize understanding of care requirements?
    a. Yes
    b. No (Ineffective Family Coping, Compromised)
13. Does the family indicate physical and emotional support for client?
    a. Yes (Family Coping, Potential for Growth)
    b. No
14. Does the family or primary caregiver indicate interest in a support group?
    a. Yes (Family Coping, Potential for Growth)
    b. No
15. Does the patient exhibit re-experience of traumatic events (flashbacks or nightmares)?
    a. Yes (Posttrauma response)
    b. No
16. Does the patient exhibit vagueness about traumatic event?
    a. Yes (Posttrauma Response)
    b. No
17. Is there evidence of positive communication and community participation in planning for predicted community stressors?
    a. Yes (Potential for Enhanced Community Coping)
    b. No
18. Is there evidence of community conflict and deficits in community participation?
    a. Yes (Ineffective Community Coping)
    b. No

Conceptual Information

To understand coping, one must first understand the concept of stress because coping is the system's attempt to adapt to stress. An understanding of these concepts and their interrelationships is crucial for the promotion of well-being. Research has clearly demonstrated that undue stress can be related to major health problems if inappropriate coping is present.[1]

Stress has been defined as the body's nonspecific response to any demand placed upon it.[1] These demands can be any situation that would require the system to adapt. For the individual, this situation could include anything from getting out of bed in the morning to experiencing the loss resulting from a major environmental disaster. Stress is life.

The body's physiologic response to stress involves activation of the autonomic nervous system. The symptoms of this activation can include sweating, tachycardia, tachypnea, nausea, and tremors. This process has been labeled the *general-adaptation syndrome (GAS)*[4] and occurs in three stages: alarm reaction, resistance, and exhaustion. The alarm stage mobilizes the system's defense forces by initiating the autonomic nervous system response. The system is prepared for "fight or flight." In the resistance stage, the system fights back and adapts, and normal functioning returns. If the stress continues and all attempts of the system to adapt fail, exhaustion occurs, and the system is at risk for experiencing major disorganization.

Four levels of psychophysiologic stress responses have been described.[4] The first level comprises the day-to-day stressors that all systems experience as a part of living. This stress calls upon the self-regulating processes of the system for adaptation. Intrasystem coping mechanisms are used, and the system does not require assistance from outside sources to adapt. Level 2 responds to less-routine or new experiences encountered by the system. The system experiences a mild alarm reaction that is not prolonged. The individual system might experience a mild increase in heart rate, sensations of bladder fullness and increased frequency of urination, temporary insomnia, tachypnea, anxiety, fear, guilt, shame, or frustration. Some outside assistance may be necessary to facilitate adaptation. This assistance could be in the form of identifying stressors and strengths or encouraging the individual to solve problems. Level 3 consists of the moderate amount of stress that occurs when a persistent stress is encountered or when a new situation is perceived as threatening. Emergency adapting processes are activated. The individual would experience tachycardia, palpitations, tremors, weakness, cool pale skin, headache, oliguria, vomiting, constipation, and increased susceptibility to infections. This level of stress usually requires assistance from a professional helper. This assistance can include identifying problems and coping strengths, teaching, performing tasks for the client, or altering the environment to facilitate coping. When the system cannot adapt to a stressful situation with assistance, a severe degree of stress is experienced. This is labeled level 4. This occurs when all coping strategies are exhausted. Intervention at this level requires the assistance of professionals who have the skills to assist with the development of unique coping strategies.

Since stress is life itself, adaptation to reduce the effects on the system is imperative. To begin this process, it is important to understand those factors that can influence the system's ability to respond to stress. Stress can arise from biophysical, chemical, psychosocial, and cultural sources. The basic health of the affected system improves the ability to respond to these stressors. Response to the biophysical-chemical stressors can be improved by improving the condition of the biologic system. This would include proper nutrition, appropriate amounts of rest, appropriate levels of exercise, and reduced exposure of the system to toxic chemicals.[1]

The literature[1] indicates that a great deal of psychosocial-cultural stress evolves from a philosophy of life that is impossible to fulfill. This would indicate that a great deal of stress arises from the perception of events, not in the events themselves. This is compounded by the social and cultural influences on the system. The sociocultural influences could include the cultural attitudes about age, body appearance, and family roles and the social approaches to assistance for working mothers, advancement in employment status, and so on. The system's beliefs about these social-cultural stressors can affect the degree to which the stressors affect the system. If the stressor is perceived as unnatural or impossible to adapt to, the system's stress level will be increased. Response to the psychosocial-cultural stressors can be improved with attitude assessment and interventions that reduce the physiologic response to psychosocial stressors.

Coping has been defined as behavior (conscious and unconscious) that a system uses to change a situation for the better or to manage the stress-resultant emotions.[5] These kinds of behaviors can occur on the biologic, psychologic, and social levels. Effective coping uses biologic, psychologic, and social resources in attempts to manage the situation.

A coping model has been presented[3] that addresses the biologic, psychologic, and sociocultural aspects of this process. The model indicates that systems have *generalized resistance resources* (GRRs) to facilitate coping. GRRs are those characteristics of the system that can facilitate effective tension management. Genetic characteristics that provide increased resistance to the effects of stressors are considered physical and biochemical GRRs. These GRRs can include levels of immunity, nutritional status, and the adaptability of the neurologic system. Valuative and attitudinal GRRs describe consistent features of the system's coping behavior. This could include personality characteristics and the system's perception of the stressor. The more flexible, rational, and long term these are, the more effective they are as GRRs. Interpersonal-relational GRRs include social support systems and can provide an important resource in managing stress. Finally, those cultural supports that facilitate coping are referred to as macrosociocultural GRRs. *Macrosociocultural GRRs* could include religions, rites of passage, and governmental structures.

In 1979, Kobasa introduced the concept of hardiness to the literature on coping.[6,7] She described the hardy individual as having three characteristics that provide him or her with the ability to cope effectively with stress. The first characteristic is commitment or a purpose and involvement in life. Challenge is the second characteristic of the hardy individual. Challenge is the belief that the changes in life can be meaningful opportunities for personal growth. The third characteristic is control. Control has three components: cognitive control, decisional control, and repertoire of coping skills. Kobasa and other authors proposed that the hardy individual would remain healthier and experience less disabling psychologic stress.

An understanding of the concept of hardiness can facilitate the nurse's assessment of the client's potential ability to cope with life's stresses. Based on this assessment, the nurse can then develop interventions that support or develop commitment, challenge, and control for the client. These interventions might include providing the client with as much control as possible in the situation, facilitating his or her positive orientation with reframes, and assisting in the development of a variety of coping strategies.[6]

Wagnild and Young have questioned the validity of hardiness as a concept.[8] The concern of these authors evolves from their observation that the tools utilized to measure the various components of hardiness do not provide clear distinctions between the identified concepts and other influencing variables. Wagnild and Young conclude that it is important to continue the research related to a hardiness concept, and, until a more precise understanding of what constitutes this concept is developed, it will be difficult to apply it to therapeutic interventions.[8] From a clinical perspective hardiness is a useful concept to consider when interacting with the client system for it provides a model for understanding client response and presents fertile content for clinical nursing research related to psychosocial aspects of coping.

Effective coping can occur when the system has a strong physiologic base combined with adequate psychosociocultural support. This implies that any intervention that addresses coping behavior should address each of these areas. Interventions that have been applied to this process include therapeutic touch, kinesiology, meditation, relaxation training, hypnosis, family therapy, nutritional counseling, massage, and physical exercise.

Developmental Considerations

The number of resources available to the system greatly affects its ability to cope with stressors. Thus there is a need to maximize physical, cognitive, and psychosocial development. Cross-cultural research has identified those characteristics that are common to individuals who are perceived as mature and capable of coping effectively. These characteristics include an ability to anticipate consequences; calm, clear thinking; potential fulfillment; problem solving that is orderly and organized; predictability; purposefulness; realisticness; reflectiveness; strong convictions; and implacability.[9] The development of these characteristics is maximized in environments that provide children with a loving, warm environment; respect and acceptance for personal interests, ideas, needs, and talents; stable role models; challenges that foster development of competence and responsibility; opportunities to explore all of their feelings; a variety of experiences; opportunities for age-appropriate problem solving and the knowledge that they must live with the consequences of their decisions; opportunities to develop commitments to others; and encouragement in the development of their own standards, values, and goals.[9]

According to developmental stages, there are some specific etiologies and symptom clusters.

INFANT

Interactions with significant others are the primary source of the infant's response to trauma or stress. If the significant other is supportive and consistent, the effects of the event on the infant are minimized. Events that separate infants from their significant others also pose a threat to this age group. Primary symptoms are disruptions in physiologic responses.

The chronic diseases place this age group at special risk. Since the development of coping behavior is limited at this age, the primary caregivers (usually the parents) provide the child with the support to cope. If the caregivers cannot provide the proper supports, then the child is affected. Chronic illness in the child places an extreme stress on the family and can result in divorce. Support for the parents is crucial in supporting the child's coping.

TODDLER AND PRESCHOOLER

Responses of significant others are still the primary supports for the child in this age group. Thus, as for the infant, the response of significant others or separation from these persons can have an effect on the toddler and preschooler. In addition, threats to body integrity pose a special threat to this age group. Traumatic events that inflict physical damage on these children place the child at greatest risk. Regression is the primary symptom and coping behavior. This can be frustrating to caregivers who expect the child to assist in a time of crisis with age-appropriate developmental behavior when the child

may regress to a very dependent stage. Other methods used by young children in coping include denial, repression, and projection. Coping may be more difficult because adults may not recognize that young children can experience crisis and will, therefore, not provide assistance with the coping process.[10]

SCHOOL-AGE CHILD

Symptoms include problems with school performance, withdrawal from family and peers, behavioral regression, physical problems related to anxiety, and aggressive behavior to self or others. Coping behavior includes that used by the younger child, only in a more effective manner. This age group may find a great deal of support from siblings during crisis. Situations that can precipitate crisis in this age group include school entry, threats to body image, peer problems, and family stress such as divorce or death of a loved one.[10]

Chronic disease or disability also affects the adjustment of this age group. Again, the primary support for adaptation comes from the primary caregivers, usually the parents.

ADOLESCENT

The adolescent demonstrates more adultlike coping behavior. Symptoms of stress include anxiety, increased physical activity, increased daydreaming, increased apathy, change in mood cycles, alteration in sleeping patterns, aggressive behavior directed at self or others, and physical symptoms associated with anxiety. Crisis-producing situations can include role changes, peer difficulties, threats to body integrity, rapidly changing body functioning, conflict with parents, personal failures, sexual awareness, and school demands.[10]

Response to traumatic events is similar to that of adults. Etiologies of crisis-producing events, for this age group, are also similar to those for adults. Specific events that place this age group at greater risk are those that affect the peer group and could have effects on body image or sexual functioning. Coping behavior is adultlike. This age group may find support from peers especially useful in facilitating coping. Coping may also be affected by limited life experience and impulsive behavior.

Illnesses that threaten body image could result in difficulties in adjustment. Peers again provide a primary support system and can have a great impact on the adolescent's acceptance. Educating significant peers about the client's situation could facilitate their acceptance of the client and in turn facilitate the client's adjustment to the change in health status. Adjustment could also be facilitated by involving the client in a support group composed of peers with similar alterations.

YOUNG ADULT

Symptoms of problems with coping include changes in performance of roles at home and at work, aggressive behavior directed at the self or others, and physical symptoms associated with anxiety and denial. Changes in role performance might include loss of interest in sexual relationships or withdrawal from the community. Situations that might tax the coping abilities of the young adult include balancing increasing role responsibilities, dealing with threats to the self or to body integrity, leaving home, and making career choices.[10]

Alterations in health status that affect the ability of role performance place this age group at risk for impaired adjustment. This could include loss of ability to function in job responsibilities. Behavior can include regression, but this does not necessarily indicate that the client is experiencing impaired adjustment.

ADULT

Coping resources have broadened for this age group due to past successful coping experiences and the possible addition of adult children as supports during crisis. Symptoms of difficulties with coping are similar to those of the young adult. Age-related stressors include loss, such as significant others and physical functioning; role changes such as job loss and the leaving of adult children; aging parents; career pressures; and cultural role expectations.[10]

OLDER ADULT

Symptoms of extreme stress in this age group may be overlooked and attributed to senility. These symptoms include withdrawal, decreased functioning, increased physical complaints, and aggressive behavior. Coping behavior is affected by decreased function of hearing, vision, and mobility as well as loss of support systems and other resources. These problems can be balanced by life experience that has provided the individual with many situations of successful coping to fall back on during stressful times. Situations that place this age group at risk are multiple losses, decreased physical functioning, increased dependence, retirement, relocation, and loss of respect due to cultural attitudes.

The effects of multiple losses related to alteration in health status and the loss of support systems place the older adult at risk for impaired adjustment. In the absence of illness affecting cognitive functioning, the older adult can assume responsibility for making decisions related to alterations in health status. This ability combined with life experience can facilitate creative problem solving with the support of health care personnel.[11]

The following is a presentation of the developmental framework of the family life cycle as described by Carter and McGoldrick.[12]

Between families: The unattached young adult—the process of this level is accepting parent-child separation. The individual must separate from his or her family of origin and develop intimate peer relationships and a career.

The joining of families through marriage: The newly married couple—the process of this level involves commitment to a new system. The individuals form a marital system and realign relationships with extended families and friends to include spouse.

The family with young children: The task faced is to accept a new generation of members into the system. The marital system adjusts to make space for the child(ren) and assumes parent roles. Another realignment takes place to include parenting and grandparenting roles.

The family with adolescents: The family task is to increase flexibility of family boundaries to include children's independence. The parent-child relationships shift to allow the adolescents to move in and out of the system. The parents refocus on midlife marital and career issues, and there is a beginning shift toward concerns for the older generation.

The family in later life: Accepting the shifting of generational roles is the task of this stage. The system maintains individual and couple functioning and interests in conjunction with physiologic decline. There is an exploration of new role options with more support for a more central role for the middle generation. The system also makes room for the wisdom and experience of the elderly and to support the older generation without overprotecting them. This stage will also include coping with the deaths of significant others and preparation for death.

Specific problems can arise in family coping when the family developmental cycle or expectations do not correspond with the developmental tasks of individual family members. There are three stages that are nodal points in family development.

The joining of families through marriage requires a commitment to a new system. If the separation from the parents is not successful, then the new family does not have an opportunity to form its own identity, combining the experiences both bring into this new relationship. Symptoms of unsuccessful resolution of this stage could result in the marital partners returning home to their parents when conflict arises or an ongoing struggle over loyalties to families of origin.

The second major shift occurs when children enter the system. The new role of parent is assumed, and the couple's boundaries must be opened to accept the child. Unsuccessful resolution of this stage could result in physical or emotional abuse of the child. If there is a developmental delay in the parents and they are not ready to assume the responsibilities that accompany parenthood, family dysfunction can occur.

A family with adolescents is faced with the task of increasing flexibility to include children's independence. This may require a major shift in family rules. This is also influenced by the parents' perception of the adolescent and the environment. If the adolescent is seen as being competent, and the environment that the adolescent interacts in is seen as safe, then it will be much easier for the family to provide the necessary shifts in relationships. When this stage is not resolved successfully, the adolescent may enhance behavior that highlights his or her differences with the family to force separation, or the frequency and intensity of family conflict may increase. Unsuccessful resolution of this stage may indicate that the family has overly rigid boundaries to the external world and individual boundaries that are overly permeable.

Application of the concept of coping at the aggregate or community level is in the process of development. Additional research is needed to identify and validate community-based diagnoses. Successful communities are healthy communities.[13,14]

NOTE: For the individual diagnoses in this chapter, the mental health nursing actions serve as the generic nursing actions. This change is due to the fact that the nature of the diagnoses in this chapter basically call for the skills, knowledge, and expertise of a psychiatric-mental health nursing specialist.

APPLICABLE NURSING DIAGNOSES

Adjustment, Impaired

DEFINITION

The state in which the individual is unable to modify his or her lifestyle or behavior in a manner consistent with a change in health status.[15]

NANDA TAXONOMY: EXCHANGING 5.1.1.1.1

DEFINING CHARACTERISTICS[15]

1. Major defining characteristics
   a. Verbalization of nonacceptance of health status change
   b. Nonexistent or unsuccessful ability to be involved in problem solving or goal setting

2. Minor defining characteristics
   a. Lack of movement toward independence
   b. Extended period of shock, disbelief, or anger regarding health status change
   c. Lack of future-oriented thinking

RELATED FACTORS[15]

1. Disability requiring change in lifestyle
2. Inadequate support systems
3. Impaired cognition
4. Sensory overload
5. Assault to self-esteem
6. Altered locus of control
7. Incomplete grieving

RELATED CLINICAL CONCERNS

1. Alzheimer's disease
2. Head injury sequelae
3. Any new diagnosis for the patient
4. Couvade syndrome
5. Postpartum depression or puerperal psychosis
6. Personality disorders
7. Substance use or abuse disorders
8. Psychotic disorders

HAVE YOU SELECTED THE CORRECT DIAGNOSIS?

Ineffective Individual Coping   This diagnosis results from the client's inability to cope appropriately with stress. Impaired Adjustment is the client's inability to adjust to a specific disease process. If the client's behavior is related to the adjustment to a specific disease process, the diagnosis would be Impaired Adjustment; however, if the behavior is related to coping with general life stressors, the diagnosis would be Ineffective Individual Coping.

Powerlessness   This diagnosis would be appropriate as a primary or codiagnosis if the client demonstrates the belief that personal action cannot affect or alter the situation. Impaired Adjustment may result from Powerlessness. If this is the situation, then the appropriate primary diagnosis would be Powerlessness.

Sensory-Perceptual Alteration   This diagnosis can affect the individual's ability to adjust to an alteration in health status. If it is determined that perceptual alterations are affecting the client's ability to adapt, then the appropriate primary diagnosis would be Sensory-Perceptual Alteration.

Altered Thought Process   This diagnosis can inhibit the client's ability to adapt effectively to an alteration in health status. If the inability to adapt to the alteration is related to an alteration in thought processes, then the appropriate primary diagnosis would be Altered Thought Process.

Dysfunctional Grieving   Grieving can have a strong effect on the client's ability to adjust to an alteration in health status. The differentiation is complicated by the fact that a normal response to an alteration in health status can be grief. If, however, the client is not reporting a sense of loss, then the appropriate diagnosis would be Impaired Adjustment. If the client reports a sense of loss with the appropriate defining characteristics, then the appropriate diagnosis would be Grieving. If the grieving is prolonged or exceptionally severe, then an appropriate codiagnosis with Impaired Adjustment would be Dysfunctional Grieving.

EXPECTED OUTCOMES

1. Will verbalize increased adaptation to change in health status by (date) and/or
2. Will return-demonstrate measures necessary to increase independence by (date)

TARGET DATES

Adjustment to a change in health status will require time; therefore, an acceptable initial target date would be no sooner than 7 to 10 days following the date of diagnosis.

NURSING ACTIONS/INTERVENTIONS WITH RATIONALES

Adult Health

ACTIONS/INTERVENTIONS	RATIONALES
• Establish a therapeutic relationship with patient and significant others by showing empathy and concern for patient, calling patient by name, answering questions honestly, involving patient in decision making, etc.	A therapeutic relationship promotes cooperation in the plan of care and gives patient a person to talk with.
• Explain the disease process and prognosis to patient.	Knowledge of disease process and limitations are necessary for adjustment.
• Encourage patient to ask questions about health status by allowing opportunity and by asking patient to share his or her understanding of the situation.	Increasing knowledge and understanding leads to improved coping and adjustment.
• Encourage patient to express feelings about disease process and prognosis by sitting with the patient for 30 min once a shift at (times). Use techniques such as active listening, reflection, and asking open-ended questions.	Verbalization of feelings leads to understanding and adjustment.
• Identify previous coping mechanisms, and assist patient to find new ones.	Determines what coping strategies have been successful and provides an opportunity to try new strategies.
• Help patient find alternatives or modification in previous lifestyle behavior by using assistive devices, changing level of participation in activities, learning new behaviors, etc.	Helps patient continue to have satisfaction in activities and provides a sense of control in lifestyle.
• Encourage independence in self-care activities by focusing on patient's strengths, rewarding small successes, etc.	Provides a sense of control and increases self-esteem and adjustment.
• Refer patient to psychiatric nurse practitioner (see mental health nursing actions).	Collaboration promotes holistic approach to care, and problems may need intervention by specialist.

Child Health

ACTIONS/INTERVENTIONS	RATIONALES
• Monitor for all possible etiologic factors via active listening by asking questions that are appropriate for child (who, what, where, and when) regarding first feeling of not being able to adjust.	Provides the database needed to most accurately plan care.
• Help the child to realize it is normal to need some time and assistance in adjusting to changes, e.g., the child needing assistance with ambulation following surgery.	Realistic planning increases the likelihood of compliance and increases sense of success.
• Explore the child's and family's previous coping strategies.	Previous coping strategies serve as critical information in developing interventions for the current status.
• Identify ways the child can feel better about coping with the needed adjustment, including reinforcement of desired behavior.	Effective coping can empower the child and family and thereby afford a positive adjustment.
• Assist the child and family in creating realistic goals for coping.	Realistic goals enhance success.

Continued

ACTIONS/INTERVENTIONS	RATIONALES
• Collaborate with related health team members as needed.	Collaborations with specialists serve to meet the unique needs of the patient and family.
• Provide clear and simple explanations for procedures.	Simple and clear instructions promote the child's functioning while in a stressful situation.
• Address educational needs related to health care.	Knowledge serves to empower and provides guidelines for compliance with expected behavior.
• Deal with other primary care needs promptly.	Basic primary needs require prompt attention to offer the best likelihood of minimizing adjustment difficulty.
• Provide for posthospitalization follow-up with home care as needed.	Follow-up affords long-term resolution of adjustment.
• Assist patient and family in identification of community resources that can offer support.	Identification of resources prior to discharge will encourage the patient and family to use the resources as needed and will help them cope with the changes in their lifestyle.

Women's Health

ACTIONS/INTERVENTIONS	RATIONALES
COUVADE SYNDROME	
• When counseling with expectant fathers, be alert for characteristics of couvade syndrome[16]:	Provides database that allows early intervention.
◦ Syndrome affects males only.	
◦ Wives are pregnant and usually in the third or ninth month of gestation.	
◦ Symptoms are confined to the GI or GU system; notable exceptions are toothache and skin growths.	
◦ Anxiety and affective disturbances are common—e.g., constant worrying about labor events, "I can't do this" or "I just know I will faint"—and/or overmanaging arrangements for new baby—e.g., painting nursery 3 times.	
◦ Physical findings are minimal.	
◦ Laboratory and x-ray testing yields normal results.	
◦ Patient makes no connection between his symptoms and his wife's pregnancy.	
• Provide a nonjudgmental atmosphere to allow patient (in this instance, a male with the medical diagnosis of couvade syndrome) to express concerns of:	Encourages patient to talk about feelings and allows planning of how to channel feelings into activities that will assist in preparing for fatherhood.
◦ Self-image as a father	
◦ Relationship with his father	
◦ Self-responsibility	
◦ Feelings about wife's or partner's pregnancy	
◦ Concerns about wife's or partner's safety	
• Accurately record physical symptoms described by expectant father:	Allows more effective interventions and planning.
◦ Fatigue	
◦ Weight gain	
◦ Nausea or vomiting	
◦ Headaches	
◦ Backaches	
◦ Food cravings	
• Support and guide the expectant father through the changes being experienced.	
• Assure expectant couple that:	Emphasizes that this is not necessarily unusual behavior. Assists with positive actions that support both partners and allows the male to view pregnancy realistically.
◦ Expectant fathers can suffer physical symptoms during partner's pregnancy.	

○ Pregnancy affects both partners.
○ Fathers also have emotional needs during pregnancy.

POSTPARTUM AFFECTIVE DISORDERS

Postpartum Blues

This affects approximately 50–85% of all delivering women, is viewed as part of the adaptation process to childbirth, and usually resolves with normal support of family; therefore, it is not considered to be an impairment and will not be discussed here.

Postpartum Depression

Described as postpartum major affective disorder in psychiatric literature (usually occurs 2 wk to 3 mo postpartum).

- Encourage the client to express fears about the less-than-perfect infant. This can include:
  ○ Low-birth-weight infant
  ○ Different sex than that desired by parents
  ○ Fussy infant
  ○ Premature infant
  ○ Unwanted infant (could be infant as result of unwanted pregnancy and/or a result of rape)
- Continually assess the new mother's mood, observing for signs of:
  ○ Continuous crying
  ○ Insomnia not related to care of infant
  ○ Mood swings
  ○ Loss of appetite
  ○ Withdrawal
  ○ Irritability
  ○ Guilt feelings
  ○ Feeling of inability to care for self or infant or function in roles of wife and mother
  ○ Impaired memory
  ○ Lowered self-image

Nursing observations can be critical in getting these patients the professional help they need. Too often women feel this is just part of being a new mother and that they have no one who will listen. Often these signs and symptoms go unreported and unrecognized by family members.[17]

- Provide nonjudgmental atmosphere for patient to discuss problematic situations. Issues may include:
  ○ Partner's lack of sexual interest
  ○ Any illness or problems with older children
  ○ Marital status
  ○ Disappointment in experience (unwanted cesarean section, medications administered during labor, or any unexpected occurrences)
  ○ Isolation during postpartum period (unable to return to work immediately, no adults available to talk to during day, unable to complete daily activities due to fatigue, demands of infant, uncooperative partner, lack of support system, and so on)

Encourages patient to discuss feelings and verbalize disappointments or problems so that plans for coping with reality of birth experience can be initiated.

Postpartum Psychosis

The incidence of postpartum psychosis is approximately 1 in 1000 deliveries. Onset is acute and abrupt.[17]

- Obtain a complete patient history and family history, particularly regarding previous depressive or psychotic episodes. (Usually diagnosis has familial and/or genetic basis.)
- Collaborate with family members to never leave the patient alone, particularly with the infant.
- Arrange for family to take and care for the infant.

Continued

ACTIONS/INTERVENTIONS	RATIONALES
• If needed, arrange for community resources for care of the infant. • Obtain immediate assistance from mental health colleagues for mother. • Explain to family the likelihood of repetition of psychosis with subsequent pregnancies.	This diagnosis needs professional assistance immediately and is beyond the scope of practice for perinatal nursing. The main duty of the perinatal nurse is to see that no harm comes to mother or infant until mental health colleagues can assume care of mother.

Psychiatric Health

ACTIONS/INTERVENTIONS	RATIONALES
• Discuss with client his or her perception of the current alteration in health status. This should include information about the coping strategies that have been attempted and his or her assessment of what has made them ineffective in promoting adaptation.	Communicates respect for the client and his or her experience of the stressor, which promotes the development of a trusting relationship. Provides information about the client's strengths that can be utilized to promote coping and provides the nurse with an opportunity to support these strengths in a manner that promotes a positive orientation.
• Provide client with clocks and calendars to promote orientation and involvement in the environment. • Give client information about the care that is to be provided, including times for treatments, medicines, groups, and other therapy.	Maintains the client's cognitive strengths in a manner that will facilitate the development of coping strategies.[6] Promotes the client's sense of control.
• Assign client appropriate tasks during unit activities. These should be at a level that can easily be accomplished. Provide client with positive verbal support for completing the tasks. Gradually increase the difficulty of the tasks as the client's abilities increase.	Accomplishment of tasks provides the positive reinforcement that enhances self-esteem and motivates behavior. Also assists the client to develop a positive expectational set.
• Sit with client (number) minutes (number) times per day at (times) to discuss current concerns and feelings.	Communicates concern for the client and facilitates the development of a trusting relationship. Promotes the client's sense of control by communicating that his or her ideas and concerns are important.
• Provide client with familiar needed objects. These should be noted here. These should assist the client in identifying a personal space over which he or she feels some control. This space is to be respected by the staff, and the client's permission should be obtained before altering this environment.	Promotes the client's sense of control while meeting safety and security needs.
• Provide client with an environment that will optimize sensory input. This could include hearing aids, eyeglasses, pencil and paper, decreased noise in conversation areas, and appropriate lighting. (These actions should indicate an awareness of sensory deficit as well as sensory overload, and the specific interventions for this client should be noted here—e.g., place hearing aid in when client awakens and remove before bedtime (9:00 p.m.).	Appropriate levels of sensory input decreases confusion and disorganization, maximizing the client's coping abilities.
• Communicate to client an understanding that all coping behavior to this point has been his or her best effort and that asking for assistance at this time is not failure—a complex problem often requires some outside assistance to resolve.	

- Call client by the name he or she has identified as the preferred name with each interaction. Note this name on the chart.

Promotes a positive orientation while enhancing self-esteem.

- Have client dress in "street clothing." This should be items of clothing that have been brought from home and in which the client feels comfortable.

Promotes positive orientation and the client's sense of control by supporting normal daily routine and activities.

- Provide client with opportunities to make appropriate decisions related to care at his or her level of ability. This may begin as a choice between two options and then evolve into more complex decision making. It is important that this be at the client's level of functioning so that confidence can be built with successful decision-making experiences. Note here those decisions that the client has made.

Promotes the client's sense of control and enhances self-esteem when appropriate decisions are made.

- Provide client with primary care nurse on each shift. Nurse will spend 30 min once per shift at (time) developing a relationship with the client. This time could be spent answering client's questions about the hospital, about daily routines, etc., or providing the client with a backrub.

Promotes the development of a trusting relationship while promoting the client's sense of control with knowledge about the environment.

- Identify with client methods of anxiety reduction. The specific method selected by the client should be noted here. For the first 3 days the staff should remain with the client during a 30-min practice of the selected method. The method should be practiced 30 min 3 times a day at (times). (See Anxiety, Chap. 8, for specific instructions about anxiety reduction methods.)

High levels of anxiety interfere with decision making. Increased control over anxiety promotes the client's sense of control. The presence of the nurse can provide positive reinforcement, which encourages behavior. Behavioral rehearsal internalizes and personalizes the behavior.

- Provide positive social reinforcement and other behavioral rewards for demonstration of adaptation. Those things that the client finds rewarding should be listed here with a schedule for use. The kinds of behaviors that the team is to be rewarding should also be listed with the appropriate reward.

Reinforcement encourages positive behavior and enhances self-esteem.

- Assist client in identifying support systems and in developing a plan for their use. The support systems identified should be noted along with the plan for their use.

Support systems can facilitate the client's coping strategies.

- Schedule a meeting with the identified support system to assist them in understanding alterations in the client's health. Provide time to answer any questions they may have. Note the time for this meeting here and the person responsible for this meeting.

Promotes the development of a trusting relationship and provides the support system with the information that they can utilize to provide more effective support.

- Provide client with group interaction with (number) persons, (number) minutes, (number) times per day at (times). This activity should be graded with client's ability—e.g., on admission, client may tolerate 1 person for 5 min. If the interactions are brief, the frequency should be high—e.g., 5-min interactions should occur at 30-min intervals. If the client is meeting with a large client group, this may occur only once a day. The larger groups should include persons who are more advanced in adapting to their alterations and persons who may be less advanced.

Disconfirms the client's sense of aloneness and assists the client to experience personal importance to others while enhancing interpersonal relationship skills. Increasing these competencies can enhance self-esteem and promote positive orientation.

- Make available those items necessary for client to groom self. Have these items adapted as necessary to facilitate client use. List those items that are necessary here along with any assistance that is necessary from the nursing staff. Assign 1 person per day to be responsible for this assistance. Provide positive social reinforcement for client's accomplishments in this area.

Appropriate grooming enhances self-esteem. Reinforcement encourages positive behavior while enhancing self-esteem.

Continued

ACTIONS/INTERVENTIONS	RATIONALES
• Set an appointment to discuss with client and significant others effects of the loss or change on their relationship (time and date of appointment and all follow-up appointments should be listed here). Note person responsible for these meetings.	Promotes communication in the system that can serve as the basis for developing coping strategies.
• Monitor nurse's nonverbal reactions to loss or change, and provide client with verbal information when necessary to establish nurse's acceptance of the change.	Promotes the development of a trusting relationship and the development of a positive orientation.
• If nursing staff is having difficulty coping with the client's alterations, schedule a staff meeting where these issues can be discussed. An outside clinical nurse specialist may be useful in facilitating these meetings. Schedule ongoing support meetings as necessary.	Staff thoughts and feelings can be indirectly communicated to the client, which could have a negative effect on the client's developing a positive orientation.
• Utilize constructive confrontation if necessary to include I statements, relationship statements that reflect nurse's reaction to the interaction, and responses that will assist client in understanding, such as paraphrasing and validation of perceptions.	Models appropriate communication skills while providing the client with information that facilitates consensual validation.
• When a relationship has been developed, the primary care nurse will spend 30 min twice a day at (time) with the client discussing thoughts and feelings related to the alteration in health status. These discussions could include memories that have been activated by this alteration, client's fears and concerns for the future, client's plans for the future before the alteration in health status, client's perceptions of how this alteration will affect daily life, and client's perceptions of how this alteration will affect the lives of significant others.	Promotes the development of adaptive coping strategies.
• Provide client with information about care and treatment. Give information in concise terms appropriate to the client's level of understanding. Note here those areas for which client needs the most information with a plan for providing this information.	Promotes the client's sense of control. Inappropriate levels of sensory input can increase the client's confusion and disorganization.
• Do not argue with client while he or she is experiencing an alteration in thought process. (Refer to Altered Thought Process, Chap. 7, for related nursing actions.)	Arguing with these perceptions decreases the client's self-esteem and increases his or her needs to enlist dysfunctional coping behavior.
• Develop with the client a very specific behavioral plan for adapting to the alteration in health status. Note that plan here. This plan should include achievable goals so that the client will not become frustrated.	Achievement of a specific plan provides positive reinforcement and enhances self-esteem, which motivates positive behavior.
• Refer client to occupational therapy to develop the necessary adaptations to the occupational role. Note time for these meetings here.	Successful adaptation to the occupational role enhances self-esteem.
• Schedule time for the client and his or her support system to be together without interruptions. The times for these interactions should be noted here.	Provides opportunities for the support system to maintain normal relationships while the client is hospitalized.
• If client is disoriented, orient to reality as needed and before attempting any teaching activity. Provide client with clocks and calendars, and refer to day, date, and time in each interaction with this client.	Enhances the client's cognitive functioning, improving his or her ability to problem solve and to cope.
• Refer client to appropriate assistive resources as indicated. Note here those referrals made with the name of the contact person.	Establishes the client's support system in the community.

Gerontic Health

The nursing actions for gerontic patient with this diagnosis are the same as those for the adult health and mental health patient.

Home Health

ACTIONS/INTERVENTIONS	RATIONALES
• Monitor for factors contributing to impaired adjustment—e.g., psychologic, social, economic, spiritual, or environmental factors.	Provides database for intervention.
• Involve client and family in planning, implementing, and promoting reduction or elimination of impaired adjustment:	Family involvement enhances effectiveness of interventions.
○ Family conference: Discuss feelings and altered roles, and identify coping strategies that have worked in the past.	
○ Mutual goal sharing: Establish realistic goals and specify role of each family member—e.g., provide safe environment and support self-care.	
○ Communication: Clear and honest communication should be promoted among family members. If sensory impairments exist, corrective interventions are needed, e.g., eyeglasses or a hearing aid.	
• Assist client and family in lifestyle adjustments that may be required:	Family relationships can be altered by impaired adjustment. Permanent changes in behavior and family roles require evaluation and support.
○ Stress management	
○ Development and use of support networks	
○ Treatment for disability	
○ Appropriate balance of dependence and independence	
○ Grief counseling	
○ Change in role functions	
○ Treatment for cognitive impairment	
○ Provision of comfortable and safe environment	
○ Activities to increase self-esteem	
• Consult with or refer patient to appropriate assistive resources as indicated.	Utilization of existing services is efficient use of resources. Resources such as an occupational therapist, a psychiatric nurse clinician, and support groups can enhance the treatment plan.

Adjustment, Impaired

FLOWCHART EVALUATION: EXPECTED OUTCOME 1

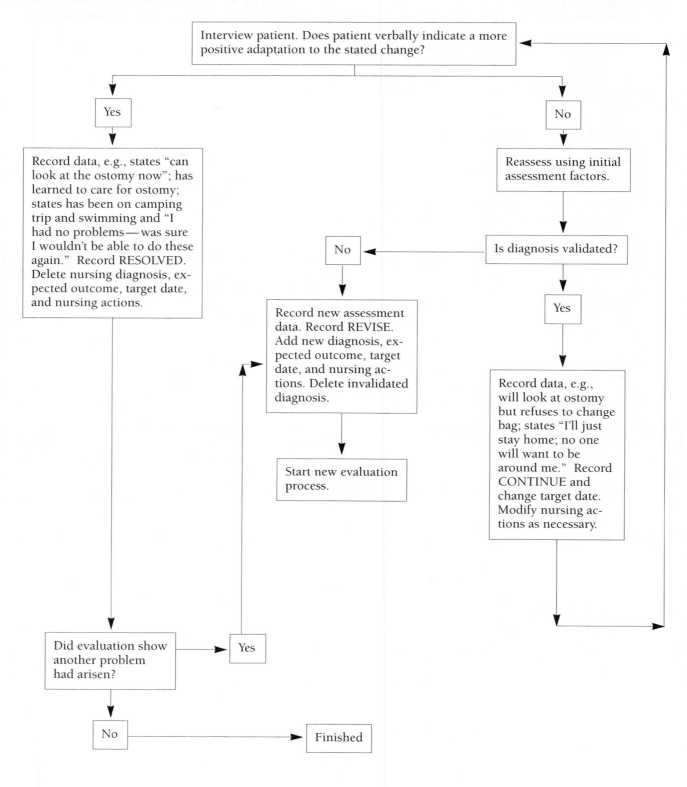

Adjustment, Impaired

FLOWCHART EVALUATION: EXPECTED OUTCOME 2

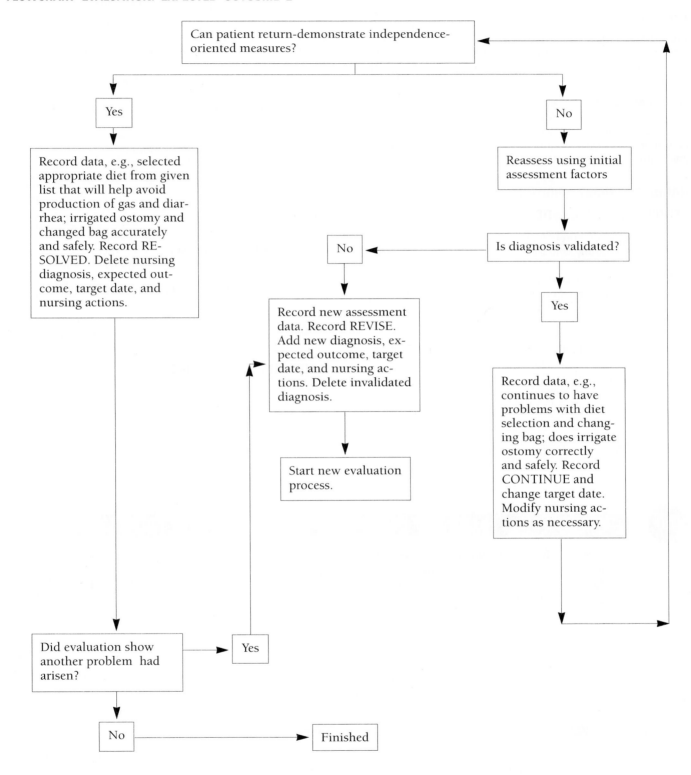

Community Coping, Ineffective and Potential for Enhanced

DEFINITION[15]

INEFFECTIVE COMMUNITY COPING A pattern of community activities for adaptation and problem solving that is unsatisfactory for meeting the demands or needs of the community.

POTENTIAL FOR ENHANCED COMMUNITY COPING A pattern of community activities for adaptation and problem solving that is satisfactory for meeting the demands or needs of the community but can be improved for management of current and future problems or stressors.

NANDA TAXONOMY: CHOOSING 5.1.3.2 AND 5.1.3.1

DEFINING CHARACTERISTICS[15]

1. Ineffective Community Coping
   a. Major defining characteristics
      None
   b. Minor defining characteristics
      (1) Community not meeting its own expectations
      (2) Deficits of community participation
      (3) Deficits in communication methods
      (4) Excessive community conflicts
      (5) Expressed difficulty in meeting demands for change
      (6) Expressed vulnerability
      (7) High illness rates
      (8) Stressors perceived as excessive
2. Potential for Enhanced Community Coping

   a. Major defining characteristics
      Deficits in one or more characteristics that indicate effective coping
   b. Minor defining characteristics
      (1) Active planning by community for predicted stressors
      (2) Active problem solving by community when faced with issues
      (3) Agreement that community is responsible for stress management
      (4) Positive communication among community members
      (5) Positive communication between community aggregates and larger community
      (6) Programs available for recreation and relaxation
      (7) Resources sufficient for managing stressors

RELATED FACTORS[15]

1. Ineffective Community Coping
   a. Deficits in social support
   b. Inadequate resources for problem solving
   c. Powerlessness
2. Potential for Enhanced Community Coping
   a. Social supports available
   b. Resources available for problem solving
   c. Community sense of power to manage stressors

RELATED CLINICAL CONCERNS

1. High incidence of violence
2. High illness rates

HAVE YOU SELECTED THE CORRECT DIAGNOSIS?

Effective Management of Therapeutic Regimen, Community This is an actual diagnosis indicating that a community has resolved its problems. Ineffective Community Coping and Potential for Enhanced Community Coping indicates that the community is either still in the throes of its problem or has just started problem solving.

EXPECTED OUTCOMES

1. Community leaders will verbally express more positive thoughts regarding the community's future by (date) and/or
2. Community will demonstrate fewer defining characteristics of ineffective coping by (date)

TARGET DATES

These diagnoses are very long term. Appropriate target dates would be expressed in terms of months or years.

NURSING ACTIONS/INTERVENTIONS WITH RATIONALES

Adult Health

Nursing actions specific for this diagnosis will require implementation in the home and community environment; therefore, the reader is referred to the Home Health nursing actions for this diagnosis.

Child Health

Same as for adult health, with acknowledgment of parents and caregivers assuming role of advocacy. Use developmentally appropriate approach. The effectiveness of interventions may depend on funding or interest of local potential supporters.

Women's Health

ACTIONS/INTERVENTIONS	RATIONALES

INEFFECTIVE COMMUNITY COPING
 	
NOTE: With early discharge of the new mother and baby, it has been noted that many communities are ineffective in having in place follow-up programs to assist these new mothers and their infants in the first critical postpartum days. Even with states' mandating "48-hour stays," there still exists a great need to support new mothers and their newborns after discharge from the hospital.
 	
• Investigate what programs are available to the new mother and her infant in the community. Different communities have different programs, such as:
  ○ Well-baby clinics
  ○ Public health department programs
  ○ Nursing centers (usually at schools of nursing in university settings)
  ○ State and federal programs such as First Steps, First Start, and maternity support programs
• Network with nursing colleagues in the community to assess how you can assist one another in providing continuity of care for these mothers and their newborns.
	Provides a coordinated flow of care for the patient. Allows for more equal distribution of scarce resources, which can eliminate the duplication of services to some while others have none.

POTENTIAL FOR ENHANCED COMMUNITY COPING **NOTE**: Many private nursing agencies and acute care hospitals have or are putting into place follow-up programs to deal with the issue of early discharge of the new mother and her infant. These programs include both telephone follow-up, postpartum after-care centers, and home visits.[18–21] Telephone Follow-Up • Call discharged mother within 36–48 h after discharge. Allow mother time to answer questions and expand on her answers if necessary. (Sometimes this takes some leading and directed questioning by the nurse.)	Provides follow-up contact with the new mother and her family. This contact can provide important information and monitoring, reinforcement of previous education, emotional and professional support to new parents, and referral to appropriate professional services if needed.

Continued

ACTIONS/INTERVENTIONS	RATIONALES

• Provide a nonjudgmental atmosphere that allows the new mother and/or father to verbalize concerns and needs.
• Ask for descriptions of infant's color, cord, circumcision (if appropriate), feeding patterns, stool patterns, and number of wet diapers.
• Ask mother to describe feeding sessions. If breast-feeding:
  ○ How often and how long does infant nurse?
  ○ Does infant nurse on both sides?
  ○ How do mother's breasts look (cracked, bleeding, or sore)?
  ○ Does infant latch on correctly?
  ○ What does the infant's stool look like, and how many wet diapers are there in a 24-h period?
  If formula feeding:
  ○ How often does infant feed?
  ○ How many ounces does infant take?
  ○ Is infant tolerating formula (not spitting excessively or having projectile vomiting)?
  ○ What is the color of the stool and pattern? How many wet diapers?
• Discuss potential for injury to infant, covering the following topics:
  ○ Use of approved car seat
  ○ Smoking in presence of infant or in a home where infant is
  ○ Use of proper bedding and proper positioning of infant in bed (on back or side)
  ○ Environmental safety ("childproofing" the house)
• Ask mother how she is feeling (tired, overwhelmed, out of sorts, etc.). Inquire about her physical well-being:
  ○ Episiotomy
  ○ Incision (if C-section)
  ○ Any alterations in involution (lochia-rubra, serosa, or alba)
  ○ Breasts
  ○ Stools (diarrhea or constipation)
  ○ Any signs and symptoms of infection (increased temperature, increased tenderness of uterus [abdomen], foul-smelling lochia)
• Instruct mother and/or father to call primary health care provider if any signs of infection are noted.
• If concerns are noted, make arrangements for mother, father, and infant to return to postpartum follow-up center or clinic and/or schedule a home visit by a nurse. If concerns are urgent, recommend that mother, father, and infant go to the emergency room and/or their primary health care provider immediately.	

Follow-up Clinic and/or Home Visit • Assess interaction between parents and parents with newborn. If siblings are present, assess their interaction with parents and new baby. • Assess mother for physical and psychologic well-being. (See above for physical well-being. See Adjustment, Impaired, for psychological well-being.)	Provides a creative solution to the early discharge of new mothers and their infants from the acute care system after birth. Allows for continuation of quality nursing care and monitoring of the postpartum progress of the mother and her infant.

- Assess home for social economic needs and make appropriate referrals, such as:
  - Enough to eat
  - Cleanliness
  - Assistance for new mother in home
  - Transportation
- Assess infant for physical well-being. (See above.)
- Document findings, and place them in mother and infant's charts when returning to hospital. Send copy of documentation to primary health care provider for both mother and infant.

Psychiatric Health

Refer to Home Health actions and interventions for these care plans.

Gerontic Health

ACTIONS/INTERVENTIONS	RATIONALES
INEFFECTIVE COMMUNITY COPING	
• Discuss examples of ineffective coping in order to begin problem solving.	Increases awareness of problems in the community and stimulates interest.
• Clarify questions related to coping that arise from problem-solving sessions.	Helps identify strategies that may increase coping skills.
• Identify fiscal resources available to the community for problem solving.	Local, regional, state, or federal programs may have funds dedicated to address problems related to aging.
• Identify local leaders (formal as well as informal) who have power within the community and gain their perspective.	
• Encourage use of community services to network for problem solving, such as radio or TV stations who offer to air public service announcements, newspapers to publish letters to the editors, or libraries to make available access to community internets.	Conserves money. Also increases likelihood of reaching the target audience in the community.
POTENTIAL FOR ENHANCED COMMUNITY COPING	
• Encourage participation in community activities.	Older adults are more likely to be involved in organized activities, such as senior citizens' groups. They are also more likely to vote and actively support or campaign for government candidates.
• Enlist older adults in community setting in problem-solving meetings.	Can provide historical perspective on the community and its growth pattern and needs.
• Consult with organized community resources such as RSVP or AARP groups for problem solving and future planning.	Provides a wealth of life experiences for problem solving within the community.
• Consider using phone trees, computer connections, or letter writing for older adults with decreased mobility who can still add to community life and growth.	Time is an important factor in community growth and planning, and older adults may have more time to assist the community. Activities such as those mentioned may be possible even for those with limited mobility.

Home Health

ACTIONS/INTERVENTIONS	RATIONALES

• Involve community groups in problem identification and program development:
  ○ Identify local needs for addressing problems or stressors.
  ○ Encourage participation in the community process.
	Involvement at the local level enhances community development and communication.

• Identify community strengths and weaknesses:
  ○ Develop strategies to enhance strengths and correct weaknesses.
  ○ Identify resources needed and resources available.
	Community recognition of strengths, weaknesses, and resources enhances the potential.

• Develop collaborative relationships within the community to promote development of the community.
• Utilize strategies identified for enhanced community coping to identify factors leading to Ineffective Community Coping:
  ○ Develop strategies to correct the deficits.
  ○ Develop plan with community involvement to correct deficits.
	Supportive relationships enhance the success of the plan.

Community Coping, Ineffective and Potential for Enhanced

FLOWCHART EVALUATION: EXPECTED OUTCOME 1

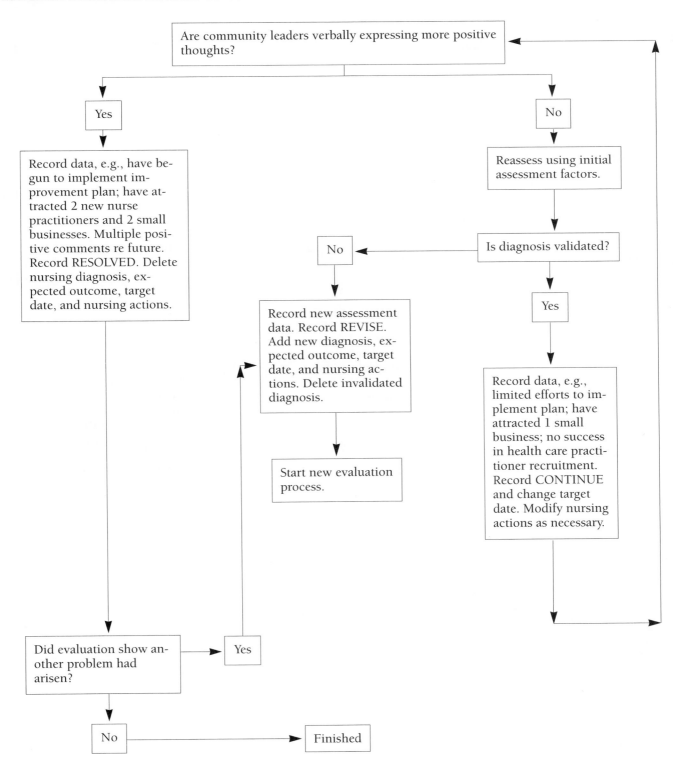

Community Coping, Ineffective and Potential for Enhanced

FLOWCHART EVALUATION: EXPECTED OUTCOME 2

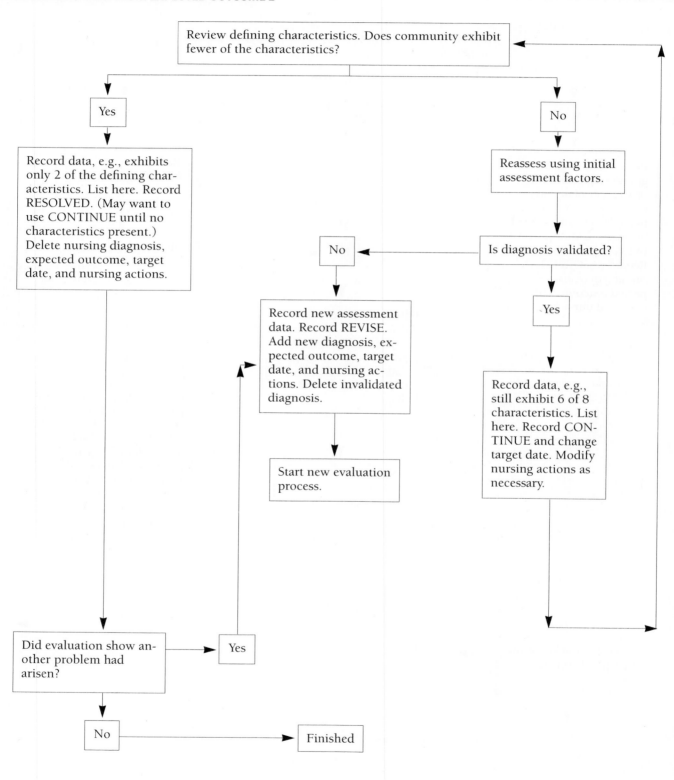

Family Coping, Ineffective, Compromised and Disabling

DEFINITION[15]

COMPROMISED A usually supportive primary person (family member or close friend) is providing insufficient, ineffective, or compromised support, comfort, assistance, or encouragement, which may be needed by the client to manage or master adaptive tasks related to his or her health challenge.

DISABLING Behavior of significant person (family or other primary person) that disables his or her own capacities and the client's capacities to effectively address tasks essential to either person's adaptation to the health challenge.

NANDA TAXONOMY: CHOOSING 5.1.2.1.1 AND 5.1.2.1.2

DEFINING CHARACTERISTICS[15]

1. Compromised
   a. Subjective:
      (1) Client expresses or confirms a concern or complaint about significant other's response to his or her health problems.
      (2) Significant person describes preoccupation with personal reaction (e.g., fear, anticipatory grief, guilt, or anxiety) to client's illness, disability, or to other situational or developmental crises.
      (3) Significant person describes or confirms an inadequate understanding or knowledge base that interferes with effective assistive or supportive behaviors.
   b. Objective:
      (1) Significant person attempts assistive or supportive behaviors with less than satisfactory results.
      (2) Significant person withdraws or enters into limited or temporary personal communication with the client at the time of need.
      (3) Significant person displays protective behavior disproportionate (too little or too much) to the client's abilities or need for autonomy.
2. Disabling
   a. Neglectful care of the client in regard to basic human needs and/or illness treatment
   b. Distortion of reality regarding the client's health problem, including extreme denial about its existence or severity
   c. Intolerance
   d. Rejection
   e. Abandonment
   f. Desertion
   g. Carrying on usual routines, disregarding client's needs
   h. Psychosomaticism
   i. Taking on illness signs of client
   j. Decisions and actions by family that are detrimental to economic or social well-being
   k. Agitation, depression, aggression, or hostility
   l. Impaired restructuring of a meaningful life for self, impaired individualization, or prolonged overconcern for client
   m. Neglectful relationships with other family members
   n. Client's development of helpless, inactive dependence

RELATED FACTORS[15]

1. Compromised
   a. Inadequate or incorrect information or understanding by a primary person
   b. Temporary preoccupation by a significant person who is trying to manage emotional conflicts and personal suffering and is unable to perceive or act effectively in regard to client's needs
   c. Temporary family disorganization and role changes
   d. Other situational or developmental crises or situations the significant person may be facing
   e. Little support provided by client, in turn, for primary person
   f. Prolonged disease or disability progression that exhausts supportive capacity of significant people
2. Disabling
   a. Significant person with chronically unexpressed feelings of guilt, anxiety, hostility, despair, etc.
   b. Dissonant discrepancy of coping styles for dealing with adaptive tasks by the significant person and client or among significant people
   c. Highly ambivalent family relationships
   d. Arbitrary handling of family's resistance to treatment, which tends to solidify defensiveness as it fails to deal adequately with underlying anxiety

RELATED CLINICAL CONCERNS

1. Alzheimer's disease
2. AIDS
3. Any disorder resulting in permanent paralysis
4. Cancer
5. Any disorder of a chronic nature, for example, rheumatoid arthritis
6. Substance abuse or use
7. Somatoform disorders

HAVE YOU SELECTED THE CORRECT DIAGNOSIS?

Compromised versus Disabling Coping Compromised dysfunction reflects the family that cannot provide appropriate support to the identified patient. This problem removes a possible support system from the client. If the family dysfunction results in further dysfunction for the identified patient, then the diagnosis is Disabling. Because this diagnosis is used to describe family processes, it may be difficult at times to differentiate between compromised and disabling because there is not an identified patient or the effects of the family patterns on the client cannot be determined. When this is the situation, the diagnosis can be made as Ineffective Family Coping with no attached label.

Family Coping, Potential for Growth This diagnosis is appropriate for families that are coping well with current stressors and are in a position to enhance their coping abilities. Ineffective Family Coping describes a family that has a deficit in coping abilities that threatens the family's existence.

Altered Parenting This diagnosis refers to an inability to fulfill the parenting role. This dysfunction is circumscribed to the parent-child relationship and is time-limited when contrasted with Ineffective Family Coping.

EXPECTED OUTCOMES

1. Will initiate a plan to cope with (the identified stressor) by (date) and/or
2. Will identify the effects current coping strategies have on the family by (date)

TARGET DATES

The target dates should reflect the complexity and power of the system. Four-week intervals would be appropriate to assess for progress.

NURSING ACTIONS/INTERVENTIONS WITH RATIONALES

Adult Health

ACTIONS/INTERVENTIONS	RATIONALES
• Encourage and assist family and significant others to verbalize their needs, fears, feelings, and concerns by sitting with patient for 30 min per shift at (times) or planning a family conference. Actively listen and facilitate discussion.	Allows for identification of specific stressors and promotes creative problem solving.
• Provide accurate information about the situation.	Clarifies misconceptions and misunderstanding.
• Include family and significant others in decision making and plan of care when planning care and intervening.	Promotes active participation, motivation, and compliance.
• Assist family and significant others to identify and explore alternatives to dealing with the situation, e.g., respite care, Mom's day out, or daycare centers.	Promotes creative problem solving.
• Assist family and significant others to identify sources of community support, prior to discharge, that could assist them to cope with their feelings and to supply relief when needed.	Community resources can help strengthen family coping process and prevent isolation of family.
• Encourage family to provide time for themselves on a regular basis.	Reduces stresses and strengthens coping skills.
• Initiate referral to psychiatric clinical nurse specialists as needed.	Problems may need intervention by specialist.

Child Health

ACTIONS/INTERVENTIONS	RATIONALES
• Encourage child and family to express feelings and fears by allotting 30 min per shift, while awake, for this purpose.	Expression of concerns provides insight into views about problem and the values of the patient and family.
• Review family dynamics previous to crisis.	Knowledge of family dynamics in usual times is paramount in understanding coping dynamics during times of stress.
• Encourage family members to participate in child's care, including bathing, feeding, comfort, and diversional activity.	Family and patient input ensures individualized plan of care. Provides teaching opportunity, and increases child's security.
• Provide education to all family members regarding child's illness, prognosis, and special needs as appropriate.	Reduces anxiety, increases likelihood of compliance, and empowers family.
• Involve health team members in collaboration for care.	Increases the likelihood of a holistic plan of care for both short-term and long-term goals.
• Provide referral to appropriate community resources for support purposes.	Provides for long-term follow-up and support.
• Provide for home discharge planning at least 5 days prior to discharge.	Allows time for teaching, practice, and return-demonstration.
• Make referral for home health care as needed.	Provides for long-term follow-up and support.

Women's Health

NOTE: This diagnosis would be most likely to relate to the single mother in the area of women's health.

ACTIONS/INTERVENTIONS	RATIONALES
• Review the physical, mental, social, and economic status of the single mother, taking into account if she is widowed, divorced, single and a parent by choice, or single and a parent not by choice. (See Adjustment, Impaired.)	Provides a database that can be used to plan appropriate interventions and locate support systems for patient.
• Identify support system available to the single mother, e.g., family, friends, coworkers, or formal support groups such as church or community organizations.	
• Review patient's perception of employment status, e.g., educational level and skills, job opportunities, and opportunity for improvement of employment status.	Assists patient to realistically plan for fiscal needs of herself and infant. Allows identification of resources that could assist in improving income status.
• Identify child care requirements considering the age of children, who has legal custody of children, and child support (financial and emotional).	

• Suggest strategies for exposing children to male role models[22]:
  ◦ Assign to classes with male teachers.
  ◦ Ask for assistance from brothers or grandparents.
  ◦ Involve children in sports (coaches are usually male).
	Provides for male role modeling in the absence of a father figure.

Psychiatric Health

ACTIONS/INTERVENTIONS	RATIONALES

• Role-model effective communication by:
  ○ Seeking clarification
  ○ Demonstrating respect for individual family members and the family system
  ○ Listening to expression of thoughts and feelings
  ○ Setting clear limits
  ○ Being consistent
  ○ Communicating with the individual being addressed in a clear manner
  ○ Encouraging the sharing of information among appropriate system subgroups
	Models for the family effective communication that can enhance their problem-solving abilities.

• Demonstrate an understanding of the complexity of system problems by:
  ○ Not taking sides in family disagreements
  ○ Providing alternative explanations of behavior patterns that recognize the contributions of all persons involved in the problem, including health care providers if appropriate
  ○ Requesting the perspective of multiple family members on a problem or stressor
	Promotes the development of a trusting relationship while developing a positive orientation.

• Determine risk for physical harm, and refer patient to appropriate authorities if risk is high (child protective services, battered women's centers, or police).	Client safety is of primary concern.

• Assist family in developing behavioral short-term goals by:
  ○ Asking what changes they would expect to see when the problem is improved
  ○ Having them break the problem into several parts that combine to form the identified stressor or crisis
  ○ Setting a time limit of 1 wk to accomplish a task—e.g., "What could you do this week to improve the current situation?"
	Accomplishment of goals provides reinforcement which motivates continued positive behavior and enhances self-esteem.

• Develop with family a priority list.	Promotes the family's sense of control and promotes the development of a trusting relationship by communicating respect for the client system.
• Begin work with the presenting problem, and enlist the system's assistance in resolving concerns.	Promotes the development of a trusting relationship while enhancing the client system's sense of control.
• Include assessment data in determining how to work on the presenting problem—e.g., if behavioral controls for a child are requested, the nurse can develop a plan for teaching and implementing them in the home that includes both parents.	

• Encourage communication between family members by:
  ○ Having family members discuss alternatives to the problem in the presence of the nurse
  ○ Having each family member indicate how he or she might help resolve the problem
  ○ Having each family member indicate how he or she contributes to the maintenance of the problem or how he or she does not help the identified patient change behavior
  ○ Spending time having the family members give each other positive feedback
	Assists the family in developing problem-solving skills that will serve them in future situations.

- Support the development of appropriate subgroups by:
  - Presenting problems to the appropriate subsystems for discussion—e.g., if the problem involves a discussion of how the sexual functioning of the marital couple will change as a result of illness, this issue should be discussed with the husband and wife
  - Providing an opportunity for the children to discuss their concerns with their parents
  - Supporting appropriate generational boundaries—e.g., parent's attempts to exclude children from parental roles
- Develop direct interventions that instruct a family to do something different or not to do something. If direct interventions are not successful and reassessment indicates they were presented appropriately, this may indicate that the family system is having unusual problems with the change process and should be referred to an advanced practitioner for further care.
- Provide experiences for the family to learn how they can think differently about the problem—e.g., a job loss can be seen as an opportunity to reevaluate family goals, focus on interpersonal closeness, and enhance family problem-solving skills.
- Provide opportunities for the expression of a range of affect; this can mean laughing and crying together. This validates family members' emotions and helps them to identify the appropriateness of their affective responses. This may require that the nurse "push" the family to express feelings with the skills of confrontation or provide the feedback.[23,24]
- Develop a teaching plan to provide the family with information that will enhance their problem solving.
- Assist family with interactions with other systems by:
  - Providing information about the system
  - Maintaining open communication between nurse and other agencies or systems
  - Having family identify what their relationship is with the system and how they could best achieve the goals they have for their interactions with this system
- Provide constructive confrontation to the family about problematic coping behavior.[23] Those kinds of behavior identified by the treatment team as problematic should be listed here.
- Teach family methods to reduce anxiety and practice and discuss the use of these methods with the family (number) times per week. This should be done at least once a week until family members are using this as a coping method. This could include deep muscle relaxation, physical exercise, family games that require physical activity, or cycling. Those methods selected by the family should be listed here with the time schedule for implementation. The family should be given "homework" related to the practice of these techniques at home on a daily basis.

Promotes healthy family functioning.
Provides information on the family's ability to change at this time while promoting a positive orientation.

Promotes a positive orientation while assisting the family in developing problem-solving skills.

Validates family members' emotions and helps to identify the appropriateness of their affective responses.

Facilitates the development of support networks in the community that can be called upon in future situations.

Facilitates the development of functional coping behaviors in a warm, supportive environment.

High levels of anxiety can interfere with adaptive coping behaviors. Repeated practice of a behavior internalizes and personalizes the behavior.

Continued

ACTIONS/INTERVENTIONS	RATIONALES
• Provide family with the information about proper nutrition that was indicated as missing on the assessment. This should include time spent on discussing how proper nutrition can fit the family lifestyle. This teaching plan should be listed here. A "homework" assignment related to the necessary pattern change should be given. This should involve all of the family members. Make an assignment that has high potential for successful completion by the family.	Proper nutrition promotes physical well-being, which facilitates adaptive coping. Successful accomplishment of goals provides positive reinforcement and motivates behavior while enhancing self-esteem. romotes positive orientation.
• If a homework assignment is not completed, do not chastise the family. Indicate that the nurse misjudged the complexity of the task, and assess what made it difficult for the family to complete the task. Develop a new, less complex task based on this information. If a family continues not to complete tasks, they may need to be referred to an advanced practitioner for continued care.	
• Monitor family's desire for spiritual counseling and refer to appropriate resources. The name of the resource person should be listed here.	
• Assist family in identifying support systems and in developing a plan for their use. This plan should be recorded here.	
• Refer family to community resources as necessary for continued support.	Provides resources that can give support in the community.

Gerontic Health

ACTIONS/INTERVENTIONS	RATIONALES
• Refer patient to adult protective services if risk of physical harm is high.	Provides means for monitoring patient and family. Effective use of resources to reduce risk of harm for patient.

Home Health

NOTE: See Psychiatric Health nursing actions for detailed family-oriented interventions.

ACTIONS/INTERVENTIONS	RATIONALES
• Involve client and family in planning and implementing strategies to improve family coping: ○ Crisis management: Identify actions to identify crisis and intervene—e.g., removing individuals from situation. ○ Mutual goal setting: Identify realistic goals and specify activities for each family member. ○ Communication: Provide realistic feedback in positive manner. ○ Family conference: Each member identifies how he or she is involved, and possible interventions are considered. ○ Support for caregiver.	Family involvement and clarification of roles is necessary to enhance interventions.

ACTIONS/INTERVENTIONS	RATIONALES

• Assist family and client in lifestyle adjustments that may be required:
  ○ Stress management
  ○ Altering past ineffective coping strategies
  ○ Treatment for substance abuse
  ○ Treatment for physical illness
  ○ Appropriate use of denial
  ○ Avoiding scapegoating
  ○ Activities of daily family living
  ○ Financial concerns
  ○ Change in geographic or sociocultural location
  ○ Potential for violence
  ○ Identifying family strengths
  ○ Obtaining temporary assistance, e.g., housekeeper, sitter, or temporary placement outside home
	Changes in family roles and behaviors require long-term behavorial changes. Support is required to facilitate these lifestyle changes.

• Consult with and refer patient to assistive resources as appropriate.	Utilization of existing services is efficient use of resources. Such resources as a family therapist, protective services, a psychiatric nurse clinician, and community support groups can enhance the treatment plan.

Family Coping, Ineffective, Compromised and Disabling

FLOWCHART EVALUATION: EXPECTED OUTCOME 1

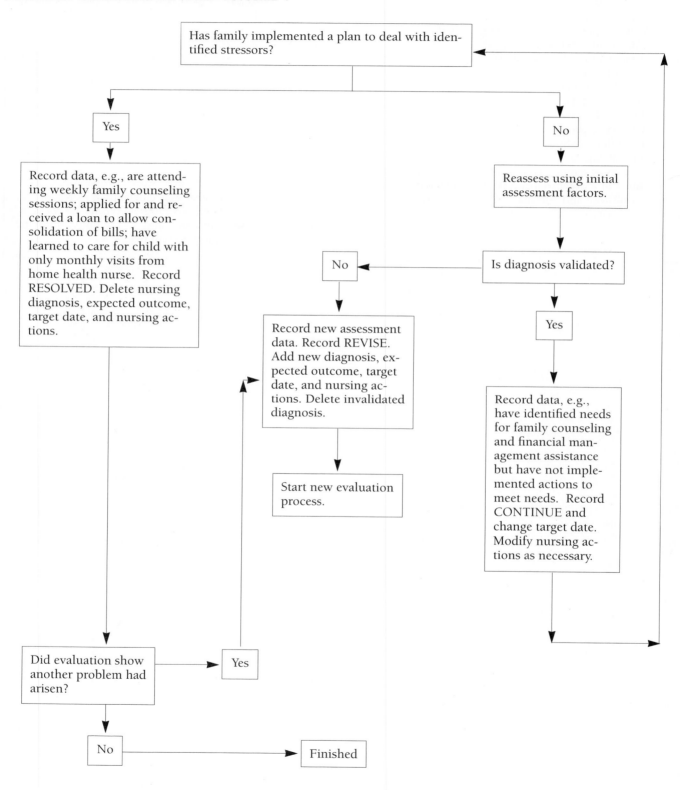

Family Coping, Ineffective, Compromised and Disabling

FLOWCHART EVALUATION: EXPECTED OUTCOME 2

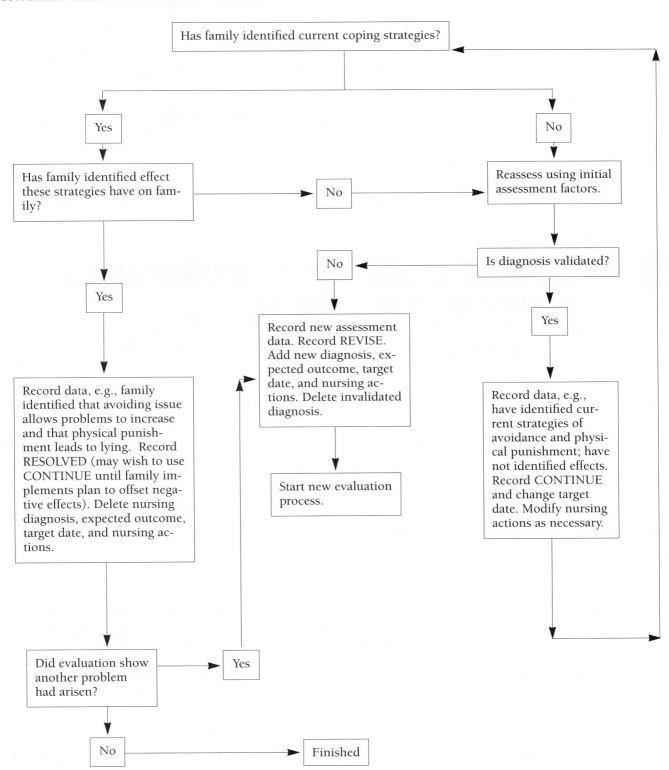

Family Coping, Potential for Growth

DEFINITION[15]

Effective managing of adaptive tasks by family member involved with the health challenge, who now is exhibiting desire and readiness for enhanced health and growth in regard to self and in relation to the client.

NANDA TAXONOMY: CHOOSING 5.1.2.2

DEFINING CHARACTERISTICS[15]

1. Major defining characteristics
   a. Family member attempting to describe growth impact of crisis on his or her own values, priorities, goals, or relationships
   b. Family member moving in direction of health-promoting and enriching lifestyle, which supports and monitors maturational processes, audits and negotiates treatment programs, and generally chooses experiences that optimize wellness

   c. Individual expressing interest in making contact on a one-to-one basis or on a mutual-aid group basis with another person who has experienced a similar situation
2. Minor defining characteristics
   None given

RELATED FACTORS[15]

Needs sufficiently gratified and adaptive tasks effectively addressed to enable goals of self-actualization to surface.

RELATED CLINICAL CONCERNS

1. Alzheimer's disease
2. AIDS
3. Any disorder resulting in permanent paralysis
4. Cancer
5. Any disorder of a chronic nature, for example, rheumatoid arthritis

HAVE YOU SELECTED THE CORRECT DIAGNOSIS?

Ineffective Family Coping and Altered Family Process   Family Coping, Potential for Growth, addresses the family that is currently handling stresses well and that is in a position to enhance their coping abilities. The other nursing diagnoses related to family functioning address various aspects of family dysfunction. If any dysfunction is present, Family Coping, Potential for Growth, would not be the diagnosis of choice.

EXPECTED OUTCOMES

1. Will verbalize satisfaction with current progress toward family goals by (date) and/or
2. Will identify at least (number) community groups that can provide family with useful input and output by (date)

TARGET DATES

Depending on the family size and the commitment of each member toward growth, the target date could range from weeks to months. A reasonable initial target date would be 2 weeks.

NURSING ACTIONS/INTERVENTIONS WITH RATIONALES
Adult Health

ACTIONS/INTERVENTIONS	RATIONALES
• Provide opportunities for family and significant others to discuss patient's condition and treatment modalities by scheduling at least 1 family session every other day.	Promotes understanding, open communication, creative problem solving, and growth.
• Include family and significant others in planning and providing care as care is planned and implemented.	Promotes active participation, motivation, and compliance. Provides a teaching opportunity and an opportunity for family to practice in a supportive environment.
• Provide instruction as needed in supportive and assistive behavior for patient.	Understanding and knowledge base are needed to adapt to situations. Reduces anxiety.
• Answer questions clearly and honestly.	Promotes a trusting relationship.
• Refer family and significant others to support groups and resources as indicated.	Coordination and collaboration organize resources and decrease duplication of services. Provides a broader range of networked resources.

Child Health

ACTIONS/INTERVENTIONS	RATIONALES
• Identify how the child views the current crisis by using play, puppetry, etc. • Identify family and child's previous and current coping patterns. • Assist child in identifying ways the current crisis or situation can enhance his or her coping for future needs. • Identify appropriate health team members who can assist in providing support for growth potential. • Offer educational instruction to meet patient's and family's needs related to health care. • Allow for sufficient time while in hospital to reinforce necessary skills for care, e.g., ROM exercises.	The impact of the crisis on the child is basic data needed for planning care. Family coping behaviors serve as reference data to understand the child's response and behavior. Will also provide needs assessment data for planning of teaching. Viewing current situation for beneficial outcomes can assist in creating a positive outcome. Specialists may best assist patient in positive resolution of crisis. Knowledge serves to empower the patient and family and assists in reducing anxiety. Learning in a supportive environment provides reinforcement of desired content.

Women's Health

ACTIONS/INTERVENTIONS	RATIONALES
• Encourage participation of significant others in preparation for birth, e.g., spouse, boyfriend, partner, children, in-laws, grandparents, and others who are important to the individual. • Discuss childbirth and the changes that will occur in the family unit. • Encourage patient to list family lifestyle adjustments that need to be made. Involve significant others in discussion and problem-solving activities regarding family adjustments to the newborn, e.g., child care, working, household responsibilities, social network, or support groups. • Encourage woman and partner (significant other) to attend childbirth education classes or parenting classes in preparation for the birthing experience.	Enhances support system for patient and promotes positive anticipation of birth. Provides directions for anticipation of birth and allows more long-range planning that can prevent crises. Provides basic information that assists in easing labor experience. Promotes a more positive birth experience and reduces anxiety.

Psychiatric Health

ACTIONS/INTERVENTIONS	RATIONALES
• Talk with family to identify their goals and concerns. • Assist family in identifying strengths. • Refer family to appropriate community support groups. • Teach family those skills necessary to provide care to an ill member. • Talk with family about the role flexibility necessary to cope with an ill member and how this may be affecting their family. • Provide family with information about normal developmental stages and anticipatory guidance related to these stages.	Promotes development of a trusting relationship by communicating respect and concern for the family. Promotes a positive orientation. Provides support networks in the community. Provides family with an increased repertoire of behavior that they can use to effectively cope with the situation. Assists family in anticipatory planning for the necessary adjustments that could evolve from the present situation. Anticipatory planning increases their opportunities for successful coping, which enhances self-esteem. Promotes sense of control and increases opportunities for successful coping.

Continued

ACTIONS/INTERVENTIONS	RATIONALES
• Discuss with family normal adaptive responses to an ill family member, and relate this to their current functioning.	Promotes family's strengths.
• Support appropriate family boundaries by providing information to the appropriate family subgroup.	Promotes healthy family functioning.
• Model effective communication skills for family by using active listening skills, I messages, problem-solving skills, and open communication without secrets.	Effective communication improves problem-solving abilities.
• Spend 1 h with family on a weekly basis providing them with the opportunity to practice communication skills and to share feelings (if this is an identified goal).	Behavioral rehearsal provides opportunities for feedback and modeling of new behaviors by the nurse.
• Arrange 1-h appointments with client weekly for 1 mo to assess progress on the established goals. The need for continued follow-up can be decided at the end of the last scheduled visit.	Provides opportunities for the nurse to give positive reinforcement and promotes positive orientation.
• Accept family's decisions about goals for care.	Promotes family's sense of control.
• Discuss with family the role nutrition has in health maintenance, and develop a family nutritional plan. Consult with nutritionist as necessary.	Nutrition impacts coping abilities.
• Discuss with family the role exercise has in improving ability to cope with stress and assist in the development of a family exercise plan. Consult with physical therapist as necessary.	Exercise improves physical stamina and increases the production of endorphins.

Gerontic Health

The nursing actions for gerontic patient with this diagnosis are the same as those for the adult health and mental health patient.

Home Health

NOTE: See Psychiatric Health nursing actions for specific family-oriented activities.

ACTIONS/INTERVENTIONS	RATIONALES
• Involve client and family in planning and implementing strategies to enhance health and growth: 　◦ Family conference: Identify family strengths. 　◦ Mutual goal setting: Establish family goals, and identify specific activities for each family member. 　◦ Communication: Enhance family discussions and support.	Family involvement in planning enhances growth and implementation of the plan.
• Assist family and client in lifestyle adjustments that may be required: 　◦ Provide information related to health promotion. 　◦ Provide information related to expected growth and development milestones, both individual and family. 　◦ Assist in development and use of support networks.	Support enhances permanent behavioral changes.
• Consult with and refer patient to assistive resources as appropriate.	Community services provide a wealth of resources to enhance growth—e.g., service organizations such as Lion's Club, Altrusa, etc., colleges and universities, or recreational facilities.

Family Coping, Potential for Growth

FLOWCHART EVALUATION: EXPECTED OUTCOME 1

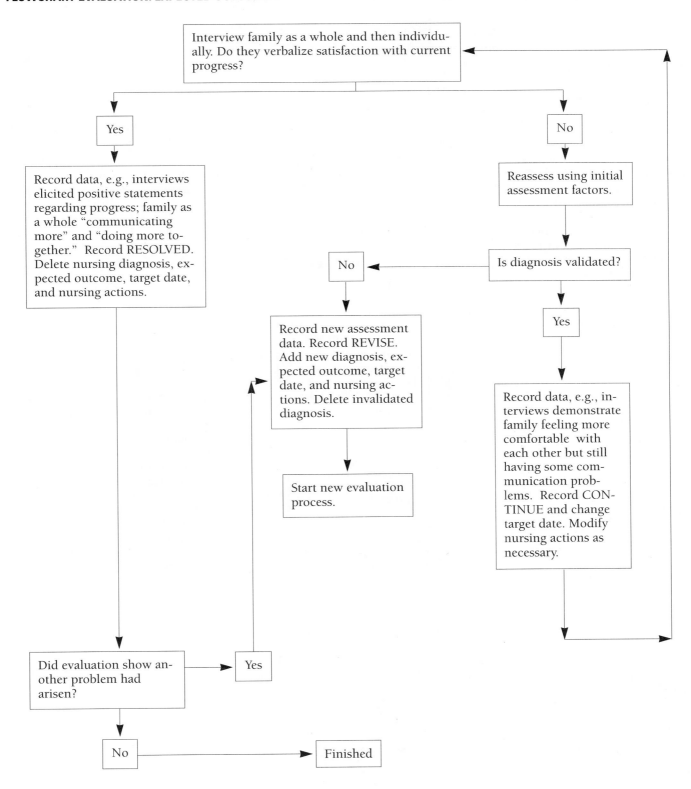

Family Coping, Potential for Growth

FLOWCHART EVALUATION: EXPECTED OUTCOME 2

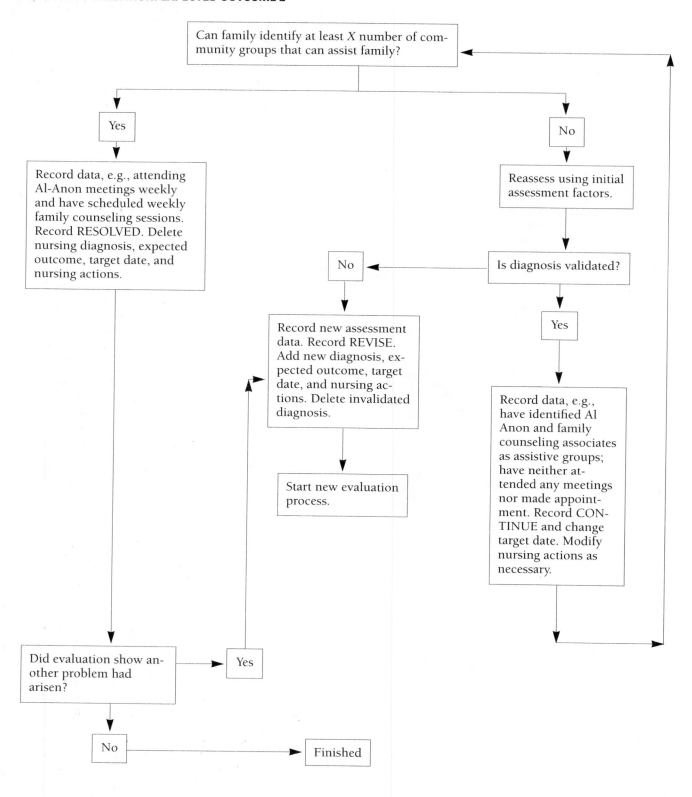

Individual Coping, Ineffective

DEFINITION[15]

INEFFECTIVE INDIVIDUAL COPING Impairment of adaptive behaviors and abilities of a person in meeting life's demands and roles.

DEFENSIVE COPING The state in which an individual repeatedly projects falsely positive self-evaluation based on a self-protective pattern that defends against underlying perceived threats to positive self-regard.

INEFFECTIVE DENIAL The state of a conscious or unconscious attempt to disavow the knowledge or meaning of an event to reduce anxiety or fear to the detriment of health.

NANDA TAXONOMY: CHOOSING 5.1.1.1, 5.1.1.1.2, AND 5.1.1.1.3

DEFINING CHARACTERISTICS[15]

1. Ineffective Individual Coping
   a. Major defining characteristics
      (1) Verbalization of inability to cope or inability to ask for help*
      (2) Inability to meet role expectations
      (3) Inability to meet basic needs
      (4) Inability to problem solve*
      (5) Alteration in societal participation
      (6) Destructive behavior toward self or others
      (7) Inappropriate use of defense mechanisms
      (8) Change in usual communication patterns
      (9) Verbal manipulation
      (10) High illness rate
      (11) High rate of accident
   b. Minor defining characteristics
      None given
2. Defensive Coping
   a. Major defining characteristics
      (1) Denial of obvious problems or weaknesses
      (2) Projection of blame or responsibility
      (3) Rationalizing of failures
      (4) Hypersensitivity to slight or criticism
      (5) Grandiosity
   b. Minor defining characteristics
      (1) Superior attitude toward others
      (2) Difficulty establishing or maintaining relationships

      (3) Hostile laughter or ridicule of others
      (4) Difficulty in reality testing perceptions
      (5) Lack of follow-through or participation in treatment or therapy
3. Ineffective Denial
   a. Major defining characteristics
      (1) Delays seeking or refuses health care attention to the detriment of health
      (2) Does not perceive personal relevance of symptoms or danger
   b. Minor defining characteristics
      (1) Uses home remedies (self-treatment) to relieve symptoms
      (2) Does not admit fear of death or invalidism
      (3) Minimizes symptoms
      (4) Displaces source of symptoms to other organs
      (5) Unable to admit impact of disease on life pattern
      (6) Makes dismissive gestures or comments when speaking of distressing events
      (7) Displaces fear of impact of the condition
      (8) Displays inappropriate affect

RELATED FACTORS[15]

1. Ineffective Individual Coping
   a. Situational crises
   b. Maturational crises
   c. Personal vulnerability
2. Defensive Coping
   a. None given
3. Ineffective Denial
   a. None given

RELATED CLINICAL CONCERNS

1. Eating disorders
2. Substance abuse or use disorders ˙
3. Psychotic disorder
4. Somatoform disorders
5. Dissociative disorders
6. Adjustment disorders
7. A diagnosis with a terminal prognosis
8. Chronic illnesses or disabilities
9. Any condition that can cause alterations in body image or function

---

*Critical.

HAVE YOU SELECTED THE CORRECT DIAGNOSIS?

Anxiety Ineffective Individual Coping would be used if the client demonstrates both an inability to cope appropriately and anxiety. If the client is demonstrating anxiety with appropriate coping, then the diagnosis would be Anxiety. Ineffective Individual Coping would only be used if the client could not adapt to the anxiety.

Risk for Violence If the aggressive behavior of the client poses the threat of physical or psychologic harm, the most appropriate diagnosis would be Risk for Violence. If the client's risk for violence is assessed to be very low, then this would be the secondary diagnosis with Ineffective Individual Coping being the primary diagnosis. In this situation the diagnosis of Risk for Violence would serve as a reminder to care providers to remain alert to the potential for this behavior.

Sensory-Perceptual Alteration If coping abilities are affected by alterations in sensory input, then Sensory-Perceptual Alteration would be the most appropriate primary diagnosis.

Altered Thought Process This diagnosis can affect the individual's ability to cope. If these alterations are present with Ineffective Individual Coping, then the primary diagnosis should be Altered Thought Process. Effective problem solving is inhibited as long as this disruption in thinking is present.

Dysfunctional Grieving If the client's behavior can be related to resolving a loss or change, then the appropriate diagnosis is Dysfunctional Grieving. The loss can be actual or perceived. If the client demonstrates an inability to manage this process, then the appropriate diagnosis would be Ineffective Individual Coping.

Powerlessness This diagnosis can produce a personal perception that would result in Ineffective Individual Coping. If one perceives that one's own actions cannot influence the situation, then Powerlessness would be the primary diagnosis.

EXPECTED OUTCOMES

1. Will describe implementation of a plan to cope with the identified stressors by (date) and/or
2. Will return-demonstrate at least (number) new coping strategies by (date)

TARGET DATES

A realistic target date, considering assessment and teaching time, would be 7 days from the date of the diagnosis.

NURSING ACTIONS/INTERVENTIONS WITH RATIONALES

Adult Health

ACTIONS/INTERVENTIONS	RATIONALES
• Assist patient to identify and explore specific situations that are creating stress and possible alternatives for dealing with the situation by allowing at least 1 h per shift for interviewing and teaching.	Identification of problem area is first step in problem solving and promotes creative problem solving.
• Help the patient to evaluate which methods he or she has used that have not been successful or have been only partially successful.	Allows for strengthening of effective coping methods and elimination of ineffective ones.
• Monitor for and reinforce behavior suggesting effective coping continuously.	Strengthens and enhances coping skills. Increases confidence to risk new coping strategies.
• Maintain consistency in approach and teaching whenever interacting with patient.	Reduces stress. Promotes trusting relationship.

- Encourage participation in care by assisting patient to maintain activities of daily living to degree possible.
- Encourage support from family and significant others by allowing participation in care, encouraging questions, and allowing expression of feelings.
- Teach relaxation techniques such as meditation, exercise, yoga, deep breathing, or imagery. Have patient practice for 10 min twice a shift at (times).
- Assist patient to identify and use available support systems before discharging from hospital.
- Initiate referral to psychiatric clinical nurse specialist as needed.

Promotes self-care, enhances coping, builds self-esteem, and increases motivation and compliance.
Broadens support network. Builds self-esteem in support systems.

Reduces stress and provides alternative coping strategies.

Broadens support network to reach short-term and long-term goals.
Specialized skills may be needed to intervene in significant problem areas.

Child Health

ACTIONS/INTERVENTIONS	RATIONALES
• Establish a trusting relationship with the child and respective family by allowing time (30 min) per shift, while awake, for verbalization of concerns and their perception of the situation.	Promotes communication and allows gathering of data that enhances care planning.
• Identify need for collaboration with related health team members.	Specialist, e.g., mental health, may best be able to deal with the problem.
• Reinforce appropriate behavior of choosing or coping by verbal praise.	Positive reinforcement will enhance learning of coping mechanisms.
• Assist the patient and family in setting realistic goals.	Realistic goals enhance success, which increases coping ability.
• Provide appropriate attention to primary nursing needs.	Meeting of primary care needs allows patient to focus energy on coping.
• Offer education to provide clarification of information as needed, regarding any health-related needs.	Provides basic knowledge needed to avoid future crises. Increases options for coping choices.
• Determine appropriate developmental baseline behavior versus actual coping behavior.	Baseline data will provide valuable information for comparative follow-up.
• Administer medications as ordered, including sedatives.	Relaxation assists in decreasing anxiety. Conserves energy to deal with crisis.
• Set aside time each shift (specify) to deal with how child and parents feel about the defensive behavior. This may require art, puppetry, or related expressive dynamics.	Acting out or expressing feelings provides valuable data that increase the likelihood of a successful plan of care.
• Provide feedback with support for progress. When progress is not occurring, provide reflective referral back to child and parent as applicable.	Feedback serves to clarify and allows for reviewing the specific coping activity with reteaching as needed.
• Provide ongoing information regarding child's health status, which could affect defensive behavior by child or parents.	Factors related to coping may well be influenced by residual effects from illness. Misinformation or lack of information can also be detrimental to positive coping.
• Throughout defensive coping period, monitor and ensure child's safety.	Basic standard of care.
• Determine disciplinary plans for all to abide by with safety in mind.	Structured limit setting will provide security and safety.
• Provide appropriate reality confrontation according to readiness of child and parents.	Reality confrontation helps keep perspective on here and now and is a useful approach to initiate coping with current situation.
• Provide for discharge planning with reinforcement of value of follow-up appointments as needed.	Attaching value to follow-up increases the likelihood of satisfactory attendance for appointments and other follow-up activities.
• Identify, along with patient and family, resources to assist in coping, including support groups.	Support groups provide empowerment and a sense of shared concern.

Women's Health

ACTIONS/INTERVENTIONS	RATIONALES
• Identify groups at high risk for ineffective individual coping, e.g., single parents, minority women, women with superwoman syndrome, and lesbians.	Provides database that allows for early recognition, planning, and action.
• Identify situations that place patients at risk for ineffective individual coping—e.g., unwanted or unplanned pregnancy, unhappy home situation (marriage), demands at work, or demands of children or spouse. (See Adjustment, Impaired, for Postpartum Depression.)	
• Assist patient in identifying typical stressful times—e.g., at home, at work, in social situations, or during an average day.	
• Assist patient in identifying lifestyle adjustments that may be made to lower stress levels—e.g., planning for divorce or planning for job change (either part-time or unemployment for a period of time).	Supports patient in identification and planning of strategies to reduce stress.
• Assist patient in identifying factors that contribute to ineffective coping—e.g., depression, guilt (blaming self), assuming helplessness, passive acceptance of traditional feminine role, anger toward self and others (aggressive behavior, suicide threats, or substance abuse), or failure to make time for self (relaxation, pleasure, or self-care).	Identification of factors that contribute to the situation is the first step in learning positive rather than negative skills.
• Assist patient in developing problem-solving skills to modify stressors—e.g., using 12-step plans (as developed by Alcoholics Anonymous) or planning time for self-rewarding activities such as exercise or long, quiet baths.	Assists patient in planning positive actions and in communicating her needs to others.
• Assist patient in identifying negative and positive responses to stressors—e.g., pressures at work such as being constantly interrupted or becoming defensive when challenged.	
• Assist patient in developing an individual plan of stress management—e.g., relaxation techniques or assertiveness training.	
• Involve significant others in discussion and problem-solving activities.	
• Provide a nonjudgmental atmosphere that allows the patient to discuss her feelings about the pregnancy, including such areas as lifestyle, children, or support systems.	
• Explore patient's use of what she perceives are contraceptives,[25] e.g., pills, intrauterine device, diaphragm, withdrawal, feminine hygiene products, douching, foams (spermicides), or rhythm.	Provides basis for planning lifestyle options.
• Explore patient's lack of contraceptive use due to[26]: ignorance—"It won't happen to me" syndrome; guilt—"If I use the pill, then I am not good"; spontaneity; excitement due to risk, loneliness, crisis, or pressure, or uncertainty in sex role relationships or self-image.	Provides health care personnel information to plan care that enhances likelihood of successful compliance.

Psychiatric Health

ACTIONS/INTERVENTIONS	RATIONALES
• Determine client's functional abilities and developmental level for the adaptation of all future interventions. (The results of this assessment should be noted here.)	Cognitive abilities can impact the client's ability to develop appropriate coping behaviors.
• Discuss with the client his or her perception of the current crisis and stressors. This should include information about the coping strategies that the client has attempted and his or her assessment of what has made them ineffective in resolving this stressor or crisis.	Promotes the development of a trusting relationship by communicating respect for the client.
• Assist client in developing an appropriate time frame for the resolution of the situation. (Often when experiencing a crisis, an individual has the perception that resolution must take place immediately.) This could include, as appropriate to the client's situation:	"De-catastrophizes" the client's perceptions of the situation.[27]
◦ Informing client that any difficulty that has taxed his or her resources as much as this one has will take an extended time to resolve because it must be complex	
◦ Informing the client that a situation as important as this one is to the individual's future deserves a well-thought-out answer and that a decision should not be made hastily	
◦ Assisting the client in determining the source of the time pressure and the appropriateness of this time frame	
◦ Assisting the client in developing an appropriate perspective on the time frame (One question that could be useful is "What would be the worst that could happen if this problem is not resolved by [put client's stated time frame here]?")	
• Provide a quiet, nonstimulating environment or an environment that does not add additional stress to an already overwhelmed coping ability. (Potential environmental stressors for this client should be listed here with the plan for reducing them in this environment).	Inappropriate levels of sensory stimuli can increase confusion and disorganization.
• Sit with client (number) minutes (number) times per day at (specify times here) to discuss current concerns and feelings.	Communication of concerns in a supportive environment can facilitate the development of adaptive coping behaviors. Continues the development of a trusting relationship.
• Assist client with setting appropriate limits on aggressive behavior. (See Risk for Violence, Chap. 9, for more detailed nursing actions if this diagnosis develops.)	
• Decrease environmental stimulation as appropriate (this might include a secluded environment).	Inappropriate levels of environmental stimuli can increase disorganization and confusion, increasing the risk for acting-out behavior.
• Providing client with appropriate alternative outlets for physical tension. (This should be stated specifically and could include walking, running, talking with a staff member, using a punching bag, listening to music, or doing a deep muscle relaxation sequence.) Strategies should be employed (number) times per day at (times) or when increased tension is observed. These outlets should be selected with the client's input.	Physical activity decreases the tension that is related to anxiety. Appropriate control of behavior promotes the client's sense of control and enhances self-esteem.
• Orient client to date, time, and place. Provide clocks, calendars, and bulletin boards. Make references to this information in daily interactions with the client. The frequency needed for this client should be noted here, e.g., every 2 h, every day, or 3 times a day.	Orientation enhances the client's coping abilities.

Continued

ACTIONS/INTERVENTIONS	RATIONALES
• Provide client with familiar or needed objects. These should be noted here.	Promotes the client's sense of control while meeting security needs.
• Provide client with an environment that will optimize sensory input. This could include hearing aids, eyeglasses, pencil and paper, decreased noise in conversation areas, or appropriate lighting. (These interventions should indicate an awareness of sensory deficit as well as sensory overload.) The specific interventions for this client should be noted here—e.g., place hearing aid in when client awakens and remove before bedtime (9:00 p.m.).	Inappropriate levels of sensory stimuli can increase confusion and disorganization.
• Provide client with achievable tasks, activities, and goals (these should be listed here). These activities should be provided with increasing complexity to give client an increasing sense of accomplishment and mastery.	Accomplishment of these goals provides reinforcement and encourages positive behavior while enhancing self-esteem.
• Communicate to client an understanding that all coping behavior to this point has been his or her best effort and that asking for assistance at this time is not failure. A complex problem often requires some outside assistance to resolve.	Assists client to maintain self-esteem, diminishes feelings of failure, and promotes a positive orientation.
• Provide client with opportunities to make appropriate decisions related to care at his or her level of ability. This may begin as a choice between two options and then evolve into more complex decision making.	
• It is important that decision making be at the client's level of functioning so that confidence can be built with successful decision-making experience.	Promotes the client's sense of control.
• Provide client with a primary care nurse on each shift.	Promotes the development of a trusting relationship.
• When relationship has been developed with primary care nurse, this person will sit with client (minutes—begin with 30 and increase as client's ability to concentrate improves) per shift to discuss concerns about sexual issues, fears, and anxieties.	Promotes development of a trusting relationship. Discussion of concerns in a supportive environment promotes the development of alternative coping behaviors.
• Provide constructive confrontation for client about problematic coping behavior.[23] Those kinds of behavior identified by the treatment team should be listed here.	Assists client in reality testing of coping behaviors.
• Provide client with information about care and treatment. Give information in concise terms appropriate to the client's level of understanding.	Promotes the client's sense of control. Inappropriate level of sensory stimuli increases confusion and disorganization.
• Identify with client methods for anxiety reduction. Those specific methods selected should be listed here.	High levels of anxiety decrease the client's coping abilities and interfere with the learning of new behaviors.
• Assist client with practice of anxiety reduction techniques, and remind him or her to implement these techniques when level of anxiety is increasing.	Repeated practice of a behavior internalizes and personalizes the behavior.
• Provide client with opportunities to test problem solutions either by role-playing or by applying them to graded real-life experiences.	Behavioral rehearsal helps to facilitate the client's learning new skills through the use of feedback and modeling by the nurse.
• Assist client to revise problem solutions if they are not effective. (This will assist patient to learn that no solution is perfect or final and that problem solving is a process of applying various alternatives and revising them as necessary.)	Promotes positive orientation and enhances the client's self-esteem by turning disadvantages into advantages.[27]
• Allow client to discover and develop solutions that best fit his or her concerns. The nurse's role is to provide assistance and feedback and to encourage creative approaches to problem behavior.	Promotes the client's sense of control and development of new behaviors. Enhances the client's problem-solving behaviors and improves self-esteem.

- Teach client these skills that facilitate problem solving such as assertive behavior, goal setting, relaxation, evaluation, information gathering, requesting assistance, and early identification of problem behavior. Those skills that are identified by the treatment team as being necessary should be listed here with the teaching plan. This should include a schedule of the information to be provided and identification of the person responsible for providing the information.

Increases repertoire of coping behaviors, decreasing all-or-none thinking.[27]

- Spend (number) minutes 2 times per day at (times) with client role-playing and practicing problem solving and implementation of developed solutions. This will be the responsibility of the primary care nurse.

Repeated practice of a behavior internalizes and personalizes the behavior.

- Assist client in identifying those problems he or she cannot control or resolve and in developing coping strategies for these situations. This may involve alteration of the client's perception of the problem.

Increases the client's opportunities for success in early problem-solving attempts. This success provides reinforcement, which motivates positive behavior and enhances self-esteem.

- Monitor client's desire for spiritual counseling, and refer client to appropriate resources.

Increases the resources available to the client.

- Provide positive social reinforcement and other behavioral rewards for demonstration of adaptive problem solving. (Those things that the client finds rewarding should be listed here with a schedule for use. The kinds of behavior that are to be rewarded should also be listed.)

Reinforcement encourages positive behavior and enhances self-esteem.

- Assist client in identifying support systems and in developing a plan for their use.

Decreases the client's sense of social isolation.

- The following interventions relate to the client who is experiencing problems related to organic brain dysfunction:

Inappropriate levels of sensory stimuli increase confusion and disorganization.

  ○ Maintain a consistent environment; do not move furniture or personal belongings.
  ○ Remove hazardous objects from the environment such as loose rugs or small items on the floor.

Client safety is of primary concern.

  ○ Provide environmental cues to assist client in locating important places such as the bathroom, own room, or the dining room.
  ○ Do not argue with client about details of recent past.

The client cannot remember this information, and arguing increases the client's level of frustration, which can participate aggressive behavior.

  ○ Avoid situations that result in aggressive behavior by redirecting client's attention.

Prevention provides the safest approach to aggression.

  ○ Provide a constant daily routine and a homelike atmosphere, to include personal belongings, music, social mealtimes with assistance with meal preparation. This action can often provide appetite cues to client and stimulate memories.

Appropriate levels of sensory stimuli can increase orientation and organization.

  ○ Provide group experiences that explore current events, seasonal changes, reminiscences, and organizing life experiences.

Promotes the client's orientation and maximizes cognitive abilities.

- The following interventions relate to the client who is experiencing Defensive Coping:

Promotes the development of a trusting relationship.

  ○ Approach client in a positive, nonjudgmental manner.
  ○ Focus any feedback on client's behavior.

Communicates acceptance of the client while providing information on coping behaviors that create problems.

  ○ Provide an opportunity for client to share his or her perspectives and feelings.

Promotes the development of a trusting relationship by communicating acceptance of the individual. This relationship will decrease the need for defensive coping.

  ○ Use I statements—e.g., "I feel angry when I see you breaking the window."

Provides modeling of more effective coping behaviors.

Continued

ACTIONS/INTERVENTIONS	RATIONALES
○ Develop a trusting relationship with the client before using confrontation or requesting major changes in behavior.[28,29]	Trusting relationships decrease need for defensive coping and increase the client's ability to respond to this information constructively.
○ Provide positive reinforcement for client when issues are addressed (those things that are reinforcing for this client should be noted here).	Reinforcement encourages positive behavior while enhancing self-esteem.
○ When client's defenses increase, reduce anxiety in situation. (See Anxiety, Chap. 6, for precise information on anxiety control.)	Anxiety increases the client's use of familiar coping behaviors and makes it difficult to practice new behaviors.
○ Determine the kinds of behavior by staff members that increase client's defensive coping, and note them here with a plan to decrease them.	Provides an environment that is supportive of the client's learning new coping behaviors.
○ Be clear and direct with client.	Inappropriate levels of sensory stimuli can increase confusion and disorganization.
○ If defensive coping is related to alteration in self-concept, refer to the appropriate nursing diagnosis for interventions.	High levels of anxiety inhibit the client's ability to learn new behaviors.
○ Reduce or eliminate environmental stressors or threats.	
○ Arrange time for client to be involved in activity that he or she enjoys and that provides him or her with positive emotional experiences. Note activity and time for this activity here.	Promotes positive orientation.
• The following interventions are for the client experiencing Denial:	High levels of anxiety increase the client's use of familiar coping behaviors and make it difficult to practice new behaviors.
○ Determine if current use of denial is appropriate in the current situations.	
○ If denial is determined to be inappropriate, initiate the following interventions:	Communicates acceptance of the client, promoting the development of a trusting relationship.
(1) Provide a safe, secure environment.	
(2) Allow client time to express feelings.	
(3) Provide a positive, nonjudgmental environment.	Promotes positive orientation.
(4) Develop a trusting relationship with client before presenting threatening information.	A trusting relationship decreases the client's need to enlist dysfunctional coping behaviors.
(5) Present information in a clear, concise manner.	Inappropriate levels of sensory stimuli can increase the client's confusion and disorganization.
○ Determine which kinds of staff behavior reinforce denial, and note them here with alternative behavior.	Models appropriate coping behavior while decreasing direct threats to the client's self-system.
○ Utilize I messages, and reflect on client's behavior.[24]	
○ Present client with information that demonstrates inconsistencies between thoughts and feelings, between thoughts and behavior, and between thoughts about others and their perceptions of the situation.	Places in question the client's current coping behaviors and facilitates the examining of options and alternatives.[27]
○ Arrange for client to participate in a group that will provide feedback from peers regarding the stressful situation.	Assists client to experience personal importance to others while enhancing interpersonal relationship skills. Increasing the client's competencies can enhance self-esteem and promote positive orientation.
○ Present client with differences between his or her perceptions and the nurse's perceptions with I messages.	Assists client in questioning the evidence that he or she has been using to support ineffective coping behaviors without directly challenging them. This decreases the need for client to use ineffective coping behaviors.[27]
○ Do not agree with client's perceptions that are related to denial.	Would support and reinforce ineffective coping behaviors.
○ Schedule time for client and support system to discuss issues related to the current problem. (Note this time here with the name of the staff person responsible for this session.)	Support system understanding promotes the continuation of new coping behaviors after discharge.
○ Assist support system in learning constructive ways of coping with the client's denial.	

○ Schedule time for client to be involved in positive esteem-building activity. (This activity should be selected with client input.)

○ Provide positive feedback for client addressing concerns in a direct manner. (Note here those things that are rewarding for the client.)

Feedback encourages positive behavior and enhances self-esteem.

○ Determine needs that are being met with denial. Establish and present client with alternative kinds of behavior for meeting those needs. Note alternatives here.

Gerontic Health

ACTIONS/INTERVENTIONS	RATIONALES
• Discuss with patient any recent life changes that may have affected his or her coping, such as loss of a loved one, relocation, loss of best friend, or loss of a pet.[30]	Recent or multiple losses may significantly impact usual coping skills.

Home Health

NOTE: See Psychiatric Health nursing actions for detailed interventions.

ACTIONS/INTERVENTIONS	RATIONALES
• Involve client and family in planning and implementing strategies to improve individual coping: ○ Family conference: Identify problem and role each family member plays. ○ Mutual goal setting: Set realistic goals. Specify activities for each family member. Establish evaluation criteria. ○ Communication: Use accurate and honest feedback in a positive manner. • Assist family and client in lifestyle adjustments that may be required: ○ Stress management ○ Development and use of support networks ○ Alteration of past ineffective coping strategies ○ Treatment for substance abuse ○ Treatment for physical illness ○ Activities to increase self-esteem: Exercise or stress management ○ Temporary assistance: Babysitter, housekeeper, or secretarial support • Identify signs and symptoms of illness. • Point out hazards and benefits of home remedies, self-diagnosis, and self-prescribing. • Consult with and refer patient to assistive resources as appropriate.	Family involvement enhances effectiveness of interventions. Permanent changes in behavior and family roles require support and accurate information. Utilization of existing services is efficient use of resources. Resources such as a psychiatric nurse clinician, family therapist, and support groups can enhance the treatment plan.

Individual Coping, Ineffective; Defensive Coping; and Ineffective Denial

FLOWCHART EVALUATION: EXPECTED OUTCOME 1

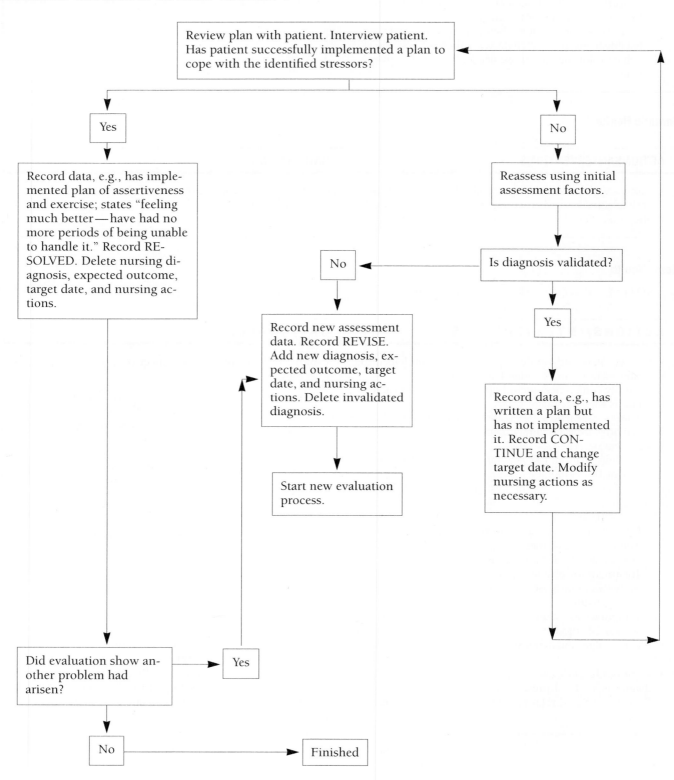

Individual Coping, Ineffective; Defensive Coping; and Ineffective Denial

FLOWCHART EVALUATION: EXPECTED OUTCOME 2

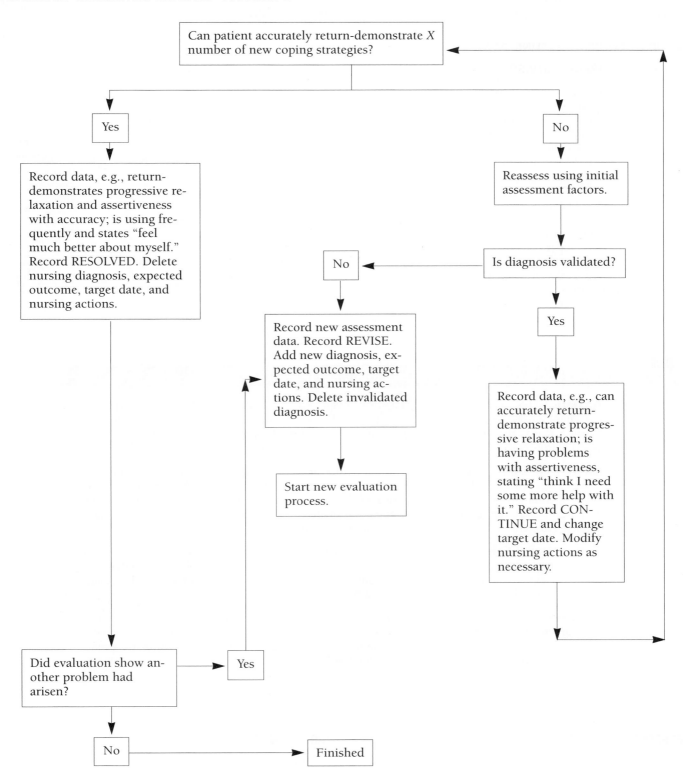

Posttrauma Response

DEFINITION[15]

The state of an individual's experiencing a sustained painful response to an overwhelming traumatic event(s).

NANDA TAXONOMY: FEELING 9.2.3

DEFINING CHARACTERISTICS[15]

1. Major defining characteristics
   a. Reexperience of the traumatic event, which may be identified in cognitive, affective, and/or sensory motor activities (flashbacks, intrusive thoughts, repetitive dreams or nightmares, excessive verbalization of the traumatic event, or verbalization of survival guilt or guilt about behavior required for survival)
2. Minor defining characteristics
   a. Psychic or emotional numbness (impaired interpretation of reality, confusion, dissociation or amnesia, vagueness about traumatic event, or constricted affect)
   b. Altered lifestyle (self-destructiveness such as substance abuse, suicide attempt, or other acting-out behavior, difficulty with interpersonal relationships, development of phobia regarding trauma, poor impulse control or irritability and explosiveness)

RELATED FACTORS[15]

1. Disasters
2. Wars
3. Epidemics
4. Rape
5. Assault
6. Torture
7. Catastrophic illness or accident

NOTE: Groups at risk for this diagnosis are veterans, specific ethnic or religious groups such as Japanese-Americans who were relocated during World War II, and Holocaust survivors.

RELATED CLINICAL CONCERNS

1. Rape victim
2. Multiple injuries (motor vehicle accident)
3. Victims of assault and torture[31]
4. Posttraumatic stress disorder
5. Multiple personality disorder

STOP

HAVE YOU SELECTED THE CORRECT DIAGNOSIS?

Anxiety   This may be the initial diagnosis given to the individual. As the relationship with the client progresses, it may become evident that the source of the anxiety is a traumatic event. If this is the case, then the diagnosis of Posttrauma Response would be added. As long as the symptoms of Anxiety are predominant, this would be the primary diagnosis.

Altered Thought Process   Some of the symptoms of Posttrauma Response are similar to those of Altered Thought Process. If these alterations are present in the client who has experienced a traumatic event, then the primary diagnosis would be Posttrauma Response. If the disruption in thinking persists after intervention has begun for Posttrauma Response, then Altered Thought Process should be reconsidered as a diagnosis.

Dysfunctional Grieving   This is the appropriate diagnosis if the client's behavior is related to resolving a loss or change and this loss or change is not the result of an overwhelming traumatic event. If it is the result of a traumatic event, then this is the most appropriate diagnosis for the behavior the client is demonstrating.

Rape-Trauma Syndrome   This diagnosis is the correct diagnosis if the individual's symptoms are related to a rape. If the symptoms are related to another overwhelming traumatic event or if the rape occurred in conjunction with another overwhelming traumatic event, then the appropriate diagnosis would be Posttrauma Response.

EXPECTED OUTCOMES

1. Will demonstrate return to pretrauma behavior by (date) and/or
2. Will report decrease in signs and symptoms of posttrauma response by (date)

TARGET DATES

Due to the highly individualized and personalized response to trauma, target dates will have to be highly individualized and based on initial assessment. A reasonable initial target date would be 7 days.

NURSING ACTIONS/INTERVENTIONS WITH RATIONALES

Adult Health

ACTIONS/INTERVENTIONS	RATIONALES
• Establish a therapeutic relationship by actively listening, calling the person by name, showing empathy and concern, not belittling feelings, etc.	Promotes trust and open expression of feelings.
• Avoid prolonged waiting periods for patient for routine procedures.	This tactic may have been one used by the torturer and standard care procedures, e.g., drawing blood or ECG, may be perceived as torture because of the memories they evoke.[31]
• Encourage patient to express feelings about the event by actively listening, asking open-ended questions, reflection, etc.	Provides database for planning interventions.
• Help patient to see the event realistically by clarifying misconceptions and looking at both sides of the situation.	Provides objective view. Promotes problem solving.
• Prior to discharge, help patient identify support groups for people who have previously experienced the same or similar traumatic events.	Enhances coping methods. Promotes use of community resource networks to help meet short- and long-term goals and advocate for the patient.
• Initiate a psychiatric nursing consultation as needed.	Situation may require specialized skills to intervene.
• Help patient to identify diversional activities to activate when he or she feels he or she is going to reexperience the event.	Provides alternative coping strategy.
• Orient patient to reality as needed.	Helps patient focus on here and now rather than on past events.
• Engage patient in social interactions with nurses or with other support groups as appropriate.	Decreases isolation. Encourages communication. Provides diversional activity.
• Teach patient relaxation and stress management techniques prior to discharge.	Reduces stress and promotes alternative coping methods.

Child Health

ACTIONS/INTERVENTIONS	RATIONALES
• Monitor for details surrounding the incident causing posttrauma response.	Circumstances surrounding the event may provide clues as to how the child may be internalizing people, places, and objects as symbols or reminders.

• Allow for developmental needs in encouraging child to express feelings about trauma:
  ○ Play for infants
  ○ Puppets or dolls for toddlers
  ○ Stories or play for preschoolers
	Appropriate methods should help to resolve the emotions surrounding the incident and avoid further traumatization.

• Deal appropriately with other primary nursing needs, e.g., nutrition or rest.	Allows focusing of energy on dealing with the crisis.
• Provide for one-to-one care and continuity of staff.	Enhances trust.
• Encourage patient and family to note positive outcomes of experience, e.g., being able to deal with crisis.	Potential for growth exists in crisis management.
• Review previous coping skills.	Coping may be enhanced by consideration of previous skills within framework of current situation.
• Address educational needs according to situation, e.g., rights of the individual or related follow-up.	Knowledge provides empowerment and enhances decision making.
• Allow for visitation by family and significant others.	Family visitation offers opportunity for reassurance and promotes resuming daily routines and relationships.
• Refer patient appropriately for continuity and follow-up after discharge from hospital.	Continuity and follow-up will foster likelihood of resolution of major conflicts.

Continued

ACTIONS/INTERVENTIONS	RATIONALES
• Provide for diversional activity of child's choice. • Allow for potential sleep disturbances. Provide favorite toy or security object. Offer adequate comforting such as by holding infant on waking. • Provide for follow-up for delayed posttrauma response up to 2 years after the trauma. • Reassure child that he or she is not being punished and is not responsible for trauma.	Promotes relaxation. Recurrent nightmares may occur as a result of the trauma. Delayed response can be noted long after the initial event and must be included in the planning of care.[32] Depending on the cognitive level and coping ability, the child may associate the event as being caused by something "wrong" that he or she did or said.

Women's Health

This nursing diagnosis will pertain to the woman the same as to any other adult. The reader is referred to Rape Trauma Syndrome (Chap. 10) and to the other nursing actions in this section.

ACTIONS/INTERVENTIONS	RATIONALES
• Assign a primary care nurse to the client, and assign the same staff member to the client each day on each shift. • Begin appropriate anxiety-reducing interventions if this is a significant problem for the client. (See Anxiety, Chap. 8, for detailed intervention strategies and assessment criteria.) • Discuss with client his or her perception of the current situation and stressors. This should include information about the coping strategies that the client has attempted and his or her assessment of what has made them ineffective in resolving this situation. • Provide a quiet, nonstimulating environment or an environment that does not add additional stress to an already overwhelmed coping ability. (Potential environmental stressors for this client should be listed here with the plan for reducing them in this environment.) • Sit with client (number) minutes (number) times a day at (times) to discuss the traumatic event. Person responsible for this activity should be listed here. This should be the nurse who has established a relationship with the client. • Assist client with setting appropriate limits on aggressive behavior (see Risk for Violence, Chap. 9, for nursing actions if this is an appropriate diagnosis) by: ○ Decreasing environmental stimulation as appropriate (this might include a secluded environment or a time-out). ○ Providing client with appropriate alternative outlets for physical tension (this should be stated specifically and could include walking, running, talking with staff member, using a punching bag, listening to music, or doing a deep muscle relaxation sequence) (number) times per day at (times) or when increased tension is observed. These outlets should be selected with the client's input. Those outlets that the client selects should be listed here.	Promotes the development of a trusting relationship. Provides the client with increased repertoire of coping behaviors to cope with intense emotional experiences. Promotes the client's sense of control while communicating respect for the client's experience. Inappropriate levels of sensory stimuli can increase confusion and disorganization. Promotes the development of a trusting relationship while providing the client with an opportunity to review and attach meaning to the client's experience.[28] Inappropriate levels of sensory stimuli can increase confusion and disorganization, which increases the risk for aggressive behavior. Physical activity decreases physical tension and increases the production of endorphins, which can increase the feeling of well-being. This also provides the client with opportunities to practice new coping behaviors in a supportive environment.

- ○ Talking with client about past situations that resulted in loss of control, and discuss alternative ways of coping with these situations. (Persons responsible for this discussion should be noted here. This will not be accomplished in one discussion; the time and date for the initial discussion should be noted with the times and dates for follow-up discussions.)

    Increases the client's coping options and assists with cognitive appraisal of past coping behaviors.[27]

- Once the symptoms have been identified and linked to the traumatic event, the primary nurse will sit with the client (number) minutes (begin with 30 and increase as the client's ability to concentrate improves) per shift to discuss the traumatic event. These discussions should include:

    Promotes the client's positive orientation.

    - ○ The uniqueness of the situation, noting that one could not plan for the behavior that might be needed to endure this situation
    - ○ Ways of evaluating behavior, noting that usual moral and ethical standards may be inappropriate for the unique situation of a traumatic event

    Assists the client to evaluate and gain perspective on behavior while moving away from all-or-none thinking.[27]

    - ○ Details of the event as the individual remembers them and the thoughts and feelings that occur with these memories

    Assists the client in attaching meaning to the experience.

    - ○ Meaning of life since the event and the implications that has for the future

    Promotes positive orientation while assisting the client to review cognitive distortions.[27]
    Inhibits automatic behavioral responses.[27]

- If feelings become extreme such as with rage or despondency, then the client should focus on thoughts rather than feelings about the event.

- Provide constructive confrontation for client about problematic coping behavior.[23] Those kinds of behavior identified by the treatment team as problematic should be listed here with the selected method of confrontation.

    Assists the client to gain a perspective on the experience and to label cognitive distortions that inhibit effective coping.[27]

- Provide client with information about care and treatment.

    Promotes the client's sense of control.

- Provide client with opportunities to make appropriate decisions related to care at his or her level of ability. This may begin as a choice between two options and then evolve into more complex decision making. It is important that the decision making be at the client's level of functioning so that confidence can be built with successful decision-making experiences. Those decisions that the client has made should be noted.

    Success in this activity provides positive reinforcement and promotes the client's utilizing alternative coping behaviors while enhancing self-esteem.

- Provide positive social reinforcement and other behavioral rewards for demonstration of adaptive problem solving and coping. Those things that the client finds rewarding should be listed here with a schedule for use. Those kinds of behavior that are to be rewarded should also be listed.

    Reinforcement encourages positive behavior and enhances self-esteem.

- Assist client in identifying support systems and in developing a plan for their use. This plan should be noted here.

    Support system understanding promotes their appropriate support of the client.

- Inform significant others of the relationship between the client's behavior and the traumatic event. Discuss with them their thoughts and feelings about the client's behavior. The person responsible for these discussions should be noted here, along with the schedule for the discussion times. This should also include information about the importance of supporting the client in discussing the event and how this might be facilitated. The concerns that significant others have about their response to this sharing should be discussed as well as planning for the types of information they might be exposed to.

    Support system understanding promotes their appropriate support of the client.

Continued

ACTIONS/INTERVENTIONS	RATIONALES

• When client develops a degree of comfort discussing the traumatic event, meetings between the client and significant others should be scheduled. Content of these meetings should include:
  ○ Opportunities for the client to share thoughts and feelings about the event
  ○ Opportunities for the significant others to share their thoughts and feelings about client's behavior
  ○ Sharing of thoughts and feelings related to other events in the relationship as they surface as important topics of discussion during the meetings
  ○ Sharing of caring thoughts and feelings with each other
	Promotes the development of adaptive coping within the support system.

• Arrange for client to attend support group meetings with others who have experienced similar traumas. The times and days for these meetings should be noted here with any special arrangements that are needed to facilitate client's attendance, e.g., transportation to group meeting place. This could include veterans' groups, groups for survivors of natural disasters, and victims' groups.	Decreases the sense of social isolation and decreases feelings of deviance. Consensual validation from other group members enhances self-esteem, providing increased emotional resources for coping.
• Schedule client involvement in unit activities. Note here the client's responsibilities in these activities with times that the client will be involved in the activity.	Decreases social isolation and provides opportunity to practice new coping skills in a supportive environment.

Gerontic Health

The nursing actions for a gerontic patient with this diagnosis are the same as those given for the adult health and mental health patient.

Home Health

NOTE: See Psychiatric Health nursing actions for detailed interventions. If family violence is involved, refer to Chapter 9.

ACTIONS/INTERVENTIONS	RATIONALES
• Monitor for factors contributing to Posttrauma Response.	Provides database for early recognition and intervention.

• Teach client and family appropriate monitoring of signs and symptoms of Posttrauma Response:
  ○ Flashbacks
  ○ Nightmares
  ○ Survival guilt
  ○ Confusion
  ○ Amnesia
  ○ Constricted affect
  ○ Substance abuse
  ○ Suicide attempt
  ○ Poor impulse control
	Permits early intervention.

• Assist client and family in lifestyle adjustments that may be required:
  ○ Recognition of feelings
  ○ Prevention of harm to self or others
  ○ Treatment of substance abuse
  ○ Provision of safe environment
  ○ Development and use of support network
	Lifestyle changes require long-term changes in behavior. Support facilitates these changes.

- ○ Prevention of further trauma
- ○ Role changes
- ○ Treatment of injuries
- Involve client and family in planning and implementing strategies to reduce or eliminate Posttrauma Response:
  - ○ Family conference: Identify family members' response to traumatic event.
  - ○ Communication: Share caring thoughts and feelings.
  - ○ Mutual goal setting: Set realistic goals, and specify activities for each individual. Establish evaluation criteria.
- Consult with assistive resources as indicated.

Family involvement in planning enhances the effectiveness of the interventions.

Utilization of existing services is efficient use of resources. Patient's attending support groups specific to the precipitating event—e.g., rape crisis, Vietnam vets—and a psychiatric nurse clinician or a family therapist can enhance the treatment plan.

Posttrauma Response

FLOWCHART EVALUATION: EXPECTED OUTCOME 1

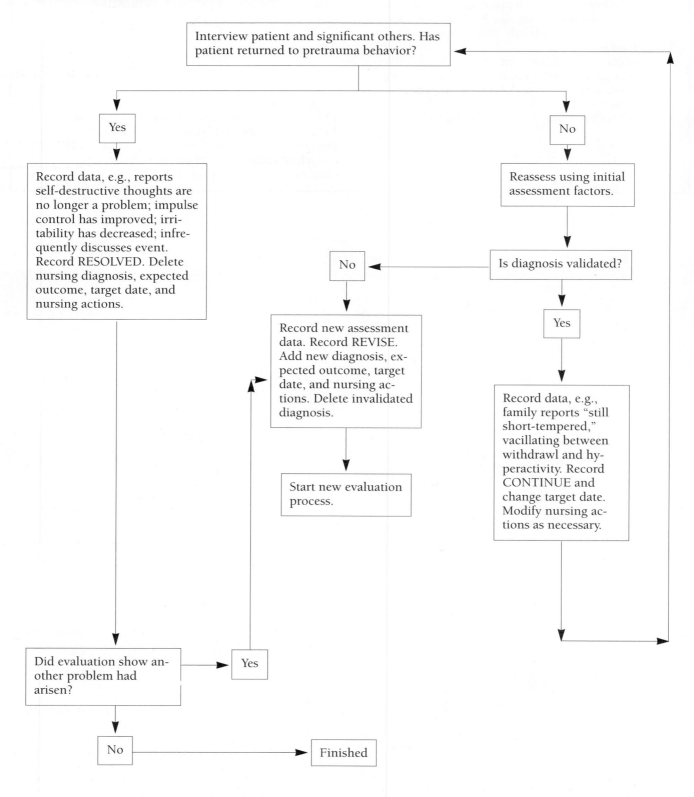

Posttrauma Response

FLOWCHART EVALUATION: EXPECTED OUTCOME 2

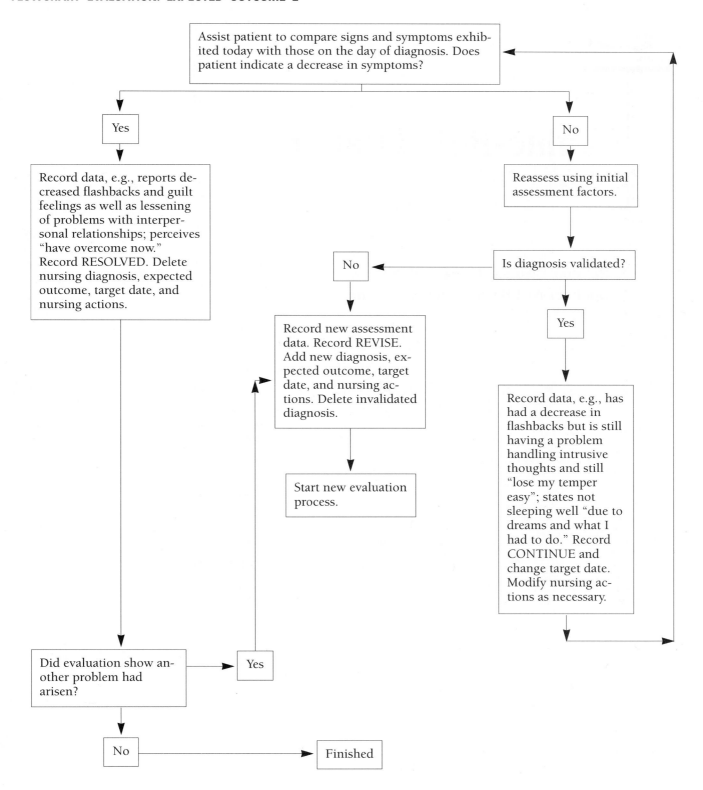

Assist patient to compare signs and symptoms exhibited today with those on the day of diagnosis. Does patient indicate a decrease in symptoms?

Yes

No

Record data, e.g., reports decreased flashbacks and guilt feelings as well as lessening of problems with interpersonal relationships; perceives "have overcome now." Record RESOLVED. Delete nursing diagnosis, expected outcome, target date, and nursing actions.

Reassess using initial assessment factors.

Is diagnosis validated?

No

Yes

Record new assessment data. Record REVISE. Add new diagnosis, expected outcome, target date, and nursing actions. Delete invalidated diagnosis.

Start new evaluation process.

Record data, e.g., has had a decrease in flashbacks but is still having a problem handling intrusive thoughts and still "lose my temper easy"; states not sleeping well "due to dreams and what I had to do." Record CONTINUE and change target date. Modify nursing actions as necessary.

Did evaluation show another problem had arisen?

Yes

No

Finished

Value-Belief Pattern

Pattern Description

The nurse may care for patients who, because of health alterations, experience disturbances in their individual value-belief systems. A person's value-belief system is the core of his or her existence, his or her interconnectedness with his or her spiritual side as well as his or her interconnectedness with his or her environment. This value-belief system gives meaning and purpose to life. Some call this faith: "Faith carries us forward when there is no longer reason to carry on. It enables us to exist during the in-between times: between meanings, amid dangers of radical discontinuity, even in the face of death. Faith is a sine qua non of life, a primal force we cannot do without."[12] Faith can be in many things, a superior being, the environment, self, family, or community. The nurse may care for patients who, because of their faith or value-belief system, cope and even increase their spiritual well-being when faced with health alterations. Other patients the nurse cares for may experience disturbances in their individual value-belief system or faith because of health alterations. These alterations may take a form ranging from being disturbed to being demolished. These disturbances can be manifested by the inability to practice formal religious directions, such as attending church or following a specific diet, to being totally unable to manage their own spiritual needs and live within a certain spiritual structure. Conversely, religion can affect physical or emotional well-being if the practice of the religion results in spiritual distress. An individual's value-belief system can contribute to alterations in health just as alterations in health can contribute to disturbances in the individual's values and beliefs. The nurse must individualize care to help enhance and support faith while minimizing spiritual distress when meeting the specific needs of the individual patient within his or her value-belief system.

The value-belief pattern looks specifically at how the individual not only retains faith and enhances his or her value-belief system in times of stress but also at how physical illness can interfere with the individual's ability to practice religion and maintain beliefs, values, and spiritual life, as well as how a person's judgment and interpretation of, or the meaning of life (faith) for himself or herself can affect or interfere with health care practices.

Pattern Assessment

1. Does the patient express anger toward a supreme being regarding his or her current condition?
   a. Yes (Spiritual Distress)
   b. No (Spiritual Well-Being)
2. Does the patient verbalize conflict about personal spiritual beliefs?
   a. Yes (Spiritual Distress)
   b. No (Spiritual Well-Being)
3. Does the patient indicate positive thoughts about spirituality?
   a. Yes (Potential for Enhanced Spiritual Well-Being)
   b. No (Spiritual Distress)
4. Does the patient indicate comfort with self?
   a. Yes (Potential for Enhanced Spiritual Well-Being)
   b. No

Conceptual Information

The faith, belief, or value system of a person can be described as the predominating force (spirituality) which provides the vital direction to that person's existence. This predominating force can be a faith in a supreme being or God, a belief in one's self, or a belief in others. By this, it is conceptualized that each person must find his or her place in the world, nature, and in relationships with other beings. This faith, belief, or value system is exhibited by the individual in the form of organized religion, attitudes, and actions related to the individual's sense of what is right, cultural beliefs, and the individual's internal motivations.

All persons have some philosophical orientation to life that assists them in constructing their reality, regardless of whether or not they practice a formal religion. Spirituality is interwoven into a person's cultural background, beliefs, and individual value system. This spirituality is what gives life meaning and allows the person to function in a more total manner. These beliefs and values influence a person's behavior and attitudes toward what is right and what is wrong, and with the lifestyle he or she practices. Many authors[3,4] stress that not only must the nurse take into consideration the patient's beliefs and value system but the nurse must also recognize his or her beliefs and values. The nurse must know about or develop resources to assist with understanding the different beliefs and religious practices of groups encountered in practice settings. Further understanding and assessment of a patient's beliefs can be ascertained by asking questions such as "How do you practice your religion?" or "Which beliefs and practices are important to you?"[5]

Studies have shown that the value of specific rituals such as prayer to the individuals who practice them is not affected by the fact that they can or cannot be proven scientifically.[6] The impact of values and beliefs is best described by the following quote[4]:

> When as much emphasis is placed on the symbolic and intuitive as on the analytical, consciousness develops more fully. The expansion of consciousness is what life and, therefore, health is all about and health can coexist with illness and even encompass it as a meaningful aspect.

This can be seen in those individuals who consider suffering, illness, and even death as having "meaning in life" or as "God's will."

Many individuals believe that the only value of life, and the source of strength and power, is the will of the individual and that there is no need for assistance from the outside. This focus has been described[6] as "a person's authority within himself." This focus may actually revolve around work, physical activity, or self[6]—"I can do anything I want to when I want to do." Three predominant indicators have been listed[7] that must be considered when judging the value of continued life: mental capacity, physical capacity, and pain. This would indicate that life, in and of itself, is not intrinsically valuable to the possessor of it; instead, it is the quality of conscious life that is important.

In one phenomenologic study[8] of spirituality, the constituents of spirituality, as reported by the study subjects, were described and included (1) realization of humanity of self or valued other; (2) event of nonhuman intervention; (3) receiving divine intervention; (4) visceral knowing; (5) willingness to sacrifice; (6) physical sensations; (7) a personal experience; (9) a reality experience; (10) not easily explained; and (11) different from or more than daily experience. In 1981 Fowler[1] described his faith development theory, which was influenced by the work of Piaget and Kolberg. Fowler describes faith as not always religious in its content or context but "a person's or group's way of moving into the force field of life. It is our way of finding coherence in and giving meaning to the multiple forces and relations that make up our lives." Fowler described the experience of spirituality in different stages of the life cycle. He states that one transitions from one stage to another, some fast and some slow, and that it is not a simple change of mind or even a conscious movement from one phase to another and that it can be a long and painful process. Six states of faith are recognized by Fowler:

1. *Intuitive-projective*: Experiencing the work as a child, fluid and full of novelty, with a rudimentary awareness of self as the center of the universe. Preoperational reasoning and judgment are employed by people in this stage. There is no reasoning or logic to thought; therefore, the capacity for taking the role or perspective of others is extremely limited.
2. *Mythic-literal*: People in this stage can separate real from unreal on the basis of experience, and therefore the world becomes more linear and orderly than in stage 1. This is accompanied by a private world of speculation, fantasy, and wonder. Bounds of the social world widen, and the questioning of "good and evil" is begun. Often these thoughts, which can be reassuring, hopeful, or full of terror and fear, are symbolized in dreams and daydreams.[1,9]
3. *Synthetic-conventional*: One begins to structure the world and the environment in interpersonal terms. The individual constructs an image of self as seen by others and becomes aware that others are performing the same operations in their relationships. This is a conformist stage, where peers and their values become most important. Influences from earlier stages are carried "within" as reference points by which beliefs, values, and actions are values, and actions are validated and sanctioned.
4. *Individuative-reflexive*: One begins to construct and maintain his or her own identity, autonomy, and faith, without relying on others. The sense of self is now reciprocal with a faith outlook or worldview that negotiates between self and significant others. One knows he or she is different from others, and his or her views and faith are vulnerable to challenge and change.
5. *Paradoxical-consolidative*: Many previous dimensions that were formally suppressed or ignored are integrated. One becomes open to the voices of one's most inner self. A coming to terms with one's social unconsciousness; the myths, norms, ideal images, and prejudices that have, until now, formed one's life. One can see injustice because of an expanded awareness of the demands of justice and the implications of those demands.
6. *Universalizing*: The individual at this stage becomes a disciplined activist. He or she exhibits qualities that shake the usual criteria of normalcy. He or she leads and embraces strategies of nonviolent suffering and of ultimate respect for life. "They often become martyrs to the visions they incarnate."[2]

Another study[10] provides insights regarding the interactive process of caring as it relates to spiritual needs. Trust, meaningful support systems, and a respect for personal beliefs were identified by participants as central to care.

Because of the conscious, subconscious, and unconscious components of the value-belief system, nurses must be continually alert for disruptions in the system. There is a need to be aware that every individual expresses disruptions in spirituality differently.[11] Some withdraw, some become more religious, and some become angry and defiant. Nurses need to be cognizant of not only the patient's spiritual beliefs but also the stage of spiritual development in which the patient and nurse are. This will affect and determine not only the needs and concerns of the patients but also how the nurse will approach the patient to care for those needs and concerns. This awareness of and respect for the impact and influence values and beliefs have on the patient cannot be overemphasized in planning and providing high-quality care for the patient.

Developmental Considerations

The geographic, social, political, and home environment in which one lives has a major effect on how a person develops, how he or she will view health, and how spirituality, values, and beliefs are formulated. The values a person holds influence all facets of life. How one perceives the world about him or her, as well as his or her basic philosophy, guides all interactions with others and ultimately reflects a person's individuality.

Fowler, in describing his developmental stages of faith, states that he has found, regardless of chronologic age, adults and adolescents in stages 2 and 3 and some adults in all stages. But persons are usually found in the various stages as shown in the parentheses at the end of each developmental stage in the following narrative.

INFANT

The infant is totally dependent on the parents and those about him or her and is busy building trust or mistrust.[12] Unable at this age to form values or distinguish spirituality, the infant is a mirror image of those about him or her. The parent's method of interaction, communication, and fulfillment of the emotional and physiologic needs of the infant form the basis for value development (Fowler's stage 1).

TODDLER AND PRESCHOOLER

The toddler imitates those about him or her: parents, siblings, and other adults. The toddler develops by mimicking observed behavior and receiving either positive or negative reinforcement. Values begin to form as the toddler starts to become aware of others and to interact with those around him or her. Values become known to individuals through the process of social cognition, which begins in early childhood. This arises not from objects or the subject but from the interaction between the subject and those objects[13] (Fowler's stage 1).

SCHOOL-AGE CHILD

The school-age child begins to be influenced by peers outside the family structure and begins to question and make choices. The school-age child actively participates in his or her own moral development. Individual reasoning develops through various stages, beginning in the school-age years.[14] Play is the major mechanism of learning throughout the school-age years (Fowler's stage 2).

ADOLESCENT

The adolescent searches for his or her own identity and begins to practice values that are separate and yet congruent with his or her family units. The adolescent is constantly questioning, trying, and searching for the "truth of life" and for his or her identity in the scheme of things. He or she sees values as being either "black or white," and there can be no overlapping. The adolescent is still struggling with his or her own independence and formulating his or her own values, beliefs, and spirituality (Fowler's stages 2 and 3).

YOUNG ADULT

Young adults are constantly examining, reformulating, and changing their values, beliefs, and spirituality. Often they change completely the values and beliefs they developed during adolescence, although it is important to note that they often keep the basic values and beliefs they learned during their young years with their families (Fowler's stages 3 and 4).

ADULT

Adults usually strengthen the values and beliefs they have formed according to their life experiences. The adult is continually exploring and trying to see if his or her value system fits within his or her lifestyle. They are busy teaching children the values and beliefs that they wish their children to adopt for their lives (Fowler's stages 4 and 5).

OLDER ADULT

Older adults find great solace in their spirituality and the values and beliefs they have formed through a lifetime. In general, the older adult continues to use the values, beliefs, and spiritual patterns adopted in adulthood[5] (Fowler's stages 5 and 6).

APPLICABLE NURSING DIAGNOSES

Spiritual Distress (Distress of Human Spirit)

DEFINITION

Disruption in the life principle that pervades a person's entire being and that integrates and transcends one's biologic and psychosocial nature.[15]

NANDA TAXONOMY: VALUING 4.1.1

DEFINING CHARACTERISTICS[15]

1. Major defining characteristics
   a. Expresses concerns with meaning of life or death and/or belief systems*
   b. Expresses anger toward God
   c. Questions meaning of suffering
   d. Verbalizes inner conflict about beliefs
   e. Verbalizes concern about relationship with deity
   f. Questions meaning of own existence
   g. Unable to participate in usual religious practices
   h. Seeks spiritual assistance
   i. Questions moral or ethical implications of therapeutic regimen
   j. Gallows humor
   k. Displaces anger toward religious representatives
   l. Describes nightmares or sleep disturbances
   m. Alteration in behavior or mood evidenced by anger, crying, withdrawal, preoccupation, anxiety, hostility, apathy, and so forth
2. Minor defining characteristics
   None given

RELATED FACTORS[15]

1. Separation from religious or cultural ties
2. Challenged belief and value system, for example, due to moral or ethical implications of therapy, due to intense suffering

RELATED CLINICAL CONCERNS

1. Cancer
2. Severe head injury, for example, brain death
3. Chronic illnesses, for example, rheumatoid arthritis or multiple sclerosis
4. Mental retardation
5. Burns
6. Sudden infant death syndrome (SIDS)
7. Stillbirth or fetal demise
8. Infertility

---

*Critical.

HAVE YOU SELECTED THE CORRECT DIAGNOSIS?

Ineffective Individual Coping Many individuals use religion or beliefs as a means of bargaining in unwanted life situations or denying their role in the situation by blaming it on a superior being. Others will find their source of strength and hope from their beliefs in a superior being or God and are able to live fully functional lives despite physical handicaps. If the patient mentions any of the defining characteristics of this diagnosis, then the primary diagnosis is Spiritual Distress, which must be attended to before trying to intervene for Ineffective Individual Coping.

EXPECTED OUTCOMES

1. Will verbalize sense of spiritual peace by (date) and/or
2. Will describe at least (number) support systems to use when spiritual conflict arises by (date)

TARGET DATES

Because of the largely subconscious nature of spiritual beliefs and values, it is recommended that the target date be at least 5 days from the date of diagnosis.

NURSING ACTIONS/INTERVENTIONS WITH RATIONALES

Adult Health

ACTIONS/INTERVENTIONS	RATIONALES
• Assist patient to identify and define his or her values, particularly in relation to health and illness, through the use of value clarification techniques such as sentence completion, rank-ordering exercises, and completion of health value scales.	Clarifies values and beliefs and helps patient understand the impact of values and beliefs on health and illness.
• Demonstrate respect for and acceptance of the patient's value and spiritual system by not judging, moralizing, arguing, or advising changes in values or religious practices.	Spiritual values and beliefs are highly personal. A nurse's attitude can positively or negatively influence the therapeutic relationship.
• Adapt nursing therapeutics as necessary to incorporate values and religious beliefs, e.g., diet, administration of blood or blood products, or rituals.	Maintains and respects patient's preferences during hospitalization.
• Schedule appropriate rituals as necessary, e.g., baptism, confession, or communion.	Provides comfort for patient.
• Arrange visits from needed support persons, e.g., pastor, rabbi, priest, or prayer group, as needed.	Promotes comfort and reduces anxiety.
• Provide privacy for religious practices and rituals as necessary.	Allows for expression of religious practices.
• Encourage family to bring significant symbols to patient, e.g., Bible, rosary, or icons, as needed.	Promotes comfort.
• Plan to spend at least 15 min twice a day at (times) with patient to allow verbalization, questioning, counseling, and support on a one-to-one basis.	Promotes mutual sharing and builds a trusting relationship.
• Assist patient to develop problem-solving behavior through practice of problem-solving techniques at least twice daily at (times) during hospitalization.	Involves patient in self-management activities. Increases motivation.

Child Health

ACTIONS/INTERVENTIONS	RATIONALES
• Support the patient in attaining or maintaining spiritual integrity according to specific identified needs and developmental level. Remember to pay attention to the parental dyad's value-beliefs preferences: 　∘ Allow for appropriate privacy. 　∘ Allow time for self-reflection. 　∘ Allow time for prayer and practice of worship as permitted. 　∘ Support the child in expressing feelings about spiritual distress and related factors through using open-ended questions and providing time for this at least twice a day at (times). 　∘ Act as advocate for the child and family when they are expressing differing beliefs from that of the staff, institution, or significant others.	Openness affords trust as the child grapples with the meaning of such stressors as illness and death.
• Answer value-belief-related questions honestly according to patient's developmental level and after conferring with parents.	Sensitivity to needs within legal domains regarding appropriate standards of care honors the child's rights and attaches value to the family's cultural wishes.

Women's Health

ACTIONS/INTERVENTIONS	RATIONALES
• Allow mother and family to express feelings at the less-than-perfect pregnancy outcome.[16] 　∘ Stillborn or infant death: 　　(1) Provide time for the mother and family to see, hold, and take pictures of infant if so desired. 　　(2) Provide quiet, private place where mother and family can be with infant. 　　(3) Arrange for religious practices requested, e.g., baptism or other rituals. 　　(4) Contact religious or cultural leader as requested by the mother or family. 　　(5) Refer patient to appropriate support groups within the community.	Allows family to receive religious and social support as a means of coping.
∘ Spontaneous abortion: 　　(1) Provide patient with factual information regarding etiology of spontaneous abortion. 　　(2) Encourage verbal expressions of grief. 　　(3) Allow expression of feelings such as anger. 　　(4) Contact religious or cultural leader as requested by patient. 　　(5) Provide referrals to appropriate support groups within the community.	Assists in reducing guilt, blame, etc. Provides information and support for family.
∘ Less-than-perfect baby, e.g., sick baby or infant with anomaly: 　　(1) Provide quiet, private place for mother and family to visit with infant. 　　(2) Encourage verbalization of fears and asking of any question by providing time for one-to-one interactions at least twice a day at (times). 　　(3) Encourage touching and holding of infant by mother and family.	

Continued

ACTIONS/INTERVENTIONS	RATIONALES
(4) Teach methods of caring for the infant, e.g., special feeding techniques.	
(5) Teach methods of coping with the stress connected with caring for the infant, e.g., planned alone time for relaxation techniques.	
(6) Assign one staff member to care for both mother and infant.	
(7) Contact religious or cultural leader as requested by mother or family.	
(8) Provide patient with information and referrals to appropriate support groups and community agencies.	Provides support and information and assists with coping.
• Provide support for the woman facing an unwanted pregnancy.	
○ Encourage questions and verbalization of patient's life expectations by providing at least 15 min of one-to-one time at least twice a day at (times).	Provides information about choices and consequences of each choice, which can assist with decision making. Gives long-term support by providing referrals.
○ Provide information on options available to patient, e.g., adoption, abortion, or keeping baby.	
○ Assist patient in identifying lifestyle adjustments that each decision could entail, e.g., dealing with guilt or finances.	
○ Involve significant others and include patient's religious or cultural leader, if so desired by patient, in discussion and problem-solving activities regarding lifestyle adjustments.	
• Assist patient facing gynecologic surgery to express her perceptions of lifestyle adjustments:	Provides support and gives preoperative information, which assists with postoperative recovery.
○ Provide explanation of surgical procedure and perioperative nursing care.	
○ Provide factual information as to physiologic and psychologic reactions she may experience.	
○ Allow patient to grieve loss of body image, e.g., inability to have a child.	
○ Involve significant others in discussion and problem-solving activities regarding life cycle changes that could affect self-concept and interpersonal relationships, e.g., hot flashes, sexual relationships, or ability to have children.	
• Participate with patient in religious support activities, e.g., praying or reading religious literature aloud.	Demonstrates visible support for the role these activities play in the patient's life.

Psychiatric Health

ACTIONS/INTERVENTIONS	RATIONALES
• Remove items from the environment that increase problem behavior (list specific items for each client, e.g., Bible or religious pictures).	Environment will assist the client in demonstrating appropriate coping behaviors, which increases opportunities for succeeding with new coping behaviors. Success provides reinforcement, which encourages positive behavior and enhances self-esteem.
• Restrict visitors who increase problem behavior for the client. Discuss with family and other frequent visitors the necessity of not discussing the problem ideas with the client.	Promotes the client's sense of control.
• Request consultation from religious leader who has had education and experience in assisting clients to cope with this type of spiritual distress.	Meets the client's spiritual needs in a constructive manner.

- **Do not** discuss with client belief systems that are related to problem behavior (state here specifically what that content is).
- **Do not** argue with client about religious belief system or behaviors that evolve from this system.
- **Do not** joke with client about belief system or behavior that evolves from this system.
- Spend time with client when themes of conversation are not related to the problem behavior.

- Limit topics of conversation to daily activities or situations that do not include religious beliefs.

- Provide activities that decrease client time alone to reflect on the problem beliefs. Suggested activities include:
  - Physical exercises such as walks, bicycle riding, swimming, or exercise classes
  - Group activities such as board games, meal preparation, sports, or arts and crafts

These discussions only serve to reinforce client's misconceptions.

This would reinforce the dysfunctional belief system.

Protects the client's self-esteem at a time when it is most vulnerable.
Presence of the nurse at this time provides reinforcement for this behavior, which encourages the positive behavior and enhances self-esteem.
Environmental structure helps client to focus away from problem areas, which supports his or her efforts to enlist more appropriate coping behaviors.
Provides the client with opportunities to practice alternative coping behaviors in a supportive environment.

Gerontic Health

ACTIONS/INTERVENTIONS	RATIONALES
• Encourage use of reminiscence to aid patient in examining life.[17]	Assists patient in finding meaning in life experiences and ego integrity.
• Discuss with patient possible sources of spiritual distress, and use problem-solving process as indicated.	Enables patient to identify problem areas and potential correctable measures to ameliorate distress.

Home Health

ACTIONS/INTERVENTIONS	RATIONALES

• Involve client and family in planning, implementing, and promoting spiritual well-being through:
  ○ Arranging family conferences to discuss spiritual values
  ○ Assisting with mutual goal setting for the client and family to enhance spiritual well-being of the client and family such as personal prayer, interactions with clergy, family, and nurses to find meaning during illness[18]
  ○ Assigning family members to specific tasks that assist in maintaining spiritual well-being, e.g., support person for client, companionship in meeting mutual goals, prayer, meditation, reading scripture, etc.[16]
  ○ Interviewing designed to provide opportunities for expression of spiritual needs.[18]
	Family and client involvement enhances the effectiveness of the interventions.

• Assist client to identify factors contributing to spiritual distress, e.g., significant life experiences, treatment prescribed by health care team, or inability to perform spiritual rituals.	Identification of contributing factors provides the opportunity for planning designed to decrease these factors.
• Assist client and family in lifestyle adjustments that may be required, e.g., diet, environmental changes, or hygiene practices.	Lifestyle changes require change in behavior. Self-evaluation and support facilitate these changes.
• Refer patient to appropriate assistive resources as indicated.	Challenges to one's value system may require long-term follow-up. Use of the network of existing community services provides for effective utilization of resources.

Spiritual Distress (Distress of the Human Spirit)

FLOWCHART EVALUATION: EXPECTED OUTCOME 1

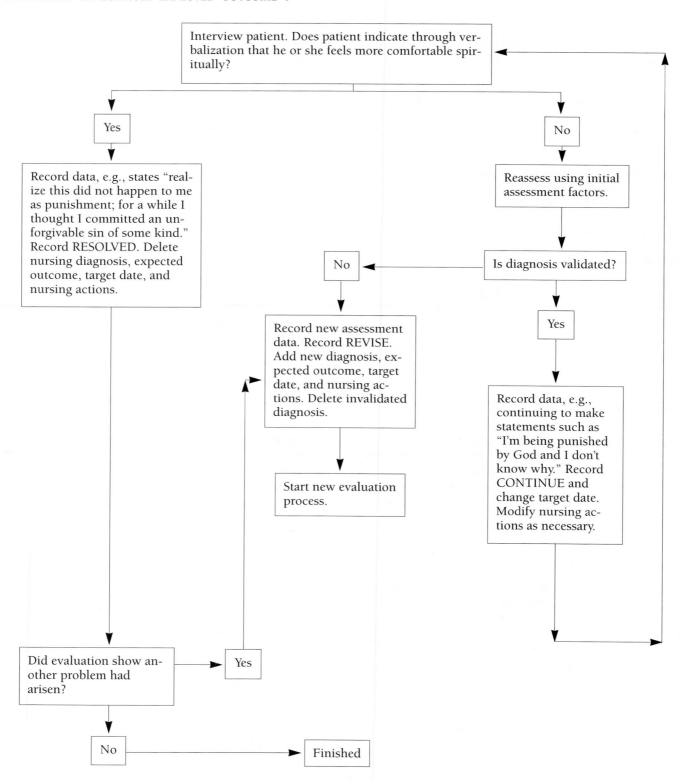

Spiritual Distress (Distress of the Human Spirit)

FLOWCHART EVALUATION: EXPECTED OUTCOME 2

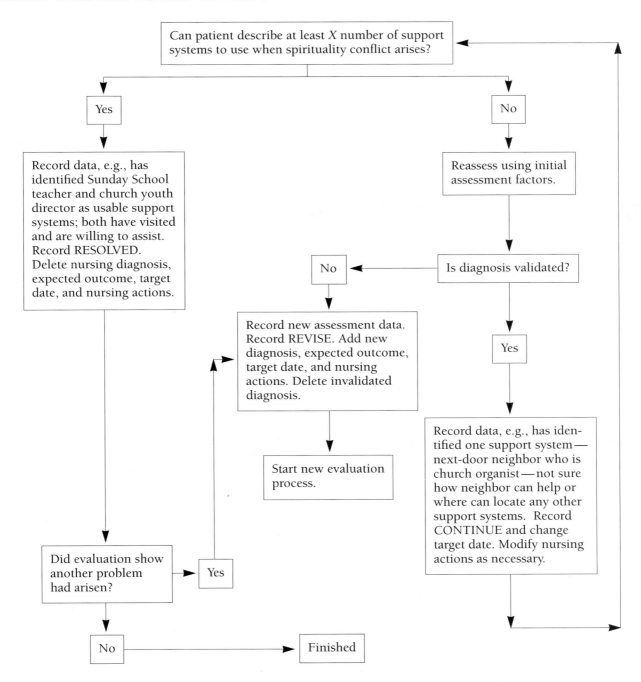

Can patient describe at least X number of support systems to use when spirituality conflict arises?

Yes

Record data, e.g., has identified Sunday School teacher and church youth director as usable support systems; both have visited and are willing to assist. Record RESOLVED. Delete nursing diagnosis, expected outcome, target date, and nursing actions.

No

Reassess using initial assessment factors.

Is diagnosis validated?

No

Record new assessment data. Record REVISE. Add new diagnosis, expected outcome, target date, and nursing actions. Delete invalidated diagnosis.

Start new evaluation process.

Yes

Record data, e.g., has identified one support system—next-door neighbor who is church organist—not sure how neighbor can help or where can locate any other support systems. Record CONTINUE and change target date. Modify nursing actions as necessary.

Did evaluation show another problem had arisen?

Yes

No

Finished

Spiritual Well-Being, Potential for Enhanced

DEFINITION[15]

Spiritual well-being is the process of an individual's developing or unfolding of mystery through harmonious interconnectedness that springs from inner strengths.

NANDA TAXONOMY: VALUING 4.2

DEFINING CHARACTERISTICS[15]

1. Inner Strengths
   a. A sense of awareness, self-consciousness, sacred source, unifying force inner core, and transcendence
2. Unfolding Mystery
   a. One's experience about life's purpose and meaning, mystery, uncertainty, and struggles
3. Harmonious Interconnectedness
   a. Relatedness, connectedness, harmony with self, other, higher power or God, and the environment

RELATED FACTORS[15]

None given

RELATED CLINICAL CONCERNS[15]

1. Any terminal diagnosis
2. Any chronic disease diagnosis

HAVE YOU SELECTED THE CORRECT DIAGNOSIS?

Spiritual Distress This diagnosis indicates that the patient is experiencing significant problems with spirituality. Potential for Enhanced indicates that the patient is making progress in resolving any such problems.

EXPECTED OUTCOMES

1. Will verbally express satisfaction with state of spirituality by (date) and/or
2. Will exhibit majority (number percent) of defining characteristics for diagnosis by (date)

TARGET DATES

The target date for this diagnosis will be highly individualized. An appropriate initial date to check progress would be 10 to 14 days.

NURSING ACTIONS/INTERVENTIONS WITH RATIONALES

Adult Health

ACTIONS/INTERVENTIONS	RATIONALES
• Establish a trusting relationship.	A trusting relationship assists the patient to express his or her feelings to the nurse.
• Provide in-depth spiritual assessment.	These are all spiritual care practices that enhance spirituality.[19-21]
• Convey technical competence.	
• Act as facilitator among family, clergy, and other providers.	
• Be present: Touch, make eye contact, and use facial expressions.	
• Treat the patient as a unique individual.	
• Inquire about religion, values, relationships, transcendence, affective feeling, communication, and spiritual practices.	Spirituality is expressed in all these areas.[22]
• Support and enhance patient's spirituality.	
• Pray for and with patient.	These are all spiritual care practices.
• Read Bible with the patient.	
• Refer patient to chaplain, clergy, or spiritual advisor.	
• Provide patient with religious materials.	
• Serve as a therapeutic presence.	
• Listen and talk to patient.	

- If possible, allow patient to interact with and/or "care" for other patients.

- Encourage patient to talk about and reflect on hopes, dreams, God, faith, religious beliefs, social support, acceptance, health, forgiveness, hopelessness; provide privacy, and personal time for reflection; assure presence of higher being.
- Encourage family and friends' interactions with patient to express love and concern for the patient.
- Have patient express his or her health and well-being through connectedness: intrapersonally, interpersonally, and transpersonally.

- Advocate for patient's spiritual beliefs with the health team.
- Show respect and support for patient beliefs and values.[21]
- Demonstrate compassion and acceptance. Be sensitive to patient's spiritual needs.

- Assist patient to meet own spiritual needs. Assist patient to use spiritual resources to meet personal situation.
- Encourage patient to keep significant symbols nearby.

- Inform patient or family where chapel or prayer room is located.
- Be willing to cooperate with and/or facilitate the administration of the patient's rituals.
- Nurse should determine own values and spirituality.

Provides expansion of personal boundaries through connectedness. Provides a sense of wholeness and well-being. Person may be "ill" and still be "healthy" in terms of spirituality, as spirituality provides the patient with the capacity for health through transcendence of ordinary boundaries and various modes of connectedness.[23] Solitude may liberate the spirit and lead to true knowledge of self, peace and joy, and an appreciation of life on a more profound level.[24]

Expressions of self-transcendence may differ across individuals and life phases in general.[23] Interactions within the person and with the environment generate conflicts that can provide the impetus for development through self-transcendence. Making meaning of life is integral to human development and enhancement of health.[25]

Shows respect and support for patient's beliefs and values.[21]
Spiritual nursing care needs to be based on a more universal concept of inspiring rather than focusing around religious concepts.[26] However, depending on the patient's beliefs, religious concepts may be integral to care.

Significant symbols can be a source of consolation and spiritual support.[24]
A patient's spiritual needs are complex and individual.[21]

Shows respect for patient's spiritual values and needs.[24]

Awareness of nurse's own feelings is helpful in guiding and/or controlling his or her actions.[21]

Child Health

Consider all actions given for Adult Health, but modify them to be developmentally appropriate. When infant or child is incapable of expressing spiritual preferences or indices, refer child to parents or staff or advocacy as deemed appropriate.

ACTIONS/INTERVENTIONS	RATIONALES
• Allow 30 min each shift for expression of feelings about current health status, and/or offer structured observation of infant, child, or parents to offer insight into thoughts relevant to current status.	Feelings regarding current status will provide opportunity to discover the spiritual factors valued.
• Allow for component of play therapy to provide spiritual data.	Play facilitates meaningful interaction for children and may best afford insights into thought processes.
• Abide by family's wishes in times of spiritual need and as part of regular care to degree possible.	Trust will be afforded to enhance current spiritual well-being when it is shown to have value.
• Incorporate spirituality into local support system by encouraging donations of time, reading materials, videos, art supplies, etc., with age-appropriate materials for all levels of development.	Valuing of community potentials increases likelihood of spiritual support, especially for young.

Women's Health

ACTIONS/INTERVENTIONS	RATIONALES
NOTE: All the actions under Spiritual Distress can apply here as well as the following: • Allow the woman and her family to direct the spiritual care needed when possible. • Be available and willing to call whatever spiritual advisor the woman and family wish. • Provide quiet, noninterruptive space for discussion, prayer, or communication with spiritual advisor. • Allow patient and family to participate in rituals as requested when possible. • Be open to spiritual awareness in both the patient's life and in the nurse's own life. This could be accomplished through participating in a dream-telling group.[9] • Assess how patient views her "sense of fit" in her world.[27] • Assess the patient's sources of strength and relationships that are important to her.[27] • Encourage the woman to give voice to her story.[27] • Encourage time for self-reflection and making connections.	By allowing the patient to express her own beliefs and values, strengths, and relationships, great insight into how health care providers can give high-quality care to the whole person can emerge. This can form the basis of care or support to our patients.

Psychiatric Health

Refer to Adult Health interventions.

Gerontic Health

ACTIONS/INTERVENTIONS	RATIONALES
• Determine availability of religious services or ceremonies for the patient. • Coordinate, as needed, transportation to formal services or visits from religious representatives. • Provide time for religious activities or personal time for meditation or contemplation. • Establish ongoing relationship with patient that fosters trust and sharing. • Encourage life review or reminiscing to assist the older patient in identification of past stressors and coping skills. • Discuss how aging has changed the patient, from their perspective, and what those changes have meant to the patient. • Discuss spiritual care needs with patient, and identify preferred spiritual advisor, counselor, or resource for the patient. • Offer opportunities to pray with older patient, if you are comfortable in so doing.	If the patient attends religious services, he or she may need information about what services are offered. The number of active, participating church members is highest in the older adult group. Aging physical changes may interfere with access to services. Depending on the care setting and care needs, it may be difficult to incorporate activities or personal time, and the patient may be hesitant to make his or her need known. Provides an opportunity to gradually reveal self and nurture spiritual growth for the caregiver and the care recipient. Offers insight into coping ability and needs. Enhances self-worth and problem-solving skills the older patient possesses. Promotes developmentally appropriate reflection. Clergy are frequently used as personal counselors by older adults. Health-related prayer is considered a source of comfort to many older patients.

Home Health

ACTIONS/INTERVENTIONS	RATIONALES

• Involve client and family in planning and implementing strategies to enhance spiritual well-being:
  ○ Identify values and beliefs.
  ○ Develop lifestyle choices that support values and beliefs.
  ○ Explore meaning of spirituality to self and family.
  ○ Identify actions and behaviors that express spirituality.
	Family involvement enhances effectiveness of intervention.

Spiritual Well-Being, Potential for Enhanced

FLOWCHART EVALUATION: EXPECTED OUTCOME 1

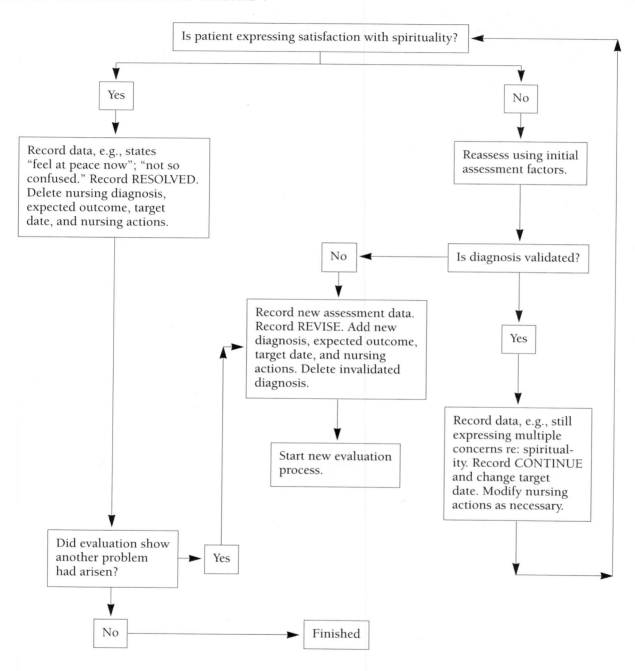

Spiritual Well-Being, Potential for Enhanced

FLOWCHART EVALUATION: EXPECTED OUTCOME 2

NANDA's Diagnostic Label Qualifiers

From the North American Nursing Diagnosis Association, *Nursing Diagnoses: Definitions and Classification: 1995–1996* Philadelphia, 1994, page 104.

Acute: Severe but of short duration.

Altered: A change from baseline.

Chronic: Lasting a long time; recurring; habitual; constant.

Decreased: Lessened; lesser in size, amount, or degree.

Deficient: Inadequate in amount, quality, or degree; defective; not sufficient; incomplete.

Depleted: Emptied wholly or in part; exhausted of.

Disturbed: Agitated; interrupted; interfered with.

Dysfunctional: Abnormal, incomplete functioning.

Excessive: Characterized by an amount or quantity that is greater than is necessary, desirable, or useful.

Increased: Greater in size, amount, or degree.

Ineffective: Not producing the desired effect.

Impaired: Made worse, weakened; damaged; reduced; deteriorated.

Intermittent: Stopping and starting again at intervals; periodic; cyclic.

Potential for enhanced: (for use with wellness diagnoses) Made greater; to increase in quality or more desired.

References

Chapter 1

1. Gordon, M: Nursing Diagnoses: Process and Application, ed. 3. Mosby–Year Book, St Louis, 1994.
2. Iyer, PW, Taptich, BJ, and Bernocchi-Losey, D: Nursing Process and Nursing Diagnosis, ed 3. WB Saunders Company, Philadelphia, 1995.
3. Doenges, ME, and Moorhouse, MF: Nurse's Pocket Guide: Nursing Diagnosis with Interventions, ed 4. FA Davis, Philadelphia, 1993.
4. Alfaro, R: Applying Nursing Diagnosis and Nursing Process: A Step-by-Step Guide. JB Lippincott Co, Philadelphia, 1990.
5. American Nurses Association: Nursing: A Social Policy Statement. Author, Kansas City, MO, 1980.
6. American Nurses Association: Standards of Clinical Nursing Practice. Author, Kansas City, MO, 1991.
7. Board of Nurse Examiners for the State of Texas: Standards of Nursing Practice. Texas Nurse Practice Act. Author, Austin, TX, 1994.
8. Brider, P: Who killed the nursing care plan? Am J Nurs 91:35, 1991.
9. Joint Commission of Accreditation of Healthcare Organizations: Accreditation Manual for Hospitals. Author, Chicago, 1994.
10. Carroll-Johnson, R: Reflections on the ninth biennial conference. Nurs Diagn 1:50, 1991.
11. Kozier, BB, Erb, GH, and Olivieri, R: Fundamentals of Nursing, ed 5. Addison-Wesley Nursing, Redwood City, CA, 1995.
12. North American Nursing Diagnosis Association: Definitions and Classifications, 1995–1996. Author, Philadelphia, 1994.
13. Tartaglia, MJ: Nursing diagnosis: Keystone of your care plan. Nursing 15:34, 1985.
14. Kieffer, JS: Nursing diagnosis can make a critical difference. Nurs Life 4:18, 1984.
15. Bolander, VB: Sorensen and Luckmann's Basic Nursing: A Psychophysiologic Approach, ed 3. WB Saunders Company, Philadelphia, 1994.
16. Cox, HC: Developing Nursing Care Plan Objectives: A Programmed Unit of Study. Texas Tech University Health Sciences Center School of Nursing, Continuing Education Program, Lubbock, TX, 1982.
17. Weed, LM: Medical records that guide and teach. N Engl J Med 27:593, 1986.
18. Lampe, S: FOCUS Charting, ed 4. Creative Nursing Management, Minneapolis, 1988.
19. Siegrist, L, Deltor, R, and Stocks, B: The PIE System: Planning and documentation of nursing care. Quality Review Bulletin, June, 1986.
20. Burks, LJ, and Murphy, J: Charting by Exception. John Wiley and Sons, New York, 1988.
21. Flynn, JM, and Heffron, PB: Nursing From Concept to Practice, ed 2. Appleton & Lange, Norwalk, CT, 1988.
22. Yura, H, and Walsh, MB: The Nursing Process: Assessing, Planning, Implementing, Evaluating, ed 5. Appleton-Century-Crofts, East Norwalk, CT, 1988.
23. Gordon, M: Manual of Nursing Diagnosis: 1991–1992. Mosby, St Louis, 1991.
24. Roy, C, Sr: Historical perspective of the theoretical framework for the classification of nursing diagnosis. In Kim, MJ, and Moritz, DA (eds): Classification of Nursing Diagnosis: Proceedings of the Third and Fourth National Conferences. McGraw-Hill, St Louis, 1982, p. 235.
25. Roy, C, Sr: Framework for Classification System Development: Progress and Issues. In Kim, MI, McFarland, GK, and McLane, AM (eds): Classification of Nursing Diagnosis: Proceedings of the Fifth National Conference. McGraw-Hill, St Louis, 1984, p. 29.
26. Kritek, PB: Report of the Group Who Worked on Taxonomies. In Kim, MJ, McFarland, GK, and McLane, AM (eds): Classification of Nursing Diagnosis: Proceedings of the Fifth National Conference. McGraw-Hill, St Louis, p 46, 1984.
27. Newman, MA: Looking at the whole. Am J Nurs 84:1496, 1984.
28. North American Nursing Diagnosis Association: Taxonomy I With Complete Diagnoses. Author, St Louis, 1987.
29. Doenges, ME, Moorhouse, MF, and Geissler, AC: Nursing Care Plans: Guidelines for Planning and Documenting Patient Care, ed 3. FA Davis, Philadelphia, 1993.
30. Doenges, ME, and Moorhouse, MG: Application of Nursing Process: An Interactive Text. FA Davis, Philadelphia, 1992.

Chapter 2

1. Rogers, ME: An Introduction to the Theoretical Basis for Nursing. FA Davis, Philadelphia, 1970.
2. Kneeshaw, M, and Lunney, M: Nursing diagnosis: Not for individuals only. Geriat Nsg 37:246, 1989.
3. Rosenstock, I: Historical origins of the health belief model. In Becker, M (ed): The Health Belief Model and Personal Behavior. Charles B. Slack, Thorofare, NJ, 1974.
4. Ridenour, N: Health beliefs, preventive behavioral intentions and knowledge of gonorrhea: Predictors of recidivism? In Monograph 1983, Proceedings of 2nd Annual Sigma Theta Tau Conference, The World of Work: Research in Nursing Practice. Sigma Theta Tau, Indianapolis, 1983.
5. Fleury, J: The application of motivational theory to cardiovascular risk reduction. Image: J of Nsg Scholar 24:229, 1992.
6. Janz, NK: The health belief model in understanding cardiovascular risk factor reduction behaviors. Cardiovascular Nursing 24:39, 1988.
7. Pender, NJ: Health Promotion in Nursing Practice, ed 2. Appleton-Century-Crofts, East Norwalk, CT, 1987.
8. Brubaker, B: Health promotion: A linguistic analysis. Adv Nurs Sci 5:1, 1983.
9. Department of Health and Human Services: Healthy People 2000: National Health Promotion and Disease Prevention Objectives. US Government Printing Office, Washington, DC, 1990.
10. Health and Human Services: Put prevention into practice. Waldorf, MD: American Nurses Association, 1994.
11. Shortridge, L, and Valanis, B: The epidemiological model applied in community health nursing. In Stanhope, M, and Lancaster, J (eds): Community Health Nursing: Process and Practice for Promoting Health, ed 3. Mosby, St Louis, 1992.
12. Gleit, C, and Tatro, S: Nursing diagnosis for healthy individuals. Nurs Health Care 32:151, 1981.
13. Popkess-Vawter, S: Wellness nursing diagnoses: To be or not to be? Nurs Diagn, 2:19, 1991.
14. Knollmueller, RN: Prevention Across the Life Span: Healthy People for the 21st Century. Washington, DC: American Nurses Publishing, 1993.
15. Schuster, CS, and Ashburn, SS: The Process of Human Development: A Holistic Life-Span Approach, ed 3. Lippincott, New York, 1992.

16. Preventive Services Task Force: Guide to Clinical Preventive Services. Williams & Wilkins, Baltimore, 1989.

17. American Academy of Pediatrics. Committee of Infectious Diseases: 1994 Red Book: Report of the Committee on Infectious Diseases, ed 23, Author, Elk Grove Village, IL, 1994.

18. Centers for Disease Control: Recommended childhood immunization schedule—United States, 1995. Morb Mort Weekly Report 44:RR-5, 1, 1995.

19. American Family Physician: AAFP updates childhood immunizations schedule. Am Fam Phys 51:2031, 1995.

20. Centers for Disease Control: Progress toward elimination of *Haemophilus influenzae* type b disease among infants and children—United States, 1987–1993. Morb Mort Weekly Report 43:8, 144, 1994.

21. Centers for Disease Control: *Haemophilus b* conjugate vaccines for prevention of *Haemophilus influenzae* type b disease among infants and children two months of age and older. Recommendations of the immunization practices advisory committee (ACIP). Morb Mort Weekly Report 40:RR-1, 1, 1991.

22. Centers for Disease Control: General recommendations on immunization: Recommendations of the advisory committee on immunization practices (ACIP). Morb Mort Weekly Report 43:RR-1, 1, 1994.

23. Centers for Disease Control: Hepatitis B virus: A comprehensive strategy for eliminating transmission in the United States through universal childhood vaccination. Morb Mort Weekly Report, 40:RR-13, 1991.

24. Baron, M, and Tafuro, P: The extremes of age: The newborn and the elderly. Nurs Clin North Am, 20:181, 1985.

25. Schuster, CS: Normal physiological parameters through the life cycle. Nurse Pract 2:25, 1977.

26. Devore, N, Jackson, V, and Peining, S: TORCH infections. Am J Nurs 83:1600, 1983.

27. Immunizations Practices Advisory Committee: Measles prevention: Recommendations of the immunizations practices advisory committee. Morb Mort Weekly Report 38:1, 1989.

28. American College of Physicians: Guide for Adult Immunization, ed 3. Author, Philadelphia, 1994.

29. Centers for Disease Control: Youth risk behavior surveillance—United States, 1993. Morb Mort Weekly Report 44:SS-1, 1995.

30. Centers for Disease Control: Update on adult immunization. Morb Mort Weekly Report 40:RR-12, 1991.

31. Immunizations Practices Advisory Committee: Pneumococcal polysaccaride vaccine. Morb Mort Weekly Reports 38:64, 1989.

32. Shapiro, E, et al: The protective efficacy of polyvalent pneumococcal-polysaccharide vaccine. N Engl J Med 325:1453, 1991.

33. Centers for Disease Control: Adult immunization: A report by the national vaccine advisory committee. Department of Health and Human Services, Atlanta, 1994.

34. Zimmerman, RK, and Clover, RD: Adult immunizations—A practical approach for clinicians: Part I. Am Family Practice 51:4, 859, 1995.

35. Zimmerman, RK, and Clover, RD: Adult immunizations—A practical approach for clinicians: Part II. Am Family Practice 51:4, 1139, 1995.

36. Centers for Disease Control: Prevention and control of influenza: Part I, Vaccines. Recommendations of the Advisory Committee on Immunization Practices (ACIP). Morb Mort Weekly Report 43:RR-6, 1, 1994.

37. Centers for Disease Control: Prevention and control of influenza: Part II, Antiviral agents. Recommendations of the Advisory Committee on Immunization Practices (ACIP). Morb Mortal Weekly Report 43:RR-15, 1, 1994.

38. Gergen, PJ, McQuillan, GM, Keily, M, Ezzati-Rice, TM, Sutter, RW, and Virella, G: A population-based serologic survey of immunity to tetanus in the United States. N Engl J Med 332:12, 761, 1995.

39. Yoshikawa, T: Tuberculosis in aging adults. J Am Ger Soc 40, 178, 1992.

40. North American Nursing Diagnosis Association: Nursing Diagnoses: Definitions & Classification: 1995–1996. Author, Philadelphia, 1994.

41. Wright, SM: Validity of the human energy assessment form. W J of Nurs Res 13(5):635–647, 1991.

42. Krieger, D: The Therapeutic Touch: How to Use Your Hands to Help or Heal. Prentice-Hall, Englewood Cliffs, NJ, 1979.

43. Krieger, D: Living the Therapeutic Touch: Healing as a Lifestyle. Prentice-Hall, Englewood Cliffs, NJ, 1987.

44. Dossey, FM, Keegan, L, Guzzetta, CE, and Kolkmeier, LG: Holistic Nursing: A Handbook for Practice. Aspen Publishers Inc, Gaithersburg, MD, 1988.

45. Whitis, G, and Iyer, P: Patient Outcomes in Pediatric Nursing. Springhouse Corp, Springhouse, PA, 1995.

46. McCoy, PA, and Votroubek, W: Pediatric Home Care: A Comprehensive Approach. Aspen Publishers Inc, Gaithersburg, MD, 1990.

47. Miller, L: Psychotherapy of epilepsy: Seizure control and psychosocial adjustment. J Cog Rehab 12(1):14–30.

48. Gatts et al: Reducing crying and irritability in neonates using a continuously controlled early environment. J Perinatology 15(2): 215–221, 1995.

49. Alexander, C, and Steefel, L: Biofeedback: Listen to the body. RN, 51–52, August, 1995.

50. Talton, CW: Touch—of all kinds—is therapeutic. RN, 61–64, February, 1995.

51. Morrelli, I: Interview with author on use of therapeutic touch during labor. 1995.

52. Erickson, HC, Tomlin, EM, and Swain, MP: Modeling and Role-Modeling: A Theory and Paradigm for Nursing. Prentice-Hall, Englewood Cliffs, NJ, 1983.

53. Becker, R, and Selden, G: The Body Electric. William Morrow, New York, 1985.

54. Thie, J: Touch for Health. Devorss & Company, Marina del Rey, CA, 1979.

55. Quinn, J, and Strelkauskas, A: Psychoimmunologic effects of therapeutic touch on practitioners and recently bereaved recipients: A pilot study. Adv in Nurs Sci 15(4): 13–26, 1993.

56. Snyder, M: Independent Nursing Interventions, ed 2. Delmar Publishers, Albany, NY, 1992.

57. Kunz, L, and Kunz, B: The Practitioner's Guide to Reflexology. Prentice-Hall, Englewood Cliffs, NJ, 1985.

58. Wright, L, and Leahey, M: Nurses and Families, ed 2. FA Davis, Philadelphia, 1994.

59. Thie, J: Touch for Health. Devorss & Company, Marina del Rey, CA, 1979.

60. Anderson, R, and Anderson, K: Success and failure attributions in smoking cessations among men and women. Am Assoc Occup Health Nurs J 38:180, 1990.

61. Wewers, M, and Gonyon, D: Cigarette craving during the immediate postcessation period. Appl Nurs Res 2:46, 1989.

62. Frost, C: Implications of smoking bans in the workplace. Am Assoc Occup Health Nurs J 39:270, 1991.

63. Daughton, DM, Andrews, CE, Orona, CP, Patil, KD, and Rennard, SI: Total indoor smoking ban and smoker behavior. Prev Med 21:670, 1992.

64. Volden, C, Langemo, D, Adamson, M, and Oeschsel, L: The relationship of age, gender, and exercise practices to measures of health, lifestyle, and self-esteem. Appl Nurs Res 3:20, 1990.

65. Brown, J, and March, S: Use of botanicals for health purposes by members of a prepaid health plan. Res Nurs Health 14:330, 1991.

66. Watzlawick, P, Weakland, J, and Fisch, R: Change: Principles of Problem Formation and Problem Resolution. WW Norton, New York, 1974.

67. Rendom, DC, Davis, DK, Giorella, EC, and Tranzillo, MJ: The right to know, the right to be taught. J Gerontol Nurs 12:33, 1986.

68. Briasco, M: Indoor air pollution: Are employees sick from their work? Am Assoc Occup Health Nurs J 38:375, 1990.

69. Kipen, HM, Hallman, W, Kelly-McNeil, K, and Fiedler, N: Measuring chemical sensitivity prevalence: A questionnaire for population studies. Am J Pub Health 85:574, 1985.

70. Bonheur, B, and Young, S: Exercise as a health-promoting lifestyle choice. Appl Nurs Res 4:2, 1991.

71. Rosenkoetter, M: Health promotion: The influence of pets on life patterns in the home. Holist Nurs Pract 5:42, 1991.

72. Centers for Disease Control: Recommendations for the prevention of HIV transmission in health-care setting. Morb Mort Weekly Report 36:1, 1987.

73. Centers for Disease Control: Update: Universal precautions for prevention of transmission of human immunodeficiency virus, hepatitis B virus, and other bloodborn pathogens in health-care settings. Morb Mort Weekly Report 37:377, 1988.

74. Centers for Disease Control: Recommendations for preventing transmission of human immunodeficiency virus and hepatitis B virus to patients during exposure-prone invasive procedures. Morb Mort Weekly Report 40:1, 1991.

75. Benenson, A: Control of communicable disease in man (15th ed). American Public Health Association, Washington, DC, 1990.

76. Dooley, S, et al: Guidelines for preventing the transmission of tuberculosis in health-care settings, with special focus on HIV-related issues. Morb Mort Weekly Report 39:RR-17, 1990.

77. Centers for Disease Control: Tuberculosis control laws—United States, 1993. Recommendations of the Advisory Council for the Elimination of Tuberculosis (ACET). Morb Mort Weekly Report 42:RR-15, 1993.

78. Mace, N, and Rabin, P: The 36-hour Day: A Family Guide. Johns Hopkins University Press, Baltimore, 1991.

79. Evans, L, and Strumpf, N: Myths about elder restraint. Image 22:124, 1990.

80. Kilpack, V, et al: Using research-based interventions to decrease patient falls. Appl Nurs Res 4:68, 1991.

81. Hogue, CC: Managing falls: The current basis for practice. In Funk, SG, Tournquist, EM, Champagne, MT, and Wiese, RA (eds): Key Aspects of Elder Care. Springer Publishing Company, New York, 1992, pp. 41–56.

82. Jech, AO: Preventing falls in the elderly. Geriat Nsg 13:43, 1992.

83. Williams, J: Employee experiences with early return to work programs. Am Assoc Occup Health Nurs 39:64, 1991.

84. National Immunization Campaign: Community Leader's Guide for the National Immunization Campaign. Author, Washington, DC, 1991.

85. Buckley, K, and Kulb, NW: High risk maternity nursing manual. Williams & Wilkins, Baltimore, 1993.

86. Mandeville, LK, and Troiano, NH: High-risk intrapartum nursing. JB Lippincott Co, Philadelphia, 1992.

87. Stainton, MC: Supporting family functioning during a high-risk pregnancy. Am J Maternal/Child Nurs 19(1):24–28, 1994.

88. Hagey, R, and McDonough, P: The problem of professional labeling. Nurs Outlook 32:151, 1984.

89. Edel, M: Noncompliance: An appropriate nursing diagnosis? Nurs Outlook 33:183, 1985.

90. Breunig, K, et al: Noncompliance as a nursing diagnosis: Current use in clinical practice. In Hurley, M (ed): Classification of Nursing Diagnosis: Proceedings of the Sixth Conference. Mosby, St Louis, 1986.

91. Keeling, A, Utz, SW, Schuster, G, and Boyle, A: Noncompliance revisited: A disciplinary perspective of a nursing diagnosis. Nurs Diagnosis 4:91, 1993.

92. Beauchamp, T, and Childress, J: Principles of Biomedical Ethics, ed 4, Oxford University Press, New York, 1994.

93. Cooper, M: Chronic illness and nursing's ethical challenge. Holist Nurs Pract 5:10, 1990.

94. Thorne, S: Constructive noncompliance in chronic illness. Holist Nurs Pract 5:62, 1990.

95. Benner, PE, and Wrubel, J: The Primacy of Caring: Stress and Coping in Health and Illness. Addison-Wesley, Menlo Park, CA, 1989.

96. Gadow, S: Covenant without cure: Letting go and holding on in chronic illness. In Watson, J, and Ray, M (eds): The Ethics of Care and the Ethics of Cure: Synthesis in Chronicity. National League for Nursing, New York, 1988.

97. Watson, J: Nursing, Human Science and Human Care: A Theory of Nursing, National League for Nursing, New York, 1991.

98. Clark, AL: Culture and Childbearing. FA Davis, Philadelphia, 1981.

99. Hoffman, L: A co-evolutionary framework for systemic family therapy? In Hansen, JC, and Keeney, BP (eds): Diagnosis and Assessment in Family Therapy. Aspen Systems, Rockville, MD, 1983.

100. Kontz, M: Compliance redefined and implications for home care. Holist Nurs Pract 3:54, 1989.

101. Smith, F, and Knice-Ambinder, M: Promoting medication compliance in clients with chronic mental illness. Holist Nurs Pract 4:70, 1989.

103. Gravey, E, and Oseasohn, C: Multiple drug regimens: Medication compliance among veterans 65 years and older. Res Nurs Health 14:51, 1991.

103. Jones, S, Jones, P, and Katz, J: A nursing intervention to increase compliance in otitis media patients. Appl Nurs Res 4:68, 1989.

104. Mandeville, LK, and Troiano, N: High-Risk Intrapartum Nursing. JB Lippincott Co, Philadelphia, 1992.

Chapter 3

1. Potter, PA, and Perry, AG: Instructors' Manual for Fundamentals of Nursing: Concepts, Process and Practice, ed 3. Mosby–Year Book, St Louis, 1993.

2. Flynn, JM, and Heffron, PB: Nursing: From Concept to Practice, ed 2. Appleton & Lange, Norwalk, CT, 1988.

3. Mitchell, PH, and Loustau, A: Concepts Basic to Nursing Practice. McGraw-Hill, New York, 1981.

4. Murray, RB, and Zentner, JP: Nursing Assessment and Health Promotion Strategies Through the Life Span, ed 5. Appleton & Lange, Norwalk, CT, 1993.

5. May, KA, and Mahlmeister, LR: Comprehensive Maternity Nursing: Nursing Process and the Childbearing Family. JB Lippincott Co, Philadelphia, 1990.

6. Frigerio, C, Schutz, Y, Whitehead, R, and Jdequien, E: A New Procedure to Assess the Energy Requirements of Lactation in Gambian Women. Am J Clin Nutr 54:526–533.

7. Kemp, M, et al: Factors that contribute to pressure sores in surgical patients. Res Nurs Health 13:293, 1990.

8. Guyton, AC: Textbook of Medical Physiology, ed 8. WB Saunders Company, Philadelphia, 1991.

9. Schuster, CS, and Ashburn, SS: The Process of Human Development: A Holistic Life-Span Approach, ed 3. JB Lippincott Co., New York, 1992.

10. Korones, SB: High-Risk Newborn Infants: The Basis for Intensive Nursing Care, ed 4. Mosby, St Louis, 1986.

11. Driscoll, J, and Heird, W: Maintenance fluid therapy during the neonatal period. In Winters, RW (ed): Principles of Pediatric Fluid Therapy, ed 2. Little, Brown & Company, Inc, Boston, 1982.

12. Brandt, PA, Chinn, PE, and Smith, ME: Current Practice in Pediatric Nursing. Mosby, St Louis, 1980.

13. McCrory, WW: Developmental Nephrology. Harvard University Press, Cambridge, MA, 1972.

14. Masiak, MJ, Naylor, MD, and Hayman, LL: Fluids and Electrolytes Through the Life Cycle. Appleton-Century-Crofts, East Norwalk, CT, 1985.

15. Stone, L, and Church, J: Childhood and Adolescence: A Psychology of the Growing Person. Random House, New York, 1968.

16. Young, C, et al: Body composition of pre-adolescent and adolescent girls. J Am Diab Assoc 53:579, 1968.

17. Chinn, P, and Leitch, C: Child Health Maintenance: Concepts in Family-Centered Care, ed 2. Mosby, St Louis, 1979.

18. Mitchell, HS, et al: Nutrition in Health and Disease, ed 17. JB Lippincott Co, New York, 1982.

19. Shafer, J: Dysgeusia in the elderly. Lancet 1:35, 1965.

20. Kopak, C: Sensory loss in the aged: The role of the nurse and the family. Nurs Clin North Am 18:373, 1983.

21. Cugini, P, et al: Methodologically critical interaction of circadian rhythm, sex and aging characterize serum aldosterone and female adenopause. J Gerontol 37:403, 1982.

22. Carnevali, DL, and Patrick, M: Nursing Management for the Elderly, ed 3. JB Lippincott Co, Philadelphia, 1993.

23. North American Nursing Diagnosis Association: Nursing Diagnosis: Definitions and Classifications: 1995–1996. Author, Philadelphia, 1994.

24. Gelenberg, AJ, Bassuk, EL, and Schoonover, SC: The Practitioner's Guide to Psychoactive Drugs. Plenum Medical Book Company, New York, 1991.

25. Townsend, M: Drug Guide for Psychiatric Nursing. FA Davis, Philadelphia, 1990.

26. Reeder, SJ, Martin, LL, and Koniak, D: Maternity Nursing: Family, Newborn and Women's Health Care, ed 17. JB Lippincott Co, Philadelphia, 1992.

27. Barger, J, and Bull, P: A comparison of the bacterial composition of breast milk stored at room temperature and stored in the refrigerator. International Journal of Childbirth Education 5:29, 1987.

28. Cunningham, AS, Jelliffe, DB, and Jelliffe, EF: Breastfeeding and health in the 1980s: A global epidemiologic review. J Pediatr 118:1, 1991.

29. Lawrence, RA: Breastfeeding: A Guide for the Medical Profession, ed 4. Mosby, St Louis, 1993.

30. Riordan, J, and Auerback, KG: Breast Feeding and Human Lactation. Jones and Bartlett, 1993.

31. Walker, M: Breastfeeding Premature Babies: Lactation Consultant Series. La Leche League International, Franklin Park, IL, 1990.

32. Mead, LJ, et al: Breastfeeding success with preterm quadruplets. J Obstet Gynecol Neonatal Nurs 21:221, 1992.

33. McCoy, R, et al: Nursing management of breastfeeding for preterm infants. J Perinat Neonatal Nurs 2:42, 1988.

34. Meier, PP, Engstrom, JL, Mangurten, HH, Estrada, E, Zimmerman, B, and Kopparthi, R: Breast feeding support services in the neonatal intensive care unit. J Obstet Gynecol Neonatal Nurs 22:338, 1993.

35. Henrikson, M, Wall, G, Lethbridge, D, and McClurg, V: Nursing diagnosis and obstetric, gynecologic and neonatal nursing: Breast feeding as an example. J Obstet Gynecol Neonatal Nurs 21:446, 1992.

36. Wong, DL: Whaley and Wong's Nursing Care of Infants and Children, ed 5. Mosby, St Louis, 1995.

37. Mandeville, LK, and Troiano, NH: High Risk Intrapartum Nursing. JB Lippincott Co, Philadelphia, 1992.
38. Beland, I, and Passos, J: Clinical Nursing: Pathophysiological and Psychosocial Approaches, ed 4. Macmillan, New York, 1981.
39. Cosgray, RE, et al: The water-intoxicated patient. Arch Psychiatr Nsg 5:308, 1990.
40. Lapierre, E, et al: Polydipsia and hyponatremia in psychiatric patients: Challenge to creative nursing care. Arch Psychiatr Nsg 2:87, 1990.
41. Boyd, MA: Polydipsia in the chronically mentally ill: A review. Arch Psychiatr Nsg 3:166, 1990.
42. Olds, SB, London, ML, and Ladewig, PA: Maternal Newborn Nursing: A Family-Centered Approach. Addison-Wesley Publishing Co Inc, Redwood City, CA, 1992.
43. Bailey, C: Fit or Fat? Houghton Mifflin, Boston, 1978.
44. Orr, E: Breast feeding after a cesarean. Int J Childbirth Ed 9:26, 1994.
45. Niefert, MR, and Secat, JM: Milk yield and prolactin rise with simultaneous breast pump. Ambulatory Pediatric Association Meeting Abstracts, Washington, DC, May, 1985.
46. Frantz, KB: Managing Nipple Problems (Reprint No. 11). LaLeche League International, Franklin Park, IL, 1982.
47. Niefert, MR, and Secat, JM: Lactation insufficiency: A rational approach. Birth 16:182, 1989.
48. Walker, M: Management of selected early breastfeeding problems seen in clinical practice. Birth 16:148, 1989.
49. Anderson, GC, et al: Development of sucking in term infants from birth to four hours postbirth. Res Nurs Health 5:21, 1982.
50. Metheney, N, et al: Detection of Inadvertent Respiratory Placement of Small-Bore Feeding Tubes. Heart Lung 19:631, 1990.
51. Metheney, N, et al: Effectiveness of Auscultory Method in Predicting Feeding Tube Location. Nurs Res 39:266, 1990.
52. Nursing Mothers' Council of the Boston Association for Childbirth Education: Breastfeeding Your Baby. Avery, Garden City, NY, 1989.
53. Grams, M: Breastfeeding Source Book. Achievement Press, Sheridan, WY, 1990.
54. Garner, D, and Garfinkel, P (eds): Handbook of Psychotherapy for Anorexia Nervosa and Bulima. Guilford Press, New York, 1985.
55. Erickson, HC, and Kinney, C: Modeling and Role-Modeling: Theory, Research, and Practice. Author, Austin, 1990.
56. Haber, J, et al: Comprehensive Psychiatric Nursing, ed 4. Mosby–Year Book, St Louis, 1992.
57. Wilson, HS, and Kneisl, CR: Psychiatric Nursing, ed 4. Addison-Wesley Publishing Co Inc, Redwood City, CA, 1992.
58. Watzlawick, P, Weakland, J, and Fisch, R: Change: Principles of Problem Formation and Problem Resolution. WW Norton & Co Inc, New York, 1974.
59. Maas, M, Buckealter, K, and Hardy, M: Nursing Diagnoses and Interventions for the Elderly. Addison-Wesley Nursing, Fort Collins, CO, 1991.

Chapter 4

1. Bruya, MA: Elimination status. In Mitchell, PH, and Loustau, A (eds): Concepts Basic to Nursing, ed 3. McGraw-Hill, New York, 1981.
2. Bartucci, MR: Assessment of the renal system. In Phipps, WJ, et al (eds): Medical-Surgical Nursing: Concepts and Clinical Practice, ed 5. Mosby, St Louis, 1995.
3. Flynn, JM, and Heffron, PB: Nursing: From Concept to Practice, ed 2, Appleton & Lange, Norwalk, CT, 1988.
4. Kelly, MA: Nursing Diagnosis Source Book. Appleton-Century-Crofts, East Norwalk, CT, 1985.
5. Gettrust, KV, and Brabec, PD: Nursing Diagnosis in Clinical Practice: Guides for Care Planning. Delmar Publishers, New York, 1992.
6. Sherman, S: Urinary Incontinence in Community Dwelling Elders in Urban and Rural Areas. Unpublished Thesis. Texas Tech University Health Sciences Center School of Nursing, Lubbock, TX, 1990.
7. Burgio, K, Mathews, K, and Engel, B: Prevalence, incidence and correlates of urinary incontinence in healthy, middle-aged women. J Urol 196:1255, 1991.
8. Clay, E: Urinary continence/incontinence. Habit retraining: A tested method to regain urinary control. Geriatr Nur 1:252, 1980.
9. Murray, RB, and Zentner, JP: Nursing Assessment and Health Promotion through the Life Span, ed 5. Appleton & Lange, Norwalk, CT, 1993.
10. Schuster, CS, and Ashburn, SS: The Process of Human Development: A Holistic Life-Span Approach, ed 3. JB Lippincott Co, Philadelphia, 1992.
11. Carnevali, DL, and Patrick, M: Nursing Management for the Elderly, ed 3. JB Lippincott Co, Philadelphia, 1993.
12. Burggraf, V, and Stanley, M: Nursing the Elderly: A Care Plan Approach. JB Lippincott Co, St Louis, 1989.
13. Matteson, MA, and McConnell, ES: Gerontological Nursing: Concepts and Practices. WB Saunders Company, Philadelphia, 1988.
14. Mobily, PR, and Kelley, LS: Iatrogenesis in the elderly: Factors of immobility. J Gerontol Nurs 17:9, 1991.
15. North American Nursing Diagnosis Association: Nursing Diagnoses: Definitions and Classification: 1995–1996. Author, Philadelphia, 1994.
16. Fogel, CI, and Wood, NF: Health Care of Women: A Nursing Perspective. Mosby, St Louis, 1981.
17. Schmelzer, M: Effectiveness of wheat bran in preventing constipation of hospitalized orthopaedic surgery patients. Orthop Nurs 9:55, 1990.
18. Heather, C, et al: Effect of bulk forming cathartic on diarrhea in tube fed patients. Heart Lung 20:409, 1991.
19. Black, JM, and Matassarin-Jacobs, E: Luckmann's and Sorensen's Medical-Surgical Nursing: A Psychophysiological Approach, ed 4. WB Saunders Company, Philadelphia, 1993.
20. Haber, J, et al: Comprehensive Psychiatric Nursing, ed 4. Mosby, St Louis, 1992.
21. Wilson, HS, and Kneisl, CR: Psychiatric Nursing, ed 4. Addison-Wesley Publishing Co Inc, Redwood, CA, 1992.
22. Jacobson, N, and Margolin, G: Marital Therapy. Brunner/Mazel, New York, 1979.
23. Hawkins, JW, and Grovine, B: Postpartum Nursing: Health Care of Women. Springer Publishing Co Inc, New York, 1985.

Chapter 5

1. Potter, PA, and Perry, AG: Instructor's Manual for Use with Fundamentals of Nursing: Concepts, Process, and Practice, ed 3. Mosby–Year Book, St Louis, 1993.
2. Kelly, MA: Nursing Diagnosis Source Book. Appleton-Century-Crofts, East Norwalk, CT, 1985.
3. Mitchell, PH: Motor status. In Mitchell, PH, and Loustau, A (eds): Concepts Basic to Nursing. McGraw-Hill, New York, 1981.
4. Lentz, M: Selected aspects of deconditioning secondary to immobilization. Nurs Clin North Am 16:729, 1980.
5. Pardue, N: Immobility. In Flynn, JM, and Heffron, PB (eds): Nursing: From Concept to Practice, ed 2. Appleton & Lange, Norwalk, CT, 1988.
6. Murray, RB, and Zentner, JP: Nursing Assessment and Health Promotion Strategies through the Life Span, ed 5. Appleton & Lange, Norwalk, CT, 1993.
7. Schuster, CS, and Ashburn, SS: The Process of Human Development: A Holistic Life-Span Approach, ed 3. JB Lippincott Co, Philadelphia, 1992.
8. Noble, E: Essential Exercises for the Childbearing Year, ed 3. Houghton Mifflin, Boston, 1988.
9. Duncan, J, Gordon, N, and Scott, C: Women walking for health and fitness: How much is enough? J Am Med Assoc 266:3295, 1991.
10. North American Nursing Diagnosis Association: Nursing Diagnoses: Definitions and Classification: 1995–1996. NANDA, Philadelphia, 1994.
11. Buckley, K, and Kulb, NW: High Risk Maternity Nursing Manual. Williams & Wilkins, Baltimore, 1993.
12. Creasy, RK, and Resnik, R: Maternal-Fetal Medicine: Principles and Practice. WB Saunders Company, Philadelphia, 1994.
13. Gabbe, SG, Niebyl, JR, and Simpson, JL: Obstetrics: Normal and Problem Pregnancies. Churchill Livingstone Inc, New York, 1994.
14. Eganhouse, DJ, and Burnside, SM: Nursing assessment and responsibilities in monitoring the preterm pregnancy. J Obstet Gynecol and Neonatal Nurs 21:355–363, 1992.
15. Fuchs, A, Fuchs, F, and Stubblefield, PG: Preterm Birth: Causes, Prevention, and Management. McGraw-Hill, New York, 1993.
16. Knuppel, RA, and Drukker, JE: High Risk Pregnancy: A Team Approach. WB Saunders Company, Philadelphia, 1993.
17. Mandeville, LK, and Troiano, NH: High-Risk Intrapartum Nursing. JB Lippincott Co, Philadelphia, 1992.
18. Tucker, SM, Canobbio, MM, Paquette, EV, and Wells, MF: Patient Care Standards: Nursing Process, Diagnosis and Outcome. Mosby–Year Book, St Louis, 1992.
19. Stainton, MC: Supporting family functioning during a high risk pregnancy. MCN: Am J Matern Child Nurs 19:24–28, 1994.

20. Erickson, HC, and Kinney, CK: Modeling and Role-Modeling: Theory, Research & Practice. Society for Advancement of Modeling and Role-Modeling, Austin, 1990.
21. Wilson, JS, and Kneisl, CR: Psychiatric Nursing, ed 4. Addison-Wesley Publishing Co Inc, Redwood, CA, 1992.
22. Haber, J, et al: Comprehensive Psychiatric Nursing, ed 4. Mosby–Year Book, St Louis, 1992.
23. Dossey, BM, et al: Holistic Nursing: A Handbook for Practice. Aspen, Gaithersburg, MD, 1995.
24. Clark, C: Wellness Nursing. Springer Publishing Co Inc, New York, 1986.
25. Wright, LM, and Leahey, M: Nurses & Families: A Guide to Family Assessment and Intervention. FA Davis, Philadelphia, 1994.
26. Maas, M, Buckwalter, KC, and Hardy, MA: Nursing Diagnosis and Interventions for the Elderly. Addison-Wesley Publishing Co Inc, Redwood City, CA, 1991.
27. Townsend, MC: Drug Guide for Psychiatric Nursing. FA Davis, Philadelphia, 1990.
28. Association of Women's Health, Obstetric, and Neonatal Nurses: Second Stage Labor Nursing Management Protocol. Author, Washington, DC, 1994.
29. Andrews, CM, and Chranowski, M: Maternal position, labor, and comfort. Appl Nurs Res 3:7–13, 1990.
30. Gilliss, C, et al: Toward a Science of Family Nursing. Addison-Wesley Publishing Co Inc, Menlo Park, CA, 1989.
31. Eliopoulos, C: Manual of Gerontologic Nursing. Mosby, St Louis, 1995.
32. Doenges, ME, and Moorhouse, MF: Nurse's Pocket Guide: Nursing Diagnoses with Interventions. FA Davis, Philadelphia, 1993.
33. Kavanagh, J, and Riegger, M: Assessment of the Cardiovascular System. In Phipps, WJ, et al (eds): Medical-Surgical Nursing: Concepts and Clinical Practice, ed 5. Mosby, St Louis, 1995.
34. Adenhold, KJ, and Roberts, JE: Phases of second stage labor. J Nurse Midwifery 36:267–275, 1991.
35. Golay, J, Vedam, S, and Sorger, L: The squatting position for the second stage of labor: Effects on labor and on maternal and fetal well-being. Birth 20:73–78, 1993.
36. Thomson, AM: Publishing techniques in the second stage of labor. J Adv Nurs 18:171–177, 1993.
37. Caldeyro-Barcia, R: The influence of maternal bearing-down efforts during second stage on fetal well-being. Birth 6:17–21, 1979.
38. Folta, A, and Metzger, B: Exercise and functional capacity after myocardial infarction. Image 21:215, 1989.
39. Kenner, C, Brueggemeyer, A, and Gunderson, LP: Comprehensive Neonatal Nursing: A Physiologic Perspective. WB Saunders Company, Philadelphia, 1993.
40. May, KA, and Mahlmeister, LR: Maternal and Neonatal Nursing: Family Centered Care. JB Lippincott Co, Philadelphia, 1994.
41. Beland, IL, and Passos, JY: Clinical Nursing: Pathophysiological and Psychosocial Approaches, ed 4. Macmillan, New York, 1981.
42. Osborn, CL: Reminiscence: When the past erases the present. J of Geront Nurs 15:6, 1989.
43. Richless, C: Current trends in mechanical ventilation. Crit Care Nurse 11:41, 1991.
44. Hazinski, MF: Nursing Care of the Critically Ill Child. Mosby, St Louis, 1992.
45. Department of Health and Human Services: Executive Summary: Guidelines for the Diagnosis and Management of Asthma. Author, Washington, DC, 1991.
46. Norton, LC, and Neureuter, A: Weaning the long-term ventilator dependent patient: Common problems and management. Crit Care Nurse 9:42, 1989.
47. Knebel, AR: Weaning from mechanical ventilation: Current controversies. Heart Lung 20:47, 1991.
48. Forrest, G: Atrial fibrillation association with autonomic dysreflexia in patients with tetraplegia. Arch Phys Med Rehabil 72:592, 1991.
49. Pine, A, Miller, S, and Alonso, J: Atrial fibrillation associated with autonomic dysreflexia. Am J Phys Med Rehabil 70:271, 1991.
50. Lindan, R, et al: Incidence and clinical features of autonomic dysreflexia in patients with spinal cord injury. Paraplegia 18:285, 1980.
51. Earnhardt, J, and Frye, B: Understanding dysreflexia. Rehabil Nurs 9:28, 1986.
52. Ceron, GE, and Rakowski-Reinhardt, AC: Action stat! Autonomic dysreflexia. Nurs 21:33, 1991.
53. Trop, C, and Bennett, C: Autonomic dysreflexia and its urological implications. J Urol 146:1461, 1991.
54. Finocchiaro, DN, and Herzfeld, ST: Understanding autonomic dysreflexia. Am J Nurs 90:56, 1990.
55. Drayton-Hargrove, S, and Reddy, M: Rehabilitation and the long term management of the spinal cord impaired adult. Nurs Clin North Am 21:599, 1986.
56. Braddom, R, and Rocco, J: Autonomic dysreflexia. A survey of current treatment. Am J Phys Med Rehabil 70:237, 1991.
57. Black, JM: Luckmann & Sorensen's Medical-Surgical Nursing: A Psychophysiologic Approach, ed 4. WB Saunders Company, Philadelphia, 1993.
58. Thompson, C: Gender differences in walking distances of people with lung disease. Appl Nurs Res 1:141, 1989.
59. Lee, R, Grayder, J, and Ross, E: Effectiveness of psychological well-being, physical status and social support on oxygen dependent COPD patients' level of functioning. Res Nurs Health 14:323, 1991.
60. Wong DL: Whaley & Wong's Nursing Care of Infants and Children, ed 5. Mosby, St Louis, 1995.
61. Fulmer, T, and Walker, K: Lessons from the elder boom in ICUs. Geriatr Nur 11:120, 1990.
62. Reeder, SJ, Martin, LL, and Koniak, D: Maternity Nursing: Family, Newborn and Women's Health Care, ed 17. JB Lippincott Co, Philadelphia, 1992.
63. Strumpf, NE, and Evans, LK: The ethical problems of prolonged physical restraint. J Gerontol Nurs 17:27, 1991.
64. Mobily, PR, and Kelley, LS: Factors of immobility. J Gerontol Nurs 17:5, 1991.
65. Penn, C: Promoting independence. J Gerontol Nurs 14:14, 1988.
66. Cunningham, S: Circulatory and Fluid-Electrolyte Status. In Mitchell, PH, and Loustau, A (eds): Concepts Basic to Nursing, ed 3. McGraw-Hill, New York, 1981.

Chapter 6

1. Hayter, J: The rhythm of sleep. Am J Nurs 80:457, 1980.
2. Roth, B: Narcolepsy and Hypersomnia. Karger, New York, 1980.
3. Lee, K: Rest status. In Mitchell, PH, and Loustau, A (eds): Concepts Basic to Nursing, ed 3. McGraw-Hill, New York, 1981.
4. Guilleminault, C: Sleep and Its Disorders in Children. Raven Press, New York, 1987.
5. Wong, DL: Whaley and Wong's Nursing Care of Infants and Children, ed 5. Mosby, St Louis, 1995.
6. Mauri, M: Sleep and the reproductive cycle: A review. Health Care Women Int 11:409, 1990.
7. Weiss, ME, and Armstrong, M: Postpartum mothers' preferences for nighttime care of the neonate. J Obstet Gynecol Neonatal Nurs 20:290, 1991.
8. Mead-Bennett, E: The relationship of primigravida sleep experience and select moods on the first postpartum day. J Obstet Gynecol Neonatal Nurs 19:146, 1990.
9. Schirmer, M: When sleep won't come. J Gerontol Nurs 9:16, 1983.
10. Sonia, AI, et al: Periodic leg movements in sleep in community dwelling elderly. Sleep 14:496, 1991.
11. North American Nursing Diagnosis Association: Nursing Diagnoses: Definitions and Classification, 1995–1996. Author, Philadelphia, 1994.
12. Wilson, HS, and Kneisl, CR: Psychiatric Nursing, ed 4. Addison-Wesley Publishing Co Inc, Redwood City, CA, 1992.
13. Fisch, R, Watzlawick, P, Weakland, J, and Segal, L: Change. Jossey-Bass, San Francisco, 1982.
14. Keane, SM, and Stella, S: Recognizing depression in the elderly. J Gerontol Nurs 15:21, 1990.

Chapter 7

1. Murray, RB, and Zentner, JP: Nursing Assessment and Health Promotion Strategies Through the Lifespan, ed 5. Appleton & Lange, Norwalk, CT, 1993.
2. North American Nursing Diagnosis Association: Nursing Diagnoses: Definitions and Classifications: 1995–1996. NANDA, Philadelphia, 1994.
3. Stringer, W, Hasso, A, Thompson, J, Hinshaw, D, and Jordan, D: Hyperventilation-induced cerebral ischemia in patients with acute brain lesions: Demonstration by xenon-enhanced CT. Am J Neuroradiol 14:475–484, 1993.

4. Muizelar, J, Marmarou, A, Wart, J, et al: Adverse effects of prolonged hyperventilation in patients with severe head injury: A randomized clinical trial. J Neurosurg 75:731–739, 1991.

5. Wolf, A, Levi, L, Marmarou, A, et al: Effect of THAM upon outcome in severe head injury: A randomized prospective clinical tract. J Neurosurg 78:54–59, 1993.

6. Jastremski. CA: Traumatic brain injury: Assessment and treatment. Crit Care Nurs Clin North Am 6:473–481, 1994.

7. Keller, C, and Williams, A: Cardiac dysrhythmias associated with CNS dysfunction. J Neurosci Nurs 25:349–355, 1993.

8. Walleck, CA: Preventing secondary brain injury. AACN Clin Issues Crit Care Nurs 3:19–28, 1992.

9. Feldman, Z, Kanter, MJ, Robertson, CS, et al: Effect of head elevation on intracranial pressure, cerebral perfusion pressure and cerebral blood flow in head injured patients. J Neurosurg 76:207, 1992.

10. Williams, A, and Coyne, SM: Effects of neck position on intracranial pressure. Am J Crit Care 2:68–71, 1993.

11. Rising, CJ: The relationship of selected nursing activities to ICP. J Neurosci Nurs 25:302–308, 1993.

12. Hickey, JV: The Clinical Practice of Neurological and Neurosurgical Nursing, ed 3. JB Lippincott Co, Philadelphia, 1991.

13. McClelland, M, Woster, PI, Sweasey, T, and Hoff, JT: Continuous midazolam/atracurium infusion for the management of increased intracranial pressure. J Neurosci Nurs 27:96–101, 1995.

14. Kerr, M, Ruday, E, Brucia, J, and Stone, K: Head-injured adults: Recommendations for endotracheal suctioning. J Neurosci Nurs 25:86–91, 1993.

15. Eisenhart, K: New perspectives in the management of adults with severe head injury. Crit Care Nurs Q 17:1–12, 1994.

16. Barsevick, A, and Llewellyn, J: A comparison of the anxiety-reducing potential of two techniques of bathing. Nurs Res 31:22–27, 1982.

17. Walleck, CA: The effect of purposeful touch on intracranial pressure. Unpublished master's thesis, University of Maryland, 1982.

18. Chestnut, R, and Marshall, L: Treatment of abnormal intracranial pressure. Neurosurg Clin North Am 2:267–284, 1991.

19. Wisner, DH, Shuster, L, and Quinn, C: Hypertonic saline resuscitation in head injury: Effects on cerebral water content. J Trauma 30:75, 1990.

20. Gilliam, EF: Intracranial hypertension: Advances in intracranial pressure monitoring. Crit Care Nurs Clin North Am 2:21–27, 1990.

21. McIntosh, T, and Morgan, A: New trends in neurodiagnostic and therapeutics. Trauma Q 8:58–73, 1992.

22. Cruz, J, Miner, ME, Allen, SJ, et al: Continuous monitoring of cerebral oxygenation in acute brain injury: Assessment of hemodynamic reserve. Neurosurgery 29:743–749, 1991.

23. Procuik, JL: Management of cerebral oxygen supply-demand balance in blunt head injury. Crit Care Nurs Aug: 38–45, 1995.

24. Bullock, R: Opportunities for neuro-protective drugs in clinical management of head injury. J Emerg Med 11:23–30, 1993.

25. Hall, E: The role of oxygen radicals in traumatic injury: Clinical implications. J Emerg Med 11:31–36, 1993.

26. Bullock, R, and Fujisawa, H: The role of glutamate antagonists for the treatment of CNS injury. J Neurotrauma 9(suppl 2):S443–S462, 1992.

27. Zimmerman, J: Therapeutic application of oxygen radical scavengers. Chest 100(suppl):189S–192S, 1991.

28. Crosby, LJ, and Parsons, LC: Cerebrovascular response of closed head-injured patients to a standardized endotracheal tube suctioning and manual hyperventilation procedure. J Neurosci Nurs 24:40–49, 1992.

29. Jaracolis, EM: Foundations of Psychiatric-Mental Health Nursing. WB Saunders Company, Philadelphia, 1994.

30. Mahoney, DF: Analysis of restraint free nursing homes. Image 33:155, 1995.

31. Wilson, H, and Kneisl, C: Psychiatric Nursing, ed 5. Addison-Wesley Publishing Co Inc, Menlo Park, CA, 1996.

32. McCloskey, J, and Blechek, G (eds): Nursing Interventions Classification. Mosby, St Louis, 1992.

33. Maxmen, JS: Psychotropic Drugs Fast Facts. WW Norton & Co Inc, New York, 1991.

34. Weinrich, S, Egbert, C, Eleazer, GP, and Haddock, KS: Agitation: Measurement, management, and intervention research. Arch Psychiatr Nurs 9:251, 1994.

35. Erickson, H, Tomlin, E, and Swain, M: Modeling and Role Modeling: A Theory and Paradigm for Nursing. RL Bryan, Columbia, SC, 1988.

36. Sullivan-Marx, E: Delirium and physical restraint in the hospitalized elderly. Image 26:295, 1994.

37. Snyder, M: Independent Nursing Interventions, ed 2. Delmar, New York, 1992.

38. Harvath, TA, Patsdaughter, CA, Bumbalo, J, and McCann, M: Dementia-related behaviors. J Psychosoc Nurs 33:35, 1994.

39. Goldsmith, SM, Hoeffer, B, and Radar, J: Problematic wandering behavior in the cognitively impaired elderly. J Psychosoc Nurs 33:6, 1994.

40. Krause, KD, and Younger, VJ: Nursing diagnoses as guidelines in the care of the neonatal ECMO patient. J Obstet Gynecol Neonatal Nurs 21:176, 1992.

41. Cox, BE: What IF? Coping with unexpected outcomes. Childbirth Instructor 1:24, 1991.

42. Parkman, SE: Helping families to say good-bye. MCN Am J Matern Child Nurs 17:14, 1992.

43. Ryan, PF, Cote-Arsenault, D, and Sugarman, LL: Facilitating care after perinatal loss: A comprehensive checklist. J Obstet Gynecol Neonatal Nurse 20:385, 1991.

44. Ladebauche, P: Unit-based family support groups: A reminder. MCH Am J Matern Child Nurse 17:18, 1992.

45. Erickson, MH: The Practical Applications of Medical & Dental Hypnosis. Brunner/Mazel, New York, 1990.

46. Keeney, BP: Aesthetics of Change. Guilford Press, New York, 1983.

47. Watzlawick, P, Weakland, J, and Fisch, R: Change. WW Norton & Co Inc, New York, 1974.

48. Aguilera, DC: Crisis Intervention: Theory and Methodology, ed 7. Mosby, St Louis, 1994.

49. Creasia, JL, and Parker, B: Conceptual Foundations of Professional Nursing Practice. Mosby–Year Book, St Louis, 1991.

50. Weinrick, S, Boyd, M, and Nussbaum, J: Continuing education: Adapting strategies to teach the elderly. J Geront Nurs 15:17, 1989.

51. Department of Health and Human Services: Acute Pain Management: Operative on Medical Procedures and Trauma. Clinical Practice Guidelines. Author, Rockville, MD, 1992.

52. Fogel, CI, and Woods, NF: Health Care of Women: A Nursing Perspective. Mosby, St Louis, 1981.

53. Gaston-Johansson, F, Fridh, G, and Turner-Norvall, K: Progression of labor pain in primiparas and multiparas. Nurs Res 37:86, 1988.

54. Maas, M, Buckwalter, KC, and Hardy, MA: Nursing Diagnosis and Interventions for the Elderly. Addison-Wesley Publishing Co Inc, Redwood, City, CA, 1991.

55. Ferrell, B, and Ferrell, B: Easing the pain. Geriatr Nurs 11:175, 1990.

56. Hofland, S: Elder beliefs: Blocks to pain management. J Geront Nurs 18:19, 1992.

57. Haber, J, et al: Comprehensive Psychiatric Nursing, ed 4. Mosby–Year Book, St Louis, 1992.

58. Puskar, KR, et al: Psychiatric nursing management of medication-free psychotic patients. Arch Psych Nurs 4:78–86, 1990.

59. Townsend, M: Nursing Diagnosis in Psychiatric Nursing, ed 3. FA Davis, Philadelphia, 1994.

60. Schwartz, MS, and Shockley, EL: The Nurse and the Mental Patient. Russell Sage Foundation, New York, 1956.

61. Buckwalter, KC, Cusack, D, Kruckeber, T, and Shoemaker, S: Family involvement with communication: Impaired residents in long-term care settings. Appl Nurs Res 4:77, 1991.

62. Friedrick, R, and Kus, R: Cognitive impairments in early sobriety: Nursing interventions. Arch Psych Nurs 5:105, 1991.

63. Gomez, G, and Gomez, E: Dementia? Or delirium? Geriatr Nurs 11:136, 1989.

64. Foreman, M: Complexities of acute confusion. Geriatr Nurs 11:136, 1990.

65. Bowman, AM: The relationship of anxiety to development of post operative delirium. J Geront Nurs 18:24, 1992.

66. Faraday, K, and Berry, M: The nurse's role in managing reversible confusion. J Geront Nurs 15:17, 1989.

Chapter 8

1. Le Mone, P: Analysis of a human phenomenon: Self-concept. Nurs Diag 126, 1991.

2. Turner, R: The self-conception in social interaction. In Gordon, C, and Gergen, KJ (eds): The Self in Social Interaction: Vol 1. Classic and Contemporary Perspectives. John Wiley & Sons, New York, 1968.

3. Gordon, C, and Gergen, KJ (eds): The Self in Social Interaction: Vol 1. Classic and Contemporary Perspectives. John Wiley & Sons, New York, 1968.

4. James, W: The self. In Gordon, C, and Gergen, KJ (eds): The Self in So-

cial Interaction: Vol 1. Classic and Contemporary Perspectives. John Wiley & Sons, New York, 1968.

5. Mead, GH: The genesis of self. In Gordon, C, and Gergen, KJ (eds): The Self in Social Interaction: Vol 1. Classic and Contemporary Perspectives. John Wiley & Sons, New York, 1968.

6. Sullivan, HS: Beginnings of the self-system. In Gordon, C, and Gergen, KJ (eds): The Self in Social Interaction: Vol 1. Classic and Contemporary Perspectives. John Wiley & Sons, New York, 1968.

7. Bruch, H: Interpersonal theory: Harry Stack Sullivan. In Burton, A (ed): Operational Theories of Personality. Brunner-Mazel, New York, 1968.

8. Perry, HS, and Gawel, ML: The Interpersonal Theory of Psychiatry. WW Norton & Co Inc, New York, 1953.

9. Glasersfeld, EV: Cybernetics, experience and the concept of self. In Gergen, KJ, and Davis, RE (eds): The Social Construction of the Person. Springer-Verlag, New York, 1985.

10. Watts, A: The Book: On the Taboo Against Knowing Who You Are. Random House, New York, 1966.

11. Jourard, S: Healthy personality and self-disclosure. In Gordon, C, and Gergen, TJ (eds): The Self in Social Interaction: Vol 1. Classic and Contemporary Perspectives. John Wiley & Sons, New York, 1968.

12. Dufault, K, and Martocchio, B: Hope: Its spheres and dimensions. Nsg Clinics of NA 20:379, 1985.

13. Vaillot, M: Hope the restoration of being. AJN 70:268, 1970.

14. McGee, R: Hope: A factor influencing crisis resolution. Adv in Nsg Sc 7:34, 1984.

15. Miller, J: Inspiring hope. AJN 85:22, 1985.

16. Watson, J: Nursing: Applying the Arts & Sciences of Human Caring. NLN Press, New York, 1994.

17. Evans, RI: The Making of Psychology. Alfred Knopf, New York, 1976.

18. Lynch, WF: Image of Hope: Imagination as Healer of the Hopeless. University of Notre Dame Press, Notre Dame, IN, 1974.

19. Bateson, G: Steps to an Ecology of Mind. Ballantine, New York, 1972.

20. Erickson, H, and Kinney, C: Modeling and Role-Modeling: Theory, Research and Practice. Society for the Advancement of Modeling & Role-Modeling, Austin, TX, 1983.

21. Santrock, JW: Life Span Development, ed 4. WC Brown, Dubuque, IA, 1992.

22. Eliopoulos, C: Manual of Gerontologic Nursing. Mosby, St Louis, 1995.

23. North American Nursing Diagnosis Association: Nursing Diagnosis: Definitions and Classification: 1995–1996. NANDA, Philadelphia, 1994.

24. Bull, M, and Lawrence, D: Mother's use of knowledge during the first postpartum weeks. J Obstet Gynecol Neonatal Nurs 14:315, 1985.

25. Reeder, SJ, Martin, LL, and Koniak, D: Maternity Nursing: Family, Newborn and Women's Health Care, ed 17. JB Lippincott Co, Philadelphia, 1992.

26. Fogel, CI, and Woods, NF: Health Care of Women: A Nursing Perspective. Mosby, St Louis, 1981.

27. Griffith-Kenney, JW: Contemporary Women's Health: A Nursing Advocacy Approach. Addison-Wesley Publishing Co Inc, Menlo Park, CA, 1986.

28. Beck, C, Reynolds, M, and Rutowski, P: Maternity blues and postpartum depression. J Obstet Gynecol Neonatal Nurs 21:287, 1992.

29. Jacobson, N, and Margolin, B: Marital Therapy. Brunner-Mazel, New York, 1989.

30. Drew, B: Differentiation of hopelessness, helplessness, and powerlessness using Erik Erikson's "Roots of Virtue." Arch Psychiatr Nurs 4:332, 1990.

31. Acorn, S, and Bampton, E: Patients' loneliness: A challenge for rehabilitation nurses. Rehabil Nurs 17:22–25, 1992.

32. Potter, PA, and Perry, AG: Basic Nursing: Theory and Practice. Mosby, St Louis, 1993.

33. Evans, RL, and Dingus, CM: Serving the vulnerable: Models for treatment of loneliness. In Hojat, M, and Crandall, R (eds): Loneliness: Theory, Research and Application. Select Press, San Rafael, CA, 1987.

34. Copel, LC: Loneliness: A conceptual model. J Psycho Nurs 26:14–19, 1988.

35. Drew, N: Combatting the social isolation of chronic mental illness. J Psycho Nurs 29:14, 1991.

36. Hoeffer, B: A causal model of loneliness among older single women. Arch Psychiatr Nurs 1:366, 1987.

37. Keeney, BP: Aesthetics of Change. Guilford Press, New York, 1983.

38. Tulman, L, and Fawcett, J: Return of functional ability after childbirth. Nurs Res 37:77, 1988.

39. Matteson, MA, and McConnell, ES: Gerontological Nursing: Concepts and Practices. WB Saunders, Philadelphia, 1988.

40. Gilliss, C, et al: Toward a Science of Family Nursing. Addison-Wesley Publishing Co Inc, Menlo Park, CA, 1989.

41. Miller, JF: Coping with Chronic Illness: Overcoming Powerlessness. FA Davis, Philadelphia, 1983.

42. Burnside, IM: Nursing and the Aged: A Self-Care Approach, ed 3. McGraw-Hill, New York, 1988.

43. Norris, J: Nursing intervention for self-esteem disturbances. Nurs Diagn 3:48, 1992.

44. King, KS, Dimond, M, and McCance, KL: Coping with relocation. Geriatr Nurs 8:258, 1987.

45. Valente, S: Deliberate self-injury: Management in a psychiatric setting. J Psychosoc Nurs Ment Health Serv 29:19, 1991.

46. Gallop, R: Self-destructive and impulsive behavior in the patient with a borderline personality disorder: Rethinking hospital treatment and management. Arch Psychiatr Nurs 6:178, 1992.

47. Reeder, D: Cognitive therapy of anger management: Theoretical and practical considerations. Arch Psychiatr Nurs 5:147, 1991.

Chapter 9

1. Turner, J: The Structure of Sociological Theory, ed 3. Dorsey Press, Homewood, IL, 1982.

2. Shibutani, R: Human Nature and Collective Behavior: Papers in Honor of Herbert Blumer. Prentice-Hall, Englewood Cliff, NJ, 1970.

3. Johnson, GB: American families: Changes and challenges. Fam Soc 72:502, 1991.

4. Clemen-Stone, S, Eigsti, DG, and McGuire, SL: Comprehensive Community Health Nursing, ed 4. Mosby, St Louis, 1995.

5. Mallinger, KM: The American family: History and development. In Nurses and Family Health Promotion: Concepts, Assessment, and Interventions. Williams & Wilkins, Baltimore, 1989.

6. Stanhope, M, and Lancaster, J: Community Health Nursing: Process and Practice for Promoting Health, ed 3. Mosby–Year Book, St Louis, 1992.

7. Murdock, G: Social Structure. Macmillan, New York, 1949.

8. North American Nursing Diagnosis Association: Nursing Diagnosis: Definition and Classification: 1995–1996. NANDA, St Louis, 1994.

9. Gennaro, S: Postpartal anxiety and depression of mothers of term and preterm infants. Nurs Res 37:82, 1988.

10. Weiss, ME, and Armstrong, M: Postpartum mothers' preferences for nighttime care of the neonate. J Obstet Gynecol Neonatal Nurs 20:290, 1991.

11. Reeder, SJ, Martin, LL, and Koniak, D: Maternity Nursing: Family, Newborn and Women's Health Care, ed 17. JB Lippincott Co, Philadelphia, 1992.

12. Chafetz, L, and Barnes, L: Issues in psychiatric caregiving. Arch Psychiatr Nurs 3:61, 1989.

13. Wilson, HS, and Kneisl, CR: Psychiatric Nursing, ed 4. Addison-Wesley Publishing Co Inc, Redwood City, CA, 1992.

14. Anderson, CM, Hogarty, GE, and Reiss, DJ: The psychoeducational family treatment of schizophrenia. In Goldstein, M (ed): New Directions for Mental Health Services. Jossey-Bass, San Francisco, 1981.

15. Baldwin, BA: Family caregiving: Trends and forecasts. Geriatr Nurs 11:172, 1990.

16. Gaynor, S: When the caregiver becomes the patient. Geriatr Nurs 10:120, 1989.

17. Krupnick, SLW, and Wade, AJ: Care Planning. Springhouse Corp, Philadelphia, 1995.

18. ACOG Committee on Ethics: Patient Choice: Maternal-Fetal Conflict. Committee Opinion, Washington, DC, 1990.

19. Chavkin, W: Mandatory treatment for drug use during pregnancy. J Am Med Assoc 266:1556, 1991.

20. Mercer, RT: The process of maternal role attainment over the first year. Nurs Res 34:198–203, 1985.

21. May, KA, and Mahlmeister, LR: Maternal & Neonatal Nursing: Family-Centered Care. JB Lippincott Co, Philadelphia, 1994.

22. Leahey, M, and Wright, L: Nurses and Families: A Guide to Family Assessment and Intervention, ed 2. FA Davis, Philadelphia, 1994.

23. Lindeman, M, Hawks, J, and Bartek, J: The alcoholic family: A nursing diagnosis validation study. Nursing Diagnosis 5:65, 1991.

24. Edwards, M, and Steinglass, P: Family therapy treatment outcomes for alcoholism. Journal of Marital and Family Therapy 21:475, 1995.

25. Stanton, D, and Todd, T: The Family Therapy of Drug Abuse and Addiction. Guilford Press, New York, 1982.

26. Mudd, SA, et al: Alcohol withdrawal and related nursing care in older adults. J Gerontol Nurs 20:17, 1994.

27. Atkinson, RM: Alcohol and substance use disorders in the elderly. In Birren, J, et al (eds): Handbook of Mental Health and Aging. Academic Press, New York, 1992.

28. Chenitz, WC, et al: Clinical Gerontological Nursing: A Guide to Advanced Practice. WB Saunders Company, Philadelphia, 1991.

29. Richter, JM: Support: A resource during crisis of role loss. J Geront Nurs 13:18, 1987.

30. Pridham, KF, Lytton, D, Chang, AS, and Rutledge, D: Early postpartum transition: Progress in maternal identity and role attainment. Res Nurs Health 14:21–31, 1991.

31. Rubin, R: Maternal Identity and the Maternal Experience. Springer Publishing Co Inc, New York, 1984.

32. Rubin, R: Cognitive style in pregnancy. AJN 3:502, 1970.

33. Gilliss, C, et al: Toward a Science of Family Nursing. Addison-Wesley Publishing Co Inc, Menlo Park, CA, 1989.

34. Patterson, G: Families. Research Press, Champaign, IL, 1971.

35. Haber, J, et al: Comprehensive Psychiatric Nursing, ed 4. Mosby–Year Book, St Louis, 1992.

36. Wong, DL: Whaley & Wong's Nursing Care of Infants and Children, ed 5. Mosby, St Louis, 1995.

37. King, KS, Dimond, M, and McCance, KL: Coping with relocation. Geriatr Nurs 8:258, 1987.

38. Griffith-Kenney, JW: Contemporary Women's Health: A Nursing Advocacy Approach. Addison-Wesley Publishing Co Inc, Menlo Park, CA, 1986.

39. Watzlawick, P, Beavin, JH, and Jackson, DP: Pragmatics of Human Communication. WW Norton & Co Inc, New York, 1967.

40. Smitherman, C: Nursing Actions for Health Promotion. FA Davis, Philadelphia, 1981.

41. Parker, B, and McFarlane, J: Identifying and helping battered pregnant women. MCH Am J Matern Child Nurs 16:161, 1991.

42. Sampselle, CM: The role in preventing violence against women. J Obstet Gynecol Neonatal Nurs 20:481, 1991.

43. Campbell, JC: A tests of two explanatory models of women's responses to battering. Nurs Res 38:18, 1989.

44. Zimbardo, P: Interview. In Evans, R: The Making of Psychology. Alfred Knopf, New York, 1976.

45. Stevenson, S: Heading off violence with verbal de-escalation. J Psychosoc Nurs Ment Health Serv 29:6, 1991.

46. Morton, P: Staff roles and responsibilities in incidents of patient violence. Arch Psychiatr Nurs 1:280, 1987.

47. Norris, M, and Kennedy, C: The view from within: How patients perceive the seclusion process. J Psychosoc Nurs Ment Health Serv 30:7, 1992.

48. Loftin, C, McDowell, D, Wiersema, B, and Cotey, T: Effects of restrictive licensing of handguns and homicide and suicide in the District of Columbia. N Engl J Med 325:1615, 1991.

49. Kellerman, A, Rivara, F, Somes, G, Reay, D, Francisco, J, Benton, J, Prodzinski, J, Flinger, C, and Hachman, B: Suicide in the home in relation to gun ownership. N Engl J Med 327:467, 1992.

50. Centers for Disease Control and the National Institute of Occupational Safety and Health: Homicide in US Workplaces: A Strategy for Prevention and Research. US Department of Health and Human Services, Morgantown, WV, 1992.

51. Roberts, C, and Quillian, J: Preventing violence through primary care intervention. Nurse Pract 17:62, 1992.

Chapter 10

1. Wood, NF: Human Sexuality in Health and Illness, ed 3. Mosby, St Louis, 1984.

2. Speroff, L, Glass, RH, and Kase, NG: Clinical Gynecologic Endocrinology and Infertility, ed 5. Williams & Wilkins, Baltimore, 1994.

3. Fogel, CI, and Woods, NF: Health Care of Women: A Nursing Perspective. Mosby, St Louis, 1981.

4. Schuster, CS, and Ashburn, SS: The Process of Human Development: A Holistic Life-Span Approach, ed 3. JB Lippincott Co, Philadelphia, 1992.

5. Biddle, BJ, and Thomas, EJ: Role Theory: Concepts and Research. Robert E. Drieger, Huntington, NY, 1979.

6. Associated Press: Study finds greater number of rape victims than supposed. Lubbock Avalanche Journal 70:A–11, April 24, 1992.

7. Molcan, KL, and Fickley, BS: Sexuality and the Life Cycle. In Poorman, SG (ed): Human Sexuality and the Nursing Process. Appleton & Lange, Norwalk, CT, 1988.

8. Ames, LB, and Ilg, FL: Child Behavior. Dell, New York, 1976.

9. Warner, CG: Rape and Sexual Assault: Management and Intervention. Aspen Systems, Germantown, MD, 1980.

10. North American Nursing Diagnosis Association. Nursing Diagnosis: Definitions and Classifications: 1995–1996. NANDA, Philadelphia, 1994.

11. Haber, J, et al: Comprehensive Psychiatric Nursing, ed 4. Mosby, St Louis, 1992.

12. McArthur, M: Reality therapy with rape victims. Arch Psychiatr Nurs 4:360, 1990.

13. Lightfoot-Klain, H, and Shaw, E: Special needs of ritually circumcised women patients. J Obstet Gynecol Neonatal Nurs 20:102, 1991.

14. Hitchcock, JM, and Wilson, HS: Personal risking: Lesbian self-disclosure of sexual orientation to professional health care providers. Nurs Res 41:178, 1992.

15. Wilson, HS, and Kneisl, CR: Psychiatric Nursing, ed 4. Addison-Wesley Publishing Co Inc, Redwood City, CA, 1992.

16. Dossey, B, et al: Holistic Nursing: A Handbook for Practice, ed 2. Aspen, Gaithersburg, MD, 1995.

17. Buczny, B: Impotence in older men: A newly recognized problem. J Geront Nurs 18:25, 1992.

18. Eliopoulos, C: Manual of Gerontological Nursing. Mosby, St Louis, 1995.

Chapter 11

1. Sutterly, D: Stress in health: A survey of self regulation modalities. Top Clin Nurs 1:1, 1979.

2. Gordon, M: Manual of Nursing Diagnosis 1986–1987. McGraw-Hill, New York, 1987.

3. Ziemer, M: Coping behavior: A response to stress. Top Clin Nurs 4:4, 1982.

4. Frain, M, and Valiga, T: The multiple dimensions of stress. Top Clin Nurs 1:43, 1979.

5. Mengel, A: Coping. Top Clin Nurs 4:80, 1982.

6. Davis, L: Hardiness. In Creasia, J, and Parker, B (eds): Conceptual Foundations of Professional Nursing Practice. Mosby, St Louis, 1991.

7. Simoni, P: Hardiness and coping approach in the workplace of the nurse. Unpublished manuscript. West Virginia University School of Nursing, Morgantown, WV, 1991.

8. Wagnild, G, and Young, H: Another look at hardiness. Image 23:257, 1991.

9. Schuster, CS, and Ashburn, SS: The Process of Human Development: A Holistic Life-Span Approach, ed 3. JB Lippincott Co, Philadelphia, 1992.

10. Smitherman, C: Nursing Actions for Health Promotion. FA Davis, Philadelphia, 1981.

11. Dixon, J, and Dixon, JP: An evolutionary-based model of health and viability. Adv Nurs Sc 6:1, 1984.

12. Carter, E, and McGolddrick, M (eds): The Changing Family Life Cycle: A Framework for Family Therapy, ed 2. Gardner Press, New York, 1988.

13. Ridenour, N: Aggregate nursing diagnoses for community health. In Carroll-Johnson, RM, and Paqvette, M (eds): Classification of Nursing Diagnoses: Proceedings of the Tenth Conference. JB Lippincott Co, Philadelphia, 1994.

14. Lunney, M, Bender, K, Ervin, N, Hickman, P, Jakob, D, Ridenour, N, and Thomas, P: Community Diagnosis: Analysis and Synthesis of the Literature. Association of Community Health Nursing Educators, Chicago, 1994.

15. North American Nursing Diagnosis Association: Nursing Diagnosis: Definition and Classification: 1995–1996. NANDA, Philadelphia, 1994.

16. Viken, RM: The modern couvade syndrome. The Female Patient 7:40, 1982.

17. May, KA, and Mahlmeister, LR: Comprehensive Maternity Nursing: Nursing Process and the Childbearing Family. JB Lippincott Co, Philadelphia, 1990.

18. Evans, C: Personal interview. Swedish Medical Center, Seattle, WA, November, 1995.

19. Evans, C: Postpartum home care in the US. J Obstet Gynecol Neonatal Nurs 24:181–186, 1995.
20. Keppler, AB: Personal interview. Evergreen Hospital, Kirkland, WA, December, 1995.
21. Keppler, AB: Postpartum care center: Follow-up care in a hospital-based clinic. J Obstet Gynecol Neonatal Nurs 24:17–21, 1995.
22. Griffith-Kenney, JW: Contemporary Women's Health: A Nursing Advocacy Approach. Addison-Wesley Publishing Co Inc, Menlo Park, CA, 1986.
23. Wilson, H, and Kneisl, C: Psychiatric Nursing, ed 4. Addison-Wesley Publishing Co Inc, Redwood City, CA, 1992.
24. Wright, LM, and Leahey, M: Nurses and Families: A Guide to Family Assessment and Intervention, ed 2. FA Davis, Philadelphia, 1984.
25. King, J: Helping patients choose an appropriate method of birth control. MCN Am J Matern Child Nurs 17:91, 1992.
26. Lightfoot-Klain, H, and Shaw, E: Special needs of ritually circumcised women patients. J of Obstet Gynecol Neonatal Nurs 20:102, 1992.
27. Reeder, C: Cognitive therapy of anger management: Theoretical and practical considerations. Arch Psychiatr Nurs 5:147, 1991.
28. Haber, J, et al (eds): Comprehensive Psychiatric Nursing, ed 4. Mosby–Year Book, St Louis, 1992.
29. Stuart, GW, and Sundeen, SJ: Principles and Practice of Psychiatric Nursing, ed 5. Mosby, St Louis, 1995.
30. Matteson, MA, and McConnell, ES: Gerontological Nursing: Concepts and Practices. WB Saunders Company, Philadelphia, 1988.
31. Laborde, JM: Torture: A nursing concern. Image 21:31, 1989.
32. Wong, DL: Whaley & Wong's Nursing Care of Infants and Children, ed 4. Mosby, St Louis, 1995.

Chapter 12

1. Fowler, J: Stages of Faith: The Psychology of Human Development and the Quest for Meaning. Harper & Row, San Francisco, 1981.
2. Fowler, J, and Keen, S: Life Maps: Conversations on the Journey of Faith. Word, Waco, TX, 1978.
3. Gordon, M: Nursing Diagnosis: Process and Application, ed 3. Mosby–Year Book, St Louis, 1994.
4. Potter, PA, and Perry, AG: Fundamentals of Nursing: Concepts, Process and Practice, ed 3. Mosby–Year Book, St Louis, 1993.
5. Corrine, BV, Valentin, M, Norontus, E, and Shirley, L: The unheard voices of women: Spiritual interventions in maternal-child health. MCN Am J Matern Child Nurs 17:141, 1992.
6. Stoll, RI: Guidelines for spiritual assessment. Am J Nurs 79:1574, 1979.
7. Bayles, MD: The value of life—By what standard? Am J Nurs 80:2226, 1980.
8. Burns, PB: Elements of spirituality and Watson's theory of transpersonal caring: Expansion of focus. In Chinn, P (ed): Anthology on Caring. National League for Nursing, New York, 1991.
9. Dombeck, MB: Dream telling: A means of spiritual awareness. Holist Nurs Pract 9:37–47, 1995.
10. Clark, CC, Cross, JR, Deane, DM, and Lowry, LW: Spirituality: Integral to quality care. Holist Nurs Pract 5:67, 1991.
11. Nagai-Jackson, MG, and Buckhardt, MA: Spirituality: Cornerstone of holistic nursing practice. Holist Nurs Pract 3:18, 1989.
12. Erickson, EH: Childhood and Society. Triad/Paladin, St Albans, England, 1978.
13. Chandler, JJ: Social cognition: A selective review of current research. In Overton, WF, and Gallagher, JM (eds): Knowledge and Development: Volume I: Research and Theory. Plenum, New York, 1977.
14. Kohlberg, L: The Philosophy of Moral Development. Harper & Row, San Francisco, 1981.
15. North American Nursing Diagnosis Association: Nursing Diagnosis: Definitions and Classification: 1995–1996. NANDA, Philadelphia, 1994.
16. Cox, BE: What if? Coping with unexpected outcomes. Childbirth Instructor 1:24, 1991.
17. Maas, M, Buckwalter, K, and Hardy, M: Nursing Diagnosis and Interventions for the Elderly. Addison-Wesley Publishing Co Inc, Redwood City, CA, 1991.
18. Reed, PG: Preferences for spiritually related nursing interventions among terminally ill and nonterminally ill hospitalized adults and well adults. App Nurs Res 4:122, 1991.
19. Taylor, EJ, Amenta, M, and Highfield, M: Spiritual care practices of oncology nurses. Oncol Nurs Forum 22:31–39, 1995.
20. Broten, PS: Spiritual care given by nurses and spiritual well being of terminally ill cancer patients. Western Michigan University, dissertation, 1991.
21. Carson, VB: Spiritual Dimensions of Nursing Practice. WB Saunders Company, Philadelphia, 1989.
22. Emblen, JD, and Halstead, L: Spiritual needs and interventions: Comparing the views of patients, nurses, and chaplains. Clin Nurs Spec 7:175–182, 1993.
23. Reed, PG: An emerging paradigm for the investigation of spirituality in nursing. Res Nurs Health 15:349–359, 1992.
24. Potter, PA, and Perry, AG: Basic Nursing: Theory and Practice. Mosby, St Louis, 1993.
25. Fitzpatrick, JJ, and Whall, AL: Conceptual Models of Nursing: Analysis and Application. Appleton & Lange, Norwalk, CT, 1989.
26. Burkhardt, MA: Spirituality: An analysis of the concept. Holist Nurs Pract 3:69–77, 1989.
27. Burkhardt, MA: Becoming and connecting: Elements of spirituality for women. Holist Nurs Pract 8:12–21, 1994.

INDEX

Page numbers followed by t indicate tables. Page numbers in italic indicate figures.